Plant and Marine-Derived Natural Product Research in Drug Discovery: Strengths and Perspective

Plant and Marine-Derived Natural Product Research in Drug Discovery: Strengths and Perspective

Editor

Noelia Duarte

MDPI • Basel • Beijing • Wuhan • Barcelona • Belgrade • Manchester • Tokyo • Cluj • Tianjin

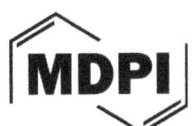

Editor
Noelia Duarte
Research Institute for
Medicines (iMED.Ulisboa)
Universidade de Lisboa
Lisbon
Portugal

Editorial Office
MDPI
St. Alban-Anlage 66
4052 Basel, Switzerland

This is a reprint of articles from the Special Issue published online in the open access journal *Pharmaceuticals* (ISSN 1424-8247) (available at: www.mdpi.com/journal/pharmaceuticals/special_issues/Plant_Marine).

For citation purposes, cite each article independently as indicated on the article page online and as indicated below:

LastName, A.A.; LastName, B.B.; LastName, C.C. Article Title. *Journal Name* **Year**, *Volume Number*, Page Range.

ISBN 978-3-0365-6811-9 (Hbk)
ISBN 978-3-0365-6810-2 (PDF)

© 2023 by the authors. Articles in this book are Open Access and distributed under the Creative Commons Attribution (CC BY) license, which allows users to download, copy and build upon published articles, as long as the author and publisher are properly credited, which ensures maximum dissemination and a wider impact of our publications.

The book as a whole is distributed by MDPI under the terms and conditions of the Creative Commons license CC BY-NC-ND.

Contents

About the Editor vii

Noélia Duarte
Special Issue on Plant and Marine-Derived Natural Product Research in Drug Discovery: Strengths and Perspective
Reprinted from: *Pharmaceuticals* **2022**, *15*, 1249, doi:10.3390/ph15101249 1

Hasan Yousefi-Manesh, Ahmad Reza Dehpour, Samira Shirooie, Fariba Bagheri, Vida Farrokhi and Seyyedeh Elaheh Mousavi et al.
Isofuranodiene, a Natural Sesquiterpene Isolated from Wild Celery (*Smyrnium olusatrum* L.), Protects Rats against Acute Ischemic Stroke
Reprinted from: *Pharmaceuticals* **2021**, *14*, 344, doi:10.3390/ph14040344 5

Elżbieta Studzińska-Sroka, Aleksandra Majchrzak-Celińska, Przemysław Zalewski, Dominik Szwajgier, Ewa Baranowska-Wójcik and Barbara Kaproń et al.
Lichen-Derived Compounds and Extracts as Biologically Active Substances with Anticancer and Neuroprotective Properties
Reprinted from: *Pharmaceuticals* **2021**, *14*, 1293, doi:10.3390/ph14121293 15

Antonio Sorlozano-Puerto, Maria Albertuz-Crespo, Isaac Lopez-Machado, Lidia Gil-Martinez, Juan Jose Ariza-Romero and Alba Maroto-Tello et al.
Antibacterial and Antifungal Activity of Propyl-Propane-Thiosulfinate and Propyl-Propane-Thiosulfonate, Two Organosulfur Compounds from *Allium cepa*: In Vitro Antimicrobial Effect via the Gas Phase
Reprinted from: *Pharmaceuticals* **2020**, *14*, 21, doi:10.3390/ph14010021 39

Marzia Vasarri, Emanuela Barletta and Donatella Degl'Innocenti
Posidonia oceanica (L.) Delile Extract Reduces Lipid Accumulation through Autophagy Activation in HepG2 Cells
Reprinted from: *Pharmaceuticals* **2021**, *14*, 969, doi:10.3390/ph14100969 57

Epole Ntungwe, Eva María Domínguez-Martín, Catarina Teodósio, Silvia Teixidó-Trujillo, Natalia Armas Capote and Lucilia Saraiva et al.
Preliminary Biological Activity Screening of *Plectranthus* spp. Extracts for the Search of Anticancer Lead Molecules
Reprinted from: *Pharmaceuticals* **2021**, *14*, 402, doi:10.3390/ph14050402 69

Ngamrayu Ngamdokmai, Tamkeen Urooj Paracha, Neti Waranuch, Krongkarn Chootip, Wudtichai Wisuitiprot and Nungruthai Suphrom et al.
Effects of Essential Oils and Some Constituents from Ingredients of Anti-Cellulite Herbal Compress on 3T3-L1 Adipocytes and Rat Aortae
Reprinted from: *Pharmaceuticals* **2021**, *14*, 253, doi:10.3390/ph14030253 81

Samira Aouichat, Miguel Navarro-Alarcon, Pablo Alarcón-Guijo, Diego Salagre, Marwa Ncir and Lazhar Zourgui et al.
Melatonin Improves Endoplasmic Reticulum Stress-Mediated IRE1 Pathway in Zücker Diabetic Fatty Rat
Reprinted from: *Pharmaceuticals* **2021**, *14*, 232, doi:10.3390/ph14030232 97

Valentina Noemi Madia, Daniela De Vita, Antonella Messore, Chiara Toniolo, Valeria Tudino and Alessandro De Leo et al.
Analytical Characterization of an Inulin-Type Fructooligosaccharide from Root-Tubers of *Asphodelus ramosus* L
Reprinted from: *Pharmaceuticals* **2021**, *14*, 278, doi:10.3390/ph14030278 111

Ana Henriques Mota, Inês Prazeres, Henrique Mestre, Andreia Bento-Silva, Maria João Rodrigues and Noélia Duarte et al.
A Newfangled Collagenase Inhibitor Topical Formulation Based on Ethosomes with *Sambucus nigra* L. Extract
Reprinted from: *Pharmaceuticals* **2021**, *14*, 467, doi:10.3390/ph14050467 121

Lupe Carolina Espinoza, Lilian Sosa, Paulo C. Granda, Nuria Bozal, Natalia Díaz-Garrido and Brenda Chulca-Torres et al.
Development of a Topical Amphotericin B and *Bursera graveolens* Essential Oil-Loaded Gel for the Treatment of Dermal Candidiasis
Reprinted from: *Pharmaceuticals* **2021**, *14*, 1033, doi:10.3390/ph14101033 147

Oluwasegun Adedokun, Epole N. Ntungwe, Cláudia Viegas, Bunyamin Adesina Ayinde, Luciano Barboni and Filippo Maggi et al.
Enhanced Anticancer Activity of *Hymenocardia acida* Stem Bark Extract Loaded into PLGA Nanoparticles
Reprinted from: *Pharmaceuticals* **2022**, *15*, 535, doi:10.3390/ph15050535 163

Javad Mottaghipisheh, Hadi Taghrir, Anahita Boveiri Dehsheikh, Kamiar Zomorodian, Cambyz Irajie and Mohammad Mahmoodi Sourestani et al.
Linarin, a Glycosylated Flavonoid, with Potential Therapeutic Attributes: A Comprehensive Review
Reprinted from: *Pharmaceuticals* **2021**, *14*, 1104, doi:10.3390/ph14111104 177

Douglas Kemboi Magozwi, Mmabatho Dinala, Nthabiseng Mokwana, Xavier Siwe-Noundou, Rui W. M. Krause and Molahlehi Sonopo et al.
Flavonoids from the Genus *Euphorbia*: Isolation, Structure, Pharmacological Activities and Structure–Activity Relationships
Reprinted from: *Pharmaceuticals* **2021**, *14*, 428, doi:10.3390/ph14050428 199

Sung Ho Lim, Ho Seon Lee, Chang Hoon Lee and Chang-Ik Choi
Pharmacological Activity of *Garcinia indica* (Kokum): An Updated Review
Reprinted from: *Pharmaceuticals* **2021**, *14*, 1338, doi:10.3390/ph14121338 233

Ana C. Gonçalves, Ana R. Nunes, Amílcar Falcão, Gilberto Alves and Luís R. Silva
Dietary Effects of Anthocyanins in Human Health: A Comprehensive Review
Reprinted from: *Pharmaceuticals* **2021**, *14*, 690, doi:10.3390/ph14070690 247

Vanessa Geraldes and Ernani Pinto
Mycosporine-Like Amino Acids (MAAs): Biology, Chemistry and Identification Features
Reprinted from: *Pharmaceuticals* **2021**, *14*, 63, doi:10.3390/ph14010063 281

Raquel Durão, Cátia Ramalhete, Ana Margarida Madureira, Eduarda Mendes and Noélia Duarte
Plant Terpenoids as Hit Compounds against Trypanosomiasis
Reprinted from: *Pharmaceuticals* **2022**, *15*, 340, doi:10.3390/ph15030340 299

About the Editor

Noelia Duarte

Noélia Duarte has a degree in Pharmaceutical Sciences (1995), M.Sc. in Pharmaceutical Chemistry (1999) and Ph.D. in Pharmacy (2008, University of Lisbon). She has been an Assistant Professor at FFUL since 2008, teaching and coordinating several 1st and 2nd cycle curricular units. She has expertise in several chromatographic and spectrophotometric techniques, including HPLC and GC, ultraviolet, infrared, nuclear magnetic resonance, and mass spectrometry (HPLC-MS/MS). Her research has been focused on the isolation and structural characterization of bioactive compounds isolated from plants and other sources, and on mass spectrometry studies applied to the identification and quantification of metabolites from plants and biological matrices. N. Duarte is author or co-author of seven book chapters, and more than 50 research papers in peer-reviewed scientific journals.

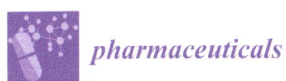

Editorial

Special Issue on Plant and Marine-Derived Natural Product Research in Drug Discovery: Strengths and Perspective

Noélia Duarte

Research Institute for Medicines (iMED.Ulisboa), Faculdade de Farmácia, Universidade de Lisboa, Av. Prof. Gama Pinto, 1649-003 Lisboa, Portugal; mduarte@ff.ulisboa.pt

For centuries, nature has been an inspirational source for the discovery of traditional remedies and drugs used in modern medicine. Natural-based treatments continue to be employed for primary health care, particularly playing a significant role in folk medicine. In addition, we are currently observing an increasing use of natural-products-based supplements from botanical and marine sources, making their standardization and scientific validation a priority to guarantee the safety of these products. Natural products and/or synthetic derivatives using their novel structures have also been of utmost importance in drug discovery and development in several clinical areas. After a period of discredit and reduced investment, we are now witnessing a renewed interest from the pharmaceutical industry and scientific community due to the urgent need to develop new drugs.

This Special Issue of *Pharmaceuticals* has assembled eleven original and six review articles dedicated to plant and marine natural products research, contributing to the scientific validation of their use and opening new perspectives in drug discovery.

Yousefi-Manesh et al. [1] studied the effect of isofuranodiene, a furanosesquiterpene isolated from *Smyrnium olusatrum* essential oil, on the oxidative stress and inflammatory response in a rat model of ischemic stroke, by assessing several biochemical markers, pathology of the hippocampi cells, and behavioral assays. Pre-treatment with isofuranodiene decreased the levels of pro-inflammatory cytokines and the lipid peroxidation indicator malondialdehyde, as markers of neuroinflammation in ischemic stroke and oxidative stress, respectively. Moreover, the pre-treated animals showed improved behavioral activity after ischemic stroke, and a faster recovery was also observed. Despite the need for further pharmacokinetic and toxicological studies, isofuranodiene may be considered a lead compound for discovering new treatments for brain ischemia.

Searching for new therapies for central nervous system (CNS) tumors, Studzińska-Sroka et al. [2] screened the biological potential of acetonic extracts of the lichens *Parmelia sulcata*, *Evernia prunastri*, and *Cladonia uncialis*, and their major metabolites salazinic acid, evernic acid, and (−)-usnic acid. The extracts and pure compounds were evaluated for their cytotoxicity against A-172 and T98G cell lines, inhibition of kynurenine pathway enzymes, and anti-inflammatory, antioxidant, and anticholinergic activities. In addition, the penetration of salazinic acid, evernic acid, and (−)-usnic acid through the blood–brain barrier (BBB) was also determined. The authors suggested that (−)-usnic acid, with its ability to cross the BBB and reduce cell proliferation, can be considered a promising lead compound for glioblastoma multiforme treatment, one of the deadliest tumors of the CNS.

Garlic (*Allium sativum*) and onion (*Allium cepa*) are two edible plants widely consumed all over the world. In recent years, several biological actions have been attributed to different organosulfur products, such as thiosulfinates and thiosulfonates, obtained from these species. Sorlozano-Puerto et al. [3] evaluated the antibacterial and anti-candidiasis activity of propyl-propane thiosulfinate and propyl-propane thiosulfonate, two volatile compounds derived from *Allium cepa*. Moreover, the ability of the compounds in gaseous phase to inhibit bacterial and yeast growth was also assessed. Propyl-propane thiosulfonate was the most promising compound showing activity against different isolates of

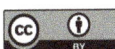

Candida spp. from human clinical samples, even at the gas phase, which, in the future, could be potentially useful in lung therapy.

Posidonia oceanica is a marine plant used in traditional medicine for the treatment of several health conditions, such as diabetes and inflammation. The aim of the study carried out by Vasarri et al. [4] was to analyze the ability of *P. oceanica* hydroalcoholic extract to trigger autophagy and reduce intracellular lipid accumulation, in an in vitro model of hepatic steatosis using the human hepatoma cell line HepG2. The authors found that the extract protected against lipid accumulation in HepG2 cells by promoting autophagy through inhibition of the mTOR pathway, offering new insights for possible complementary treatments of non-alcoholic fatty liver disease.

Ntungwe et al. [5] screened sixteen *Plectranthus* species acetone extracts for the in vitro antioxidant and antimicrobial activities against yeasts, and Gram-positive and Gram-negative bacteria. The *P. hadiensis* and *P. mutabilis* extracts showed the highest activity against *S. aureus* and *C. albicans*. Moreover, using the *Artemia salina* assay as a marker of general toxicity, *P. hadiensis* and *P.ciliatus* were selected and further tested for their cytotoxicity, showing low activities in human colon, breast, and lung cancer cell lines. 7α-acetoxy-6β-hydroxyroyleanone isolated from *P. hadiensis* was found to be twelve-fold more active than the extract in the triple-negative breast cancer cell line (MDA-MB-231S), being proposed as a promising lead compound for the development of new anti-cancer drugs.

The use of herbal compresses is widespread in traditional Thai therapies to relieve muscle pains, stress, and strains. Aiming at finding out the mechanisms of action and the bioactive constituents responsible for the anti-cellulite activity of a previous formulated herbal compress, Ngamdokmai et al. [6] presented, in their article, the preclinical effects of essential oils, extracts, and main monoterpenoid constituents on cellular lipid accumulation, triglyceride content, and vasodilatation in rat aortae. The authors concluded that the mixed oils have vasodilation activity, and all the tested samples were effective inhibitors of adipogenesis and lipolysis inducers, corroborating their application in cellulite treatment.

Melatonin was previously shown to exert a renoprotective effect in a rat model of diabesity-induced kidney injury. In their study, Aouichat et al. [7] further investigated whether melatonin could suppress the renal endoplasmic reticulum (ER) stress response and downstream unfolded protein response activation, shedding light on the beneficial effect of melatonin supplementation on ER stress-induced kidney damage under diabesity conditions.

Asphodelus L. species have been known for both food and therapeutic uses. Madia et [8] reported the isolation and identification of a polysaccharide (inulin-type fructan) from the alkaline extract of *Asphodelus ramosus* root tubers.

The goal of the study performed by Mota et al. [9] was the development of a topical ethosome-based formulation of fresh elderflower (*Sambucus nigra*) extract, to prevent its degradation and to obtain a slow release of bioactive compounds. The ethosomes were characterized in terms of their size and morphology, stability over time, entrapment capacity, and extract release profile. The extract-loaded ethosomes presented collagenase inhibition activity and very good results in the human skin compatibility assay using a semi-solid formulation.

Amphotericine B is a macrolide antibiotic clinically used to treat *Candida, Cryptoccocus,* and *Aspergillus* infections, and leishmaniasis. The intravenous administration of this antibiotic has severe side effects which have prompted the development of various formulations. The low solubility of amphotericin B also hinders its topical administration. In order to promote the diffusion of the drug through the skin in the treatment of cutaneous candidiasis, Espinoza et al. [10] developed a topical gel of amphotericin B and *Bursera graveolens* (palo santo) essential oil. The authors evaluated the physicochemical parameters, stability, in vitro release profile, and ex vivo permeation in human skin of the formulation, concluding that the topical gel of amphotericin B enriched with *B. graveolens* essential oil could be an alternative to the treatment of cutaneous candidiasis.

Consistent with the increasing use of nanotechnology for improving drug delivery, Adedokun et al. [11] compared the cytotoxic activity of *Hymenocardia acida* crude methanolic extract with the cytotoxicity of the extract loaded in PLGA nanoparticles, against human lung (H460), breast (MCF-7), and colon (HCT 116) cancer cell lines. *H. acida* extract showed to be cytotoxic against the lung cancer cell line and the solubility was improved through encapsulation. However, the encapsulated extract presented a decreased cytotoxic activity against all cell lines tested, a fact that could be due to the sustained delay in the release of the extract from the PLGA nanoparticles.

Mottaghipisheh et al. [12] reviewed the phytochemical and biological properties of the glycosylated flavone linarin (acacetin-7-O-rutinoside), which has been identified in several species of the Asteraceae, Lamiaceae, and Scrophulariaceae families. Several studies have reported promising in vitro and in vivo bioactivities, particularly on the central nervous system, arthritis, and osteoporosis disorders.

Several *Euphorbia* species have been used in traditional medicine, and have also been the source of a huge number of interesting bioactive compounds, including terpenois and flavonoids. Magozwi et al. [13] reviewed the phytochemistry, biological properties, and therapeutic potential of Euphorbia flavonoids, published in the literature from 2000 to 2020. Several bioactivities have been reported either for *Euphorbia* extracts or isolated flavonoids, particularly antiproliferative, antimicrobial, and antioxidant activities.

Garcinia indica is a species from the mangosteen family (Clusiaceae), with culinary, industrial, and therapeutic applications. The review by Lim et al. [14] highlighted recent studies regarding the in vitro and in vivo biological activities of this species, such as antioxidant, anti-inflammatory, anti-obesity, and hepato- and cardioprotective effects.

Over the last few decades, many studies have focused on the nutritional value and health-promoting properties of anthocyanins. Gonçalves [15] reviewed the chemical structure of these flavonoids, their main dietary sources, and bioavailability. They also pointed out the most recent results on the potential health benefits from the daily intake of anthocyanin-rich foods, as well as their possible pharmacological mechanisms of action.

Geraldes et al. [16] gathered and reviewed the literature on mycosporines and mycosporine-like aminoacids, summarizing their physicochemical features and biosynthesis, occurrence and distribution in nature, and phytochemical studies. They also reviewed their biological activities and biomedical and non-biomedical applications. Moreover, the authors constructed a chemical database available online for free at http://www.cena.usp.br/ernani-pinto-mycas (accessed on 14 September 2022).

Human African trypanosomiasis (sleeping sickness) and American trypanosomiasis (Chagas disease) are two protozoan neglected tropical diseases whose pharmacological therapies have serious limitations. Therefore, the discovery and development of new drugs are urgent, and natural products from plants are a promising approach to achieve this goal. In their comprehensive review, Durão et al. [17] gathered and discussed data published in the literature regarding terpenic compounds with antitrypanosomal activity against *T. brucei* and *T. cruzi*, covering the period from 2016 to 2021, and emphasizing the most promising bioactive terpenoids.

The 17 articles published in this Special Issue further strengthen the potential of natural product research for the discovery of new drugs and overall contribute to the scientific validation of their use.

Funding: This research received no external funding.

Acknowledgments: The Guest Editor is extremely grateful to all Authors for their hard work producing updated articles in a timely fashion, and also thanks to the Reviewers who carefully evaluated the submitted manuscripts.

Conflicts of Interest: The author declares no conflict of interest.

References

1. Yousefi-Manesh, H.; Dehpour, A.R.; Shirooie, S.; Bagheri, F.; Farrokhi, V.; Mousavi, S.E.; Ricciutelli, M.; Cappellacci, L.; López, V.; Maggi, F.; et al. Isofuranodiene, a natural sesquiterpene isolated from wild celery (*Smyrnium olusatrum*), protects rats against acute ischemic stroke. *Pharmaceuticals* **2021**, *14*, 344. [CrossRef] [PubMed]
2. Studzińska-Sroka, E.; Majchrzak-Celińska, A.; Zalewski, P.; Szwajgier, D.; Baranowska-Wójcik, E.; Kaproń, B.; Plech, T.; Żarowski, M.; Cielecka-Piontek, J. Lichen-derived compounds and extracts as biologically active substances with anticancer and neuroprotective properties. *Pharmaceuticals* **2021**, *14*, 1293. [CrossRef] [PubMed]
3. Sorlozano-Puerto, A.; Albertuz-Crespo, M.; Lopez-Machado, I.; Gil-Martinez, L.; Ariza-Romero, J.J.; Maroto-Tello, A.; Baños-Arjona, A.; Gutierrez-Fernandez, J. Antibacterial and antifungal activity of propyl-propane-thiosulfinate and propyl-propane-thiosulfonate, two organosulfur compounds from allium cepa: In vitro antimicrobial effect via the gas phase. *Pharmaceuticals* **2021**, *14*, 21. [CrossRef] [PubMed]
4. Vasarri, M.; Barletta, E.; Degl'innocenti, D. *Posidonia oceanica* (L.) delile extract reduces lipid accumulation through autophagy activation in hepg2 cells. *Pharmaceuticals* **2021**, *14*, 969. [CrossRef] [PubMed]
5. Ntungwe, E.; Domínguez-Martín, E.M.; Teodósio, C.; Teixidó-Trujillo, S.; Capote, N.A.; Saraiva, L.; Díaz-Lanza, A.M.; Duarte, N.; Rijo, P. Preliminary biological activity screening of *Plectranthus* spp. Extracts for the search of anticancer lead molecules. *Pharmaceuticals* **2021**, *14*, 402. [CrossRef] [PubMed]
6. Ngamdokmai, N.; Paracha, T.U.; Waranuch, N.; Chootip, K.; Wisuitiprot, W.; Suphrom, N.; Insumrong, K.; Ingkaninan, K. Effects of essential oils and some constituents from ingredients of anti-cellulite herbal compress on 3t3-l1 adipocytes and rat aortae. *Pharmaceuticals* **2021**, *14*, 253. [CrossRef] [PubMed]
7. Aouichat, S.; Navarro-Alarcon, M.; Alarcón-Guijo, P.; Salagre, D.; Ncir, M.; Zourgui, L.; Agil, A. Melatonin improves endoplasmic reticulum stress-mediated ire1α pathway in zücker diabetic fatty rat. *Pharmaceuticals* **2021**, *14*, 232. [CrossRef] [PubMed]
8. Madia, V.N.; De Vita, D.; Messore, A.; Toniolo, C.; Tudino, V.; De Leo, A.; Pindinello, I.; Ialongo, D.; Saccoliti, F.; D'Ursi, A.M.; et al. Analytical characterization of an inulin-type fructooligosaccharide from root-tubers of *Asphodelus ramosus* L. *Pharmaceuticals* **2021**, *14*, 278. [CrossRef] [PubMed]
9. Mota, A.H.; Prazeres, I.; Mestre, H.; Bento-Silva, A.; Rodrigues, M.J.; Duarte, N.; Serra, A.T.; Bronze, M.R.; Rijo, P.; Gaspar, M.M.; et al. A newfangled collagenase inhibitor topical formulation based on ethosomes with sambucus nigra l. Extract. *Pharmaceuticals* **2021**, *14*, 467. [CrossRef] [PubMed]
10. Espinoza, L.C.; Sosa, L.; Granda, P.C.; Bozal, N.; Díaz-Garrido, N.; Chulca-Torres, B.; Calpena, A.C. Development of a topical amphotericin b and bursera graveolens essential oil-loaded gel for the treatment of dermal candidiasis. *Pharmaceuticals* **2021**, *14*, 1033. [CrossRef] [PubMed]
11. Adedokun, O.; Ntungwe, E.N.; Viegas, C.; Adesina Ayinde, B.; Barboni, L.; Maggi, F.; Saraiva, L.; Rijo, P.; Fonte, P. Enhanced Anticancer Activity of Hymenocardia acida Stem Bark Extract Loaded into PLGA Nanoparticles. *Pharmaceuticals* **2022**, *15*, 535. [CrossRef] [PubMed]
12. Mottaghipisheh, J.; Taghrir, H.; Dehsheikh, A.B.; Zomorodian, K.; Irajie, C.; Sourestani, M.M.; Iraji, A. Linarin, a glycosylated flavonoid, with potential therapeutic attributes: A comprehensive review. *Pharmaceuticals* **2021**, *14*, 1104. [CrossRef] [PubMed]
13. Magozwi, D.K.; Dinala, M.; Mokwana, N.; Siwe-Noundou, X.; Krause, R.W.M.; Sonopo, M.; McGaw, L.J.; Augustyn, W.A.; Tembu, V.J. Flavonoids from the genus euphorbia: Isolation, structure, pharmacological activities and structure–activity relationships. *Pharmaceuticals* **2021**, *14*, 428. [CrossRef] [PubMed]
14. Lim, S.H.; Lee, H.S.; Lee, C.H.; Choi, C.I. Pharmacological Activity of Garcinia indica (Kokum): An Updated Review. *Pharmaceuticals* **2021**, *14*, 1338. [CrossRef] [PubMed]
15. Gonçalves, A.C.; Nunes, A.R.; Falcão, A.; Alves, G.; Silva, L.R. Dietary effects of anthocyanins in human health: A comprehensive review. *Pharmaceuticals* **2021**, *14*, 690. [CrossRef] [PubMed]
16. Geraldes, V.; Pinto, E. Mycosporine-like amino acids (Maas): Biology, chemistry and identification features. *Pharmaceuticals* **2021**, *14*, 63. [CrossRef] [PubMed]
17. Durão, R.; Ramalhete, C.; Madureira, A.M.; Mendes, E.; Duarte, N. Plant Terpenoids as Hit Compounds against Trypanosomiasis. *Pharmaceuticals* **2022**, *15*, 340. [CrossRef] [PubMed]

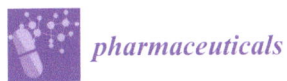

Article

Isofuranodiene, a Natural Sesquiterpene Isolated from Wild Celery (*Smyrnium olusatrum* L.), Protects Rats against Acute Ischemic Stroke

Hasan Yousefi-Manesh [1,2], Ahmad Reza Dehpour [1,2], Samira Shirooie [3,*], Fariba Bagheri [1,2], Vida Farrokhi [1,2], Seyyedeh Elaheh Mousavi [1], Massimo Ricciutelli [4], Loredana Cappellacci [4], Víctor López [5], Filippo Maggi [4,*] and Riccardo Petrelli [4]

[1] Department of Pharmacology, School of Medicine, Tehran University of Medical Sciences, Tehran 1417613151, Iran; hasanyousefimanesh@gmail.com (H.Y.-M.); dehpour@yahoo.com (A.R.D.); f.bagheri.3223@gmail.com (F.B.); vida.farrokhi@yahoo.com (V.F.); semousavi@sina.tums.ac.ir (S.E.M.)
[2] Experimental Medicine Research Center, Tehran University of Medical Sciences, Tehran 1417613151, Iran
[3] Pharmaceutical Sciences Research Center, Health Institute, Kermanshah University of Medical Sciences, Kermanshah 6734667149, Iran
[4] School of Pharmacy, University of Camerino, 62032 Camerino, Italy; massimo.ricciutelli@unicam.it (M.R.); loredana.cappellacci@unicam.it (L.C.); riccardo.petrelli@unicam.it (R.P.)
[5] Department of Pharmacy, Faculty of Health Sciences, Universidad San Jorge, Villanueva de Gállego, 50830 Zaragoza, Spain; ilopez@usj.es
* Correspondence: shirooie@gmail.com (S.S.); filippo.maggi@unicam.it (F.M.)

Abstract: The myrrh-like furanosesquiterpene isofuranodiene (IFD) is the main constituent of wild celery (*Smyrnium olusatrum* L., Apiaceae), an overlooked vegetable that was cultivated during the Roman Empire. In the present study, we investigated the protective effects of IFD pre-treatment against oxidative stress and inflammatory response in an animal model of ischemic stroke. IFD was isolated by the crystallization of *Smyrnium olusatrum* essential oil, and its structure and purity were confirmed by NMR and HPLC analyses. Acute pre-treatment of IFD (10 mg/kg i.p.) significantly reduced the levels of the inflammatory cytokines IL-1β and TNF-α, the expression of pNF-κB/NF-κB, and the lipid peroxidation indicator MDA. Finally, IFD boosted a faster recovery and better scores in grid-walking and modified neurological severity scores (mNSS) tests. Taken together, these findings indicate IFD as a promising lead compound for the discovery of new treatments of brain ischemia.

Keywords: isofuranodiene; *Smyrnium olusatrum* L.; ischemic stroke; NF-kB; IL-1β; TNF-α

1. Introduction

Globalization has led to a change in our eating habits and the disappearance of many plants that were once eaten by older generations. Among them, the aromatic herb *Smyrnium olusatrum* L. (Apiaceae), also known as Alexanders or wild celery, represents an interesting case. *Smyrnium olusatrum* L. is a biennial plant belonging to the Apiaceae family, and is widespread in the Mediterranean basin, reaching the North African coast to the South and the British Isles to the North. It is found in shady places such as hedgerows, cliffs, and other uncultivated places, from sea level to high hills, often as a relic of kitchen gardens and monasteries. During the medieval period, *S. olusatrum* had been used as an antiscorbutic, stomachic, antiasthmatic, diuretic, and laxative remedy [1,2]. As a vegetable, *S. olusatrum* had been used until the medieval period, when it was replaced by common celery (*Apium graveolens* L.) due to changing tastes favoring tender and sweeter dishes instead of more spicy and hot ones [2]. *Smyrnium olusatrum* is a rich source of volatile sesquiterpenes containing a furan ring, among which isofuranodiene (syn. furanodiene, $C_{15}H_{20}O$, IFD) is the most abundant [3]. This compound is also a key marker of other medicinal and aromatic plant species such as *Commiphora myrrha* (Nees) Engl.,

Curcuma wenyujin Y.H. Chen and C. Ling, *Eugenia uniflora* L., *Chloranthus japonicus* Siebold and *Vepris unifoliolata* Baill.) Labat [1,3]. It has also been found in some marine organisms, such as corals [4]. It is noteworthy that our group has recently proven that IFD may exert neuritogenic, anti-inflammatory, and anticancer activities, as well as insecticidal and acaricidal properties [5–9]. In recent years, researchers' increasing interest towards the protective role of natural substances, especially those contained in fruits, vegetables, and medicinal plants, against ischemic stroke has been observed. Thus, natural products are playing a notable role in discovering new therapeutic treatments for stroke.

Ischemic stroke is one of the most complicated, destructive, and fatal neurological disorders [10]. This disease is the second highest cause of death, and the third most common factor of disability worldwide [11]. From an economic perspective, stroke has a burden of approximately GBP 2.4 billion for informal care costs and GBP 2.1 billion for indirect costs such as benefit payments and productivity reduction, because of death and disability within the global health economy [11]. One of the most critical roles in the pathogenesis of ischemic stroke is played by inflammatory processes [12]. These processes will raise the amount of different inflammatory factors in several parts of the central nervous system (CNS), especially in the brain. During the reperfusion phase, which occurs after stroke alleviation, the production of reactive oxygen species (ROS) starts to increase due to hypoxia caused by disruption of the brain blood flow [13]. ROS generation can lead to overexpression of cell survival programs that relieve tissue injury caused by ischemia. However, this overexpression may cause oxidative stress that can advance to cell apoptosis and death [14]. The brain has a high concentration of peroxidizable lipids; therefore, it can be a suitable target for reactive oxygen species. Malondialdehyde (MDA), as the final product of lipid peroxidation, can cause cell toxicity and death. The amount of MDA produced is one of the most important biomarkers for measuring the brain's oxidative stress level [15]. TNF-α and IL-1β progress the inflammatory response by releasing Essential Amino Acids (EAA), nitric oxide (NO), and free oxygen radicals, and increase stroke-induced tissue injury [16]. NF-κB is another factor that overexpresses after ischemic-reperfusion occurs in stroke. NF-κB causes tissue damage, apoptosis, and neuronal death in some brain regions such as the hippocampus, and triggers many inflammatory pathways and mediators [17]. Strokes may cause physical and behavioral disabilities, such as motor impairments. Most of these complications are caused by neuronal and tissue injury in the brain cortex's motor regions and damage in subcortical projection pathways. Therefore, strokes may lead to a reduction in movement speed, ability, and control [18].

In the present work, we evaluated for the first time the neuroprotective effects of IFD against oxidative stress and inflammatory conditions in a rat model of ischemic stroke. For this purpose, the efficacy of IFD against bilateral carotid artery (BCA) occlusion injury was determined by evaluating the levels of pro-inflammatory cytokines (IL-1β and TNF-α) and MDA, a marker of lipid peroxidation, and the expression of pNF-κB/NF-κB in the rat brain. In addition, the effect of IFD treatment on rat behavior after brain stroke induction was determined by the grid-walking and modified neurological severity scores (mNSS) tests.

2. Results

2.1. IFD Shortened the Behavioral Recovery Period after the Brain Stroke

Two behavioral tests, namely mNSS and grid-walking, have been performed to evaluate rat neurological functioning after ischemic stroke. Statistically significant differences were observed in the grid-walking test and motor scores in the mNSS test between the IFD-treated rats and the non-treated stroke group (the control group) ($p < 0.05$). As shown in Figure 1A,B, IFD pre-treated rats had a faster recovery and better scores in the grid-walking and mNSS tests, whereas rats from the control group that received no treatment showed a lower rate of amelioration and higher scores in both tests compared with the sham group ($p < 0.01$). Moreover, there are no significant differences between the pre-treated group and the positive control group. It was noticed from this test that IFD improved the outcomes on the brain ischemic reperfused group.

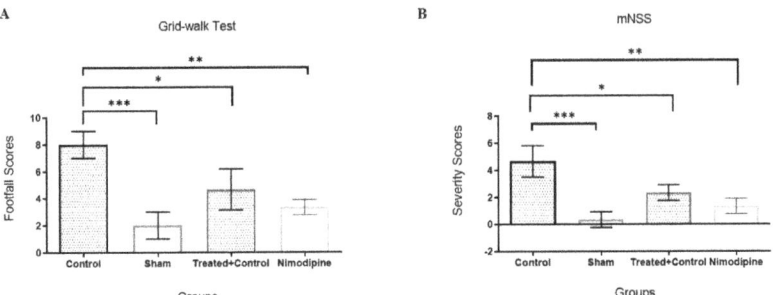

Figure 1. Behavioral tests in rats. (**A**): Grid-walking test, (**B**): modified neurological severity scores (mNSS) test. Data are mean ± SEM. * $p < 0.05$, ** $p < 0.01$, *** $p < 0.001$.

2.2. Effects of IFD on Inflammatory Cytokines and Oxidative Stress in Ischemic Brains

As shown in Figure 2A–C, 24 h after BCA occlusion, pro-inflammatory cytokines such as TNF-α and IL-1β, and MDA, as a lipid peroxidation marker, were assessed via ELISA assay. BCA occlusion (control group) showed increased levels of TNF-α, IL-1β, and MDA when compared with the sham group ($p < 0.001$). On the other hand, pre-treatment with IFD reversed these effects significantly compared to the control group ($p < 0.01$ and $p < 0.001$, respectively). In addition, MDA in the pre-treated group and the positive control group did not have a significant difference.

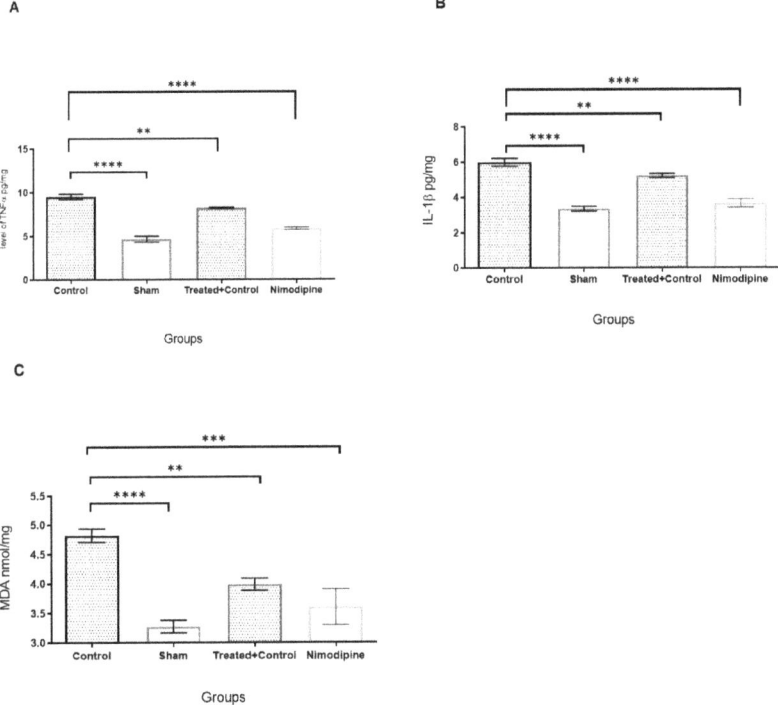

Figure 2. IFD pre-treatment reduced inflammatory cytokines and oxidative stress 24 h after ischemic stroke. (**A**): TNF-α, (**B**): IL-1β and (**C**): MDA levels of the brain tissues of the sham, control, IFD treatment + ischemic stroke, and Nimodipine as a positive control. All values are shown as mean ± SEM. ** $p < 0.01$, *** $p < 0.001$, **** $p < 0.0001$.

2.3. The Anti-Inflammatory Effects of IFD May Be Mediated through pNF-κB Protein Downregulation

The results of the Western blot analysis showed that BCA occlusion increased the phosphorylation of NF-κB p65 (active form) in the control group when compared with the sham group ($p < 0.001$). Of note, pre-treatment with IFD reduced its phosphorylated form significantly in respect to the control group ($p < 0.01$) (Figure 3A,B).

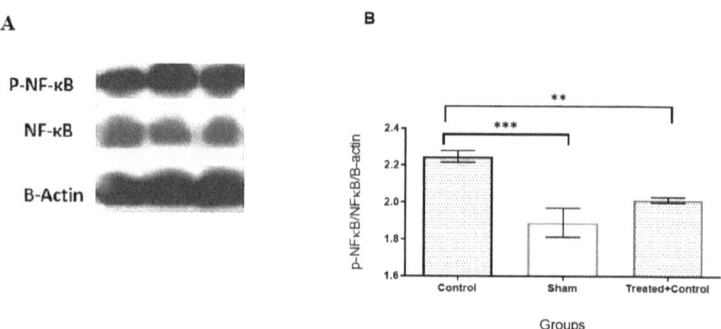

Figure 3. (**A**). Western blot of NF-κB phosphorylation in brain tissues of groups. (**B**). IFD pre-treatment reduced phosphorylation of NF-κB in animals 24 h after reperfusion. Data are shown as mean ± SEM. ** $p < 0.01$, *** $p < 0.001$.

3. Discussion

IFD has attracted the attention of many researchers and academics in recent years due to its anticancer, analgesic, neuritogenic, anti-inflammatory, hepatoprotective, antiprotozoal, and insecticidal properties [5,7,8,19–22].

In the present study, we highlighted for the first time the neuroprotective effects of IFD on an acutely pre-treated ischemic stroke rat model by measuring biochemical markers, pathology of the hippocampi cells, and behavioral assays. Li et al. have indicated that IFD has anti-inflammatory effects on liver injury induced by d-galactosamine/lipopolysaccharide in rats, by reducing inflammatory cytokines such as IL6, IL-1β, and TNF-α, decreasing the marker of peroxidation of lipids, MDA, and providing hepatoprotection by a reduction in aminotransferase levels [6]. Previous research has indicated that compounds with a similar structure to IFD prevented inflammation and reduced the expression of pro-inflammatory cytokines [23,24]. Owing to its hydrophobic nature and small size, IFD can cross the blood–brain barrier, exerting its effect in neurons [5]. This effect enhances the neuroprotective potential of IFD, making it valuable for the treatment of brain disorders.

According to the biochemical assessments in our study, the acute pre-treatment with IFD significantly reduced the levels of the inflammatory cytokines IL-1β and TNF-α, which are both important mediators of neuroinflammation in ischemic stroke, and decreased the lipid peroxidation indicator MDA, as a marker of oxidative stress. In addition, IFD ameliorated the behavioral effects, improving the sensorimotor reflexes and reducing the injury's score severity. NF-κB has an important role in impairment during brain ischemia. For example, hypoxia, ROS, and other inflammatory mediators activate NF-kB signaling, increase phosphorylation, and activate the NF-κB p65 subunit [25]. During cerebral ischemic-reperfusion, NF-κB is involved in many processes, e.g., apoptosis and inflammation, by regulating gene expression [26]. NF-κB hyperactivity, as an initial factor of inflammation in the brain, leads to apoptosis of the hippocampus neurons and elevates cytokine expressions such as IL-6, IL-8, and TNF-α in neurons, endothelial and glial cells [27]. In addition, NF-κB increases the expression of pro-apoptotic genes such as P53, iNOS, and COX-2 in glial and neuronal cells [28]. Our findings showed that pre-treatment with IFD reduced phosphorylation and activation of NF-κB in the rat brains' prefrontal cortex compared with the control group. This result supports the hypothesis that IFD is able to prevent the inflammatory cascade and apoptosis of neurons. These results are partly supported by our previous study in which IFD was found to mimic the neuroactivity of NGF for neuronal survival, development, and differentiation [5].

It is worth mentioning that IFD is present in high quantities in all the parts of *S. olusatrum*, and it can be easily collected in the EO obtained by hydrodistillation. Wild celery represents today an ideal and rich source for the extraction of IFD. In this regard, Maggi et al. led an intense campaign to isolate EO from roots, basal leaves, flowers, and green or ripe fruits of wild celery, highlighting high IFD levels in different plant organs [1–3]. In detail, EO from basal leaves contained up to 37.2% IFD, the EO from roots contained up to 46.6% IFD, whereas the EO obtained from fruits (green and ripe) contained up to 31.5% and 20.7% IFD, respectively. Lastly, the EO from the flowers contained a maximum of 56.2% IFD. This research has laid the foundations for IFD extraction's scalability from *S. olusatrum*, highlighting the flowers as the best candidate due to the high concentration of the target molecule. The isolation and purification of a bulk amount of IFD can be easily carried out by crystallization or, alternatively, flash chromatography [5].

4. Materials and Methods

4.1. Purification and Analysis of IFD

The plant material (inflorescences) used was from a wild population of *S. olusatrum* growing in Pioraco, central Italy (N 43°10′41″; E 12°59′27″, 440 m a.s.l.), collected in April 2018. A herbarium specimen was deposited in the *Herbarium Camerinensis* of the University of Camerino, under the codex CAME 25677. Fresh inflorescences were hydrodistilled for 4 h using a Clevenger-type apparatus in order to obtain a yellowish essential oil with a yield of 1.8% on a dry weight basis. Afterward, crude crystals of IFD ($C_{15}H_{20}O$) were obtained by adding analytical grade hexane (300 mL) to 10 g of flower essential oil and storing the mixture at −20 °C for 6 days. Once all crude crystals had been filtered out, they were recrystallized (3 times) using hot methanol, obtaining pure white crystals of IFD (yield = 75%) (Figure 1). Accurate 1D (^{1}H NMR and ^{13}C NMR) and 2D (COSY, TOCSY, and HMBC) NMR studies were carried out on a Bruker Avance III 500 MHz spectrometer (Billerica, MA), and comparison with the data reported in the literature helped us to confirm the IFD's structure [7,22]. The purity of IFD (~99%) was assessed by HPLC using an HP-1100 series (Agilent Technologies, Palo Alto, CA, USA) LC system equipped with a diode array detector (DAD). The separation was accomplished on a Kinetex© PFP (100A, 100 × 4.6 mm i.d., 2.6 µm), thermostatted at 40 °C using H_2O (Milli-Q SP Reagent Water System, Millipore, Bedford, MA, USA) and CH_3CN (Carlo Erba Acetonitrile for HPLC Plus gradient, Milan, Italy) as mobile phases A and B, respectively. The gradient elution (1.0 mL/min) was set as follows: 0–15 min (40% B), 15–30 min (60% B). IFD was diluted in CH_3CN and injected (5 µL) into HPLC using disposable Minisart SRP4 filters, with a pore width of 0.45 µm (Chromafil PET-20/25, Sartorius Stedim Biotech GmbH, Goettingen, Germany). The peak of IFD eluted at a retention time of 22.432 min (Figure 1) and was monitored at different wavelengths (220, 230, and 254 nm). The presence of curzerene, an artifact of IFD [1], has been excluded (Figure 4).

4.2. Animals and Experimental Groups

Twenty-eight male adult Wistar rats (8–10 weeks old) weighing 220–260 g were obtained from the Animal Center in Tehran University, Department of Pharmacology. Rats were maintained under standard laboratory conditions (temperature: 24 ± 1 °C, humidity: 60–65%, light/dark cycle: 12 h) with free access to standard animal food and water. All procedures were conducted in accordance with the guidelines of the Animal Ethics Committee of Tehran University of Medical Sciences (ethical approval number is 989843). They also complied with the NIH guide for the care and use of laboratory animals (NIH Publication No. 80-23; revised 1978).

The rats were randomly divided into four groups:

1. Sham group (saline injection as vehicle and surgery without induction of BCA occlusion and treatment).
2. Control group (saline injection as vehicle and induction of BCA occlusion without treatment).
3. Treated + control group (pre-administration of IFD + BCA occlusion model induction).
4. Positive control group (pre-administration of Nimodipine + BCA occlusion model induction).

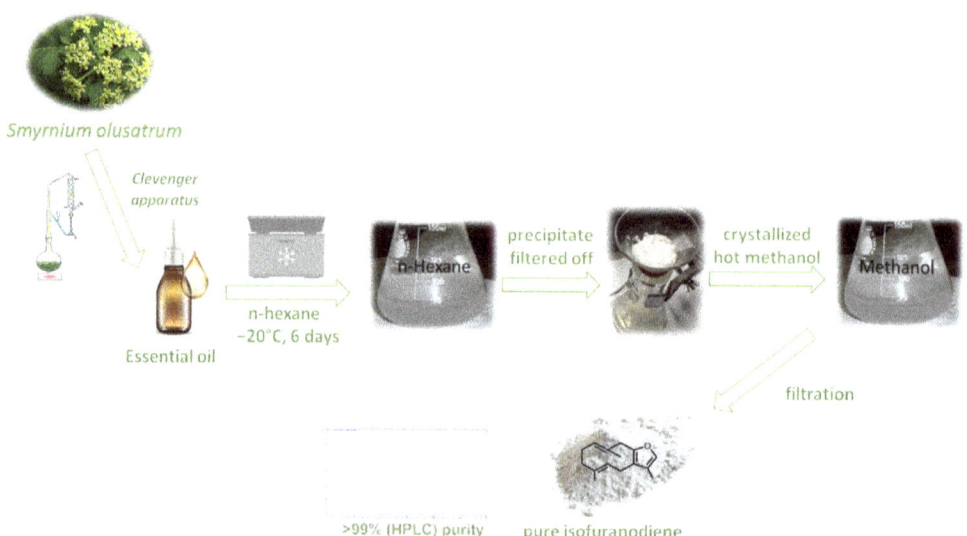

Figure 4. Isolation and purification of isofuranodiene.

4.3. Induction of Ischemic Stroke

The rats were anesthetized with an intraperitoneal injection of Ketamine (45 mg/kg); then, after incision of the rat neck, carotid arteries were occluded by a clamp. After 30 min occlusion, the clamp was removed and 60 min reperfusion was performed [12].

4.4. Treatments

The number of rats in each group was 7. Rats in treated groups received a single dose of 10 mg/kg of IFD (dissolved in saline as a vehicle, i.p.). This dose was chosen according to the minimum dose with high efficacy. This dose was revealed to be safe, as shown in a previous study [6]. Rats in the positive control group received a single dose of 10 mg/kg of Nimodipine (i.p.) for 30 min before BCA occlusion induction.

4.5. Behavioral Tests

Twenty-four hours after brain stroke induction, the grid-walking and modified neurological severity scores (mNSS) tests were used to assess the behavioral deficiency and remission caused by IFD treatment in rats. For the grid-walking test, a grid floor (45 × 45 cm) with holes measuring 1 cm across and 2.5 cm in height was used, and an assessment of the modified neurological severity score was performed. Our scoring system was based on the animals' footfall. The animals were allowed to walk freely on the grid floor for 1 min, and then video recording was started and analyzed by blind researchers. Each time the rat's claws touched the floor it was scored two, and every time they pulled their paw before touching the floor it was scored one. Higher scores indicated more severe injuries [29]. The mNSS test evaluates the function of motor and sensory reflexes. For each inability to carry out the test, one point was scored. The scale was graded from 0 (normal function) to 18 (maximum inability) [30].

4.6. Molecular Assays

The whole-brain homogenates were centrifuged at 12,000 rpm for 15 min, and the supernatants were assessed for amounts of inflammatory mediators such as TNFα (no. CSB-E11987r) and IL-1β (no. CSB-E08055r) using an R&D systems ELISA kit. In addition, the amount of MDA in the homogenates was evaluated using the lipid peroxidation assay with an MDA assay kit (no. KA3736).

4.7. Western Blotting

The changes in the expression of pNF-kB/NF-kB in the prefrontal cortex of the rat brain were evaluated by the Western blot assay. Following centrifuging at 12,000 rpm for 20 min at 4 °C, 10 mg of protein was determined on 10% SDS-PAGE gel and transferred onto polyvinylidene difluoride (PVDF) membranes (Millipore, Germany). Five percent non-fat skim milk was used in order to obstruct membranes in 120 min. Then, membranes were incubated overnight with these primary antibodies: β-actin, NF-kB, and pNF-kB. All of the antibodies were purchased from Santa Cruz Biotechnology (Santa Cruz, CA, USA). Tris-Buffered Saline with Tween 20 (TBST) was used for washing the membranes 3 times; then, they were incubated with secondary antibodies at room temperature for 1 h. The BM chemiluminescence Western blot kit (Roche, Mannheim, Germany) was used to detect bands, whereas the software ImageJ (Version 1.52t, Wayne Rasband (NIH), Bethesda, MD, USA) was used to evaluate their optimal density. The relative amount of pNF-kB/NF-kB was determined using GraphPad Prism 6 (San Diego, CA, USA).

4.8. Statistical Analysis

In this study, all analyses were carried out with Graph Pad Prism version 9 and SPSS software (version 22) (SPSS Inc., Chicago, IL, USA). One-way analysis of variance (ANOVA) followed by Tukey's post hoc test was used to evaluate multiple groups' differences. A p-value less than 0.05 was determined as a statistically significant level.

5. Conclusions

In conclusion, IFD, a natural sesquiterpene obtainable in great amounts from wild celery by a scalable procedure, exerts protective effects against brain ischemia by suppressing NF-κB-activation and reducing pro-inflammatory cytokines. Our data demonstrate the neuroprotective properties of IFD, suggesting that it may be effective in stroke therapy. Moreover, IFD may be considered a lead compound for discovering new treatments of brain ischemia. However, further pre-clinical studies such as pharmacokinetics and toxicological studies are needed in order to confirm the use of IFD as a promising compound to manage severe problems in ischemic stroke.

Author Contributions: Conceptualization, methodology, writing—original draft preparation, funding acquisition, H.Y.-M.; methodology, data curation, formal analysis, A.R.D., S.S., F.B., V.F., S.E.M., M.R.; methodology, data curation, formal analysis, revising and editing, L.C.; conceptualization, methodology, data curation, formal analysis, writing—original draft preparation, V.L., F.M.; conceptualization, methodology, data curation, formal analysis, funding acquisition, revising and editing, R.P. All authors have read and agreed to the published version of this manuscript.

Funding: This study has been supported by the Tehran University of Medical Sciences (TUMS) and a grant from the Italian Ministry of Health to R.P. (PRIN 2017CBNCYT_005).

Institutional Review Board Statement: This study was performed in accordance with Iranian regulations, and approval was obtained from the Animal Ethics Committee of Tehran University of Medical Sciences (ethical approval number is 989843, approved on 10 January 2020).

Informed Consent Statement: Not applicable.

Data Availability Statement: The data supporting the findings of this study are available on request from the corresponding authors upon reasonable request.

Conflicts of Interest: The authors declare no conflict of interest.

References

1. Maggi, F.; Barboni, L.; Papa, F.; Caprioli, G.; Ricciutelli, M.; Sagratini, G.; Vittori, S. A forgotten vegetable (*Smyrnium olusatrum* L., Apiaceae) as a rich source of isofuranodiene. *Food Chem.* **2012**, *135*, 2852–2862. [CrossRef]
2. Quassinti, L.; Bramucci, M.; Lupidi, G.; Barboni, L.; Ricciutelli, M.; Sagratini, G.; Papa, F.; Caprioli, G.; Petrelli, D.; Vitali, L.A.; et al. In vitro biological activity of essential oils and isolated furanosesquiterpenes from the neglected vegetable *Smyrnium olusatrum* L. (Apiaceae). *Food Chem.* **2013**, *138*, 808–813. [CrossRef]
3. Maggi, F.; Papa, F.; Giuliani, C.; Maleci Bini, L.; Venditti, A.; Bianco, A.; Nicoletti, M.; Iannarelli, R.; Caprioli, G.; Sagratini, G.; et al. Essential oil chemotypification and secretory structures of the neglected vegetable *Smyrnium olusatrum* L. (Apiaceae) growing in central Italy. *Flavour Fragr. J.* **2015**, *30*, 139–159. [CrossRef]
4. Giordano, G.; Carbone, M.; Ciavatta, M.L.; Silvano, E.; Gavagnin, M.; Garson, M.J.; Cheney, K.L.; Mudianta, I.W.; Russo, G.F.; Villani, G.; et al. Volatile secondary metabolites as aposematic olfactory signals and defensive weapons in aquatic environments. *Proc. Natl. Acad. Sci. USA* **2017**, *114*, 3451–3456. [CrossRef] [PubMed]
5. Mustafa, A.M.; Maggi, F.; Papa, F.; Kaya, E.; Dikmen, M.; Öztürk, Y. Isofuranodiene: A neuritogenic compound isolated from wild celery (*Smyrnium olusatrum* L., Apiaceae). *Food Chem.* **2016**, *192*, 782–787. [CrossRef] [PubMed]
6. Li, W.; Shi, J.; Papa, F.; Maggi, F.; Chen, X. Isofuranodiene, the main volatile constituent of wild celery (*Smyrnium olusatrum* L.), protects d-galactosamin/lipopolysacchride-induced liver injury in rats. *Nat. Prod. Res.* **2016**, *30*, 1162–1165. [CrossRef]
7. Benelli, G.; Pavela, R.; Canale, A.; Nicoletti, M.; Petrelli, R.; Cappellacci, L.; Galassi, R.; Maggi, F. Isofuranodiene and germacrone from *Smyrnium olusatrum* essential oil as acaricides and oviposition inhibitors against *Tetranychus urticae*: Impact of chemical stabilization of isofuranodiene by interaction with silver triflate. *J. Pest. Sci.* **2017**, *90*, 693–699. [CrossRef]
8. Brunetti, A.; Marinelli, O.; Morelli, M.B.; Iannarelli, R.; Amantini, C.; Russotti, D.; Santoni, G.; Maggi, F.; Nabissi, M. Isofuranodiene synergizes with Temozolomide in inducing glioma cells death. *Phytomedicine* **2019**, *52*, 51–59. [CrossRef] [PubMed]
9. Kavallieratos, N.G.; Boukouvala, M.C.; Ntalli, N.; Kontodimas, D.C.; Cappellacci, L.; Petrelli, R.; Ricciutelli, M.; Benelli, M.; Maggi, F. Efficacy of the furanosesquiterpene isofuranodiene against the stored-product insects *Prostephanus truncatus* (Coleoptera: Bostrychidae) and *Trogoderma granarium* (Coleoptera: Dermestidae). *J. Stored Prod. Res.* **2020**, *86*, 101553. [CrossRef]
10. Zhao, M.; Deng, X.; Gao, F.; Zhang, D.; Wang, S.; Zhang, Y.; Zhao, J. Ischemic stroke in young adults with moyamoya disease: Prognostic factors for stroke recurrence and functional outcome after revascularization. *World Neurosurg.* **2017**, *103*, 161–167. [CrossRef]
11. Johnson, C.O.; Nguyen, M.; Roth, G.A.; Nichols, E.; Alam, T.; Abate, D.; Adebayo, O.M. Global, regional, and national burden of stroke, 1990–2016: A systematic analysis for the Global Burden of Disease Study 2016. *Lancet Neurol.* **2019**, *18*, 439–458. [CrossRef]
12. Yousefi-Manesh, H.; Rashidian, A.; Hemmati, S.; Shirooie, S.; Sadeghi, M.A.; Zarei, N.; Dehpour, A.R. Therapeutic effects of modafinil in ischemic stroke; possible role of NF-κB downregulation. *Immunopharmacol. Immunotoxicol.* **2019**, *41*, 558–564. [CrossRef]
13. Nabavi, S.F.; Sureda, A.; Sanches-Silva, A.; Pandima Devi, K.; Ahmed, T.; Shahid, M.; Vacca, R.A. Novel therapeutic strategies for stroke: The role of autophagy. *Crit. Rev. Clin. Lab. Sci.* **2019**, *56*, 182–199. [CrossRef] [PubMed]
14. Granger, D.N.; Kvietys, P.R. Reperfusion injury and reactive oxygen species: The evolution of a concept. *Redox Biol.* **2015**, *6*, 524–551. [CrossRef] [PubMed]
15. Elsayed, W.M.; Abdel-Gawad, E.H.A.; Mesallam, D.I.; El-Serafy, T.S. The relationship between oxidative stress and acute ischemic stroke severity and functional outcome. *Egypt J. Neurol. Psychiatr. Neurosurg.* **2020**, *56*, 1–6. [CrossRef]
16. Clausen, B.H.; Wirenfeldt, M.; Høgedal, S.S.; Frich, L.H.; Nielsen, H.H.; Schrøder, H.D.; Lambertsen, K.L. Characterization of the TNF and IL-1 systems in human brain and blood after ischemic stroke. *Acta Neuropathol. Commun.* **2020**, *8*, 1–17. [CrossRef] [PubMed]
17. Nabavi, M.S.; Habtemariam, S.; Daglia, M.; Braidy, N.; Loizzo, M.; Tundis, R.; Nabavi, F.S. Neuroprotective effects of ginkgolide B against ischemic stroke: A review of current literature. *Curr. Top. Med. Chem.* **2015**, *15*, 2222–2232. [CrossRef]
18. De Oliveira, J.L.; Ávila, M.; Martins, T.C.; Alvarez-Silva, M.; Winkelmann-Duarte, E.C.; Salgado, A.S.I.; Martins, D.F. Medium-and long-term functional behavior evaluations in an experimental focal ischemic stroke mouse model. *Cogn. Neurodyn.* **2020**, *14*, 473–481. [CrossRef]
19. Lu, J.J.; Dang, Y.Y.; Huang, M.; Xu, W.S.; Chen, X.P.; Wang, Y.T. Anticancer properties of terpenoids isolated from Rhizoma Curcumae–a review. *J. Ethnopharmacol.* **2012**, *143*, 406–411. [CrossRef]
20. Germano, A.; Occhipinti, A.; Barbero, F.; Maffei, M.E. A pilot study on bioactive constituents and analgesic effects of MyrLiq®, a *Commiphora myrrha* extract with a high furanodiene content. *BioMed Res. Int.* **2017**, 380435. [CrossRef]
21. Petrelli, R.; Ranjbarian, F.; Dall'Acqua, S.; Papa, F.; Iannarelli, R.; Kamte, S.L.N.; Vittori, S.; Benelli, G.; Maggi, F.; Hofer, A.; et al. An overlooked horticultural crop, *Smyrnium olusatrum*, as a potential source of compounds effective against African trypanosomiasis. *Parasitol. Int.* **2017**, *66*, 146–151. [CrossRef] [PubMed]
22. Pavela, R.; Pavoni, L.; Bonacucina, G.; Cespi, M.; Kavallieratos, N.G.; Cappellacci, L.; Petrelli, R.; Maggi, F.; Benelli, G. Rationale for developing novel mosquito larvicides based on isofuranodiene microemulsions. *J. Pest. Sci.* **2019**, *92*, 909–921. [CrossRef]

23. Matsuda, H.; Ninomiya, K.; Morikawa, T.; Yoshikawa, M. Inhibitory effect and action mechanism of sesquiterpenes from Zedoariae Rhizoma on D-galactosamine/lipopolysaccharide-induced liver injury. *Bioorg. Med. Chem. Lett.* **1998**, *8*, 339–344. [CrossRef]
24. Morikawa, T.; Matsuda, H.; Ninomiya, K.; Yoshikawa, M. Medicinal foodstuffs. XXIX. Potent protective effects of sesquiterpenes and curcumin from Zedoariae Rhizoma on liver injury induced by D-galactosamine/lipopolysaccharide or tumor necrosis factor-α. *Biol. Pharm. Bull.* **2002**, *25*, 627–631. [CrossRef]
25. Howell, J.A.; Bidwell III, G.L. Targeting the NF-κB pathway for therapy of ischemic stroke. *Therap. Del.* **2020**, *11*, 113–123. [CrossRef] [PubMed]
26. Latanich, C.A.; Toledo-Pereyra, L.H. Searching for NF-κB-based treatments of ischemia reperfusion injury. *J. Invest. Surg.* **2009**, *22*, 301–315. [CrossRef] [PubMed]
27. Zhou, J.; Li, M.; Jin, W.F.; Li, X.H.; Zhang, Y.Y. Role of NF-κB on neurons after cerebral ischemia reperfusion. *Int. J. Pharmacol.* **2018**, *14*, 451–459. [CrossRef]
28. Campos-Esparza, M.R.; Sánchez-Gómez, M.V.; Matute, C. Molecular mechanisms of neuroprotection by two natural antioxidant polyphenols. *Cell Calcium* **2009**, *45*, 358–368. [CrossRef] [PubMed]
29. Chen, S.F.; Hsu, C.W.; Huang, W.H.; Wang, J.Y. Post-injury baicalein improves histological and functional outcomes and reduces inflammatory cytokines after experimental traumatic brain injury. *Br. J. Pharmacol.* **2008**, *155*, 1279–1296. [CrossRef] [PubMed]
30. Zhou, Y.X.; Wang, X.; Tang, D.; Li, Y.; Jiao, Y.F.; Gan, Y.; Li, P.Y. IL-2mAb reduces demyelination after focal cerebral ischemia by suppressing CD8+ T cells. *CNS Neurosci. Ther.* **2019**, *25*, 532–543. [CrossRef]

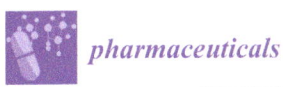

Article

Lichen-Derived Compounds and Extracts as Biologically Active Substances with Anticancer and Neuroprotective Properties

Elżbieta Studzińska-Sroka [1,*], Aleksandra Majchrzak-Celińska [2], Przemysław Zalewski [1], Dominik Szwajgier [3], Ewa Baranowska-Wójcik [3], Barbara Kaproń [4], Tomasz Plech [5], Marcin Żarowski [6] and Judyta Cielecka-Piontek [1]

- [1] Department of Pharmacognosy, Poznan University of Medical Sciences, Święcickiego 4, 60-781 Poznan, Poland; pzalewski@ump.edu.pl (P.Z.); jpiontek@ump.edu.pl (J.C.-P.)
- [2] Department of Pharmaceutical Biochemistry, Poznan University of Medical Sciences, Święcickiego 4, 60-781 Poznan, Poland; majchrzakcelinska@ump.edu.pl
- [3] Department of Biotechnology, Microbiology and Human Nutrition, University of Life Sciences in Lublin, Skromna 8, 20-704 Lublin, Poland; dominik.szwajgier@up.lublin.pl (D.S.); ewa.baranowska@up.lublin.pl (E.B.-W.)
- [4] Department of Clinical Genetics, Medical University of Lublin, Radziwiłłowska 11, 20-080 Lublin, Poland; barbara.kapron@umlub.pl
- [5] Department of Pharmacology, Medical University of Lublin, Chodźki 4a, 20-093 Lublin, Poland; tomasz.plech@umlub.pl
- [6] Department of Developmental Neurology, Poznan University of Medical Sciences, Przybyszewski 49, 60-355 Poznan, Poland; zarowski@ump.edu.pl
- * Correspondence: elastudzinska@ump.edu.pl

Abstract: Lichens are a source of chemical compounds with valuable biological properties, structurally predisposed to penetration into the central nervous system (CNS). Hence, our research aimed to examine the biological potential of lipophilic extracts of *Parmelia sulcata*, *Evernia prunastri*, *Cladonia uncialis*, and their major secondary metabolites, in the context of searching for new therapies for CNS diseases, mainly glioblastoma multiforme (GBM). The extracts selected for the study were standardized for their content of salazinic acid, evernic acid, and (−)-usnic acid, respectively. The extracts and lichen metabolites were evaluated in terms of their anti-tumor activity, i.e., cytotoxicity against A-172 and T98G cell lines and anti-IDO1, IDO2, TDO activity, their anti-inflammatory properties exerted by anti-COX-2 and anti-hyaluronidase activity, antioxidant activity, and anti-acetylcholinesterase and anti-butyrylcholinesterase activity. The results of this study indicate that lichen-derived compounds and extracts exert significant cytotoxicity against GBM cells, inhibit the kynurenine pathway enzymes, and have anti-inflammatory properties and weak antioxidant and anti-cholinesterase properties. Moreover, evernic acid and (−)-usnic acid were shown to be able to cross the blood-brain barrier. These results demonstrate that lichen-derived extracts and compounds, especially (−)-usnic acid, can be regarded as prototypes of pharmacologically active compounds within the CNS, especially suitable for the treatment of GBM.

Keywords: (−)-usnic acid; evernic acid; salazinic acid; secondary metabolites; lichen extracts; biological activity

1. Introduction

Secondary metabolites of lichens are polyphenolic compounds, constituting a group of natural substances with unique chemical structures and interesting biological properties. Phenolic compounds are effective against different neoplasms, which are one of the most important medical problems. Central nervous system (CNS) tumors are especially challenging, with glioblastoma multiforme (GBM) being one of the most deadly cancers. A growing body of evidence shows that natural bioactive molecules may serve well as an alternative approach to the treatment and control of GBM [1]. This prompted us to undertake further research on lichen-derived substances as important novel remedies useful in GBM therapy.

The research on lichen-derived compounds has recently been intensified, leading to the acquisition of data on their various mechanisms resulting in anticancer activity [2], as well as their anti-inflammatory, antioxidant, and neuroprotective properties [3]. Lichens grow in all continents, but *Parmelia sulcata (Parmeliaceae)*, *Evernia prunastri (Parmeliaceae)*, and *Cladonia uncialis (Cladoniaceae)* are species especially abundant in the northern hemisphere [4]. Their biological potential is attributed largely to lipophilic phenolic compounds, namely salazinic acid, evernic acid, and (−) - usnic acid, respectively [5,6]. The cytotoxic properties of salazinic acid and *P. sulcata* extracts, as well as evernic acid and *E. prunastri* lipophilic extracts, have been confirmed on various cancer cell lines [7–10]. Moreover, moderate antioxidant activity of salazinic acid [11] and *P. sulcata* extracts [10,12] has been reported. Evidence also exists for neuroprotective and anti-inflammatory properties of evernic acid, which can especially be important in the context of Parkinson's disease [13,14]. The derivatives of dibenzofurans, including usnic acids (right and left-handed isomer) are known for their strong anticancer properties [15]. Among other research, their activity against tumors developing in the CNS (neuroblastoma, GBM) [16–18] was also reported. The literature indicates the anti-inflammatory potential and the anti-neurodegenerative effect [14] of these compounds. The right-handed isomer is more often studied, while data on the left-handed isoform are limited. There are also no studies on the anti-tumor activity of *C. uncialis*.

Current literature also indicates that lichen-derived compounds, as well as their synthetic derivatives, can enhance the effects of currently used anticancer drugs. For instance, the co-treatment of lobarstin, a secondary metabolite isolated from *Stereocaulon alpinum*, enhanced toxicity of temozolomide when used in GBM T98G cells [19]. In another study, the ketamine derivatives of (+)-usnic acid had significant cytotoxicity against human GBM-astrocytoma cell line U87MG, and a novel N-heterocyclic derivative of (+)-usnic acid was found to be even more active than temozolomide [20]. These findings justify further studies exploring the possible applications of lichenochemicals in brain tumor treatment.

In addition to the lichen-derived compounds, the biological potential of lichen-derived extracts has largely remained unexplored. Lichen extracts are a source of a plethora of compounds including pulvinic acid derivatives, terpenes, carotenoids, depsides, depsidones, depsones, anthraquinones, and xanthones [21]. Such a high diversity of compounds, often acting synergistically, makes the extracts very attractive for investigation. Moreover, there is growing evidence that crude lichen extracts often have greater in vitro or/and in vivo activity as compared to pure compounds [22].

Our previous study indicated the anticancer and neuroprotective potential of physodic acid and the acetone extract from *Hypogymnia physodes* [23], encouraging us to undertake further work aimed at examining the biological potential of selected lichen-derived extracts and their dominant secondary metabolites in the context of their potential application in GBM treatment and the protection of the brain tissue. Thus, in this study we evaluated the cytotoxic, anti-inflammatory, antioxidant, and anticholinergic properties of lichen acetone extracts from *P. sulcata*, *E. prunastri*, and *C. uncialis* as well as their most important components, salazinic acid, evernic acid and (−)-usnic acid (Figure 1), respectively. Using the in vitro PAMPA-BBB model, the penetration of the tested lichen compounds through the blood-brain barrier (BBB) was also determined.

Salazinic acid   Evernic acid   (-)-Usnic acid

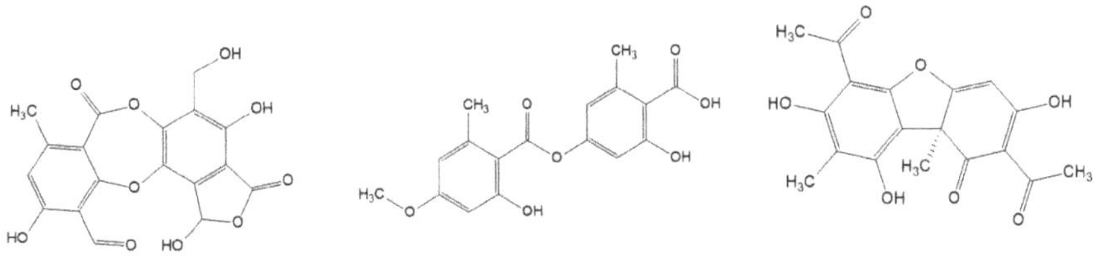

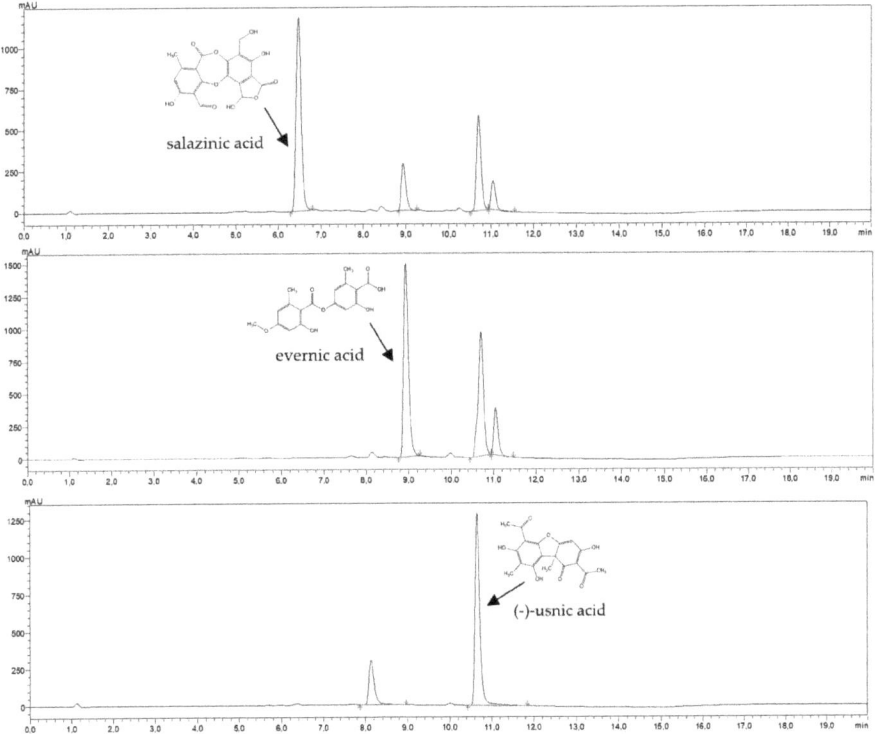

Figure 1. The chemical structures of lichen-derived substances—salazinic acid, evernic acid and (−)-usnic acid—investigated in this study.

2. Results

2.1. Phytochemicals Analysis

2.1.1. Quantitative Analysis of Extracts' Components

The content of the species-specific compounds in the lichen acetone extracts was determined using HPLC analysis. The best separation of the *P. sulcata, E. prunastri,* and *C. uncialis* acetone extracts was obtained with gradient elution (acetonitrile and 0.5% formic acid) on 5 µm core–shell particles. The components of the lichen extracts were separated in less than 11 min. As presented in Figure 2, the method was selective for salazinic acid (t_R = 6.5 min), evernic acid (t_R = 8.9 min), and (−)-usnic acid (t_R = 10.6 min).

Figure 2. The chromatograms of acetone extract from *P. sulcata, E. prunastri,* and *C. uncialis*, showing the identified compounds, i.e., salazinic acid, evernic acid, and (−)-usnic acid, respectively. The compounds were characterised by t_R = 6.5 min, 8.9 min, and 10.6 min, respectively.

The HPLC analysis revealed that the acetone extracts of *P. sulcata* contained 23.05% of salazinic acid, *E. prunastri* extracts contained 66.63% of evernic acid, while *C. uncialis* extracts contained 30.65% of (−)-usnic acid.

2.1.2. Total Polyphenols Content

The total polyphenols content was determined in the lichen extracts using the spectrophotometric Folin–Ciocalteau method. The tested acetone extracts (*P. sulcata*, *E. prunastri*, *C. uncialis*) were characterized by a different content of phenolic compounds. The highest content of the phenolic compounds was measured for *E. prunastri* extract (276.95 ± 3.87 mg GAE/g of extract), as compared to *P. sulcata* and *C. uncialis* extracts, which demonstrated lower content of polyphenols (130.5 ± 0.3 mg GAE/g of extract and 71.0 ± 0.3 mg GAE/g of extract, respectively).

2.2. Biological Activity

2.2.1. Anti-Tumor Activity

Cytotoxic Activity against GBM Cells

The viability assay showed the dose-dependent cytotoxicity of the tested lichen-derived compounds and extracts in regard to GBM cells. Generally, both A-172 and T98G cells reacted in a similar manner to the treatments (Figure 3). Salazinic acid reduced cell viability only at the highest tested concentration (100 µM), while *P. sulcata* extract diminished the percentage of living cells at 50 µg/mL and 100 µg/mL concentration in both cell lines (also 25 µg/mL concentration reached statistical significance in the A-172 cell line). Evernic acid reduced A-172 cell viability at 10 µM concentration; in the T98G cell line, however, it was only mildly cytotoxic—only the highest tested concentration led to ~ 20% reduction in cell viability. *E. prunastri* extract significantly reduced A-172 cell viability at 25 µg/mL concentration, but the highest tested concentration still allowed the survival of more than one fourth of the seeded cell population. In contrast, in the T98G cell line, 50 µg/mL *E. prunastri* extract decreased viability to 60.50 ± 0.71%, but 100 µg/mL concentration was completely cytotoxic. As far as (−)-usnic acid is concerned, all the tested concentrations up to 100 µg/mL in A-172 and 50 µg/mL in the T98G cell line were generally not cytotoxic. In regard to the *C. uncialis* extract, it significantly reduced cell viability even at 1 µg/mL, while the highest tested concentration of this extract led to almost complete cell death, i.e., only 8.33 ± 1.15% and 11.67 ± 0.58% of A-172 and T98G cells, respectively, were still alive and metabolically active. The IC_{50} values of all the analyzed lichen-derived compounds and extracts are presented in Table 1.

Table 1. The IC_{50} of the analyzed lichen-derived compounds/extracts established after 48 h treatment of A-172 and T98G cell lines.

Lichen-Derived Compound/ Extract	A-172		T98G	
	IC_{50} (µg/mL)	IC_{50} (µM)	IC_{50} (µg/mL)	IC_{50} (µM)
Salazinic acid	>38.8	>100.0	>38.8	>100.0
P. sulcata extract	73.6 ± 7.3	-	89.8 ± 5.1	-
Evernic acid	>33.2	>100.0	>33.2	>100.0
E. prunastri extract	73.8 ± 5.5	-	61.0 ± 1.1	-
(−)-Usnic acid	31.5 ± 0.8	91.4 ± 2.0	13.0 ± 1.3	37.8 ± 3.8
C. uncialis extract	11.0 ± 4.6	-	3.9 ± 2.2	-

IC_{50} ± SEM was calculated from the results obtained in three independent experiments with four measurements per assay, for each point in the concentration curve.

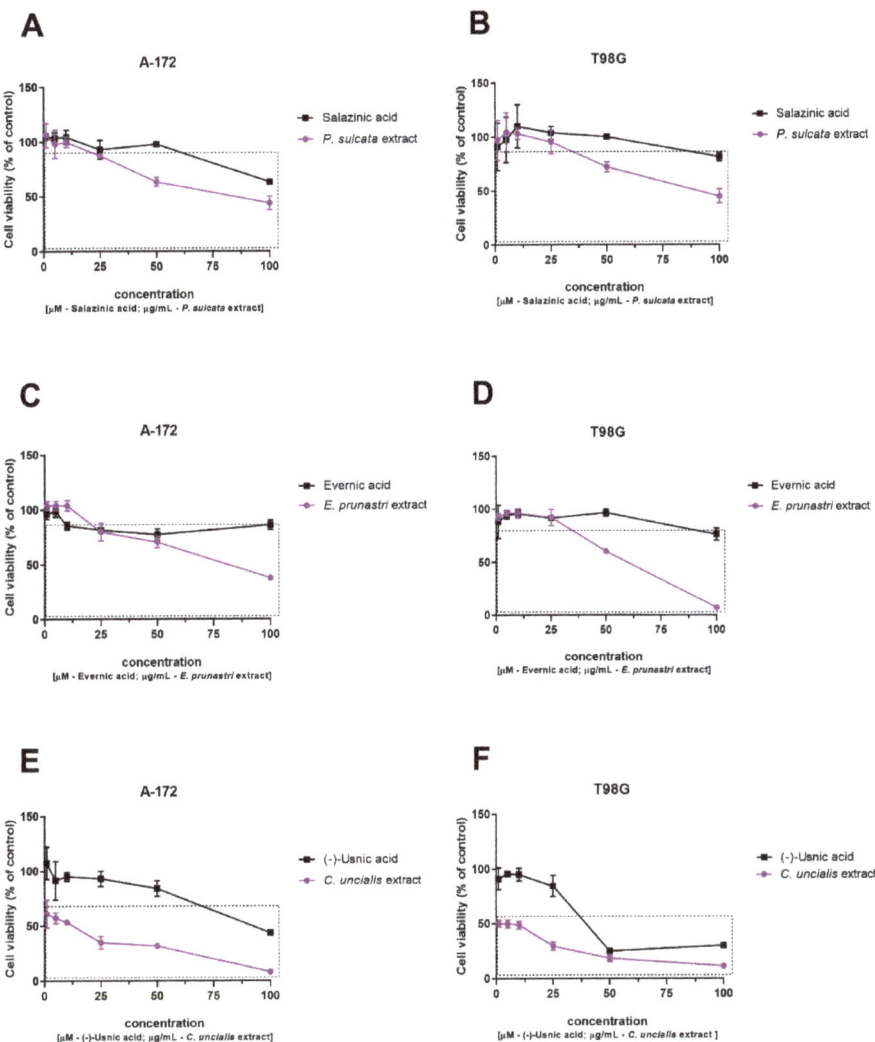

Figure 3. The cytotoxicity evaluation of salazinic acid and *P. sulcata* acetone extract in A-172 cell line (**A**) and T98G cell line (**B**), of evernic acid and *E. prunastri* acetone extract in A-172 cell line (**C**) and T98G cell line (**D**), and of (−)-usnic acid and *C. uncialis* acetone extract in A-172 cell line (**E**) and T98G cell line (**F**), based on 48 h MTT test. DMSO-treated cells (control) were assigned as 100% cell viability. Statistically significant difference in cell viability between the cells exposed to the analyzed lichen-derived compound or extract as compared to the control cells is indicated with a rectangle. The mean values ± SEM from three independent experiments with four measurements per assay are presented.

Inhibition of the Kynurenine Pathway Enzymes: Indoleamine 2,3-Dioxygenases 1 (IDO1), Indoleamine 2,3-Dioxygenases 2 (IDO2), and Tryptophan 2,3-Dioxygenase (TDO)

The kynurenine pathway plays a role in the development of GBM and is regarded as a possible molecular target for GBM treatment [24]. Thus, our next goal was to analyze if the lichen-derived compounds and extracts possess inhibitory properties related to kynurenine pathway enzymes, indoleamine 2,3-dioxygenases 1 (IDO1), indoleamine 2,3-dioxygenases 2 (IDO2), and tryptophan 2,3-dioxygenase (TDO). Our results show that out of the investigated lichen-derived compounds, only salazinic acid did not exhibit any inhibition effect against IDO1, IDO2, and TDO enzymes (Table 2). The other lichen-derived compounds and extracts, similarly to epacadostat (the reference drug with IC_{50} = 17.4 ± 1.1 nM), turned out to be IDO1 selective inhibitors. Evernic acid and (−)-usnic acid, assayed in a fixed concentration of 100 µg/mL, displayed ability to reduce the activity of IDO1 by 32.84 ± 1.93% and 21.62 ± 0.85%, respectively. The most effective inhibitory activity was shown by C. uncialis extract, that inhibited IDO1 by 54.82 ± 3.51%. The extracts obtained from E. prunastri and P. sulcata reduced the activity of the tested enzyme by 43.06 ± 1.97% and 20.47 ± 1.23%, respectively (Table 2).

Table 2. Effect of the investigated lichen extracts and reference compounds on the activity of indoleamine-2,3-dioxygenase (IDO1, IDO2) and tryptophan-2,3-dioxygenase (TDO).

Lichen-Derived Compound/Extract	Inhibition (%)		
	IDO1	IDO2	TDO
Salazinic acid	-	-	-
P. sulcata extract	20.5 ± 1.2	-	-
Evernic acid	32.8 ± 1.9	-	-
E. prunastri extract	43.1 ± 2.0	-	-
(−)-Usnic acid	21.6 ± 0.9	-	-
C. uncialis extract	54.8 ± 3.5	-	-
epacadostat	95.6 ± 2.8	-	-

"-"—not active (i.e., inhibitory effect was lower than 10%). Concentration of examined samples was 100 µg/mL. The mean values ± SEM from three independent measurements are presented.

2.2.2. Anti-Inflammatory Activity
Inhibition of Cyclooxygenase-2 (COX-2)

Cyclooxygenase-2 (COX-2), the enzyme involved in both initiation and resolution of inflammation [25], has been implicated in tumorigenesis and progression of GBM [26]. Overexpression of COX2 appears also during natural or pathological aging of the brain [27]. The results of our study indicate that all the tested lichen-derived compounds and extracts exerted anti-COX-2 effects. As shown in Table 3, the most potent anti-COX-2 activity was shown by P. sulcata extract (65.9 ± 4.1%) and salazinic acid (60.3 ± 3.0%). (−)-Usnic acid and evernic acid were also characterized by strong anti-inflammatory activity, inhibiting COX-2 to 59.3 ± 3.5% and 50.7 ± 2.1%, respectively. The anti-COX-2 activity of the other analyzed extracts, namely E. prunastri and C. uncialis extracts were weaker, though still noticeable.

Table 3. Inhibition of cyclooxygenase-2 (COX-2) enzyme by the extracts of P. sulcata, E. prunastri, and C. uncialis as well as their major secondary metabolites: salazinic acid, evernic acid and (−)-usnic acid.

Lichen-Derived Compound/Extract	Equivalent Concentration of Acetylsalicylic Acid (mg/mL)	COX-2 Inhibition (%)
Salazinic acid	12.9 ± 0.1	60.3 ± 3.0
P. sulcata extract	13.0 ± 0.8	65.9 ± 4.1
Evernic acid	10.9 ± 1.8	50.7 ± 2.1
E. prunastri extract	10.0 ± 0.2	35.9 ± 2.8
(−)-Usnic acid	12.9 ± 1.5	59.3 ± 3.5
C. uncialis extract	10.4 ± 0.1	45.9 ± 1.9

Concentration of examined samples: see Section 4. The mean values ± SEM from three independent experiments with four measurements per assay are presented.

Anti-Hyaluronidase Activity

Hyaluronidase is an enzyme responsible for maintaining the homeostasis of hyaluronan in the extracellular matrix. Upregulation of this enzyme activity is observed in chronic inflammatory conditions [28]. In addition, hyaluronidase, responsible for generating smaller fragments of hyaluronidase (HA), may be crucial for the correct functioning of the CNS [29]. Therefore, we determined the effect of lichen-derived compounds and extracts on hyaluronidase activity. The results presented in Figure 4 show that in the tested concentration range, lichen-derived compounds and extracts, excluding *C. uncialis* extract ($IC_{50} > 0.75$ mg/mL), demonstrate the ability to inhibit hyaluronidase (Figure 4). In fact, the inhibitory properties of salazinic acid and evernic acid were similar to those obtained for β-escin, used as a standard. In addition, we noticed the pronounced difference between the extracts' activity and the activity of pure compounds. The inhibitory potential was more pronounced for the examined extracts.

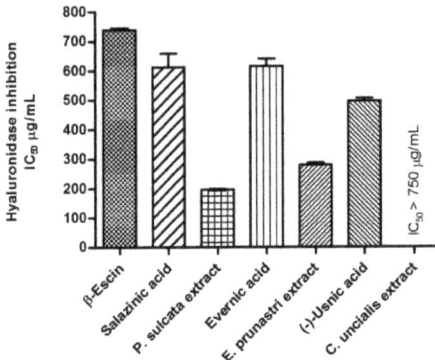

Figure 4. Inhibition of hyaluronidase by lichen-derived substances and extracts as well as by β-escin (served as a standard in this assay). Results are presented as IC_{50} mean values (mg/mL) ± SEM (five measurements; $n = 5$ for lichen-derived compounds; and $n = 6$ for β-escin) obtained in two independent experiments.

2.2.3. Impact on Reactive Oxygen Species (ROS) Homeostasis

The disruption of CNS homeostasis may be caused by oxidative stress [30]. However, in cancer cells ROS are able to trigger programmed cell death and ROS generation is an important mechanism of chemo- and radio-therapy [31]. Therefore, it is important to determine how lichen-derived compounds and extracts influence ROS homeostasis. In this context, assessment of the antioxidant activity of *P. sulcata*, *E. prunastri*, *C. uncialis* acetone extracts, and salazinic acid, evernic acid (−)-usnic acid isolated from these lichens, was undertaken using two different spectroscopic methods. The well-known DPPH method assesses the free radical scavenging ability of a sample in vitro, while the CUPRAC method shows the ability of the tested substances to reduce cations of metals. As displayed in Table 4, only *P. sulcata* and *E. prunastri* extracts were able to scavenge the DPPH radical and reduce Cu^{2+} ions measured in the assumed concentration range. In the DPPH test, the *P. sulcata* extract was more active than the *E. prunastri* extract. The CUPRAC method showed that *E. prunastri* extract reduced metal ions more strongly than *P. sulcata* extract. It is worth mentioning that the detected activity of *E. prunastri* was only 3–4 times lower than resveratrol, which is considered as a potent antioxidant. None of the tested lichen-derived compounds showed antioxidant activity in the performed experimental models and concentrations.

Table 4. Antioxidant activity of lichen extracts and compounds measured using DPPH and CUPRAC analysis.

Lichen-Derived Compound/Extract	DPPH IC$_{50}$ (µg/mL)	CUPRAC IC$_{0.5}$ (µg/mL)
Salazinic acid	>750.0	>250.0
P. sulcata extract	669.3 ± 11.8	175.4 ± 1.0
Evernic acid	>750.0	>250.0
E. prunastri extract	1926.3 ± 33.2	103.4 ± 1.4
(−)-Usnic acid	>750.0	>250.0
C. uncialis extract	>2500.0	>312.5
resveratrol	25.1 ± 0.1	29.7 ± 0.1

IC$_{50}$—the IC$_{50}$ values, i.e., the concentration of an antioxidant necessary to halve the initial DPPH$^{\bullet}$ concentration (for lichen-derived substances the highest concentration was 750.0 µg/mL, for extracts 2500.0 µg/mL); IC$_{0.5}$ values, i.e., the concentration of an antioxidant necessary to achieve the absorbance of 0.5 in the CUPRAC analysis (for lichen-derived substances the highest concentration was 250.0 µg/mL, for extracts 312.5 µg/mL). The mean values ± SEM from three measurements are presented (n = 3).

Effect on Antioxidant Enzyme Activity

Superoxide dismutase (SOD), glutathione reductase (GR), and glutathione peroxidase (GPx) are the main endogenous enzymatic defense systems of human cells [32]. Therefore, we checked the influence of the lichen-derived compounds and extracts on SOD, GR, and GPx using in vitro spectroscopic methods. In regard to SOD, the present study showed that both lichen-derived compounds and extracts have the capacity to inhibit the activity of this enzyme (Table 5). The highest inhibitory activity was detected for E. prunastri extract, as it inhibited more than half of SOD activity (53.4% ± 2.4%) (Table 5). P. sulcata extract and its major constituent salazinic acid, as well as evernic acid and (−)-usnic acid, inhibited SOD activity by ~20%. The weakest, although still noticeable SOD inhibitory activity was exerted by C. uncialis extract (12.8% ± 1.0%).

Table 5. Effect of lichen extracts and compounds on SOD activity.

Lichen-Derived Compound/Extract	SOD Inhibition (%)
Salazinic acid	19.4 ± 0.3
P. sulcata extract	22.0 ± 1.3
Evernic acid	21.2 ± 0.0
E. prunastri extract	53.4 ± 2.4
(−)-Usnic acid	19.6 ± 0.6
C. uncialis extract	12.8 ± 1.0

Concentration of examined sample in the reaction mixture: 537.6 µg/mL reaction mixture. The mean values ± SEM from three measurements are presented (n = 3).

The inhibitory effect of lichen substances on GR and GPx enzymes was also determined in our study. The results show that the most potent inhibitory effect was demonstrated by E. prunastri extract, which inhibited both GR and GPx. Interestingly GPx was inhibited only in 20.0 ± 2.1% by evernic acid, contrasted to 92.4 ± 4.3% by the E. prunastri extract, evernic acid. Both enzymes (GP and GPx) were also inhibited by (−) - usnic acid, but more weakly than by the E. prunastri extract. Quite potent inhibition against GPx was also presented by the PS extract, which did not inhibit the GR at all. Salazinic acid and C. uncialis extract showed no activity (Table 6).

Table 6. Effect of lichen extracts and compounds on GR and GPx activity.

Lichen-Derived Compound/Extract	GR Inhibition under Reaction Conditions (%)	GR Inhibitory Activity (nMol Depleted NADPH/min Incubation)	GPx Inhibition under Reaction Conditions (%)	GPx Inhibitory Activity (nMol Depleted NADPH/min Incubation)
Salazinic acid	-	-	-	-
P. sulcata extract	-	-	47.1 ± 0.7	93.9 ± 5.2
Evernic acid	-	-	20.0 ± 2.1	39.9 ± 1.0
E. prunastri extract	91.1 ± 7.2	3551.2 ± 264.4	92.4 ± 4.3	184.2 ± 30.2
(−)-Usnic acid	18.2 ± 2.2	710.2 ± 42.3	13.7 ± 2.3	27.3 ± 1.3
C. uncialis extract	-	-	-	-

"-"—not active; concentration of examined sample in the reaction mixture: 444.4 µg/mL (GR), 243.9 µg/mL (GPx).

2.2.4. Anticholinergic Activity

Cholinesterases are a group of enzymes responsible by the hydrolysis of acetylcholine, playing a fundamental role in neurosynaptic communication. Increased activity of these enzymes has also been noted in brain tumors [33]. Thus, to investigate the anticholinesterase effect (anti-AChE and anti-BChE) of *P. sulcata*, *E. prunastri*, *C. uncialis* and isolates of salazinic acid, evernic acid and (−)-usnic acid, the modified Elman's method was used. Our results indicated the diversified activity of the tested extracts and compounds. The extract of *C. uncialis* only, weakly inhibited AChE. BChE, an enzyme with lower substrate specificity [34], was inhibited by most of the tested substances (Table 7). The greatest inhibition of BChE was shown by evernic acid.

Table 7. Inhibition of AChE and BChE by lichen substances expressed as equivalent reference concentration.

Lichen-Derived Compound/Extract	Equivalent Reference Concentration (µg/mL)									
	Neostygmine		Magniflorine		Donepezil		Eserine		Rivastigmine	
	AChE	BChE	AChE	BChE	AChE	BChE	AChE	BChE	AChE	BChE
Salazinic acid	-	13.6 ± 0.1	-	43.2 ± 0.2	-	7.9 ± 0.3	-	9.0 ± 0.1	-	70.9 ± 0.3
P. sulacata extract	-	8.1 ± 0.0	-	26.2 ± 0.6	-	4.8 ± 0.1	-	5.4 ± 0.6	-	42.9 ± 0.1
Evernic acid	-	16.5 ± 0.2	-	52.3 ± 0.1	-	9.5 ± 0.0	-	10.9 ± 0.1	-	85.9 ± 0.1
E. prunastri extract	-	-	-	-	-	-	-	-	-	-
(−)-Usnic acid	-	-	-	-	-	-	-	-	-	-
C. uncialis extract	0.7 ± 0.1	16.5 ± 0.1	7.9 ± 0.0	52.3 ± 0.1	0.6 ± 0.1	9.5 ± 0.4	0.1 ± 0.0	10.9 ± 0.0	1.4 ± 0.0	85.9 ± 0.2

"-"—not active; concentration in the reaction mixture: 142.9 µg/mL.

2.3. Permeability through the Blood-Brain-Barrier (PAMPA-BBB)

The presence of an active compound at the site of its action is essential for achieving a biological effect. Thus, using the Parallel Artificial Membrane Permeability Assay for the Blood-Brain Barrier (PAMPA-BBB) we evaluated if lichen-derived compounds, both used as pure substances and as the components of extracts, can cross the BBB and reach the CNS. The results of our analysis revealed that the permeability of the tested compounds varied significantly. For (−)-usnic acid and evernic acid, whether it was permeated from the extract or as a pure compound, the calculated Pe proved their high permeability ($Pe > 1.5 \times 10^{-6}$ cm/s) [35,36]. We noted that (−)-usnic acid penetrated extremely strongly compared to the other tested compounds. This is indicated by the very high Pe index achieved after 1 h incubation time. Salazinic acid, the depsidone from *P. sulcata*, was characterized by the very low Pe coefficient ($Pe < 0.5 \times 10^{-6}$ cm/s). Data analysis also showed that the degree of permeation is similar, whether the compound is permeated from the extracts or as a pure substance (Table 8).

Table 8. The effective permeability (*Pe*) of salazinic acid, evernic acid, (−)-usnic acid as pure compounds and from extracts using the Parallel Artificial Membrane Permeability Assay for the Blood-Brain Barrier (PAMPA-BBB).

Lichen-Derived Compound/Extract	$Pe \times 10^{-6}$ (cm/s) $t = 1$ h	$Pe \times 10^{-6}$ (cm/s) $t = 4$ h
Salazinic acid (PC)	np	np
Salazinic acid (from PSE)	np	np
Evernic acid (PC)	5.2 ± 0.8	8.6 ± 0.4
Evernic acid (from EPE)	5.0 ± 0.7	7.2 ± 0.4
(−)-Usnic acid (PC)	92.8 ± 6.3	nd
(−)-Usnic acid (from CUE)	140.5 ± 7.3	nd

Np—classified as non-permeable (i.e., $Pe < 0.5 \times 10^{-6}$ cm/s); nd – not determined; PC—pure compound; PSE—*P. sulcata* acetone extract; EPE—*E. prunastri* acetone extract; CUE—*C. uncialis* acetone extract. Results are presented as $Pe \times 10^{-6}$ cm/s. The mean values ± SEM from three independent experiments are presented ($n = 3$).

2.4. Summary of Biological Potential of Lichen-Derived Compounds and Extracts

To summarize the results obtained, we presented the data as a star diagram (Figure 5). This chart allowed us to assess the total biological potential in terms of the assessed directions of activity. The highest activity among the tested compounds was characterized by (−)-usnic acid. The other two compounds were less active. Evernic acid was involved in all directions of activity presented in the graph (cytotoxic, anti-inflammatory, and antioxidant inhibitory activity). These properties were admittedly a bit weaker than those demonstrated by salazinic acid, but more diverse. Salazinic acid was, however, more potent as an anti-inflammatory agent, but it was not active in regard to IDO1 inhibition.

The analysis of the biological potential of the extracts showed that *C. uncialis* extract had the highest cytotoxic activity and the lowest anti-inflammatory and antioxidant enzyme-inhibiting activity. On the other hand, *E. prunastri* extract most strongly inhibited the antioxidant enzymes. Still, it had the weakest anti-inflammatory effect, and its cytotoxic effect on cancer cells was comparable to that of *P. sulcata* extract. However, its higher IDO1 inhibitory capacity suggests a greater antitumor potency as compared to *P. sulcata* extract. In fact, the latter exhibited the weakest properties in regard to anticancer properties.

The analysis of the charts also allowed us to observe the differences in the potency between pure compounds and the extracts. The presented figure shows that the compounds tested in the same concentration as the extracts (see Figure 5 caption) had lower activity as compared to the extracts from which they originated. The potency of the extracts was sometimes even several times higher. It is important to note that the lichen-derived extracts contain a plethora of compounds, which acting together shift the extract's properties from the ones exerted by its main components. For instance, *C. uncialis* extract and (−)-usnic acid differed in their anti-inflammatory properties, while in case of *E. prunastri* extract, its ability to inhibit antioxidant enzymes was found to be significantly enhanced due to the presence of components besides evernic acid. In turn, the extract of *P. sulcata* had high anti-inflammatory activity, especially expressed by the ability to inhibit the activity of hyaluronidase. This may indicate the synergism of the action of the substances present.

The cytotoxic activity of the extracts was slightly increased or remained at a comparable level as compared to the pure compounds. What is more, considering the amount of active substance in the tested extracts, especially for *C. uncialis* and *P. sulcata* extracts, the cytotoxic effect on GBM cells was more pronounced than for (−)-usnic and salazinic acid, respectively. To conclude, our data suggest that the lichen-derived extracts are more promising anti-GBM agents, as compared to pure lichen-derived substances.

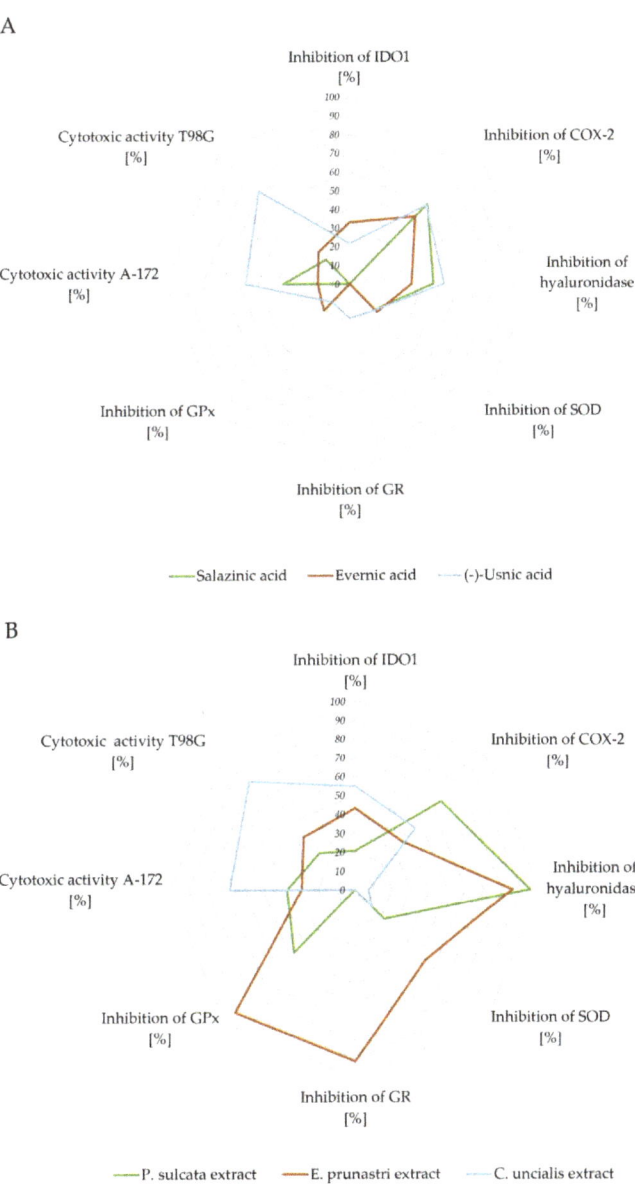

Figure 5. The biological activity of lichen-derived compounds and extracts: compounds (**A**) and extracts (**B**), expressed by the surface of area, taking into account the measured biological properties expressed in %. The graphs were made for the concentrations: inhibition of IDO1 100.0 μg/mL (**A**,**B**); inhibition of COX-2 250.0 μg/mL (**A**,**B**); inhibition of hyaluronidase 500.0 μg/mL (**A**,**B**); inhibition of SOD 537.6 μg/mL (**A**,**B**); inhibition of GR 444.4 μg/mL (**A**,**B**); inhibition of GPx 243.9 μg/mL (**A**,**B**); cytotoxicity expressed as % of cell death: A-172 100 μM (**A**), 50 μg/mL (**B**), and T98G 100 μM (**A**), 50 μg/mL (**B**).

3. Discussion

Lichens are an interesting group of organisms that draw attention due to the production of secondary metabolites with multidirectional biological properties [2,14,15,37]. We therefore selected three species of lichens, *P. sulcata*, *E. prunastri*, and *C. uncialis* for our research. Our phytochemical analysis revealed that the analyzed extracts of *P. sulcata*, *E. prunastri*, and *C. uncialis* are rich in polyphenolic compounds. Similar observations were reported by other research groups [22,38]. The HPLC method applied in order to determine the content of the dominant active compounds detected the major secondary metabolites; in *P. sulcata* extract it was salazinic acid, in *E. prunastri* extract it was evernic acid, and in *C. uncialis* it was (−)-usnic acid. The active compounds were abundant in the lichen-derived extracts. In this context, e.g. evernic acid constituted 66.63% of the *E. prunastri* extract, while salazinic acid constituted 23.05% of *P. sulcata* extract. The high content of polyphenols in non-polar lichen extracts was also confirmed by others. According to Manojlović et al. [10], salazinic acid was the dominant compound in acetone extract from *P. sulcata*. Other works indicated that evernic acid and (−)-usnic acid were the important components of acetone extracts of *E. prunastri* [6,38] and of *C. uncialis* [22,39], respectively.

Despite the growing evidence of the anticancer potential of lichen-derived substances and extracts, not much is known about their ability to influence brain tumor growth. Brain tumors are a serious therapeutic problem, the largest of which is GBM, being still one of the main challenges in clinical oncology [40]. Efforts are constantly being made to find more efficient anti-GBM therapy, as the overall survival of GBM patients rarely exceeds 15 months [41]. Since beneficial anticancer activity associated with lichen-derived compounds and extracts were previously reported in respect of various cancer cell lines, we hypothesized that *P. sulcata*, *E. prunastri* and *C. uncialis* may also decrease the viability of GBM cells. Our research confirmed the well-established role of (−)-usnic acid as a substance that decreases cancer cell viability [15]. In temozolomide-sensitive A-172 and temozolomide-resistant T98G cell line models, (−)-usnic acid was the dominant cytotoxic compound as compared to the other two lichen-derived compounds, namely, the depsidone, salazinic acid and the depside, evernic acid. Interestingly, *C. uncialis* extract even at a concentration of 1 µM, was able to significantly reduce GBM cell viability. The potential mechanisms responsible for the observed cytotoxicity can be related to pro-apoptotic properties of usnic acid, as reported for various cell line models, including colorectal adenocarcinoma (CaCo2), rhabdomyosarcoma (RD), cervical carcinoma (Hep2C), and hepatocellular carcinoma (HepG2) [2]. Data concerning the effect of usnic acid on GBM cells are, however, scarce. Only recently, the cytotoxic and genotoxic effects of (+)-usnic acid on GBM cell line U87MG cells were confirmed by Emsen et al. [17].

So far over 70 different metabolites have been identified and characterized in *E. prunastri*, and evernic acid is regarded as one of its major secondary metabolites [42]. In our study, evernic acid was cytotoxic to the A-172 cell line in a broad range of concentrations (10–100 µM); however, the cytotoxic effect was moderate – the viability dropped to ~80%, as compared to the vehicle-treated control. In the T98G cell line, the cytotoxic effects of evernic acid were observed only for the highest tested concentration (100 µM). Shcherbakova et al. found that the U-87 GBM cell line was sensitive to evernic acid, but also to *E. prunastri* extract [43]. In our study, the treatment with *E. prunastri* extract dose-dependently reduced the number of living cells. Interestingly, the temozolomide-resistant cell line, T98G, was more prone to *E. prunastri* induced cell death, as compared to the temozolomide-sensitive A-172 cell line. Furthermore, the report of Kosanić and coworkers also demonstrates that acetone extracts of *E. prunastri* and *Pseudevernia furfuraceae* possess anticancer activity against human melanoma FemX and human colon carcinoma LS174 cell lines [9].

To the best of our knowledge, *P. sulcata*, and salazinic acid were not yet tested in a model of human GBM cells; here we report their moderate cytotoxicity. Ari et al. [44] demonstrated cytotoxic effects of *P. sulcata* methanolic extracts in the C6 rat GBM cell line—cell viability significantly decreased after high doses (50 and 100 µg/mL) of the extract. In this study, *P. sulcata* extract was slightly more cytotoxic to C6 and to liver cancer Hep3B cell lines, as compared to human lung cancer A549 and PC3 cells [44].

Equally important as the cytotoxic activity of the analyzed compounds/extracts on cancer cells, is the lack of toxicity against healthy cells. Current data supports the safe profile of lichen-derived compounds and extracts in regard to normal astrocytes or neurons, supporting their neuroprotective properties [45]. For instance, in a recent study [46], evernic acid protected primary cultured neurons against 1-methyl-4-phenylpyridium (MPP+)-induced cell death, mitochondrial dysfunction, and oxidative stress, and effectively reduced MPP+-induced astroglial activation by inhibiting the NF-κB pathway. Moreover, evernic acid ameliorated 1-methyl-4-phenyl-1,2,3,6,-tetrahydropyridine-induced motor dysfunction, dopaminergic neuronal loss, and neuroinflammation in the nigrostriatal pathway in C57BL/6 mice. The neuroprotective effects of usnic acid were also reported in an acute mouse model of Parkinson's disease. It was found that 1-methyl-4-phenyl-1,2,3,6,-tetrahydropyridine-induced motor dysfunction and neuronal loss were ameliorated in the usnic acid-treated mice *versus* vehicle-treated controls [46].

Apart from the cytotoxic properties that the investigated lichen-derived compounds and extracts exerted upon cancer cells, our study also revealed that they also possess desirable inhibitory effects on indoleamine-2,3-dioxygenase 1 (IDO1). IDO1, together with IDO2 and TDO (tryptophan-2,3-dioxygenase), are responsible for the conversion of L-tryptophan into L-kynurenine (Kyn), which is the rate-limiting step of the kynurenine pathway. The downstream metabolites of the Kyn pathway play significant role in the formation of an immunosuppressive environment, due to the negative regulation of T-cell responses [47]. It has been observed that the excessive degradation of tryptophan or the accumulation of its metabolites reduces the ability of the immune system to destroy tumor cells and also increases the progression of brain tumors. Comprehensive studies on cancer patients proved that expression and activity of IDO1 is strongly correlated with pathological grades of glioma [48]. Moreover, overexpression of IDO1 correlates with poor prognosis in patients with glioma. Therefore, IDO1 has become an attractive target in the treatment of GBM. Our results showed for the first time that *C. uncialis* and *E. prunastri* extracts, in concentrations of 100 µg/mL, are able to inhibit IDO1 by $54.82 \pm 3.51\%$ and $43.06 \pm 1.97\%$, respectively. Interestingly, similarly to the results of the cytotoxicity study, both *C. uncialis* and *E.prunastri* extracts exhibited stronger IDO1 inhibitory properties than the pure compounds, used in the equivalent concentrations. Therefore, it should be assumed that it is not the dominant compound which is mostly responsible for the inhibitory activity towards IDO, and the final biological effect of the extracts depends on the action of other extract components. This is also evidenced by the analysis of the activity of *P. sulcata* extract, for which the IDO inhibitory activity was determined as 20% enzyme inhibition, while pure salazinic acid was not active. If these results could be extrapolated from the preclinical to clinical settings, the use of the above-mentioned extracts or their secondary metabolites (evernic and usnic acids) could be considered as a supplementary (add-on) therapy for GBM patients. This hypothesis needs further verification in cell-based assay for IDO inhibition and during in vivo experiments. However, previous studies proved that combination of IDO1 inhibitors with chemo- or immunotherapy led to an increased response rate when compared to classical therapies. The use of IDO1 inhibitors as add-on therapy can also be effective in inhibiting IDO-induced angiogenesis and thus reducing tumor growth and metastatic potential [49]. Due to the fact that IDO activation plays a pivotal role in the processes of cancer initiation, progression and metastasis, lichen extracts could possibly be used as dietary supplements in chemoprevention of cancer as well.

Because the inflammatory process accompanies many pathological conditions, and reveals itself in cancers and degenerative diseases of the brain tissue, we decided to examine also the anti-inflammatory potential of the tested lichen-derived compounds and extracts. Most brain tumors, including malignant glioma, show high COX-2 expression [50]. The activity of this enzyme was found to be correlated with the rate of GBM cell proliferation [51], with GBM grade [52], and poor prognosis [50]. Moreover, it has been shown that

COX-2 activity in GBM adversely affects epilepsy accompanying the disease [50]. Hence, one of the therapeutic targets to control the development of GBM and its accompanying symptoms may be COX-2. The literature indicates the anti-inflammatory properties of lichen compounds [37], including activity towards COX-2 [23,53,54]. The results of our study indicate that all the tested lichen-derived compounds and extracts showed the ability to inhibit COX-2. However, taking into account the content of test substances in the extracts calculated based on HPLC analysis, the activity of the extracts was comparable to the anti-COX-2 properties of tested compounds. The strongest inhibition of COX-2 was exerted by *P. sulcata* extract and its component—salazinic acid. The detected COX-2 inhibitory effect was higher than that of acetylsalicylic acid. The literature confirms the anti-inflammatory properties of salazinic and evernic acids, which strongly inhibited microsomal prostaglandin E2-1 synthase [53], as well as of (+)-usnic acid, which inhibited the synthesis of leukotriene B4 (LTB4) [55]. The obtained data indicate that the substances we tested, both in pure form and in extracts, can attenuate the inflammatory response induced by COX-2, which can be beneficial both in the context of brain tumors as well as neurodegenerative diseases.

Hyaluronic acid is a component of the brain's extracellular matrix. Hyaluronan particle size is associated with invasion of GBM cells and frequently-occurring therapeutic resistance [56]. Low molecular weight hyaluronan molecules, formed as the end product of degradation by hyaluronidase, are often associated with increased invasion and accelerated tumor growth [57] and increased cancer proliferation and cell adhesion [58]. From the point of view of reducing the invasiveness of the tumor, inhibition of the degradation of hyaluronic acid by the enzyme is an advantageous feature. Moreover, the activity of hyaluronidase may induce inflammation accompanying pathological changes in the brain tissue [28]. Thus, in this study, we wanted to verify whether the selected compounds and lichen extracts may affect the activity of hyaluronidase. Our results indicate that among the tested substances, those from two species, *P. sulcata* and *E. prunastri*, provide compounds capable of inhibiting hyaluronidase activity. In these two cases, in the concentration range used, the extract was more potent than the pure compound, and the activity was higher than that of β-escin, used as a standard [59]. Such results suggest that, apart from the tested compounds, the inhibition of the enzyme is also influenced by other substances contained in the extracts. On the other hand, salazinic acid, evernic acid, and (−)-usnic acid activity were similar to the reference. The anti-hyaluronidase activity of (−)-usnic acid was similar to that presented in recent literature [60].

ROS are involved in different signaling pathways to control cellular stability [61]. Their excess is related to neurodegeneration, but in relation to cancer treatment it is beneficial, as most anticancer therapies rely on ROS-induced cell death. Thus, it is important to know whether lichen-derived compounds and extracts possess antioxidant, or rather pro-oxidant properties. The results of our study show that *P. sulcata*, *E. prunastri* and *C. uncialis* extracts and their major secondary metabolites are characterized by very limited antioxidant properties. This is in line with other research data showing that extracts from *E. prunastri* and *P. sulcata* have little ability to scavenge ROS [12,38]. However, in our study the observed ability of these extracts to reduce copper ions was noticeable. The reducing properties of *E. prunastri* were only three times lower than that of resveratrol, used as a standard [62]. Other researchers have studied the antioxidant effect of some lichen-derived substances. In a study by Kosanić et al. [9], *E. prunastri* extract and evernic acid showed weak free radical scavenging activity in the DPPH test, compared to the standard. Salazinic acid and usnic acid were, in turn, assessed as strong antioxidants [10,63]. Our analyzes did not confirm these results. It is worth mentioning that it has been reported that the level of antioxidant activity may vary depending on the lipophilicity of the reaction environment [64]. These observations may partially explain the discrepancies in the results.

Superoxide dismutase (SOD), glutathione reductase (GR), and glutathione peroxidase (GPx) are the main endogenous enzymatic defense systems of human cells. They play important roles in neuroprotection [65] but, in the case of an already developed CNS tumor, it was observed that a high level of these enzymes correlates with a high degree of malignancy of neoplastic cells, a shorter period of disease progression, and the development of drug resistance [66]. The literature indicates that lowering the activity of SOD, GR, and GPx may increase the effectiveness of the treatment [67]. The results of our study indicate that *P. sulcata*, *E. prunastri*, and *C. uncialis* and their major secondary metabolites inhibit the SOD enzyme, while the strongest activity was characterized by *E. prunastri* extract (53.4%). Salazinic acid, evernic acid, and usnic acid inhibited the enzyme with similar effectiveness of about 20%. GPx was most strongly inhibited by *E. prunastri* extract (92.4 ± 4.3%), while the enzyme was not inhibited by salazinic acid and *C. uncialis* extract. Therefore, probably both salazinic acid and (−)-usnic acid do not participate in the antioxidant activity of the examined extracts. GR was only inhibited by *E. prunastri* extract (91.1 ± 7.2%) and (−)-usnic acid (18.2 ± 2.2%). These results may suggest that lichen-derived compounds and extracts, in particular *E. prunastri* extract and (−)-usnic acid, may enhance the effectiveness of GBM therapies.

Another therapeutic target in CNS diseases is acetylcholine-metabolizing cholinesterases. As their activity is increased in neurodegenerative diseases, inhibition of these enzymes positively affects patients with degenerative changes in the CNS, e.g., Alzheimer's disease. Increased AChE and BChE activity was also observed in brain tumors, including GBM [68]. Our study found only a small or no inhibitory effect of the studied lichen-derived compounds and extracts on the activity of cholinesterases. Only the extract of *C. uncialis* showed the activity against AChE, compared to the reference substance. A similarly low inhibitory activity of lichens secondary metabolites against both AChE and BChE was confirmed in our other studies [23] as well as by other authors [69].

Due to the blood-brain barrier (BBB), which limits the penetration of most anticancer drugs into the CNS, standard GBM treatment is limited to surgical resection, followed by radiotherapy in combination with temozolomide [70]. Therefore, it is important to know if a molecule with therapeutic properties can penetrate into the CNS. One of the methods of obtaining such data is the PAMPA-BBB analysis, which allows collecting preliminary data on whether the studied molecule can show the ability to diffuse passively through the BBB. Very little is known about the ability of lichen-derived compounds and extracts to penetrate into the CNS. Our most recent study demonstrated that physodic acid is characterized by a high permeability coefficient, meaning it can reach the CNS via passive diffusion [23]. In this study we showed that evernic acid and especially (−)-usnic acid, reaching a very high P_e value after 1 h of incubation, can also penetrate the BBB well. Thus, taking into account our observations on the penetration and strong cytotoxicity of (−)-usnic acid, we can suppose that the ability of this compound to penetrate the CNS is high enough to have a cytotoxic effect on neoplastic cells. It has to be noted that evernic and usnic acids can penetrate via the BBB both as single substances and as active ingredients of the extracts. In contrast, our study showed that salazinic acid is incapable of penetration through the tested type of biological barrier, regardless of whether it was a component of the extract or a pure compound. The analysed lichen-derived compounds selected for the study differed in chemical structure, which would explain the differences in BBB permeation.

4. Materials and Methods

4.1. Plant Material

The examined lichens were manually collected: *C. uncialis*, Jastrzębsko Stare, Greater, VI 2015, Poland, *E. prunastri* from the maple bark, West Pomeranian, XI 2015, *P. sulcata*, Podlesice, Silesian region, VIII 2015, Poland, and authenticated by Dr Daria Zarabska-Bożejewicz (The Institute for Agricultural and Forest Environment of the Polish Academy of Sciences in Poznan). Voucher specimens (CUES 2015.06; EPES 2015.11; PSES 2015.08) have been deposited in the herbarium of the Department of Pharmacognosy at Poznan University of Medical Sciences.

4.2. Solvents and Chemicals

Formic acid, sodium carbonate, sodium hydroxide, DMSO, acetone, ammonium acetate, copper (II) chloride were purchased from Avantor Performance Materials Poland S.A. (Gliwice, Poland). The Folin–Ciocalteu phenol reagent was from Merck (Darmstadt, Germany). HPLC grade water, HPLC grade acetonitrile, acetate buffer were from JT Baker–Avantor Performance Materials B.V. (Deventer, The Netherlands), tannic acid from Roth GmbH (Karlsruhe, Germany). Salazinic acid, evernic acid, and (−)-usnic acid were isolated and identified in the Department of Pharmacognosy of Poznan University of Medical Sciences. Atranorin was purchased from ChromaDex ((Los Angeles, CA, USA). All other chemicals were from the Sigma–Aldrich Chemical Co. (Taufkirchen, Germany).

4.3. Preparation of Extract

Dried, cleaned and fragmented thalli of *P. sulcata*, *E. prunastri*, *C. uncialis* (5.0 g) were sonicated at 35 °C for 6 × 30 min with acetone (100 mL × 6) in an ultrasonic bath. The extracts were filtered using Whatman filterpaper No. 1 and concentrated by evaporation using a rotary evaporator under vacuum at 35–40 °C to afford a solid residue (*P. sulcata* 435 mg, with yield of 8.71%; *E. prunastri* 429 mg, with yield of 8.24%; *C. uncialis* 71.52 mg, with yield of 1.43%).

4.4. HPLC Analysis

Analysis was performed on (Thermo Scientific UltiMate 3000 UHPLC, Waltham, MA USA) system. The separation was achieved on Kinetex C18 column (100 × 2.1 mm, 5 µm) with mobile phase consisting of acetonitrile and 0.5 % formic acid with a flow rate of 0.3 mL/min. The gradient elution started from 5% of acetonitrile to 100% during 10 min. After that step, isocratic elution with 100% acetonitrile proceeded for 2 min. During the final 5 min, the concentration of acetonitrile decreased to the initial condition (5%). The detection wavelength was 254 nm, and the temperature was 40 °C. The method was validated for salazinic acid, evernic acid, and (−)-usnic acid [23].

4.5. Total Phenolic Content (TPC)

TPC was determined using the Folin–Ciocalteu method [71]. 0.1 mL of DMSO/acetone extracts from *P. sulcata*, *E. prunastri*, *C. uncialis*, prepared at concentrations of 10 mg/mL, 2 mg/mL, and 5 mg/mL, respectively, were mixed with 4.0 mL of distilled water and with 0.5 mL of Folin–Ciocalteu's reagent. Immediately afterwards, 20% sodium carbonate was added (2.0 mL), and subsequently, the samples were supplemented with distilled water (a total volume of 10 mL). The samples were incubated for 30 min at room temperature (in the dark). The absorbance was measured at 760 nm (spectrophotometer UV/VIS, Lambda 35, Elmer–Perkin, Waltham, MA, USA). The blank contained the DMSO instead of the examined sample. The results were presented as mg of gallic acid equivalent (GAE) per g of a dry extract ± SEM (to prepare the calibration curve of gallic acid, 0.2–0.8 mg/mL concentrations of gallic acid were used).

4.6. Determination of Cytotoxicity of Lichen-Derived Substances

4.6.1. Compounds/Extracts

Stock solutions in dimethylsulfoxide DMSO (Sigma-Aldrich, St. Louis, MO, USA), (10 mM for compounds and 10 mg/mL for extracts) were prepared and stored at −20 °C. For the experiments, the stock solutions were diluted ex tempore to the final selected concentration with complete cell culture medium.

4.6.2. Cell Culture and Assessment of Cell Viability

Human glioblastoma A-172 and T98G cell lines were purchased from the American Type Culture Collection (ATCC, Manassas, VA, USA), and the European Collection of Authenticated Cell Cultures (ECACC, Salisbury, UK), respectively. The cells were grown at 37 °C in 95% humidified and 5% CO_2 atmosphere. Media recommended by the provider were used to cultivate the cells: ATCC-formulated Dulbecco's modified Eagle's medium (DMEM) (Sigma Aldrich, St. Louis, MO, USA), and ATCC-formulated Eagle's Minimum Essential Medium (EMEM) (Sigma-Aldrich, St. Louis, MO, USA) were used for A-172 and T98G cells, respectively. Moreover, the media were supplemented with 10% fetal bovine serum (FBS) (Biowest, France) and 1% antibiotics (penicillin and streptomycin) solution (Sigma-Aldrich, St. Louis, MO, USA). The medium for the T98G cell line was additionally supplemented with 2 mM glutamine, 1% non-essential amino acids, and 1% sodium pyruvate (all obtained from Sigma Aldrich, St. Louis, MO, USA). For the experiments, the amount of FBS was reduced to 5%. All experiments were carried out 24 h after the cells were seeded on 96-well plates.

The effect of the tested compounds and extracts on GBM cell viability was assessed by measuring the ability of cells to metabolize 3-(4,5-dimethylthiazol-2-yl)-2,5-diphenyl-tetrazolium bromide (MTT), as previously described [72]. In brief, 1×10^4 cells per well were seeded on 96-well plates. After 24 h incubation, they were treated with varying concentrations of lichen-derived compounds (1, 5, 10, 25, 50 and 100 µM) and extracts (1, 5, 10, 25, 50 and 100 µg/mL). Cells treated with medium containing the respective concentrations of DMSO (Sigma-Aldrich, St. Louis, MO, USA) were used as a control. After 48 h incubation the cells were washed with phosphate-buffered saline (PBS) buffer and incubated for 4 h in the presence of PBS containing 0.5 mg/mL MTT salt (Merck, Darmstadt, Germany). Next, the formazan crystals were dissolved in acidic isopropanol. In order to enhance dissolution of formazan crystals the plates were shaken on the orbital shaker for 30 min. Finally, the absorbance was measured at $\lambda = 570$ nm and $\lambda = 690$ nm on the microplate reader (Tecan Infinite M200). All the experiments were repeated three times with at least four measurements per assay.

4.7. Inhibition of Indoleamine 2,3-Dioxygenase (IDO1)

Inhibitory effects of the investigated extracts and standards (salazinic acid, evernic acid, (−)-usnic acid), as well as the reference IDO1 inhibitor (epacadostat) were determined using Universal IDO1/IDO2/TDO Inhibitor Screening Assay Kit from BPS Bioscience, Inc. (San Diego, CA, USA). This colorimetric assay is based on the measurement of the ability of IDO1, IDO2 and TDO to convert L-tryptophan into N-formylkynurenine (NFK). The experiments were performed according to the manufacturer's guidelines. The final concentration of the compounds and extracts in the reaction mixture was 100 µg/mL. The amount of NFK was measured spectrophotometrically at 320 nm using an Epoch BioTek microplate reader (BioTek Instruments, Inc., Winooski, VT, USA). The samples were run in triplicate and the results were expressed as mean ± SEM.

4.8. Effect on Cyclooxygenase-2 (COX-2) Activity

For the assay, reagents from Cayman COX Activity Assay Kit (Chemical, Ann Arbor, MI, USA, No. 760151) were prepared strictly as suggested by the producer and were combined with COX-2 enzyme (Human recombinant, Cayman No. 60122, pre-diluted 100-fold using 100 mM, pH 8.0 Tris buffer). A volume of 0.01 mL of the studied sample, dissolved in pure DMSO to obtain 5 mg/mL, was mixed with 0.12 mL of Tris buffer (100 mM, pH 8.0), 0.01 mL hemin, shaken and left for 5 min at 25 °C followed by addition of 0.02 mL colorimetric substrate and 0.02 mL arachidonic acid solution. To start the reaction, 0.02 mL of COX-2 solution was added. The increase of absorbance during incubation at room temperature was recorded at 590 nm. Negative (blank) sample (buffer instead of studied sample) and positive sample (COX-2 inhibitor DuP-697) were run simultaneously. Background of studied samples (0.01 mL of sample mixed with 0.19 mL buffer) was also measured and included in the calculations. Each sample was run in at least 4 repeats. Inhibition of the enzyme activity was expressed in % (indicates by how many % the activity has been reduced in relation to the negative or blank sample for which the maximum activity was assumed as 100%, under the conditions used in the method). Also, inhibition of enzyme activity was expressed as acetylsalicylic acid equivalent concentration (mg/mL). For this purpose, acetylsalicylic acid solutions were prepared at 14 concentrations (0.2–10.0 mg/mL) and analyzed similarly to tested samples.

4.9. Anti-Hyaluronidase Activity

Inhibition of hyaluronidase (HA) was determined by a method described by Studzińska-Sroka et al. [23]. Briefly, 25 µL of incubation buffer (50 mM, pH 7.0, with 77 mM NaCl and 1 mg/mL of albumin), 25 µL of enzyme (30 U/mL of acetate buffer pH 7.0), 10 µL solutions of the tested extracts (1.25–7.5 mg/mL) or lichen substances (0.625–5.0 mg/mL), and 15 µL of acetate buffer (pH 4.5) were mixed (the final concentrations were: 0.125–0.75 mg/mL). After incubation at 37 °C for 15 min, 25 µL of HA (0.3 mg/mL in acetate buffer) was added. Subsequently, the plate was incubated for 45 min (37 °C). After this time, 200 µL of 2.5% CTAB in 2% NaOH was put in. The turbidance of the reaction mixture was measured as the absorbance at 600 nm (Multiskan GO 1510, Thermo Fisher Scientific, Vantaa, Finland) after 10 min of incubation at room temperature. β-escin was used as the positive control (6.0–10.0 mg/mL, with the final concentration 0.6–1.0 mg/mL). All experiments were carried out three times and the average from $n = 5$ (lichen substances) or $n = 6$ (lichen extracts and β-escin) measurements was calculated. The percentage of inhibition was calculated by using the equation below.

$$\% \text{ inhibition activity} = \frac{(T_s - TE_{blank})}{(TH_{blank} - TE_{blank})} \times 100\% \tag{1}$$

where: T_S = absorbance of sample; TE_{blank} = absorbance of the enzyme + examined substance; TH_{blank} = absorbance of the HA + examined substance.

4.10. Antioxidant Activity

4.10.1. DPPH and CUPRAC analysis

Two methods were used to test the antioxidant activity: DPPH and CUPRAC. The DPPH assay was effected according to Kikowska et al. (2018) [73], with slight modifications. Briefly, 25.0 µL of examined extracts or compounds were prepared at different concentrations (within the range 1.25–20 mg/mL, for each extract, and with two different concentrations: 3 mg/mL, and 6 mg/mL, for salazinic acid, evernic acid and (−)-usnic acid). Each was mixed with 175.0 µL of DPPH• solution (3.9 mg DPPH in 50.0 mL of MeOH); the reached final assay concentrations were: 156.25 µg/mL to 2500 µg/mL, for extracts, and 375 µg/mL to 750 µg/mL, for lichen compounds. The samples were then shaken and incubated in the dark (30 min) at room temperature. Next, the absorbance was measured at 517 nm. The control blank contained 25.0 µL of DMSO and 175.0 µL of DPPH• solution. For calculating the scavenging % of DPPH• free radicals, the following formula was used:

$$\text{DPPH scavenging activity (\%)} = [(A_0 - A_1)/A_0] \times 100\%, \tag{2}$$

where A_0 is the absorbance of the control and A_1 is the absorbance of the sample. The IC_{50} values, i.e., (a concentration of antioxidant necessary to halve the initial DPPH• quantity), were used to compare the quality of the antioxidant potency of the studied extracts. The lower absorbance of the reaction mixture indicated a higher free radical scavenging activity. For the investigated substances, two independent experiments were carried out and the average from $n = 3$ measurements was calculated.

To measure the antioxidant capacity of the lichen extracts and compounds the CUPRAC assay was used [23]. The CUPRAC reagent was freshly prepared before the analysis and composed of equal parts of acetate buffer (pH 7.0), 7.5 mM neocuproine (Sigma-Aldrich, St. Louis, MO, USA) solution in 96% ethanol, and 10 mM $CuCl_2xH_2O$ solution. The samples (50 µL) dissolved in DMSO at different concentrations (78 µg/mL–1250 µg/mL, for extracts, and 125–1000 µg/mL, for compounds), were mixed with the CUPRAC reagent (150 µL) (the final assay concentrations were: 19 µg/mL – 312 µg/mL, for extracts, and 31 µg/mL–250 µg/mL, for compounds). After shaking and incubating in the dark at room temperature for 30 min, the absorbance was read at 450 nm. Resveratrol was used as a standard (25–400 µg/mL; the final assay concentrations were 6.25–100 µg/mL). The results were expressed as the $IC_{0.5}$, the concentration at which the absorbance was 0.5. For the investigated substances, two independent experiments were carried out and the average from $n = 3$ measurements was calculated.

4.10.2. Effect on Antioxidant Enzymes Activity

Effect on Superoxide Dismutase Activity (SOD)

Sample (50 µL, 5 mg/mL of pure DMSO) was mixed with 10 µL SOD (0.24 U), 160 µL nitrobluetatrazolium solution (0.0025 M), 205 µL phosphate buffer (0.2 M, pH 7.5), 30 µL xanthine (150 mM in 1 M NaOH) and 0.01 mL xanthine oxidase (0.065 U, Sigma Aldrich X4875). The change in the absorbance at 550 nm was measured in tested samples vs. controls without the studied sample after 20 min of incubation and the effect on the enzyme was calculated using the equation [74]:

$$\text{Inhibition [\%]} = 100 - 100 \times \frac{(\text{Abs. 30 min} - \text{Abs. 0 min})}{(\text{Abs. control. 30 min} - \text{Abs. control 0 min})} \quad (3)$$

Effect on Glutathione Reductase (GR) Activity

Sample (20 µL, 5 mg/mL of pure DMSO) was mixed with 10 µL of EDTA solution and 12 µL of GSSG solution and incubated for 5 min at 25 °C; 4 µL of NADPH solution and was then added (all reagents were dissolved in 0.1 mM sodium phosphate buffer, pH 7.6), and the initial absorbance (340 nm) was recorded. The reaction was then started by addition of 2 U glutathione reductase (2 µL, Sigma Aldrich no G3664), 177 µL of 0.1 mM sodium phosphate buffer, and the absorbance was recorded after 5 min of incubation at 25 °C. Concentrations of reagents in the final mixture (805 µL) were as follows: 0.5 mM EDTA, 10 mM GSSG and 10 mM NADPH. Blank sample was prepared with buffer instead of the sample and background was measured (mixture containing studied sample and buffer only). One unit of enzyme activity has been defined as nMol of NADPH consumed/min·mL sample, in comparison with nMol of NADPH consumed/min in blank (reagent) sample [75].

Effect on Glutathione Peroxidase (GPx) Activity

Sample (20 µL, 5 mg/mL of pure DMSO) was mixed with 8 µL of EDTA solution, 10 µL of glutathione reductase (0.2 U Sigma G3664), 4 µL of GSH solution, 10 µL of glutathione peroxidase (0.04 U Sigma G6137), 22 µL of H_2O_2 and 332 µL of 50 mM sodium phosphate, pH 7.0). To start the reaction, 4 µL of NADPH solution (N5130) was added and the decrease in the absorbance (340 nm) was read after 10 min of incubation at 25 °C. All solutions were prepared in 50 mM buffer and concentrations of reagents in the final mixture were as follows: 1mM EDTA, 0.2 U glutathione reductase, 2 mM GSH, 0.04 U glutathione peroxidase, 1.5 mM H_2O_2 and 0.8 mM NADPH. Blank sample was prepared with buffer instead of the studied sample and background was measured (mixture containing studied sample and buffer only). One unit of enzyme activity was defined as nMol of NADPH consumed/min·mL sample, in comparison with nMol of NADPH consumed/min in blank (reagent) sample [76].

4.11. Anti-Cholinesterase Activity

Ellman's colorimetric method was used [77] with modifications described previously [78]. Tested sample (10 µL) at concentration 5 mg/mL was mixed with 20 µL of AChE (or BChE) solution (0.28 U/mL) and completed after 5 min with 35 µL of ATChI (or BTCh) (1.5 mmol/L), 175 µL of 0.3 mmol/L DTNB (containing 10 mmol/L NaCl and 2 mmol/L $MgCl_2$) and 110 µL with Tris-HCl buffer (50 mmol/L, pH 8.0). Samples containing 10 µL of Tris-HCl buffer instead of the studied sample were run in the same way ("blank" samples). The increase in the absorbance due to the spontaneous hydrolysis of the substrate was monitored using "blank" samples containing ATCh (or BTCh) and DTNB completed to 350 µL with Tris-HCl buffer. All samples were incubated at 22 °C (30 min; incubation time was determined after optimization experiments, details not shown), and the absorbance was measured (405 nm, 96-well microplate reader, Tecan Sunrise, Grödig, Austria). The "false-positive" effect of studied compounds was measured according to Rhee et al. [79] with minor modifications, as described previously [78]: after mixing of the substrate with the enzyme and buffer, the "false-positive" sample was left for incubation. Then, a studied sample and DTNB were added, followed by an immediate measurement of the absorbance.

Reference cholinesterase inhibitors were used for the calculations of results (eserine, neostigmine, magniflorine, rivastigmine and donepezil). For this purpose, for each compound, 16 dilutions in pure DMSO were prepared (2.57–41.14 µg/mL). These solutions (10 µL) were tested as described above and calibration curves were produced.

Each sample was analyzed in at least eight repeats, and all solutions used in a set of analyses were prepared in the same buffer. For calculations, the background of the sample (10 µL mixed with 340 µL of Tris buffer) was measured at 405 nm and subtracted during calculations. Then, the absorbance of the test sample was subtracted from the absorbance of the "blank" sample.

4.12. Permeability through the Blood-Brain-Barrier (PAMPA-BBB)

To evaluate the effective permeability (P_e) of the salazinic acid, evernic acid, (−)-usnic acid as pure compounds and from the extracts (*P. sulcata* acetone extract, *E. prunastri* acetone extract, *C. uncialis* acetone extract, respectively), Parallel Artificial Membrane Permeability Assay (PAMPA) for the Blood-Brain Barrier (BBB) was used (Pion Inc., Billerica, MA, USA). The stock solutions of acetone extracts from *C. uncialis*, *E. prunastri* and *P. sulcata* and from (−)-usnic acid, evernic acid, salazinic acid, were prepared with DMSO (the concentrations of salazinic acid, evernic acid, and (−)-usnic acid reached were 2.5 mg/mL for pure compounds and extracts). Next, the donor solution was prepared (5 µL of stock solution/1000 µL of Prisma buffer, pH = 7.4 (Prisma HT, Pion Inc.). Subsequently, each filter membrane of the acceptor plate wells was coated with 5 µL BBB-1 lipid solution (Pion Inc.), and 180 µL of the donor solution was added to the donor wells. The acceptor well was filled with 200 µL BSB (Brain Sink Buffer, Pion Inc.). The plate was incubated for 1 h or 4 h at 37 °C. After incubation, the donor and acceptor concentrations of examined substances were determined using the HPLC. Effective permeability (P_e) of the compounds was calculated by using the following equation.

$$P_e = -\frac{\ln\left(1 - \frac{C_A}{C_{eq}}\right)}{S \times \left(\frac{1}{V_D} + \frac{1}{V_A}\right) \times t} \qquad (4)$$

where P_e is the effective permeability coefficient (cm/s), V_D = donor volume, V_A = acceptor volume, C_{eq} = equilibrium concentration and $C_{eq} = \frac{C_D \times V_D + C_A \times V_A}{V_D + V_A}$, S = membrane area, and t = incubation time (in seconds) [35,36].

Compounds with P_e ($\times 10^{-6}$ cm/s) > 1.5 are classified as high permeation predicted, while P_e ($\times 10^{-6}$ cm/s) < 1.5 are classified as low permeation predicted. Samples were analyzed in triplicate and the average is reported.

4.13. Statistical Analysis

Results were expressed as means ± SEM. The median effect concentrations (IC_{50} or $IC_{0.5}$ values) were determined using a concentration–response curve. Statistical differences were calculated using the unpaired t-test with two-tailed distribution, with significant differences considered at $p < 0.05$.

5. Conclusions

To conclude, our study shows that lichen-derived compounds and extracts exert cytotoxic activity against GBM cells, inhibit the enzymes involved in the kynurenine pathway, COX-2, and hyaluronidase, and have very mild antioxidant properties, making them good candidates for adjuvant anti-GBM therapeutics. Usnic acid, with its ability to cross the BBB and reduce GBM cell proliferation, can be regarded as a prototype for compounds with activity within the CNS, in particular for GBM treatment. Lichen-derived compounds and extracts should also be further evaluated as neuroprotective agents.

Author Contributions: Conceptualization, E.S.-S. and J.C.-P.; methodology, E.S.-S., A.M.-C., P.Z., D.S., E.B.-W., B.K. and T.P.; validation, P.Z.; formal analysis, E.S.-S., A.M.-C., P.Z., D.S., E.B.-W. and B.K.; investigation, E.S.-S., A.M.-C., P.Z., D.S., E.B.-W. and B.K.; resources, J.C.-P., A.M.-C., D.S., E.B.-W. and T.P.; data curation, E.S.-S., A.M.-C., P.Z., D.S., E.B.-W. and B.K.; writing—original draft preparation, E.S.-S., A.M.-C., P.Z., J.C.-P. and T.P.; writing—review and editing, E.S.-S., A.M.-C., J.C.-P., T.P., D.S. and M.Ż.; visualization, E.S.-S., A.M.-C. and J.C.-P.; supervision, P.Z. and E.S.-S.; project administration, E.S.-S., P.Z. and J.C.-P.; funding acquisition, J.C.-P. and T.P. All authors have read and agreed to the published version of the manuscript.

Funding: This research was funded by the grant OPUS from the National Science Centre, Poland UMO- 2020/37/B/NZ7/03975. The cytotoxicity evaluation was funded by Poznan University of Medical Sciences. The IDO1/IDO2/TDO inhibition studies were financed from statutory fund (DS.544) of the Medical University of Lublin (Poland).

Institutional Review Board Statement: Not applicable.

Informed Consent Statement: Not applicable.

Data Availability Statement: Data is contained within the article.

Conflicts of Interest: The authors declare no conflict of interest.

References

1. Majchrzak-Celińska, A.; Kleszcz, R.; Stasiłowicz-Krzemień, A.; Cielecka-Piontek, J. Sodium Butyrate Enhances Curcuminoids Permeability through the Blood-Brain Barrier, Restores Wnt/β-Catenin Pathway Antagonists Gene Expression and Reduces the Viability of Glioblastoma Cells. *Int. J. Mol. Sci.* **2021**, *22*, 11285. [CrossRef] [PubMed]
2. Solárová, Z.; Liskova, A.; Samec, M.; Kubatka, P.; Büsselberg, D.; Solár, P. Anticancer potential of lichens' secondary metabolites. *Biomolecules* **2020**, *10*, 87. [CrossRef] [PubMed]
3. Zhao, Y.; Wang, M.; Xu, B. A comprehensive review on secondary metabolites and health-promoting effects of edible lichen. *J. Funct. Foods* **2021**, *80*, 104283. [CrossRef]
4. Purvis, O.W.; Coppins, B.J.; Hawksworth, D.L.; James, P.W. *The Lichen Flora of Great Britain and Irleande*; Natural History Museum: London, UK, 2019.
5. Stojanovic, G.; Stojanovic, I.; Smelcerovic, A. Lichen depsidones as potential novel pharmacologically active compounds. *Mini. Rev. Org. Chem.* **2012**, *9*, 178–184. [CrossRef]
6. Maslać, A.; Maslać, M.; Tkalec, M. The impact of cadmium on photosynthetic performance and secondary metabolites in the lichens *Parmelia sulcata*, *Flavoparmelia caperata* and *Evernia prunastri*. *Acta Bot. Croat.* **2016**, *75*, 186–193. [CrossRef]
7. Alexandrino, C.A.F.; Honda, N.K.; Matos, M.d.F.C.; Portugal, L.C.; Souza, P.R.B.d.; Perdomo, R.T.; Guimarães, R.d.C.A.; Kadri, M.C.T.; Silva, M.C.B.L.; Bogo, D. Antitumor effect of depsidones from lichens on tumor cell lines and experimental murine melanoma. *Rev. Bras. Farmacogn.* **2019**, *29*, 449–456. [CrossRef]
8. Ari, F.; Ulukaya, E.; Oran, S.; Celikler, S.; Ozturk, S.; Ozel, M.Z. Promising anticancer activity of a lichen, *Parmelia sulcata* Taylor, against breast cancer cell lines and genotoxic effect on human lymphocytes. *Cytotechnology* **2015**, *67*, 531–543. [CrossRef]
9. Kosanić, M.; Manojlović, N.; Janković, S.; Stanojković, T.; Ranković, B. *Evernia prunastri* and *Pseudoevernia furfuraceae* lichens and their major metabolites as antioxidant, antimicrobial and anticancer agents. *Food Chem. Toxicol.* **2013**, *53*, 112–118. [CrossRef]
10. Manojlović, N.; Ranković, B.; Kosanić, M.; Vasiljević, P.; Stanojković, T. Chemical composition of three *Parmelia* lichens and antioxidant, antimicrobial and cytotoxic activities of some their major metabolites. *Phytomedicine* **2012**, *19*, 1166–1172. [CrossRef]
11. Verma, N.; Behera, B.C.; Joshi, A. Studies on nutritional requirement for the culture of lichen *Ramalina nervulosa* and *Ramalina pacifica* to enhance the production of antioxidant metabolites. *Folia Microbiol. (Praha).* **2012**, *57*, 107–114. [CrossRef]
12. Kosanić, M.; Ranković, B.; Vukojević, J. Antioxidant properties of some lichen species. *J. Food Sci. Technol.* **2011**, *48*, 584–590. [CrossRef] [PubMed]
13. Lee, S.; Suh, Y.J.; Yang, S.; Hong, D.G.; Ishigami, A.; Kim, H.; Hur, J.-S.; Chang, S.-C.; Lee, J. Neuroprotective and Anti-Inflammatory Effects of Evernic Acid in an MPTP-Induced Parkinson's Disease Model. *Int. J. Mol. Sci.* **2021**, *22*, 2098. [CrossRef] [PubMed]
14. Fernández-Moriano, C.; Divakar, P.K.; Crespo, A.; Gómez-Serranillos, M.P. Protective effects of lichen metabolites evernic and usnic acids against redox impairment-mediated cytotoxicity in central nervous system-like cells. *Food Chem. Toxicol.* **2017**, *105*, 262–277. [CrossRef]

15. Galanty, A.; Paśko, P.; Podolak, I. Enantioselective activity of usnic acid: A comprehensive review and future perspectives. *Phytochem. Rev.* **2019**, *18*, 527–548. [CrossRef]
16. Rabelo, T.K.; Zeidán-Chuliá, F.; Vasques, L.M.; dos Santos, J.P.A.; da Rocha, R.F.; de Bittencourt Pasquali, M.A.; Rybarczyk-Filho, J.L.; Araújo, A.A.S.; Moreira, J.C.F.; Gelain, D.P. Redox characterization of usnic acid and its cytotoxic effect on human neuron-like cells (SH-SY5Y). *Toxicol. Vitr.* **2012**, *26*, 304–314. [CrossRef]
17. Emsen, B.; Aslan, A.; Türkez, H.; Joughi, A.T.; Kaya, A. The anti-cancer efficacies of diffractaic, lobaric, and usnic acid: In vitro inhibition of glioma. *J. Cancer Res Ther.* **2018**, *14*, 941–951. [CrossRef]
18. Koparal, A.T. Anti-angiogenic and antiproliferative properties of the lichen substances (−)-usnic acid and vulpinic acid. *Zeitschrift für Naturforsch. C* **2015**, *70*, 159–164. [CrossRef] [PubMed]
19. Kim, S.; Jo, S.; Lee, H.; Kim, T.U.; Kim, I.-C.; Yim, J.H.; Chung, H. Lobarstin enhances chemosensitivity in human glioblastoma T98G cells. *Anticancer Res.* **2013**, *33*, 5445–5451. [PubMed]
20. Guzow-Krzemińska, B.; Guzow, K.; Herman-Antosiewicz, A. Usnic Acid Derivatives as Cytotoxic Agents Against Cancer Cells and the Mechanisms of Their Activity. *Curr. Pharmacol. Reports* **2019**, *5*, 429–439. [CrossRef]
21. Ingelfinger, R.; Henke, M.; Roser, L.; Ulshöfer, T.; Calchera, A.; Singh, G.; Parnham, M.J.; Geisslinger, G.; Fürst, R.; Schmitt, I.; et al. Unraveling the Pharmacological Potential of Lichen Extracts in the Context of Cancer and Inflammation with a Broad Screening Approach. *Front. Pharmacol.* **2020**, *11*, 1322. [CrossRef]
22. Studzińska-Sroka, E.; Hołderna-Kędzia, E.; Galanty, A.; Bylka, W.; Kacprzak, K.; Ćwiklińska, K. In vitro antimicrobial activity of extracts and compounds isolated from *Cladonia uncialis*. *Nat. Prod. Res.* **2015**, *29*, 2302–2307. [CrossRef]
23. Studzińska-Sroka, E.; Majchrzak-Celińska, A.; Zalewski, P.; Szwajgier, D.; Baranowska-Wójcik, E.; Żarowski, M.; Plech, T.; Cielecka-Piontek, J. Permeability of *Hypogymnia physodes* Extract Component—Physodic Acid through the Blood–Brain Barrier as an Important Argument for Its Anticancer and Neuroprotective Activity within the Central Nervous System. *Cancers* **2021**, *13*, 1717. [CrossRef] [PubMed]
24. Sordillo, P.P.; Sordillo, L.A.; Helson, L. The Kynurenine Pathway: A Primary Resistance Mechanism in Patients with Glioblastoma. *Anticancer. Res.* **2017**, *37*, 2159–2171. [CrossRef]
25. Teismann, P. COX-2 in the neurodegenerative process of Parkinson's disease. *Biofactors* **2012**, *38*, 395–397. [CrossRef] [PubMed]
26. Majchrzak-Celińska, A.; Misiorek, J.O.; Kruhlenia, N.; Przybyl, L.; Kleszcz, R.; Rolle, K.; Krajka-Kuźniak, V. COXIBs and 2,5-dimethylcelecoxib counteract the hyperactivated Wnt/β-catenin pathway and COX-2/PGE2/EP4 signaling in glioblastoma cells. *BMC Cancer* **2021**, *21*, 493. [CrossRef] [PubMed]
27. Strauss, K.I. Antiinflammatory and neuroprotective actions of COX2 inhibitors in the injured brain. *Brain. Behav. Immun.* **2008**, *22*, 285–298. [CrossRef]
28. Bralley, E.; Greenspan, P.; Hargrove, J.L.; Hartle, D.K. Inhibition of hyaluronidase activity by *Vitis rotundifolia*.(Muscadine) berry seeds and skins. *Pharm. Biol.* **2007**, *45*, 667–673. [CrossRef]
29. Diao, S.; Xiao, M.; Chen, C. The Role of Hyaluronan in Myelination and Remyelination after White Matter Injury. *Brain Res.* **2021**, 147522. [CrossRef]
30. Salim, S. Oxidative Stress and the Central Nervous System. *J. Pharmacol. Exp. Ther.* **2017**, *360*, 201–205. [CrossRef]
31. Perillo, B.; Di Donato, M.; Pezone, A.; Di Zazzo, E.; Giovannelli, P.; Galasso, G.; Castoria, G.; Migliaccio, A. ROS in cancer therapy: The bright side of the moon. *Exp. Mol. Med.* **2020**, *52*, 192–203. [CrossRef]
32. Kanzaki, H.; Wada, S.; Narimiya, T.; Yamaguchi, Y.; Katsumata, Y.; Itohiya, K.; Fukaya, S.; Miyamoto, Y.; Nakamura, Y. Pathways that Regulate ROS Scavenging Enzymes, and Their Role in Defense Against Tissue Destruction in Periodontitis. *Front. Physiol.* **2017**, *8*, 351. [CrossRef] [PubMed]
33. García-Ayllón, M.S.; Sáez-Valero, J.; Muñoz-Delgado, E.; Vidal, C.J. Identification of hybrid cholinesterase forms consisting of acetyl- and butyrylcholinesterase subunits in human glioma. *Neuroscience* **2001**, *107*, 199–208. [CrossRef]
34. Pezzementi, L.; Nachon, F.; Chatonnet, A. Evolution of acetylcholinesterase and butyrylcholinesterase in the vertebrates: An atypical butyrylcholinesterase from the Medaka *Oryzias latipes*. *PLoS ONE* **2011**, *6*, e17396.
35. Chen, X.; Murawski, A.; Patel, K.; Crespi, C.L.; Balimane, P. V A novel design of artificial membrane for improving the PAMPA model. *Pharm. Res.* **2008**, *25*, 1511–1520. [CrossRef]
36. Latacz, G.; Lubelska, A.; Jastrzębska-Więsek, M.; Partyka, A.; Marć, M.A.; Satała, G.; Wilczyńska, D.; Kotańska, M.; Więcek, M.; Kamińska, K. The 1, 3, 5-triazine derivatives as innovative chemical family of 5-HT6 serotonin receptor agents with therapeutic perspectives for cognitive impairment. *Int. J. Mol. Sci.* **2019**, *20*, 3420. [CrossRef] [PubMed]
37. Studzinska-Sroka, E.; Dubino, A. Lichens as a source of chemical compounds with anti-inflammatory activity. *Herba Pol.* **2018**, *64*. [CrossRef]
38. Aoussar, N.; Rhallabi, N.; Mhand, R.A.; Manzali, R.; Bouksaim, M.; Douira, A.; Mellouki, F. Seasonal variation of antioxidant activity and phenolic content of *Pseudevernia furfuracea*, *Evernia prunastri* and *Ramalina farinacea* from Morocco. *J. Saudi Soc. Agric. Sci.* **2020**, *19*, 1–6. [CrossRef]
39. Studzińska-Sroka, E.; Tomczak, H.; Malińska, N.; Wrońska, M.; Kleszcz, R.; Galanty, A.; Cielecka-Piontek, J.; Latek, D.; Paluszczak, J. *Cladonia uncialis* as a valuable raw material of biosynthetic compounds against clinical strains of bacteria and fungi. *Acta Biochim. Pol.* **2019**, *66*, 597–603. [CrossRef]
40. Hanif, F.; Muzaffar, K.; Perveen, K.; Malhi, S.M.; Simjee, S.U. Glioblastoma Multiforme: A Review of its Epidemiology and Pathogenesis through Clinical Presentation and Treatment. *Asian Pac. J. Cancer Prev.* **2017**, *18*, 3–9. [CrossRef]

41. Brancato, V.; Nuzzo, S.; Tramontano, L.; Condorelli, G.; Salvatore, M.; Cavaliere, C. Predicting Survival in Glioblastoma Patients Using Diffusion MR Imaging Metrics—A Systematic Review. *Cancers* **2020**, *12*, 2858. [CrossRef] [PubMed]
42. Shcherbakova, A.; Strömstedt, A.A.; Göransson, U.; Gnezdilov, O.; Turanov, A.; Boldbaatar, D.; Kochkin, D.; Ulrich-Merzenich, G.; Koptina, A. Antimicrobial and antioxidant activity of *Evernia prunastri* extracts and their isolates. *World J. Microbiol. Biotechnol.* **2021**, *37*, 129. [CrossRef]
43. Shcherbakova, A.; Nyugen, L.; Koptina, A.; Backlund, A.; Shurgin, A.; Romanov, E.; Ulrich-Merzenich, G. Screening of compounds of *Evernia prunastri* (L.) for their antiproliferative activity in glioblastoma cells. *Planta Med.* **2016**, *82*, P465. [CrossRef]
44. Ari, F.; Aztopal, N.; Oran, S.; Bozdemir, S.; Celikler, S.; Ozturk, S.; Ulukaya, E. *Parmelia sulcata* Taylor and *Usnea filipendula* Stirt induce apoptosis-like cell death and DNA damage in cancer cells. *Cell Prolif.* **2014**, *47*, 457–464. [CrossRef] [PubMed]
45. White, P.A.S.; Oliveira, R.C.M.; Oliveira, A.P.; Serafini, M.R.; Araújo, A.A.S.; Gelain, D.P.; Moreira, J.C.F.; Almeida, J.R.G.S.; Quintans, J.S.S.; Quintans-Junior, L.J.; et al. Antioxidant activity and mechanisms of action of natural compounds isolated from lichens: A systematic review. *Molecules* **2014**, *19*, 14496–14527. [CrossRef]
46. Lee, S.; Lee, Y.; Ha, S.; Chung, H.Y.; Kim, H.; Hur, J.-S.; Lee, J. Anti-inflammatory effects of usnic acid in an MPTP-induced mouse model of Parkinson's disease. *Brain Res.* **2020**, *1730*, 146642. [CrossRef] [PubMed]
47. Ye, Z.; Yue, L.; Shi, J.; Shao, M.; Wu, T. Role of IDO and TDO in Cancers and Related Diseases and the Therapeutic Implications. *J. Cancer* **2019**, *10*, 2771–2782. [CrossRef] [PubMed]
48. Du, L.; Xing, Z.; Tao, B.; Li, T.; Yang, D.; Li, W.; Zheng, Y.; Kuang, C.; Yang, Q. Both IDO1 and TDO contribute to the malignancy of gliomas via the Kyn-AhR-AQP4 signaling pathway. *Signal Transduct. Target. Ther.* **2020**, *5*, 10. [CrossRef] [PubMed]
49. Mor, A.; Tankiewicz-Kwedlo, A.; Pawlak, D. Kynurenines as a Novel Target for the Treatment of Malignancies. *Pharmaceuticals* **2021**, *14*, 606. [CrossRef]
50. Qiu, J.; Shi, Z.; Jiang, J. Cyclooxygenase-2 in glioblastoma multiforme. *Drug Discov. Today* **2017**, *22*, 148–156. [CrossRef]
51. Prayson, R.A.; Castilla, E.A.; Vogelbaum, M.A.; Barnett, G.H. Cyclooxygenase-2 (COX-2) expression by immunohistochemistry in glioblastoma multiforme. *Ann. Diagn. Pathol.* **2002**, *6*, 148–153. [CrossRef] [PubMed]
52. Joki, T.; Heese, O.; Nikas, D.C.; Bello, L.; Zhang, J.; Kraeft, S.-K.; Seyfried, N.T.; Abe, T.; Chen, L.B.; Carroll, R.S. Expression of cyclooxygenase 2 (COX-2) in human glioma and in vitro inhibition by a specific COX-2 inhibitor, NS-398. *Cancer Res.* **2000**, *60*, 4926–4931.
53. Bauer, J.; Waltenberger, B.; Noha, S.M.; Schuster, D.; Rollinger, J.M.; Boustie, J.; Chollet, M.; Stuppner, H.; Werz, O. Discovery of depsides and depsidones from lichen as potent inhibitors of microsomal prostaglandin E2 synthase-1 using pharmacophore models. *ChemMedChem* **2012**, *7*, 2077. [CrossRef]
54. Bugni, T.S.; Andjelic, C.D.; Pole, A.R.; Rai, P.; Ireland, C.M.; Barrows, L.R. Biologically active components of a Papua New Guinea analgesic and anti-inflammatory lichen preparation. *Fitoterapia* **2009**, *80*, 270–273. [CrossRef]
55. Vijayakumar, C.S.; Viswanathan, S.; Reddy, M.K.; Parvathavarthini, S.; Kundu, A.B.; Sukumar, E. Anti-inflammatory activity of (+)-usnic acid. *Fitoterapia* **2000**, *71*, 564–566. [CrossRef]
56. Chen, J.-W.E.; Pedron, S.; Shyu, P.; Hu, Y.; Sarkaria, J.N.; Harley, B.A.C. Influence of Hyaluronic Acid Transitions in Tumor Microenvironment on Glioblastoma Malignancy and Invasive Behavior. *Front. Mater.* **2018**, *5*, 39. [CrossRef]
57. Monslow, J.; Govindaraju, P.; Puré, E. Hyaluronan–a functional and structural sweet spot in the tissue microenvironment. *Front. Immunol.* **2015**, *6*, 231. [CrossRef] [PubMed]
58. Tofuku, Y.; Yokouchi, M.; Murayama, T.; Minami, S.; Komiya, S. HAS3-related hyaluronan enhances biological activities necessary for metastasis of osteosarcoma cells. *Int. J. Oncol.* **2006**, *29*, 175–183. [CrossRef] [PubMed]
59. Grabowska, K.; Wróbel, D.; Żmudzki, P.; Podolak, I. Anti-inflammatory activity of saponins from roots of Impatiens parviflora DC. *Nat. Prod. Res.* **2020**, *34*, 1581–1585. [CrossRef] [PubMed]
60. Galanty, A.; Zagrodzki, P.; Gdula-Argasińska, J.; Grabowska, K.; Koczurkiewicz-Adamczyk, P.; Wróbel-Biedrawa, D.; Podolak, I.; Pękala, E.; Paśko, P. A Comparative Survey of Anti-Melanoma and Anti-Inflammatory Potential of Usnic Acid Enantiomers—A Comprehensive In Vitro Approach. *Pharmaceuticals* **2021**, *14*, 945. [CrossRef] [PubMed]
61. Rinaldi, M.; Caffo, M.; Minutoli, L.; Marini, H.; Abbritti, R.V.; Squadrito, F.; Trichilo, V.; Valenti, A.; Barresi, V.; Altavilla, D.; et al. ROS and Brain Gliomas: An Overview of Potential and Innovative Therapeutic Strategies. *Int. J. Mol. Sci.* **2016**, *17*, 984. [CrossRef]
62. Jia, B.; Zheng, X.; Wu, M.-L.; Tian, X.-T.; Song, X.; Liu, Y.-N.; Li, P.-N.; Liu, J. Increased Reactive Oxygen Species and Distinct Oxidative Damage in Resveratrol-suppressed Glioblastoma Cells. *J. Cancer* **2021**, *12*, 141–149. [CrossRef] [PubMed]
63. Cakmak, K.C.; Gülçin, İ. Anticholinergic and antioxidant activities of usnic acid-An activity-structure insight. *Toxicol. Rep.* **2019**, *6*, 1273–1280. [CrossRef] [PubMed]
64. Hoa, N.T.; Van Bay, M.; Mechler, A.; Vo, Q. V Is Usnic Acid a Promising Radical Scavenger? *ACS Omega* **2020**, *5*, 17715–17720. [CrossRef] [PubMed]
65. Krishnamurthy, P.; Wadhwani, A. Antioxidant enzymes and human health. *Antioxid. Enzym.* **2012**, *3*, 1–17.
66. Zhu, Z.; Du, S.; Du, Y.; Ren, J.; Ying, G.; Yan, Z. Glutathione reductase mediates drug resistance in glioblastoma cells by regulating redox homeostasis. *J. Neurochem.* **2018**, *144*, 93–104. [CrossRef]
67. Ramírez-Expósito, M.J.; Martínez-Martos, J.M. The Delicate Equilibrium between Oxidants and Antioxidants in Brain Glioma. *Curr. Neuropharmacol.* **2019**, *17*, 342–351. [CrossRef]

68. Barbosa, M.; Rios, O.; Velásquez, M.; Villalobos, J.; Ehrmanns, J. Acetylcholinesterase and butyrylcholinesterase histochemical activities and tumor cell growth in several brain tumors. *Surg. Neurol.* **2001**, *55*, 106–112. [CrossRef]
69. Reddy, R.G.; Veeraval, L.; Maitra, S.; Chollet-Krugler, M.; Tomasi, S.; Lohezic-Le Devehat, F.; Boustie, J.; Chakravarty, S. Lichen-derived compounds show potential for central nervous system therapeutics. *Phytomedicine* **2016**, *23*, 1527–1534. [CrossRef] [PubMed]
70. Bernardi, A.; Braganhol, E.; Jäger, E.; Figueiró, F.; Edelweiss, M.I.; Pohlmann, A.R.; Guterres, S.S.; Battastini, A.M.O. Indomethacin-loaded nanocapsules treatment reduces in vivo glioblastoma growth in a rat glioma model. *Cancer Lett.* **2009**, *281*, 53–63. [CrossRef]
71. Studzińska-Sroka, E.; Dudek-Makuch, M.; Chanaj-Kaczmarek, J.; Czepulis, N.; Korybalska, K.; Rutkowski, R.; Łuczak, J.; Grabowska, K.; Bylka, W.; Witowski, J. Anti-inflammatory Activity and Phytochemical Profile of *Galinsoga Parviflora* Cav. *Molecules* **2018**, *23*, 2133. [CrossRef]
72. Majchrzak-Celińska, A.; Zielińska-Przyjemska, M.; Wierzchowski, M.; Kleszcz, R.; Studzińska-Sroka, E.; Kaczmarek, M.; Paluszczak, J.; Cielecka-Piontek, J.; Krajka-Kuźniak, V. Methoxy-stilbenes downregulate the transcription of Wnt/β-catenin-dependent genes and lead to cell cycle arrest and apoptosis in human T98G glioblastoma cells. *Adv. Med. Sci.* **2021**, *66*, 6–20. [CrossRef] [PubMed]
73. Kikowska, M.A.; Chmielewska, M.; Włodarczyk, A.; Studzińska-Sroka, E.; Żuchowski, J.; Stochmal, A.; Kotwicka, M.; Thiem, B. Effect of pentacyclic triterpenoids-rich callus extract of *Chaenomeles japonica* (Thunb.) Lindl. ex Spach on viability, morphology, and proliferation of normal human skin fibroblasts. *Molecules* **2018**, *23*, 3009. [CrossRef] [PubMed]
74. Parschat, K.; Canne, C.; Hüttermann, J.; Kappl, R.; Fetzner, S. Xanthine dehydrogenase from *Pseudomonas putida* 86: Specificity, oxidation–reduction potentials of its redox-active centers, and first EPR characterization. *Biochim. Biophys. Acta (BBA)-Protein Struct. Mol. Enzymol.* **2001**, *1544*, 151–165. [CrossRef]
75. Moreira, P.R.; Maioli, M.A.; Medeiros, H.C.D.; Guelfi, M.; Pereira, F.T.V.; Mingatto, F.E. Protective effect of bixin on carbon tetrachloride-induced hepatotoxicity in rats. *Biol. Res.* **2014**, *47*, 1–7. [CrossRef] [PubMed]
76. Singh, R.P.; Padmavathi, B.; Rao, A.R. Modulatory influence of *Adhatoda vesica* (*Justicia adhatoda*) leaf extract on the enzymes of xenobiotic metabolism, antioxidant status and lipid peroxidation in mice. *Mol. Cell. Biochem.* **2000**, *213*, 99–109. [CrossRef] [PubMed]
77. Ellman, G.L.; Courtney, K.D.; Andres Jr, V.; Featherstone, R.M. A new and rapid colorimetric determination of acetylcholinesterase activity. *Biochem. Pharmacol.* **1961**, *7*, 88–95. [CrossRef]
78. Szwajgier, D.; Baranowska-Wójcik, E. Terpenes and phenylpropanoids as acetyl-and butyrylcholinesterase inhibitors: A comparative study. *Curr. Alzheimer Res.* **2019**, *16*, 963–973. [CrossRef]
79. Rhee, I.K.; van Rijn, R.M.; Verpoorte, R. Qualitative determination of false-positive effects in the acetylcholinesterase assay using thin layer chromatography. *Phytochem. Anal. An Int. J. Plant Chem. Biochem. Tech.* **2003**, *14*, 127–131. [CrossRef] [PubMed]

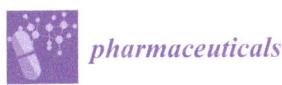

Article

Antibacterial and Antifungal Activity of Propyl-Propane-Thiosulfinate and Propyl-Propane-Thiosulfonate, Two Organosulfur Compounds from *Allium cepa*: In Vitro Antimicrobial Effect via the Gas Phase

Antonio Sorlozano-Puerto [1], Maria Albertuz-Crespo [1], Isaac Lopez-Machado [1], Lidia Gil-Martinez [2], Juan Jose Ariza-Romero [2], Alba Maroto-Tello [2], Alberto Baños-Arjona [2] and Jose Gutierrez-Fernandez [1,3,*]

1. Department of Microbiology, School of Medicine and PhD Program in Clinical Medicine and Public Health, University of Granada-ibs, Avda. de la Investigación, 11, 18016 Granada, Spain; asp@ugr.es (A.S.-P.); albertuzmaria@correo.ugr.es (M.A.-C.); isloma@correo.ugr.es (I.L.-M.)
2. DMC Research Center, Camino de Jayena, 82, 18620 Alhendín, Spain; lidiagm@domca.com (L.G.-M.); jariza@dmcrc.com (J.J.A.-R.); albamaroto@dmcrc.com (A.M.-T.); abarjona@domca.com (A.B.-A.)
3. Laboratory of Microbiology, Virgen de las Nieves University Hospital-ibs, Avda. de las Fuerzas Armadas, 2, 18012 Granada, Spain
* Correspondence: josegf@ugr.es

Abstract: Propyl-propane thiosulfinate (PTS) and propyl-propane thiosulfonate (PTSO) are two volatile compounds derived from *Allium cepa* with a widely documented antimicrobial activity. The aim of this study was to evaluate their anti-candidiasis activity and the ability of its gaseous phase to inhibit bacterial and yeast growth in vitro. The minimum inhibitory concentration of various antifungal products (including PTS and PTSO) was determined versus 203 clinical isolates of *Candida* spp. through broth microdilution assay. Additionally, the antimicrobial activity through aerial diffusion of PTS and PTSO was evaluated over the growth of a collection of bacteria and yeasts cultivated in agar plates. All yeasts were susceptible to the antifungals tested, except *C. glabrata* and *C. krusei*, that showed azole resistance. PTSO (MIC_{50} and MIC_{90} ranged from 4 to 16 mg/L and 8 to 32 mg/L, respectively) was significantly more active against yeasts than PTS (MIC_{50} and MIC_{90} ranged from 16 to 64 mg/L and 32 to 64 mg/L). Values were higher than those obtained for antifungal drugs. Gaseous phases of PTS and PTSO generated growth inhibition zones whose diameters were directly related to the substances concentration and inversely related to the microbial inoculum. The quantification of PTS and PTSO levels reached in the growth media through aerial diffusion displayed a concentration gradient from the central zone to the periphery. Only *P. aeruginosa* ATCC 27853 showed resistance, while yeasts (*C. albicans* ATCC 200955 and *C. krusei* ATCC 6258) presented the higher susceptibility to both compounds. These results suggest that PTS and PTSO display antibacterial and anti-candidiasis activity in vitro through aerial diffusion, having potential use in human therapy.

Keywords: propyl-propane-thiosulfinate; propyl-propane-thiosulfonate; antibacterial activity; antifungal activity; vapor

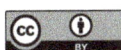

1. Introduction

In recent years, the antioxidative, hypolipidemic, hypocholesterolemia, antihypertensive, heart-protective, antithrombotic, anticancer, anti-inflammatory, immunomodulatory, and antimicrobial activities of different organosulfur products, such as thiosulfinates and thiosulfonates obtained from garlic (*Allium sativum*) and onion (*Allium cepa*), especially allicin (diallyl thiosulfinate), have been thoroughly studied [1–3].

While the precise mechanism of action has not yet been discovered, the main antimicrobial effect of these *Allium*-derived compounds has been reported to be due to its chemical reaction with thiol groups present in the main enzymes of the microbial metabolism, such as succinate dehydrogenase, alcohol dehydrogenase, thioredoxin reductase and ureases among others, via thiol-disulfide exchange reaction [4–6]. Additionally, they can react with thiols, such as glutathione, increasing the oxidized glutathione rate into a range that induces oxidative stress and cellular apoptosis [7]; they can interact with enzymes taking part of the microbial system of acetyl-CoA blocking the incorporation of acetate into fatty acids and inhibiting the development of a phospholipid bilayer of the membranes [5]; and they can inhibit RNA polymerase and, therefore, block the total synthesis of microbial RNA [8].

In onion, the most common sulfur compounds are isoalliin (S-propenyl-L-cysteine sulfoxide), methiin (S-methyl-L-cysteine sulfoxide) and propiin (S-propyl-L-cysteine sulfoxide). Propiin changes into propyl-propane thiosulfinate (PTS) due to the action of aliinase [9]. Although it is more stable than allicin, PTS is also a labile compound that, through dismutation or disproportionation reactions, changes into dipropyl disulfide and propyl-propane thiosulfonate (PTSO) [10].

In a previous study we compared the in vitro antibacterial activity of PTS and PTSO with other antibiotics. Both molecules showed broad spectrum antibacterial activity against multiresistant bacteria isolated from human clinical samples. These results contribute to the development and potential use of these compounds against human infections, such as oral, gastrointestinal, or skin infections, as well as for the treatment of urinary tract infections [11].

Candiduria is a common finding in immunosuppressed and hospitalized patients, which determines the clinical relevance of its detection and treatment. In recent decades, a remarkable increase of opportunistic candidiasis infections has been described, especially those affecting urinary tract produced by *C. albicans*, the most common among them. Nevertheless, an increase in the incidence of other different species of *Candida* has been described, some of them characterized by a higher resistance to the most common antifungals used in humans [12,13]. Therefore, in the same way as with bacteria, it would be interesting to compare the in vitro anticandidal activity of PTS and PTSO with that of other existing antifungals for potential application in medical therapy.

Both substances are volatile. Therefore, the study of their antimicrobial capacity through their gaseous phase would have great interest for the valorization of their possible use in the treatment of susceptible respiratory pathogens if PTS and PTSO reach appropriate concentrations in pulmonary epithelium administered by inhalation [3,14].

For all these reasons, the aim of this study was to evaluate anti-candidiasis activity of PTS and PTSO in vitro and the capacity of its gaseous phase to inhibit the growth of different bacteria and yeasts.

2. Results

2.1. Antifungal Susceptibility

The identification of the 203 clinical isolates of *Candida* spp. was as follows: *C. albicans* ($n = 83$), *C. glabrata* ($n = 73$), *C. krusei* ($n = 12$) and *C. tropicalis* ($n = 35$). A summary of the antifungal susceptibility data is presented in Table 1. All the isolates of *C. glabrata* and *C. krusei* were resistant to fluconazole. *C. glabrata* was also resistant to voriconazole. In the other cases, the isolates were susceptible to the assayed antifungals. Amphotericin B significantly showed more activity against *C. albicans* and *C. tropicalis* than against the two other species ($p < 0.001$), while *C. glabrata* was the species with the lowest MIC values ($p < 0.001$) to echinocandins (anidulafungin, micafungin, and caspofungin).

The behavior of PTS and PTSO was quite homogeneous, regardless of the analyzed species (Table 1). MIC_{50} and MIC_{90} values of PTS ranged from 16 to 64 mg/L for the first and from 32 to 64 mg/L for the second. The MFC_{50} and MFC_{90} ranged from 32 to 128 mg/L and 128 mg/L, respectively. On the other hand, the values of MIC_{50} and

MIC_{90} of PTSO ranged from 4 to 16 mg/L and 8 to 32 mg/L, while MFC_{50} y MFC_{90} ranged from 32 to 128 mg/L and from 64 to 128 mg/L, respectively. Considering all of the clinical isolates of *Candida* spp., the data indicated that PTSO was significantly more active than PTS ($p < 0.001$) and showed the fungicidal activity of these compounds since MIC and MFC values differed in only one dilution for both PTS (MIC_{50} = 32 mg/L and MFC_{50} = 64 mg/L; MIC_{90} = 64 mg/L and MFC_{90} = 128 mg/L) and PTSO (MIC_{50} = 16 mg/L and MFC_{50} = 32 mg/L; MIC_{90} = 32 mg/L and MFC_{90} = 64 mg/L).

Table 1. In vitro activity of different antifungal drugs, PTS, and PTSO against *Candida* spp.

Species of Yeasts (Number of Isolates)	Range of MIC (in mg/L)	MIC_{50} (in mg/L)	MIC_{90} (in mg/L)	Range of MFC (in mg/L)	MFC_{50} (in mg/L)	MFC_{90} (in mg/L)	Number of Resistant Isolates
Candida albicans (n = 83)							
Amphotericin B	0.125–0.25	0.25	0.25	1–16	4	8	0
Anidulafungin	≤0.008–0.25	0.015	0.06	0.015–>4	0.25	1	0
Micafungin	≤0.008–0.25	0.03	0.125	0.03–4	0.5	2	0
Caspofungin	≤0.008–0.25	0.06	0.06	0.06–4	0.5	2	0
Fluconazole	≤0.125–2	0.25	2	8–>64	>64	>64	0
Voriconazole	≤0.008–0.06	≤0.008	≤0.008	0.03–0.5	0.5	0.5	0
PTS	16–64	32	32	16–>128	32	128	-
PTSO	8–64	16	32	8–128	32	64	-
Candida glabrata (n = 73)							
Amphotericin B	0.06–1	0.25	0.5	1–>16	4	8	0
Anidulafungin	≤0.008–0.125	0.015	0.03	0.06–>4	0.25	0.5	0
Micafungin	≤0.008–0.06	≤0.008	0.03	0.008–4	0.06	0.25	0
Caspofungin	≤0.008–0.125	0.03	0.03	0.06–4	1	2	0
Fluconazole	0.25–>64	4	≥64	16–>64	>64	>64	73
Voriconazole	0.03–>4	0.5	≥4	2–>4	>4	>4	73
PTS	8–64	32	32	16–>128	64	128	-
PTSO	16–32	16	32	8–>128	32	64	-
Candida krusei (n = 12)							
Amphotericin B	0.25–1	0.5	1	4–16	8	16	0
Anidulafungin	≤0.008–0.06	0.015	0.03	0.125–0.5	0.25	0.5	0
Micafungin	0.06–0.25	0.125	0.125	0.5–4	0.5	1	0
Caspofungin	0.06–0.25	0.125	0.25	1–4	1	2	0
Fluconazole	8–>64	16	≥64	>64	>64	>64	12
Voriconazole	0.03–0.5	0.125	0.5	2–>4	>4	>4	0
PTS	4–32	16	32	32–>128	32	128	-
PTSO	4–16	4	8	64–>128	128	128	-
Candida tropicalis (n = 35)							
Amphotericin B	≤0.03–1	0.125	0.25	2–16	2	8	0
Anidulafungin	≤0.008–0.25	0.06	0.25	0.015–2	1	2	0
Micafungin	≤0.008–0.25	0.06	0.25	0.008–2	0.5	2	0
Caspofungin	≤0.008–0.25	0.06	0.25	0.06–4	1	4	0
Fluconazole	≤0.125–2	≤0.125	1	8–>64	>64	>64	0
Voriconazole	≤0.008–0.06	≤0.008	0.015	0.03–0.5	0.5	0.5	0
PTS	32–64	64	64	64–>128	128	128	-
PTSO	4–32	16	32	4–128	32	64	-

MIC: minimum inhibitory concentration. MFC: minimum fungicidal concentration.

2.2. Antimicrobial Activity of Vapor

PTS and PTSO inhibited growth in six of the seven microorganisms tested in the present study through its gaseous phase without coming into contact with the medium and thus, with the microorganism, except for its aerial diffusion. The vapor produced by both substances reaches the agar medium, inhibiting microbial growth in a circular area above the drop placed in the lid of the Petri dish (Figure 1). The absence of any microbial growth in the inhibition area suggests a predominant biocidal effect of these substances. Only *P. aeruginosa* ATCC 27853 showed resistance to both compounds, showing absence of inhibition halo in the majority of the concentrations and bacterial inocula used. In the case of this bacterium, halos with a diameter below 10 mm were observed only when PTSO was used at a concentration of 50 mg/mL and 25 mg/mL against a bacterial inoculum at 0.5 of McFarland scale.

As it is shown in Figure 2 and Table 2, diameters from the inhibition of growth zones were directly related to the concentration of PTS or PTSO used, and inversely related to the microbial inoculum used: the higher the concentration of PTS or PTSO were and the lower the inoculum of microorganisms were, the larger the diameter of the halo was ($p < 0.001$). Greater halos and, consequently an increased susceptibility to these compounds were observed in the case of yeasts (*C. albicans* ATCC 200955 and *C. krusei* ATCC 6258).

Considering the set of microorganisms used in this study (with the exception of *P. aeruginosa* ATCC 27853 due to the demonstrated resistance to both compounds), the antimicrobial activity of PTSO was significantly higher than that of PTS, since, for the same microbial inoculum and substance concentration, the diameters of the growth inhibition halos produced by the gas phase of PTSO were significantly larger than those obtained from PTS ($p < 0.01$, in all cases).

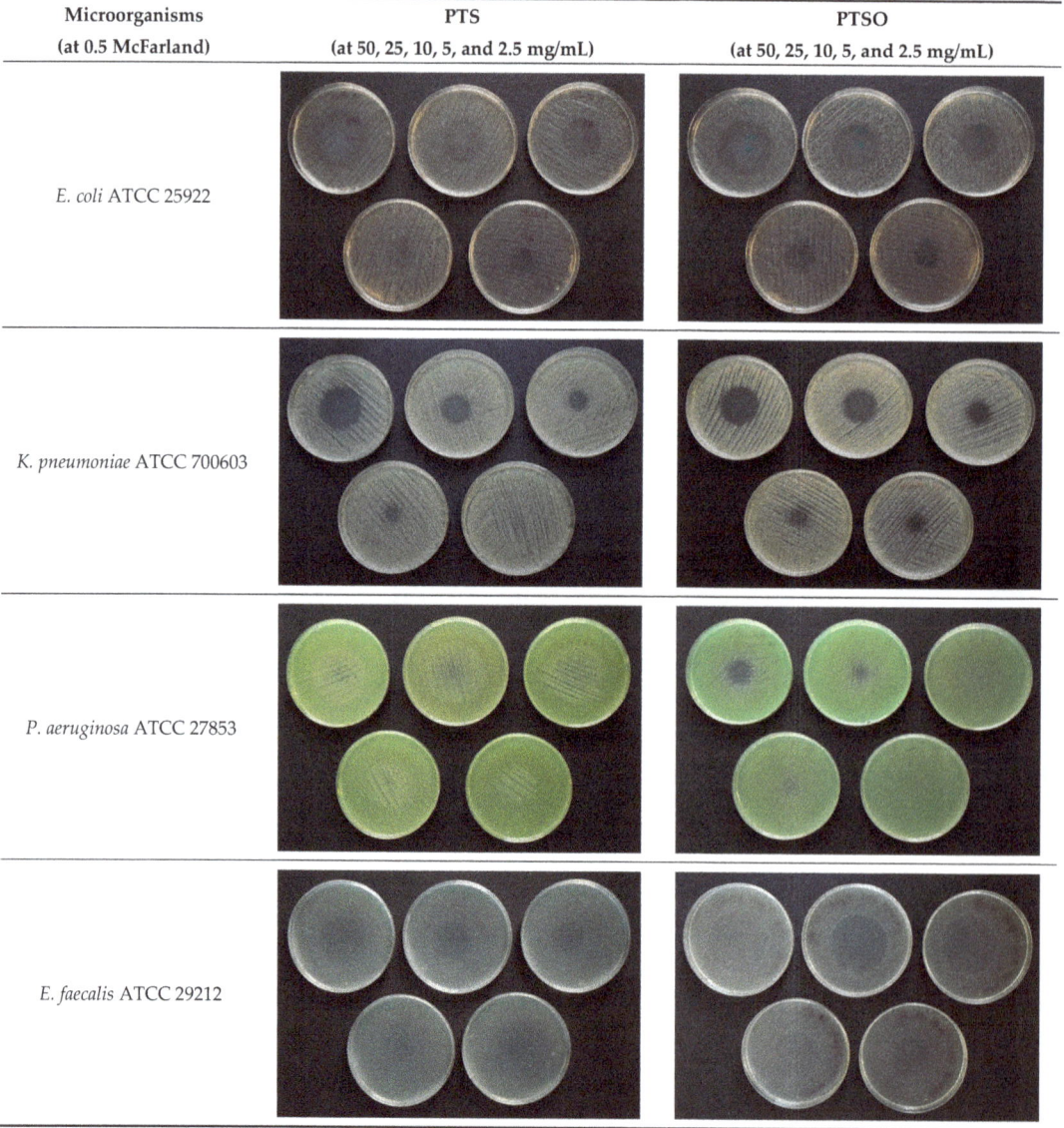

Figure 1. *Cont.*

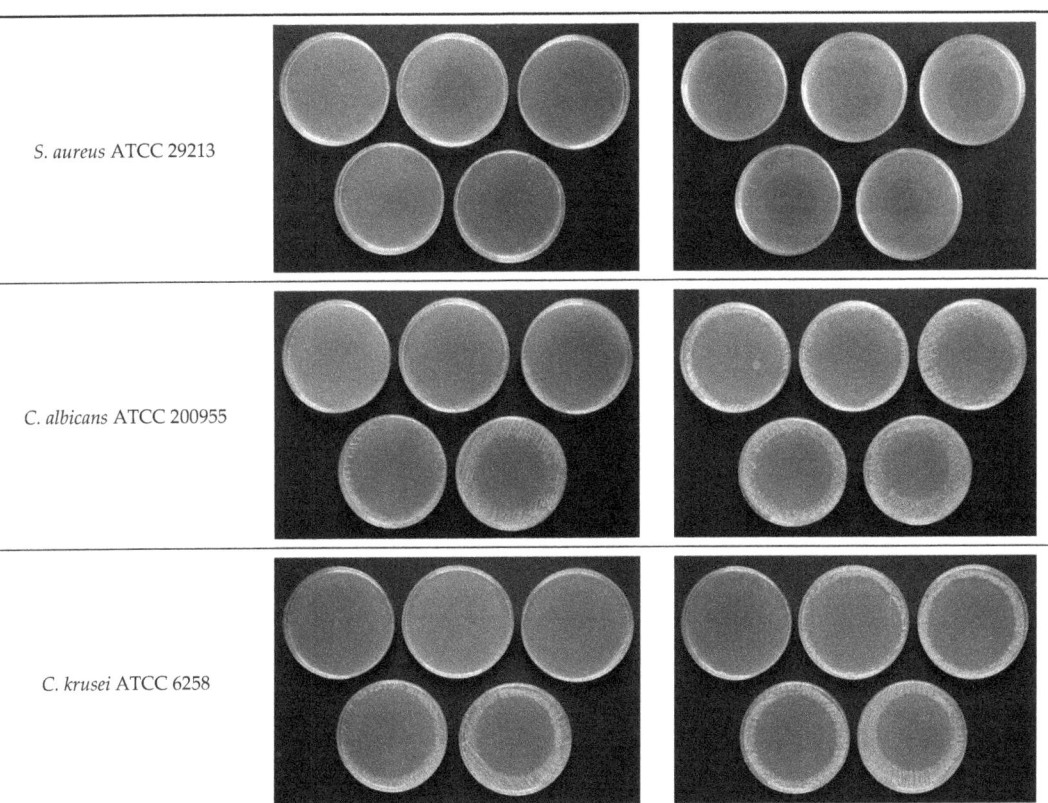

Figure 1. Antimicrobial activity of PTS and PTSO via the gas phase. Photograph showing halos of inhibition at doses of 50 mg/mL, 25 mg/mL, 10 mg/mL, 5 mg/mL, and 2.5 mg/mL (from left to right and from top to bottom). Although assays were carried out at 0.5, 1, and 2 McFarland turbidity, only the results at 0.5 McFarland are shown.

Table 3 shows the concentration of PTS and PTSO detected in the Mueller-Hinton medium by HPLC-UV. The gas phase of both compounds, deposited on the lid of the Petri dish, reached the culture medium being able to be detected and quantified. The highest concentration in all cases was reached in sample 1, which coincided with the center of the plate, located in the most vertical position just above the drop deposited on the lid. As the sample moved away from the center (samples from 2 to 6), the concentration decreased, creating a gradient from the central area of the plate (highest concentration) towards its periphery (lowest concentration). In some cases, either because the concentration of the drop was small (2.5 mg/mL) and/or because the distance to the center was higher (sample 6), the concentration reached in the medium could not be quantified because it was below the limit of detection of the HPLC-UV technique.

From the results shown in Table 3, the linear regression lines were drawn (Figure 3), relating the distance to the center of the plate (measured in mm) to the concentration that PTS or PTSO reached at a given point (in mg/L) according to each of the concentrations of the drop deposited on the lid. As it can be seen, there was a high correlation in all cases, which determined the quality of the fit.

Theoretical concentration of PTS and PTSO reached at the limit of the microbial growth inhibition zone for each microorganism and inoculum concentration is shown in Table 4. This concentration was determined by measuring the radius (in mm) of the inhibition areas obtained for each microorganism and inoculum concentration and extrapolating the results in the linear regression line for the corresponding concentrations of PTS and PTSO showed in Figure 3. The concentrations of PTSO at which microbial growth was inhibited were lower than those of PTS ($p < 0.01$), showing a greater antimicrobial activity. Furthermore, the inhibition of yeast growth compared to that of the bacteria occurred with lower concentrations, with either of the two compounds.

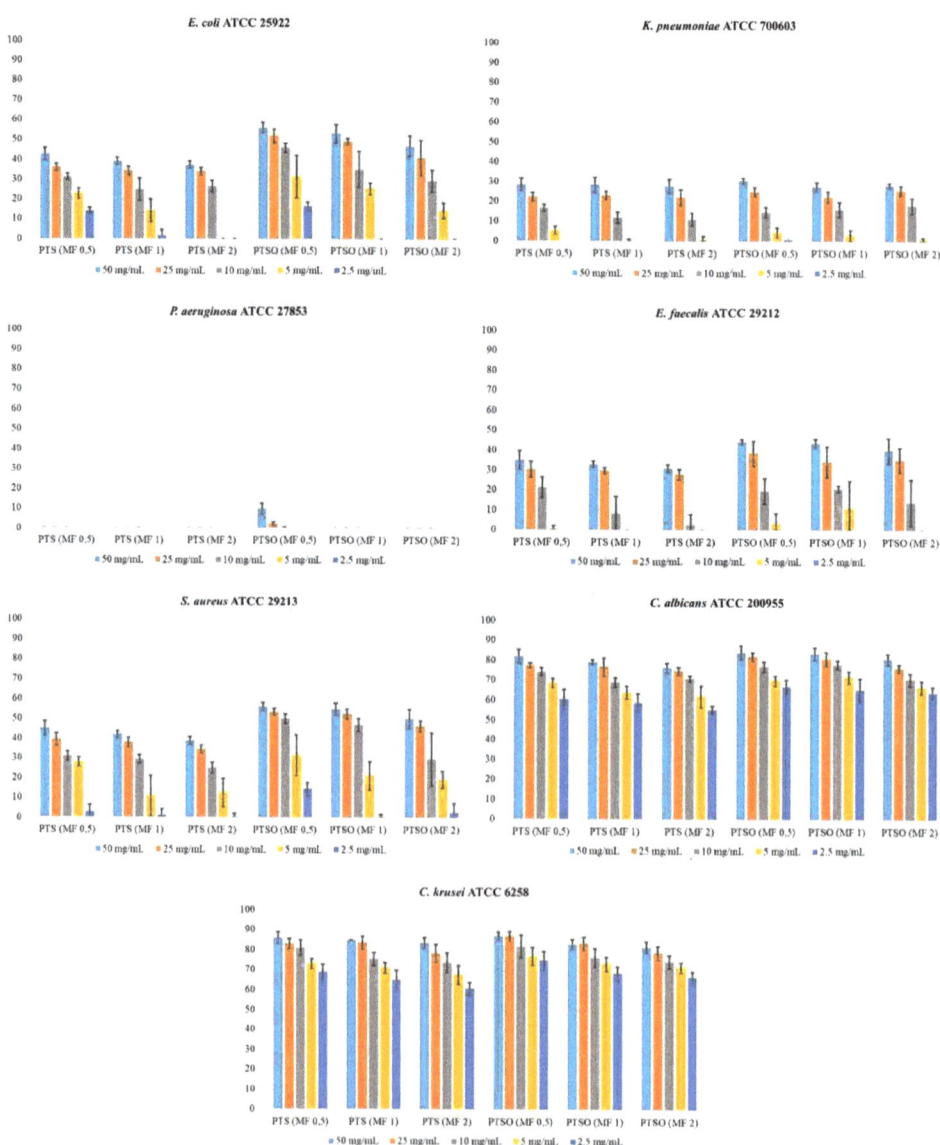

Figure 2. Average value ± standard deviation (in mm) of the growth inhibition halos for each concentration of PTS and PTSO, in the different inocula (0.5, 1, and 2 of McFarland) and for the different microorganisms. Diameters from the inhibition of growth zones were directly related to the concentration of PTS or PTSO used, and inversely related to the microbial inoculum used. Greater halos were observed in the case of yeasts. The diameters of the growth inhibition halos produced via the gas phase of PTSO were significantly larger than those obtained from PTS.

Table 2. Average diameter ± standard deviation (in mm) of the growth inhibition halos for the different PTS and PTSO concentrations, in each inoculum (0.5, 1, and 2 from McFarland) and for the different microorganisms.

Microorganisms	McFarland	PTS Concentration (Growth Inhibition in mm)						PTSO Concentration (Growth Inhibition in mm)				
		50 mg/mL	25 mg/mL	10 mg/mL	5 mg/mL	2.5 mg/mL		50 mg/mL	25 mg/mL	10 mg/mL	5 mg/mL	2.5 mg/mL
E. coli ATCC 25922	0.5	43 ± 3.2	36 ± 1.9	31 ± 1.6	23 ± 2.7	14 ± 1.6		56 ± 2.7	52 ± 3.3	46 ± 2.2	31 ± 10.8	16 ± 2.1
	1	39 ± 2.0	34 ± 2.1	25 ± 5.6	14 ± 5.7	1 ± 3.0		53 ± 4.5	49 ± 1.8	35 ± 9.2	25 ± 3.0	0
	2	37 ± 1.8	34 ± 2.0	27 ± 3.0	0	0		47 ± 5.1	42 ± 8.8	29 ± 5.5	14 ± 3.9	0
K. pneumoniae ATCC 700603	0.5	28 ± 3.3	22 ± 2.2	17 ± 1.8	5 ± 2.0	0		30 ± 1.3	25 ± 2.2	15 ± 2.5	5 ± 2.5	1 ± 0.7
	1	28 ± 3.9	23 ± 2.2	12 ± 2.8	0	0		27 ± 2.3	22 ± 2.7	16 ± 3.8	3 ± 2.7	0
	2	28 ± 3.6	22 ± 3.8	11 ± 3.3	1 ± 1.8	0		28 ± 1.2	26 ± 2.4	18 ± 3.9	1 ± 0.9	0
P. aeruginosa ATCC 27853	0.5	0	0	0	0	0		10 ± 2.7	2 ± 0.9	0	0	0
	1	0	0	0	0	0		0	0	0	0	0
	2	0	0	0	0	0		0	0	0	0	0
E. faecalis ATCC 29212	0.5	35 ± 4.6	30 ± 4.0	21 ± 5.2	1 ± 1.2	0		44 ± 1.3	38 ± 6.5	20 ± 6.3	3 ± 5.3	0
	1	33 ± 1.8	30 ± 1.6	8 ± 8.7	0	0		44 ± 2.1	34 ± 7.8	21 ± 1.6	11 ± 14.0	0
	2	31 ± 1.9	28 ± 2.7	3 ± 5.3	0	0		40 ± 6.3	35 ± 6.2	14 ± 11.6	0	0
S. aureus ATCC 29213	0.5	45 ± 3.6	39 ± 3.3	31 ± 2.4	28 ± 2.4	3 ± 3.5		56 ± 2.0	53 ± 1.8	50 ± 2.3	31 ± 10.4	14 ± 3.3
	1	42 ± 1.8	38 ± 2.5	29 ± 2.0	11 ± 10.3	1 ± 3.2		55 ± 3.1	52 ± 2.5	47 ± 3.2	21 ± 7.1	0
	2	39 ± 2.1	34 ± 2.1	25 ± 2.8	12 ± 7.1	1 ± 1.6		50 ± 4.9	46 ± 2.7	29 ± 13.5	19 ± 4.3	3 ± 4.8
C. albicans ATCC 200955	0.5	82 ± 3.4	77 ± 1.2	74 ± 1.9	69 ± 2.3	61 ± 4.9		84 ± 3.4	82 ± 2.2	77 ± 2.5	70 ± 2.4	67 ± 3.5
	1	79 ± 1.3	77 ± 4.5	69 ± 2.3	64 ± 3.3	59 ± 4.5		84 ± 3.2	81 ± 3.4	78 ± 2.1	72 ± 3.0	65 ± 5.8
	2	76 ± 2.5	75 ± 1.9	71 ± 1.5	62 ± 5.5	55 ± 1.9		81 ± 2.8	76 ± 1.9	71 ± 3.0	67 ± 3.2	64 ± 2.9
C. krusei ATCC 6258	0.5	86 ± 3.0	83 ± 2.5	81 ± 3.9	73 ± 2.5	69 ± 3.9		87 ± 2.1	87 ± 2.3	82 ± 5.6	77 ± 4.5	75 ± 4.5
	1	85 ± 0.0	84 ± 3.3	75 ± 3.2	71 ± 2.6	65 ± 5.0		83 ± 2.5	84 ± 3.2	76 ± 4.7	73 ± 3.6	69 ± 3.4
	2	84 ± 2.7	78 ± 4.5	74 ± 4.9	68 ± 4.7	61 ± 3.2		82 ± 2.8	79 ± 3.5	75 ± 3.2	72 ± 2.5	67 ± 2.8

Table 3. Concentration ± standard deviation (in mg/L) of PTS and PTSO reached in Mueller–Hinton agar for each of the samples, in relation to the initial concentration of each substance in the drop deposited on the lid of the Petri dish.

Organosulfur Compound	Initial Concentration	Sample 1	Sample 2	Sample 3	Sample 4	Sample 5	Sample 6
PTS	50 mg/mL	82.7 ± 0.1	70.8 ± 0.3	51.2 ± 0.1	30.2 ± 0.2	17.0 ± 0.3	9.4 ± 0.1
	25 mg/mL	68.6 ± 0.2	59.6 ± 0.1	42.4 ± 0.3	25.1 ± 0.2	12.4 ± 0.1	5.8 ± 0.2
	10 mg/mL	57.3 ± 0.2	48.6 ± 0.1	35.5 ± 0.1	22.1 ± 0.2	4.2 ± 0.1	<LD
	5 mg/mL	48.5 ± 0.2	36.4 ± 0.2	28.6 ± 0.3	8.5 ± 0.2	<LD	<LD
	2.5 mg/mL	<LD	<LD	<LD	<LD	<LD	<LD
PTSO	50 mg/mL	28.6 ± 0.2	26.3 ± 0.2	20.9 ± 0.2	14.8 ± 0.1	9.9 ± 0.4	4.2 ± 0.2
	25 mg/mL	23.4 ± 0.2	18.6 ± 0.2	14.8 ± 0.2	12.7 ± 0.2	8.2 ± 0.2	2.6 ± 0.1
	10 mg/mL	18.7 ± 0.1	15.8 ± 0.1	13.8 ± 0.1	12.9 ± 0.3	7.5 ± 0.1	<LD
	5 mg/mL	17.9 ± 0.1	14.8 ± 0.3	13.4 ± 0.2	7.5 ± 0.1	2.8 ± 0.3	<LD
	2.5 mg/mL	<LD	<LD	<LD	<LD	<LD	<LD

LD: Limit of detection of the HPLC-UV technique.

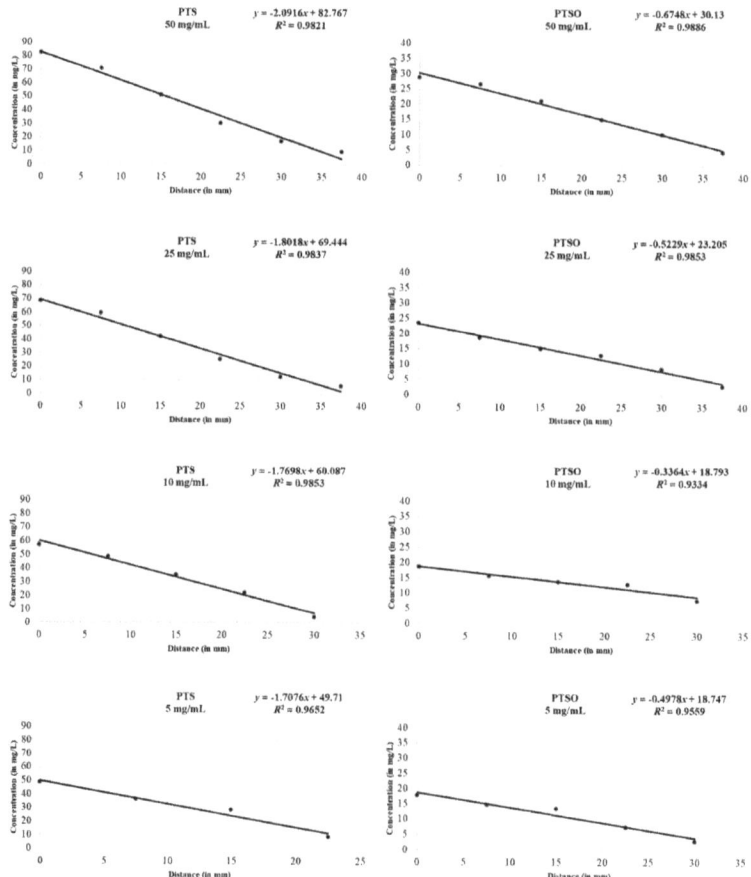

Figure 3. Relationship between the distance from the center of the Petri dish and the concentration reached via the gas phase at a defined point of the Mueller–Hinton medium for each concentration of PTS and PTSO deposited on the lid of the Petri dish. There is an inverse linear relationship between the distance to the center of the culture medium and the concentration reached via the gas phase at a given point.

Table 4. Average value ± standard deviation (in mg/L) of the concentration of PTS and PTSO reached at the limit of the microbial growth inhibition zone.

Microorganism	McFarland	Limit of the Microbial Growth	PTS Concentration				PTSO Concentration			
			50 mg/mL	25 mg/mL	10 mg/mL	5 mg/mL	50 mg/mL	25 mg/mL	10 mg/mL	5 mg/mL
E. coli ATCC 25922	0.5	Radius	21.5	18	15.5	11.5	28	26	23	15.5
		Concentration	38.1 ± 3.3	36.9 ± 1.7	32.5 ± 1.4	30.3 ± 2.3	11.3 ± 0.9	9.5 ± 0.9	11.1 ± 0.4	11.0 ± 2.7
	1	Radius	19.5	17	12.5	7	26.5	24.5	17.5	12.5
		Concentration	41.9 ± 2.1	38.5 ± 1.9	38.1 ± 5.0	37.8 ± 4.9	12.2 ± 1.5	10.4 ± 0.5	12.9 ± 1.5	12.4 ± 0.7
	2	Radius	18.5	17	13.5	0	23.5	21	14.5	7
		Concentration	43.8 ± 1.8	38.8 ± 1.8	36.5 ± 2.6	≥48.5	14.2 ± 1.7	12.2 ± 2.3	13.8 ± 0.9	15.2 ± 1.0
K. pneumoniae ATCC 700603	0.5	Radius	14	11	8.5	2.5	15	12.5	7.5	2.5
		Concentration	53.1 ± 3.4	49.4 ± 1.9	45.3 ± 1.6	45.2 ± 1.7	19.9 ± 0.5	16.7 ± 0.6	16.3 ± 0.4	17.6 ± 0.6
	1	Radius	14	11.5	6	0	13.5	11	8	1.5
		Concentration	53.2 ± 4.0	48.8 ± 2.0	49.6 ± 2.5	≥48.5	20.9 ± 0.8	17.4 ± 0.7	16.1 ± 0.6	18.0 ± 0.7
	2	Radius	14	11	5.5	0.5	14	13	9	0.5
		Concentration	53.7 ± 3.7	49.4 ± 3.4	50.4 ± 2.9	≥48.5	20.7 ± 0.4	16.5 ± 0.6	15.8 ± 0.6	≥17.9
E. faecalis ATCC 29212	0.5	Radius	17.5	15	10.5	0.5	22	19	10	1.5
		Concentration	46.2 ± 4.9	42.2 ± 3.6	41.3 ± 4.6	≥48.5	15.2 ± 0.5	13.2 ± 1.7	15.5 ± 1.1	18.0 ± 1.3
	1	Radius	16.5	15	4	0	22	17	10.5	5.5
		Concentration	48.5 ± 1.8	42.8 ± 1.4	52.9 ± 7.7	≥48.5	15.4 ± 0.7	14.3 ± 2.0	15.3 ± 0.3	16.1 ± 3.5
	2	Radius	15.5	14	1.5	0	20	17.5	7	0
		Concentration	50.5 ± 2.0	44.3 ± 2.4	57.9 ± 4.7	≥48.5	16.7 ± 2.1	14.0 ± 1.6	16.5 ± 2.0	≥17.9
S. aureus ATCC 29213	0.5	Radius	22.5	19.5	15.5	14	28	26.5	25	15.5
		Concentration	36.1 ± 3.7	34.0 ± 2.9	32.8 ± 2.1	26.1 ± 2.0	11.3 ± 0.7	9.3 ± 0.5	10.4 ± 0.4	10.9 ± 2.6
	1	Radius	21	19	14.5	5.5	27.5	26	23.5	10.5
		Concentration	39.4 ± 1.9	35.4 ± 2.2	34.2 ± 1.8	40.6 ± 8.8	11.7 ± 1.0	9.5 ± 0.7	10.9 ± 0.5	13.5 ± 1.8
	2	Radio	19.5	17	12.5	6	25	26	14.5	9.5
		Concentration	42.3 ± 2.2	38.6 ± 1.9	38.0 ± 2.5	39.1 ± 6.1	13.3 ± 1.7	11.1 ± 0.7	13.8 ± 2.3	14.0 ± 1.1
C. albicans ATCC 200955	0.5	Radius	41	38.5	37	34.5	42	41	38.5	35
		Concentration	≤5.8	≤5.8	≤4.2	≤8.5	≤4.2	≤2.6	≤7.5	≤2.8
	1	Radius	39.5	38.5	34.5	32	42	40.5	39	36
		Concentration	≤9.4	≤5.8	≤4.2	≤8.5	≤4.2	≤2.6	≤7.5	≤2.8
	2	Radius	38	37.5	35.5	31	40.5	38	35.5	33.5
		Concentration	≤9.4	≤5.8	≤4.2	≤8.5	≤4.2	≤2.6	≤7.5	≤2.8
C. krusei ATCC 6258	0.5	Radius	43	41.5	40.5	36.5	43.5	41	38.5	36.5
		Concentration	≤5.8	≤5.8	≤4.2	≤8.5	≤2.6	≤2.6	≤7.5	≤2.8
	1	Radius	42.5	42	37.5	35.5	41.5	42	38	36.5
		Concentration	≤9.4	≤5.8	≤4.2	≤8.5	≤4.2	≤2.6	≤7.5	≤2.8
	2	Radius	42	36	37	34	41	39.5	37.5	36
		Concentration	≤9.4	≤5.8	≤4.2	≤8.5	≤4.2	≤2.6	≤7.5	≤2.8

Radius: average value (in mm) of the radius of the growth inhibition halos for the 10 assays carried out with each microorganism, inoculum, concentration and organosulfur compound (see Table 2).

3. Discussion

3.1. Antifungal Susceptibility

Invasive fungal diseases of nosocomial origin or associated to health care, especially those caused by *Candida* spp., have become a major health problem as they are associated with high rates of morbidity and mortality. Although candida urinary tract infections and vulvovaginal infections are, a priori, milder processes, they have a higher incidence among the population and can be the origin of more serious and disseminated infections in patients with underlying diseases [15]. Similarly, yeast colonization of the skin and mucosal surfaces is also a risk factor for the development of invasive candidiasis in patients, especially those admitted in the intensive care unit as a consequence of risk factors such as handling by colonized healthcare personnel, central venous and urinary catheters, use of broad-spectrum antibiotics, prolonged lengths of stay, mechanical ventilation, parenteral feeding, etc. [16].

On the other hand, alongside the increase of the prevalence of yeast infections by genus *Candida*, a significant increase in the rates of resistance to antifungals commonly used in human clinics (mainly polyenes, azoles, and echinocandins) is currently described both for *C. albicans* as in other non-*albicans* species. Therefore, it is difficult to establish a preventive and therapeutic approach to these infections, which makes advisable to research new alternative therapies to conventional treatments with different and/or synergistic mechanisms of fungicide action and fewer side effects [17–20].

In this context, the thiosulfinates derived from *Allium* spp., such as allicin, have demonstrated broad antifungal activity in numerous in vitro studies against yeasts of the genus *Candida* [21–23]. In the present work, the MICs obtained for antifungals were similar to those obtained in previous research, both in our geographical area [24,25] and in more remote areas [19,26–29]. The lowest MICs were obtained for *C. albicans* and *C. tropicalis*; the highest for *C. glabrata* and *C. krusei*, especially in the case of azoles, which indicates that *Candida* species remain susceptible to commonly used antifungals and do not represent a problem for the therapeutic approach. The usual resistance of *C. glabrata* and *C. krusei* to azoles would be an exception.

Similarly, our results demonstrate that PTS and PTSO have a significant antifungal activity against different isolates of *Candida* spp. from human clinical samples, although their activity is not as strong as that of some antifungals, such as amphotericin B, echinocandins or azoles, especially if we consider the most susceptible species to them. In addition, our findings related to the antifungal effects of other organosulfur compounds against yeast isolates are in compliance with those already described in the literature [21,30,31].

In order to explain the antifungal effect of these molecules, different mechanisms of action have been proposed. The most directly associated to cell damage and decreased growth capacity of the fungus are the ability to modify essential enzymes in fungal metabolism [32], induce oxidative stress [7], alter lipids by damaging the integrity of cell membranes (including cytoplasmatic organelles, such as mitochondria or vacuoles) [33] and modify the expression of some genes [34].

Even if our preliminary results provide useful information about the potential use of PTS and PTSO for the prevention or treatment of candidiasis infections caused by multidrug resistant yeasts, further research is needed to demonstrate the effectiveness of these compounds with a wider group of fungi and in vivo models [35]. Even though these results may support their therapeutic use, the absence of cut-off points defined by international committees for this kind of substances does not allow relevant conclusions to be drawn. Further investigation regarding their pharmacokinetic and toxicological characteristics is required before considering safe clinical use.

3.2. Antimicrobial Activity of Vapor

One of the main characteristics of the organosulfur compounds obtained from plants of the genus *Allium* is their volatility, which is the main reason of the characteristic aroma that these plants exude, especially when they are mashed or crushed. Given the scarcity of volatile antimicrobials available for clinical use in humans, these molecules could be considered an alternative (alone or in combination with other antimicrobials) for the treatment of lung infections via inhalation, instead of oral or parenteral administration [3]. However, there are still few studies evaluating their antimicrobial capacity through their gas phase and their potential applicability for the treatment of infectious diseases [3,14,36].

In the present work, PTS and PTSO showed high bactericidal and fungicidal activity through their gas phase, inhibiting the growth of six of the seven microorganisms assayed (*E. coli* ATCC 25922, *K. pneumoniae* ATCC 700603, *E. faecalis* ATCC 29212, *S. aureus* ATCC 29213, *C. albicans* ATCC 200955 and *C. krusei* ATCC 6258, but not *P. aeruginosa* ATCC 27853), which might suggest that these substances are likely to be less active against *P. aeruginosa* than against other pathogens. Various studies have demonstrated that, against these bacteria and other related ones, very high concentrations of these compounds should be used to inhibit bacterial growth, which may not be feasible from a therapeutic point of view [11,37,38].

However, the microbicidal activity of these compounds was not the same against both types of microorganisms. The antifungal effect was higher than the antibacterial effect (the growth inhibition halos were significantly higher in *C. albicans* ATCC 200955 and *C. krusei* ATCC 6258 in comparison to those obtained against bacteria). The higher activity of these compounds on yeasts is also observed if we compare the results obtained in the present work on antifungal susceptibility, in terms of MIC, with a previous work of our group with clinical bacterial isolates from human origin: MIC_{50} and MIC_{90} values of PTS and PTSO are lower against yeasts than against bacteria [11]. According to some studies, it is possible that the presence of a fungal cell wall, more permeable to these compounds than the peptidoglycan wall of the bacteria, allows this cytotoxic effect at lower doses [39]. On the other hand, the gas phase of PTSO was more active than that of PTS against all the microorganisms evaluated (with the exception of *P. aeruginosa*), since the growth inhibition halos were significantly higher for PTSO than for PTS in all cases. In fact, the higher antimicrobial activity of PTSO in comparison to PTS has already been described previously by our group [11].

As shown by Leontiev et al. [14], despite of the lack of direct contact of the organosulfur compounds with the agar and with the microorganism itself, when the antimicrobial effect via the gas phase is studied, it is worth noting how clear are the microbial growth inhibition halos and how well defined are the edges. His interpretation, as well as ours, is that this could be due to the existence of a concentration gradient from the closest area of the agar to the drop, precisely at its zenith, to the periphery. In our study, the quantification of the concentration of PTS and PTSO in the agar allowed to confirm this suspicion, showing that there is an inverse linear relationship between the distance to the center of the culture medium and the concentration reached via the gas phase at a given point.

From the results obtained in the present study, as well as from previous works [3,14,40] it can be deduced that organosulfur compounds derived from *Allium* spp., such as PTS and especially PTSO could be used for the treatment of lung infections, due to its high volatility by inhalation, producing an effect directly on the lung. An advantage that would facilitate their clinical use is that these substances are perceived as innocuous as they are present naturally in food such as onion, widely consumed and included in the diet in most cultures. Among the disadvantages, we could highlight the need to improve the extraction procedures in order to preserve the biological properties of these substances avoiding their loss as a consequence of events such as heating, long-term preservation, etc. In addition, there is a need to diminish the strong impact of their smell and aroma.

However, since the microbicidal effect is directly proportional to the concentration of PTS and PTSO used, a definitive conclusion on the efficacy of this treatment cannot be drawn without evaluating the potential toxicity on human lung cells. It may be possible that the dose required to exert the expected effect in vivo is so high that it produces undesirable toxic consequences. As indicated by Reiter et al. [3], the use of lower and less toxic concentrations concomitantly with other antibiotics or antifungals could be considered if a synergistic effect is demonstrated. In this sense, it has been proven that thiosulfinates have a synergistic effect with antibiotics, such as ampicillin, piperacillin-tazobactam, levofloxacin, gentamicin, amikacin, azithromycin, vancomycin, doxycycline, or polymyxin B [41–45] and with antifungals such as azoles [22,46] or amphotericin B [21]. The potential clinical usefulness of these substances at low concentrations, via inhalation and in combination with other antimicrobials, requires further studies in vitro and with animal and/or human models.

Among the main limitations of our study, was that the methodologies used, both for the study of the antifungal effect of PTS and PTSO, as well as for the antimicrobial effect that their gas phase could exert, are not standardized. Therefore, it is not possible to establish a direct correlation between the results obtained and the potential human therapeutic use. Although their antimicrobial activity seems obvious as numerous studies have shown, international committees for the study of antimicrobial susceptibility have not yet defined cut-off points for these compounds. Thus, no final conclusion can be drawn. Furthermore, the present work has not evaluated the volatility of the organosulfur derivatives and, therefore, the possible loss of activity of PTS and PTSO over time or with increasing temperature, which other authors have described previously [36]. These factors could reduce their clinical usefulness. Finally, further studies should be focused on standardizing the methods to evaluate the antimicrobial activity, understanding how these substances are distributed or removed from the organism, determining the administration routes, and evaluating their effect in different dosages, organs and systems and evaluating the safety of their administration in humans, before safe clinical use is considered.

4. Materials and Methods

4.1. Antifungal Susceptibility Testing

4.1.1. Antifungals, PTS, and PTSO

Amphotericin B, anidulafungin, micafungin, caspofungin, fluconazole and voriconazole were purchased from Sigma-Aldrich (Madrid, Spain). PTS and PTSO are organosulfur compounds present in onion extracts (AlioCare^{TM}) which were supplied with high purity (97%) by Enzim-Orbita Agroalimentares LDA (Tavira, Portugal) and dissolved in polysorbate-80 to a final concentration of 500,000 mg/L.

4.1.2. Candida Isolates and Identification

Two hundred and three clinical isolates of *Candida* spp. obtained from urine samples processed in the Laboratory of Microbiology of the Virgen de las Nieves University Hospital (Granada, Spain) were selected. CHROMagar Orientation medium (Becton Dickinson, Franklin Lakes, NJ, USA) was used for the growth of isolates. All colonies with yeast compatible morphology were subcultured using a CHROMagar Candida medium (Becton Dickinson). Species were identified using filamentation test and ASM Vitek system (bioMérieux, Madrid, Spain) or MALDI Biotyper system (Bruker Daltonics, Billerica, MA, USA). All isolates were stored at $-40°$ C until the susceptibility study.

4.1.3. In Vitro Antifungal Assay

Standard broth microdilution method was carried out according to the guidelines of the Clinical and Laboratory Standards Institute (CLSI) [47]. A series of two-fold final dilutions of each drug, PTS, and PTSO were prepared in RPMI-1640 medium with L-glutamine but without bicarbonate. Glucose was added to a final concentration of 0.2% and pH was adjusted to 7.0 with acid morpholine propane sulfonic (0.165 M) buffer.

First, all isolates were subcultured onto Sabouraud dextrose agar. Twenty-four hours after the incubation, standard 0.5 McFarland fungal suspensions were prepared with saline solution. Microdilution testing was carried out in 96-well, flat-bottom microtiter plates with a final concentration of the yeast cell suspension equal to $1–5 \times 10^3$ cells/mL in each well. Each plate contained 10 serial two-fold dilutions of each antifungal compound, PTS or PTSO. The range of concentrations (in mg/L) assayed for each compound were as follows:

amphotericin B (0.03–16), anidulafungin (0.008–4), micafungin (0.008–4), caspofungin (0.008–4), fluconazole (0.125–64) and voriconazole (0.008–4). The concentration ranges of both PTS and PTSO were 0.25–128 mg/L. The positive controls (yeast suspension without antifungal) and negative control (RPMI medium) were added in the last two wells of the plate.

Microtiter plates were incubated at 35 °C and the minimum inhibitory concentration (MIC) values were assessed visually after 24 h (48 h in case of azoles). For amphotericin B, the MIC was determined as the lowest concentration of drug which produced a total inhibition of visual growth. For azoles and echinocandins, the MICs were defined as the lowest concentration of drug that produced ≥50% reduction of visual growth in comparison with the growth of control wells.

The clinical isolates were considered to be susceptible (S), intermediate (I) or susceptible dose-dependent (SDD, only for fluconazole), or resistant (R) to anidulafungin, micafungin, caspofungin, fluconazole and voriconazole according to the recommendations of the CLSI [48]. For amphotericin B, European Committee on Antimicrobial Susceptibility Testing (EUCAST) guidelines were followed [49]. CLSI clinical breakpoints for the susceptibility patterns of *C. albicans*, *C. tropicalis*, and *C. krusei* to anidulafungin, micafungin, and caspofungin were S ≤ 0.25 mg/L, I = 0.5 mg/L, and R ≥ 1 mg/L. Breakpoints for the susceptibility patterns of *C. glabrata* to anidulafungin and caspofungin were S ≤ 0.12 mg/L, I = 0.25 mg/L, and R ≥ 0.5 mg/L; and to micafungin were S ≤ 0.06 mg/L, I = 0.12 mg/L, and R ≥ 0.25 mg/L. CLSI clinical breakpoints for the susceptibility patterns of *C. albicans* and *C. tropicalis* to fluconazole were S ≤ 2 mg/L, SDD = 4 mg/L, and R ≥ 8 mg/L; and for *C. glabrata* SDD ≤ 32 mg/L, and R ≥ 64 mg/L. For voriconazole, S, I, and R breakpoints for *C. albicans* and *C. tropicalis* were ≤ 0.12 mg/L, 0.25–0.5 mg/L, and ≥ 1 mg/L, respectively, and for *C. krusei* ≤ 0.5 mg/L, 1 mg/L, and ≥ 2 mg/L, respectively. With regard to amphotericin B, the following cutoff values were used for all yeasts: S < 1 mg/L and R ≥ 1 mg/L. There are no cut-off points defined in CLSI or EUCAST for *C. krusei* to fluconazole neither *C. glabrata* to voriconazole. All isolates of *C. krusei* and *C. glabrata* were then considered resistant to fluconazole or voriconazole, respectively, regardless of the MICs. The values of MIC_{50} and MIC_{90} were determined as the lowest concentration of the antifungal at which 50% and 90% of the isolates were inhibited, respectively.

To determine the minimal fungicidal concentration (MFC), after mixing the contents of each well, 100 µL were inoculated onto a plate with Sabouraud dextrose agar and incubated at 35 °C for 48 h. The lowest concentrations that showed no growth after incubation gave the MFC value. MFC_{50} and MFC_{90} values were defined as the concentration of antifungal that kills 50% and 90% of the isolates, respectively.

Following the CLSI and EUCAST guidelines, *C. krusei* ATCC 6258 was used as quality control in the procedures.

4.2. Antimicrobial Activity of Gaseous PTS and PTSO

Seven microorganisms from the ATCC collection (American Type Culture Collection, Manassas, VA, USA) were used. *Escherichia coli* ATCC 25922, *Klebsiella pneumoniae* ATCC 700603, and *Pseudomonas aeruginosa* ATCC 27853 were used as representative Gram-negative bacteria. *Enterococcus faecalis* ATCC 29212 and *Staphylococcus aureus* ATCC 29213 were used as representative Gram-positive bacteria. Finally, *Candida albicans* ATCC 200955 and *Candida krusei* ATCC 6258 were used as representative yeast.

Bacteria and yeasts were grown over night at 36 ± 1 °C on sheep blood agar and Sabouraud dextrose agar plates, respectively. Colonies were suspended in 5 mL saline solution at 0.5, 1, and 2 McFarland turbidity. Bacteria were spread on Mueller-Hinton agar and yeast on Mueller–Hinton agar supplemented with 2% glucose. Drops of 20 µL of different concentrated PTS and PTSO solutions (50 mg/mL, 25 mg/mL, 10 mg/mL, 5 mg/mL, and 2.5 mg/mL) were placed in the center of a 9-cm diameter Petri dish lid and the solidified agar plates with bacteria or yeasts were placed inverted over the lid according to a previously described procedure [3,14]. Thus, the test solution and the agar itself did not come into contact except by diffusion through the air. After incubation for 24 h at 36 ± 1 °C the diameter of the inhibition zone was measured. Each trial was repeated 10 times.

In the same way as in the previous procedure but without the use of any microorganism, drops of 20 µL of different concentrations of PTS and PTSO solutions (50 mg/mL, 25 mg/mL, 10 mg/mL, 5 mg/mL and 2.5 mg/mL) were placed in the center of the Petri dishes lid and the solidified Mueller–Hinton agar plates were placed inverted over the lid. After incubation for 24 h at 36 ± 1 °C samples of the growth media with a diameter of 7.5 mm were extracted from the center of the plate to the periphery in order to determine the concentration of PTS and PTSO reached on the agar as a consequence of its evaporation (Figure 4). Each trial was repeated three times. The PTS and PTSO concentration achieved in each of the Mueller-Hinton agar samples was determined by high-performance liquid chromatography using a UV detector (HPLC-UV).

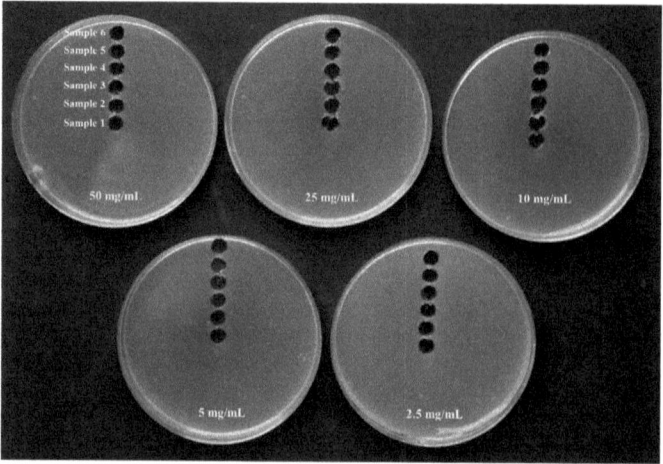

Figure 4. Procedure for obtaining samples from the Mueller–Hinton agar growth medium to establish the concentration of PTS and PTSO reached on it via the gas phase of both compounds by HPLC-UV. For each organosulfur compound and concentration, after incubation for 24 h at 36 ± 1 °C, samples with a diameter of 7.5 mm were extracted from the center of the plate to the periphery in order to determine the concentration of PTS and PTSO reached on the agar as a consequence of its evaporation.

4.3. HPLC-UV Analysis

For the analysis of PTS and PTSO in agar samples, an Agilent 1260 Infinity HPLC (Agilent Technologies Inc., Waldbron, Germany) system was used. The system is equipped with an online degasser, an autosampler, a column thermostat, a diode array detector, and a quaternary pump. The technology used to determine PTS and PTSO was previously described by our group [50,51]. The analysis was carried out in a C18 column (Zorbax Eclipse Plus 50 mm × 4.6 mm, 1.8 µm). Solvents used were 30 mM perchloric acid and MeCN (solvent A and B, respectively) dissolved in water at a flow rate of 0.85 mL min^{-1}. The injection volume was 10 µL and the gradient elution program was: 0 min, 50% B; 2.2 min, 50% B; 4.5 min, 100% B; 6.8 min, 100% B; 8 min, 50% B; 10.5 min, 50% B. The wavelength of detection was set at 200 nm. Agar samples were individually weighed and extracted in 500 µL of methanol through 5 min in vortex. The extract was filtered and directly injected into the HPLC-UV.

4.4. Statistical Analysis

In order to compare the distribution of MIC values of antifungals, PTS and PTSO in the different groups of yeasts studied, the Wilcoxon rank-sum test was used. The differences in the diameters of the growth inhibition halos and in the concentrations reached in the limits of the zone of microbial growth inhibition of the microorganisms after exposure to the gaseous phase of PTS and PTSO were compared using the Wilcoxon signed-rank test. p-values < 0.05 were considered statistically significant. Data analysis was performed using the software IBM SPSS Statistics, version 25.0. (IBM Corporation, Armonk, NY, USA).

5. Conclusions

PTS, and especially PTSO, showed antibacterial and anti-candida activity, even during their gaseous phase, which makes them potentially useful molecules for human therapy. However, it would be necessary to establish its efficacy in human trials, and to know the concentrations that they achieve in the lung tissue when they are administered by inhalation.

Author Contributions: Conceptualization: A.S.-P., J.G.-F., and A.B.-A.; methodology: A.S.-P., M.A.-C., I.L.-M., and L.G.-M.; validation: J.J.A.-R. and A.B.-A.; formal analysis: M.A.-C., I.L.-M., and L.G.-M.; investigation: A.S.-P. and M.A.-C.; resources: A.M.-T. and J.G.-F.; writing—original draft preparation: A.S.-P. and M.A.-C.; writing—review and editing: A.B.-A. and J.G.-F.; visualization: A.S.-P.; supervision: A.S.-P. and J.G.-F. All authors have read and agreed to the published version of the manuscript.

Funding: This research did not receive any specific grant from funding agencies in the public, commercial, or non-profit sectors.

Institutional Review Board Statement: Not applicable.

Informed Consent Statement: Not applicable.

Data Availability Statement: The data presented in this study are available in the main text.

Acknowledgments: We would like to acknowledge the Laboratory of Microbiology, Virgen de las Nieves University Hospital and the work of Jose Manuel Garcia-Madero in editing the text.

Conflicts of Interest: The authors declare no conflict of interest.

References

1. Borlinghaus, J.; Albrecht, F.; Gruhlke, M.C.; Nwachukwu, I.D.; Slusarenko, A.J. Allicin: Chemistry and biological properties. *Molecules* **2014**, *19*, 12591–12618. [CrossRef]
2. Chan, J.Y.; Yuen, A.C.; Chan, R.Y.; Chan, S.W. A review of the cardiovascular benefits and antioxidant properties of allicin. *Phytother. Res.* **2013**, *27*, 637–646. [CrossRef] [PubMed]
3. Reiter, J.; Levina, N.; van der Linden, M.; Gruhlke, M.; Martin, C.; Slusarenko, A.J. Diallylthiosulfinate (Allicin), a volatile antimicrobial from garlic (*Allium sativum*), kills human lung pathogenic bacteria, including MDR strains, as a vapor. *Molecules* **2017**, *22*, 1711. [CrossRef] [PubMed]
4. Ankri, S.; Mirelman, D. Antimicrobial properties of allicin from garlic. *Microbes Infect.* **1999**, *1*, 125–129. [CrossRef]
5. Focke, M.; Feld, A.; Lichtenthaler, K. Allicin, a naturally occurring antibiotic from garlic, specifically inhibits acetyl-CoA synthetase. *FEBS Lett.* **1990**, *261*, 106–108. [CrossRef]
6. Rabinkov, A.; Miron, T.; Konstantinovski, L.; Wilchek, M.; Mirelman, D.; Weiner, L. The mode of action of allicin: Trapping of radicals and interaction with thiol containing proteins. *Biochim. Biophys. Acta* **1998**, *1379*, 233–244. [CrossRef]
7. Gruhlke, M.C.; Portz, D.; Stitz, M.; Anwar, A.; Schneider, T.; Jacob, C.; Schlaich, N.L.; Slusarenko, A.J. Allicin disrupts the cell's electrochemical potential and induces apoptosis in yeast. *Free Radic. Biol. Med.* **2010**, *49*, 1916–1924. [CrossRef]
8. Feldberg, R.S.; Chang, S.C.; Kotik, A.N.; Nadler, M.; Neuwirth, Z.; Sundstrom, D.C.; Thompson, N.H. In vitro mechanism of inhibition of bacterial cell growth by allicin. *Antimicrob. Agents Chemother.* **1988**, *32*, 1763–1768. [CrossRef]
9. Keusgen, M.; Schulz, H.; Glodek, J.; Krest, I.; Krüger, H.; Herchert, N.; Keller, J. Characterization of some Allium hybrids by aroma precursors, aroma profiles, and alliinase activity. *J. Agric. Food Chem.* **2002**, *50*, 2884–2890. [CrossRef]
10. Guillamón, E. Effect of phytochemical compounds of the genus Allium on the immune system and the inflammatory response. *Ars Pharm.* **2018**, *59*, 185–196. [CrossRef]
11. Sorlozano-Puerto, A.; Albertuz-Crespo, M.; Lopez-Machado, I.; Ariza-Romero, J.J.; Baños-Arjona, A.; Exposito-Ruiz, M.; Gutierrez-Fernandez, J. In vitro antibacterial activity of propyl-propane-thiosulfinate and propyl-propane-thiosulfonate derived from *Allium* spp. against gram-negative and gram-positive multidrug-resistant bacteria isolated from human samples. *Biomed Res. Int.* **2018**, *2018*, 7861207. [CrossRef] [PubMed]

12. Singla, N.; Gulati, N.; Kaistha, N.; Chander, J. Candida colonization in urine samples of ICU patients: Determination of etiology, antifungal susceptibility testing and evaluation of associated risk factors. *Mycopathologia* **2012**, *174*, 149–155. [CrossRef] [PubMed]
13. Sobel, J.D.; Fisher, J.F.; Kauffman, C.A.; Newman, C.A. Candida urinary tract infections—Epidemiology. *Clin. Infect. Dis.* **2011**, *52*, S433–S436. [CrossRef] [PubMed]
14. Leontiev, R.; Hohaus, N.; Jacob, C.; Gruhlke, M.; Slusarenko, A.J. A comparison of the antibacterial and antifungal activities of thiosulfinate analogues of Allicin. *Sci. Rep.* **2018**, *8*, 6763. [CrossRef]
15. Miceli, M.H.; Díaz, J.A.; Lee, S.A. Emerging opportunistic yeast infections. *Lancet Infect. Dis.* **2011**, *11*, 142–151. [CrossRef]
16. Kucukates, E.; Gultekin, N.; Alisan, Z.; Hondur, N.; Ozturk, R. Identification of *Candida* species and susceptibility testing with Sensititre YeastOne microdilution panel to 9 antifungal agents. *Saudi Med. J.* **2016**, *37*, 750–757. [CrossRef]
17. Alexander, B.D.; Johnson, M.D.; Pfeiffer, C.D.; Jiménez-Ortigosa, C.; Catania, J.; Booker, R.; Castanheira, M.; Messer, S.A.; Perlin, D.S.; Pfaller, M.A. Increasing echinocandin resistance in *Candida glabrata*: Clinical failure correlates with presence of FKS mutations and elevated minimum inhibitory concentrations. *Clin. Infect. Dis.* **2013**, *56*, 1724–1732. [CrossRef]
18. Castanheira, M.; Messer, S.A.; Jones, R.N.; Farrell, D.J.; Pfaller, M.A. Activity of echinocandins and triazoles against a contemporary (2012) worldwide collection of yeast and moulds collected from invasive infections. *Int. J. Antimicrob. Agents* **2014**, *44*, 320–326. [CrossRef]
19. Cretella, D.; Barber, K.E.; King, S.T.; Stover, K.R. Comparison of susceptibility patterns using commercially available susceptibility testing methods performed on prevalent *Candida* spp. *J. Med. Microbiol.* **2016**, *65*, 1445–1451. [CrossRef]
20. Wang, E.; Farmakiotis, D.; Yang, D.; McCue, D.A.; Kantarjian, H.M.; Kontoyiannis, D.P.; Mathisen, M.S. The ever-evolving landscape of candidaemia in patients with acute leukaemia: Non-susceptibility to caspofungin and multidrug resistance are associated with increased mortality. *J. Antimicrob. Chemother.* **2015**, *70*, 2362–2368. [CrossRef]
21. An, M.; Shen, H.; Cao, Y.; Zhang, J.; Cai, Y.; Wang, R.; Jiang, Y. Allicin enhances the oxidative damage effect of amphotericin B against *Candida albicans*. *Int. J. Antimicrob. Agents* **2009**, *33*, 258–263. [CrossRef] [PubMed]
22. Khodavandi, A.; Alizadeh, F.; Aala, F.; Sekawi, Z.; Chong, P.P. In vitro investigation of antifungal activity of allicin alone and in combination with azoles against *Candida* species. *Mycopathologia* **2010**, *169*, 287–295. [CrossRef] [PubMed]
23. Khodavandi, A.; Alizadeh, F.; Harmal, N.S.; Sidik, S.M.; Othman, F.; Sekawi, Z.; Jahromi, M.A.; Ng, K.P.; Chong, P.P. Comparison between efficacy of allicin and fluconazole against *Candida albicans* in vitro and in a systemic candidiasis mouse model. *FEMS Microbiol. Lett.* **2011**, *315*, 87–93. [CrossRef] [PubMed]
24. Heras-Cañas, V.; Ros, L.; Sorlózano, A.; Gutiérrez-Soto, B.; Navarro-Marí, J.M.; Gutiérrez-Fernández, J. Isolated yeast species in urine samples in a Spanish regional hospital. *Rev. Argent. Microbiol.* **2015**, *47*, 331–334. [CrossRef]
25. Jiménez-Guerra, G.; Casanovas Moreno-Torres, I.; Gutiérrez-Soto, M.; Vazquez-Alonso, F.; Sorlózano-Puerto, A.; Navarro-Marí, J.M.; Gutiérrez-Fernández, J. Inpatient candiduria: Etiology, susceptibility to antifungal drugs and risk factors. *Rev. Esp. Quimioter.* **2018**, *31*, 323–328.
26. Aigner, M.; Erbeznik, T.; Gschwentner, M.; Lass-Flörl, C. Etest and Sensititre YeastOne susceptibility testing of echinocandins against Candida species from a single center in Austria. *Antimicrob. Agents Chemother.* **2017**, *61*, e00512-17. [CrossRef]
27. Alfouzan, W.; Al-Enezi, T.; AlRoomi, E.; Sandhya, V.; Chandy, R.; Khan, Z.U. Comparison of the VITEK 2 antifungal susceptibility system with Etest using clinical isolates of Candida species. *Rev. Iberoam. Micol.* **2017**, *34*, 171–174. [CrossRef]
28. Oz, Y.; Gokbolat, E. Evaluation of direct antifungal susceptibility testing methods of *Candida* spp. from positive blood culture bottles. *J. Clin. Lab. Anal.* **2018**, *32*, e22297. [CrossRef]
29. Siqueira, R.A.; Doi, A.M.; de Petrus Crossara, P.P.; Koga, P.; Marques, A.G.; Nunes, F.G.; Pasternak, J.; Martino, M. Evaluation of two commercial methods for the susceptibility testing of Candida species: Vitek 2® and Sensititre YeastOne®. *Rev. Iberoam. Micol.* **2018**, *35*, 83–87. [CrossRef]
30. Diba, A.; Alizadeh, F. In vitro and in vivo antifungal activity of *Allium hirtifolium* and *Allium sativum*. *Avicenna J. Phytomed.* **2018**, *8*, 465–474.
31. Shams-Ghahfarokhi, M.; Shokoohamiri, M.R.; Amirrajab, N.; Moghadasi, B.; Ghajari, A.; Zeini, F.; Sadeghi, G.; Razzaghi-Abyaneh, M. In vitro antifungal activities of *Allium cepa*, *Allium sativum* and ketoconazole against some pathogenic yeasts and dermatophytes. *Fitoterapia* **2006**, *77*, 321–323. [CrossRef] [PubMed]
32. Gruhlke, M.; Schlembach, I.; Leontiev, R.; Uebachs, A.; Gollwitzer, P.; Weiss, A.; Delaunay, A.; Toledano, M.; Slusarenko, A.J. Yap1p, the central regulator of the *S. cerevisiae* oxidative stress response, is activated by allicin, a natural oxidant and defence substance of garlic. *Free Radic. Biol. Med.* **2017**, *108*, 793–802. [CrossRef] [PubMed]
33. Li, W.R.; Shi, Q.S.; Dai, H.Q.; Liang, Q.; Xie, X.B.; Huang, X.M.; Zhao, G.Z.; Zhang, L.X. Antifungal activity, kinetics and molecular mechanism of action of garlic oil against *Candida albicans*. *Sci. Rep.* **2016**, *6*, 22805. [CrossRef] [PubMed]
34. Khodavandi, A.; Alizadeh, F.; Harmal, N.S.; Sidik, S.M.; Othman, F.; Sekawi, Z.; Chong, P.P. Expression analysis of SIR2 and SAPs1-4 gene expression in *Candida albicans* treated with allicin compared to fluconazole. *Trop. Biomed.* **2011**, *28*, 589–598.
35. Ebrahimy, F.; Dolatian, M.; Moatar, F.; Majd, H.A. Comparison of the therapeutic effects of Garcin® and fluconazole on *Candida* vaginitis. *Singap. Med. J.* **2015**, *56*, 567–572. [CrossRef]
36. Curtis, H.; Noll, U.; Störmann, J.; Slusarenko, A.J. Broad-spectrum activity of the volatile phytoanticipin allicin in extracts of garlic (*Allium sativum* L.) against plant pathogenic bacteria, fungi and Oomycetes. *Physiol. Mol. Plant Pathol.* **2004**, *65*, 79–89. [CrossRef]
37. Abubakar, E.-m.M. Efficacy of crude extracts of garlic (*Allium sativum* Linn.) against nosocomial *Escherichia coli*, *Staphylococcus aureus*, *Streptococcus pneumoniae* and *Pseudomonas aeruginosa*. *J. Med. Plant Res.* **2009**, *3*, 179–185.

38. Müller, A.; Eller, J.; Albrecht, F.; Prochnow, P.; Kuhlmann, K.; Bandow, J.E.; Slusarenko, A.J.; Leichert, L.I. Allicin induces thiol stress in bacteria through S-allylmercapto modification of protein cysteines. *J. Biol. Chem.* **2016**, *291*, 11477–11490. [CrossRef]
39. Lemar, K.M.; Turner, M.P.; Lloyd, D. Garlic (*Allium sativum*) as an anti-Candida agent: A comparison of the efficacy of fresh garlic and freeze-dried extracts. *J. Appl. Microbiol.* **2002**, *93*, 398–405. [CrossRef]
40. Shadkchan, Y.; Shemesh, E.; Mirelman, D.; Miron, T.; Rabinkov, A.; Wilchek, M.; Osherov, N. Efficacy of allicin, the reactive molecule of garlic, in inhibiting *Aspergillus* spp. in vitro, and in a murine model of disseminated aspergillosis. *J. Antimicrob. Chemother.* **2004**, *53*, 832–836. [CrossRef]
41. Abouelfetouh, A.Y.; Moussa, N.K. Enhancement of antimicrobial activity of four classes of antibiotics combined with garlic. *Asian J. Plant Sci.* **2012**, *11*, 148–152. [CrossRef]
42. Jonkers, D.; Sluimer, J.; Stobberingh, E. Effect of garlic on vancomycin-resistant enterococci. *Antimicrob. Agents Chemother.* **1999**, *43*, 3045. [CrossRef] [PubMed]
43. Ogita, A.; Nagao, Y.; Fujita, K.; Tanaka, T. Amplification of vacuole-targeting fungicidal activity of antibacterial antibiotic polymyxin B by allicin, an allyl sulfur compound from garlic. *J. Antibiot.* **2007**, *60*, 511–518. [CrossRef] [PubMed]
44. Pillai, R.; Trivedi, N.A.; Bhatt, J.D. Studies on in vitro interaction of ampicillin and fresh garlic extract against *Staphylococcus aureus* by checkerboard method. *Anc. Sci. Life* **2013**, *33*, 114–118. [CrossRef]
45. Yalindag-Ozturk, N.; Ozdamar, M.; Cengiz, P. Trial of garlic as an adjunct therapy for multidrug resistant *Pseudomonas aeruginosa* pneumonia in a critically ill infant. *J. Altern. Complement. Med.* **2011**, *17*, 379–380. [CrossRef]
46. Guo, N.; Wu, X.; Yu, L.; Liu, J.; Meng, R.; Jin, J.; Lu, H.; Wang, X.; Yan, S.; Deng, X. In vitro and in vivo interactions between fluconazole and allicin against clinical isolates of fluconazole-resistant *Candida albicans* determined by alternative methods. *FEMS Immunol. Med. Microbiol.* **2010**, *58*, 193–201. [CrossRef]
47. Clinical and Laboratory Standards Institute (CLSI). *Method for Broth Dilution Antifungal Susceptibility Testing of Yeasts*; Fourth Informational Supplement M27-S4; CLSI: Wayne, PA, USA, 2012.
48. Clinical and Laboratory Standards Institute (CLSI). *Performance Standards for Antifungal Susceptibility Testing of Yeasts*, 1st ed.; Supplement M60; CLSI: Wayne, PA, USA, 2017.
49. European Committee on Antimicrobial Susceptibility Testing (EUCAST). Antifungal Agents-Breakpoint Tables for Interpretation of MICs. Version 8.1. 2017. Available online: http://www.eucast.org/ (accessed on 24 October 2017).
50. Abad, P.; Lara, F.J.; Arroyo-Manzanares, N.; Baños, A.; Guillamón, E.; García-Campaña, A.M. High-performance liquid chromatography method for the monitoring of the *Allium* derivative propyl propane thiosulfonate used as natural additive in animal feed. *Food Anal. Methods* **2015**, *8*, 916–921. [CrossRef]
51. Abad, P.; Arroyo-Manzanares, N.; Gil, L.; García-Campaña, A.M. Use of onion extract as a dairy cattle feed supplement: Monitoring propyl propane thiosulfonate as a marker of its effect on milk attributes. *J. Agric. Food Chem.* **2017**, *65*, 793–799. [CrossRef]

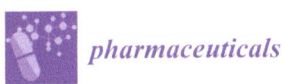

Communication

Posidonia oceanica (L.) Delile Extract Reduces Lipid Accumulation through Autophagy Activation in HepG2 Cells

Marzia Vasarri [1], Emanuela Barletta [1] and Donatella Degl'Innocenti [1,2,*]

[1] Department of Experimental and Clinical Biomedical Sciences, University of Florence, Viale Morgagni 50, 50134 Florence, Italy; marzia.vasarri@unifi.it (M.V.); emanuela.barletta@unifi.it (E.B.)
[2] Interuniversity Center of Marine Biology and Applied Ecology "G. Bacci" (CIBM), Viale N. Sauro 4, 57128 Livorno, Italy
* Correspondence: donatella.deglinnocenti@unifi.it

Abstract: *Posidonia oceanica* (L.) Delile is a marine plant traditionally used as an herbal medicine for various health disorders. *P. oceanica* leaf extract (POE) has been shown to be a phytocomplex with cell-safe bioactivities, including the ability to trigger autophagy. Autophagy is a key pathway to counteract non-alcoholic fatty liver disease (NAFLD) by controlling the breakdown of lipid droplets in the liver. The aim of this study was to explore the ability of POE to trigger autophagy and reduce lipid accumulation in human hepatoma (HepG2) cells and then verify the possible link between the effect of POE on lipid reduction and autophagy activation. Expression levels of autophagy markers were monitored by the Western blot technique in POE-treated HepG2 cells, whereas the extent of lipid accumulation in HepG2 cells was assessed by Oil red O staining. Chloroquine (CQ), an autophagy inhibitor, was used to study the relationship between POE-induced autophagy and intracellular lipid accumulation. POE was found to stimulate an autophagy flux over time in HepG2 cells by lowering the phosphorylation state of ribosomal protein S6, increasing Beclin-1 and LC3-II levels, and decreasing p62 levels. By blocking autophagy with CQ, the effect of POE on intracellular lipid accumulation was clearly reversed, suggesting that the POE phytocomplex may reduce lipid accumulation in HepG2 cells by activating the autophagic process. This work indicates that *P. oceanica* may be considered as a promising molecule supplier to discover new natural approaches for the management of NAFLD.

Keywords: *Posidonia oceanica*; autophagy; lipid accumulation; NAFLD; herbal medicine

Citation: Vasarri, M.; Barletta, E.; Degl'Innocenti, D. *Posidonia oceanica* (L.) Delile Extract Reduces Lipid Accumulation through Autophagy Activation in HepG2 Cells. *Pharmaceuticals* **2021**, *14*, 969. https://doi.org/10.3390/ph14100969

Academic Editors: Noelia Duarte and Kwang-Won Lee

Received: 19 July 2021
Accepted: 22 September 2021
Published: 24 September 2021

Publisher's Note: MDPI stays neutral with regard to jurisdictional claims in published maps and institutional affiliations.

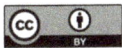

Copyright: © 2021 by the authors. Licensee MDPI, Basel, Switzerland. This article is an open access article distributed under the terms and conditions of the Creative Commons Attribution (CC BY) license (https://creativecommons.org/licenses/by/4.0/).

1. Introduction

Posidonica oceanica (L.) Delile is a marine plant belonging to the Posidoniaceae family and the only species of Posidoniaceae endemic to the Mediterranean Sea [1]. Besides the extreme ecological importance of *P. oceanica* underwater meadows, the literature tells of a millenary relationship between humans and this marine plant. Some historical sources report that in Ancient Egypt, *P. oceanica* leaves were used as an herbal medicine for various health ailments, such as sore throat and skin problems [2], but also for the treatment of inflammation and irritation and as a remedy for acne, lower limb pain, and colitis [3]. More recently, a decoction of *P. oceanica* leaves was used as an herbal medicine against diabetes and hypertension by inhabitants of coastal areas in Western Anatolia [4]. In support of this, the literature describes antidiabetic and vasoprotective effects of a hydroalcoholic extract obtained from *P. oceanica* leaves in an in vivo animal model [4].

In recent years, our group has undertaken a series of in vitro and in vivo studies that for the first time shed light on the hitherto unexplored biological mechanisms underlying the bioactive properties of a hydroalcoholic *P. oceanica* leaf extract (POE). UPLC characterization analysis showed that POE consists of 88% phenolic compounds. Of these, about 85% were represented by (+) catechins and the remaining 4% by a mixture of gallic acid (0.4%), ferulic acid (1.7%), epicatechin (1.4%), and chlorogenic acid (0.6%). The small remaining fraction (11%) remained unknown/uncharacterized (Figure 1) [5]. Moreover, POE has been shown to be consistently effective as a phytocomplex at doses nontoxic to cells [5–10].

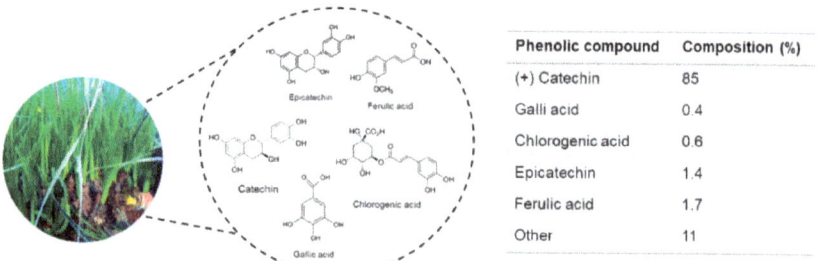

Figure 1. Phenolic composition with relative percentages of *P. oceanica* leaf extract (POE) obtained by UPLC analysis [5].

POE showed anti-inflammatory properties both in an in vitro cell model of lipopolysaccharide (LPS)-stimulated murine macrophages [8] and in different in vivo models of inflammatory pain induced by intraplantar injection of carrageenan, interleukin IL-1β, and formalin in CD-1 mice [9]. In addition, POE showed an inhibitory role on the in vitro protein glycation process by blocking the formation of advanced glycation end products (AGEs) [10], as well as the ability to inhibit the highly migratory phenotype of certain cell lines such as human fibrosarcoma HT1080 [5,6] and human neuroblastoma SH-SY5Y [7]. Further, our investigation of the mechanism of action underlying its anti-migratory role revealed that POE acts by activating a transient autophagy flux [6].

Autophagy is an evolutionarily conserved intracellular degradative process that regulates metabolism and maintains cellular homeostasis by removing aggregated, damaged and/or misfolded proteins, and damaged organelles through cytosolic sequestration and subsequent lysosomal degradation [11]. In the light of this, it is known that a deficiency in autophagy could contribute to the development or progression of several disease conditions, including non-alcoholic fatty liver disease (NAFLD) [12,13]. NAFLD is the most common liver disease in Western countries and is defined as evidence of hepatic steatosis without any cause of secondary hepatic fat accumulation, such as alcohol abuse, use of steatogenic drugs, or inherited disorders [14]. In NAFLD, cells are characterized by excessive accumulation of triglycerides and cholesterol in lipid droplets (LDs) [15]. It is generally accepted that autophagy is activated during the early phase of NAFLD in response to the acute increase in lipid availability. Autophagy may then regulate hepatocellular lipid accumulation through selective degradation of cellular lipid stores (lipophagy). However, large or chronic lipid exposure tends to deregulate the autophagy process [13,16–18]. Accumulating evidence suggests that impaired autophagy prevents the clearance of LDs, damaged mitochondria, and toxic protein aggregates, which can be produced during the progression of various liver diseases, thus contributing to the development of steatosis, steatohepatitis, fibrosis, and cancer [19,20]. This supports the possibility that autophagy may be one of the key targets for the prevention and treatment of hepatic steatosis in NAFLD [21].

Developing a treatment for patients suffering from NAFLD is challenging because of its intricate etiology, complex diagnosis, broad spectrum of stages, and presence of concomitant disorders. However, in addition to the need for lifestyle modifications, to date, herbal medicine has emerged as an alternative approach to the prevention and/or treatment of NAFLD [22]. Certain herbal extracts and natural products are considered effective in ameliorating lipid accumulation through, at least in part, activation of autophagy. Examples include Rb2, a major ginsenoside from Panax ginseng [23]; the natural polyphenol resveratrol [24–26]; the bergamot polyphenol fraction (BPF), one of the dietary polyphenols [27]; capsaicin, an extract of *Capsicum annuum* and a common food supplement [28]; and many others [22]. Some natural products have already been supported by clinical studies in the treatment of NAFLD [29], such as berberine [30], resveratrol [31], and curcumin [32], found effective in improving NAFLD parameters. Thus, the literature provides valuable information on the role of natural compounds and herbal extracts as potential candidates in the management of NAFLD.

In the light of these considerations, this work tested the ability of POE to reduce intracellular lipid accumulation in an in vitro model of hepatic steatosis using the human hepatoma cell line HepG2. The role of POE in triggering autophagy in HepG2 cells was also tested, and thus the possible correlation between POE-induced reduction of lipid accumulation and activation of an autophagic flux was verified.

2. Results and Discussion

2.1. Biochemical Composition of P. oceanica Leaf Extract (POE)

The previously developed hydroalcoholic extraction method [5] was used to recover hydrophilic compounds from *P. oceanica* leaves that were soluble enough to be readily evaluated in biological media. This method recovered 1.8 mg of dry extract per aliquot.

POE was found to be composed mainly of polyphenols and a carbohydrate fraction. By the Folin–Ciocalteau method, POE was found to contain 3.9 ± 0.4 mg/mL of polyphenols (TP) equivalent to gallic acid, while colorimetric analysis with phenol-sulfuric acid showed that POE contains 6.0 ± 1.3 mg/mL of carbohydrates (TC) equivalent to glucose. In addition, POE exhibited radical-scavenging and antioxidant activities of 9.0 ± 0.3 mg/mL and 1.0 ± 0.2 mg/mL ascorbic acid equivalents by FRAP and DPPH assays, respectively (Table 1).

Table 1. Polyphenol and carbohydrate content in POE and its antioxidant and radical-scavenging properties. All values (mg/mL) are reported as means ± SD of at least three independent extractions.

	TP	TC	Antioxidant	Radical Scavenging
Method	Folin–Ciocalteau	Phenol/sulfuric acid	Ferrozine®	DPPH
Reference control	Gallic acid	Glucose	Ascorbic acid	Ascorbic acid
POE	3.9 ± 0.4	6.0 ± 1.3	1.0 ± 0.2	9.0 ± 0.3

The data obtained are consistent with those obtained in previous work [6,8], supporting the efficiency and reproducibility of the extraction method.

2.2. Effect of POE on HepG2 Cell Viability

The viability of HepG2 cells treated with POE at dilutions of 1:100, 1:250, and 1:500 (corresponding to 36, 14, and 7.2 µg/mL dry weight of extract, respectively) was assessed using MTT assay. POE treatment, ranging from 7.2 µg/mL to 36 µg/mL concentration, did not cause any reduction in cell viability, as depicted in Figure 2. Treatment with the vehicle excluded any effect of EtOH/H_2O (70:30 v/v) on cell viability (Figure S1 in Supplementary Materials). These findings agree with the previously reported non-toxicity of POE. Indeed, the phytocomplex has already been extensively demonstrated to exert its activity without showing signs of cellular toxicity under different treatment conditions in various cell lines [5–8].

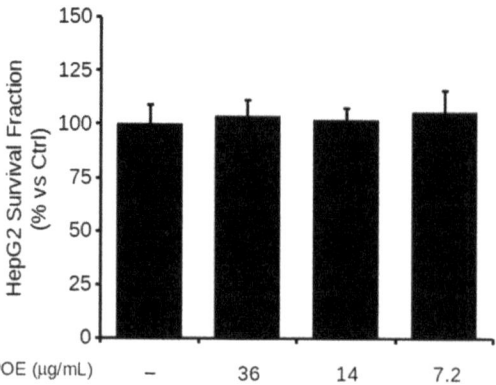

Figure 2. The effect of POE on HepG2 cell viability. MTT assay on cells untreated (−) or exposed to different POE concentrations for 24 h. Data were reported as the mean ± SD of at least three independent experiments.

For subsequent experiments, POE was therefore used at the lowest dose of 7.2 µg/mL, in agreement with previous work [6,8].

2.3. POE Activates an Autophagic Flux in HepG2 Cells

Activation of autophagy is among the newly discovered biological properties of POE [6]. In this work, this ability of POE was verified in HepG2 cells. Autophagy pathways were explored by Western blot analysis in lysates of cells treated at different time points with POE or Rapa (used as a control for autophagy activation).

Representative Western blot images in Figure 3A show that HepG2 cells underwent a transient autophagy flux over time induced by POE treatment, as well as cells treated by Rapa.

Specifically, by analyzing the mammalian target of rapamycin (mTOR) signaling pathway, the best-known autophagy-suppressive regulator, it was observed that Rapa significantly reduced the levels of the phosphorylated form of S6 (p-S6) already at 3 h (28 ± 9%), maintaining them low even at 24 h (20 ± 10%) of treatment compared to untreated control cells; POE apparently caused a reduction in p-S6 levels compared with untreated control cells as early as 3 h of treatment (90 ± 9.5%)—although the data do not show statistical significance—until it resulted in a maximum reduction in p-S6 levels at 7 h of treatment (60 ± 12%). This suggests that POE contributes to an early activation of autophagy by inhibiting the mTOR signaling pathway. However, this effect ended by 16 h, when p-S6 levels returned to baseline (97 ± 14%) (Figure 3B).

The dynamics of Beclin-1 levels were further explored, as this variation is considered a downstream event in the autophagy signaling cascade crucial for the early stage of autophagosome formation [33]. Figure 3B clearly shows that at the 7 h time point, POE caused a marked increase in Beclin-1 expression (390 ± 35%) compared to untreated control cells, supporting the observed advancement of autophagy. This effect was comparable to that induced by Rapa (483 ± 45% compared to untreated control cells). As a consequence of POE intervention on Beclin-1 expression at 7 h of treatment, the isolation membrane, a double-membrane structure encompassing cytoplasmic material, had formed to originate the autophagosome.

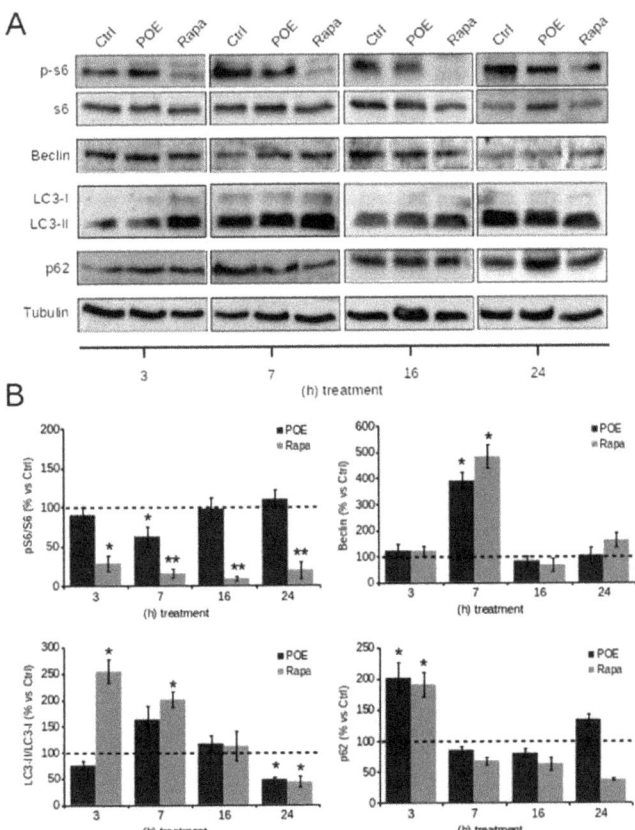

Figure 3. The effect of POE on autophagy flux activation in HepG2 cells. (**A**) Representative images of Western blot analysis of all the assayed protein markers of autophagy detected in HepG2 cells treated with POE (7.2 µg/mL), cells treated with Rapa (0.5 µM), or untreated cells (Ctrl). (**B**) Quantification of signals determined by densitometry analysis of at least three independent experiments. Error bars represent standard errors. * $p < 0.05$; ** $p < 0.01$ vs. untreated control cells (Ctrl; indicated by the dotted line). Kruskal–Wallis test. Pairwise comparisons were performed using Conover test.

Because the amount of LC3-II, the phosphatidylethanolamine-conjugated form of LC3, reveals the number of autophagosomes and autophagy-related structures, LC3 is reportedly the most widely used autophagosome marker [34]. Even though LC3-II is found in the autophagosome, it is a well-known marker of autophagosome elongation. POE-treated cells exhibit a peak in LC3-II/LC3-I expression at 7 h (162 ± 15%) similarly to Rapa-treated cells (200 ± 15%) compared to untreated control cells.

The increased expression of LC3-II further supports the evolution of autophagy in POE-treated cells. Expression levels of LC3-II/LC3-I returned to baseline from 16 h of treatment with both POE (116 ± 15%) as well as Rapa (112 ± 28%), even to the point of being down-expressed after 24 h of treatment (47 ± 5% in POE-treated cells and 42 ± 10% in Rapa-treated cells) compared to untreated control cells (Figure 3B).

The p62 protein is a ubiquitin-binding scaffold protein that co-localizes with ubiquitinated protein aggregates in many liver pathways, which is sequestered in autophagosomes upon its direct interaction with LC3 and is selectively degraded by autophagy. Thus p62 accumulates when autophagy is inhibited and decreases when autophagy flux occurs [34];

therefore, degradation of p62 is another widely used marker to monitor autophagy activity [35].

POE caused a progressive reduction in p62 levels, starting at 7 h (85 ± 5%) until 16 h of treatment (80 ± 7%), suggesting that the autophagy process was in its final step, while Rapa treatment maintained p62 levels below baseline even until 24 h (37 ± 2%). The marked decrease in p62 after POE treatment further confirmed that POE activates an autophagy flux in HepG2 cells, with a peak activation at 7 h.

These results on the role of POE in autophagy activation with maximal efficacy at 7 h of treatment are in agreement with our previous study [6].

2.4. POE Alleviates Lipid Accumulation in HepG2 Cells by Inducing Autophagy

Autophagy is a cellular recycling mechanism essential for the maintenance of normal metabolism; impaired autophagy is often linked to the pathophysiology of many diseases. In this regard, autophagy plays a key role in lipid homeostasis through the degradation of intracellular lipid droplets (lipophagy) [17,36].

In this work, the effect of POE on lipid accumulation in HepG2 cells was explored in relation to its role as an inducer of autophagy. Cells were treated with POE for 24 h, while cells treated with CQ (autophagy inhibitor) and Rapa (autophagy inducer) were used as controls.

HepG2 control cells grown in complete medium were characterized by intracellular lipid accumulation, as depicted by microscope image in Figure 4A obtained after ORO staining, while vehicle treatment excluded any effect of EtOH/H$_2$O (70:30 v/v) on lipid accumulation (data not shown).

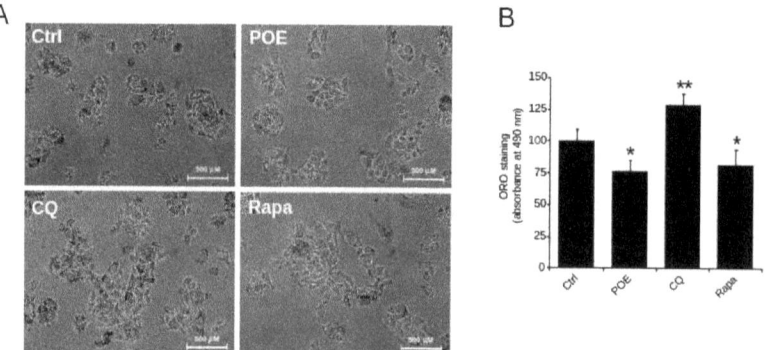

Figure 4. The effect of POE on lipid accumulation in HepG2 cells. (**A**) Representative image of ORO-stained HepG2 cells treated with POE (7.2 µg/mL), CQ (10 µM), and Rapa (0.5 µM) for 24 h. (**B**) Changes in intracellular lipid content assessed by measuring ORO absorbance at 490 nm. Data were reported as the mean ± SD of at least three independent experiments. * $p < 0.05$; ** $p < 0.01$ vs. untreated control cells (Ctrl). Tukey's HSD test.

Compared with untreated control cells, HepG2 cells treated with POE for 24 h showed a clear reduction in neutral lipid content (Figure 4A). Quantification of neutral lipids by solubilization of ORO with isopropanol, shown in Figure 4B, confirmed that POE caused an approximately 25% reduction in lipid accumulation (76 ± 8%) with respect to untreated control cells, suggesting a significant role of POE on lipid clearance.

The effect of POE was comparable to that of Rapa, which resulted in an approximately 20% reduction in lipid accumulation (81 ± 11%) compared to untreated control cells (Figure 4B); in contrast, CQ-treated cells were distinguished by an increased presence of intracellular neutral lipids (128 ± 9%) compared with untreated control cells (Figure 4B). Noteworthy, differences between treatment conditions were statistically significant.

The comparable effect of POE and Rapa suggests that POE likely intervenes in lipid accumulation through activation of an autophagic flux.

Where impaired autophagy has been shown to induce hepatosteatosis [37], autophagy activation could be an effective means of maintaining normal liver function [38].

Some pharmacological studies have demonstrated the protective effect of natural products against excessive lipid accumulation in hepatic cells through activation of the autophagic process [22].

In our in vitro experiments, POE was shown to induce an autophagy flux in HepG2 cells in a time-dependent manner and to reduce intracellular lipid accumulation.

Thus, in the present study, it was tested whether POE-induced lipid elimination occurs in an autophagy-dependent manner. HepG2 cells were treated with POE for 7 h, a time point found to be relevant for POE-induced autophagy activation, and then supplemented with CQ for up to 24 h (POE + CQ).

The microscopy image shown in Figure 5A depicts a clear increase in lipid accumulation in POE + CQ cells compared with POE-treated cells. Quantification of intracellular neutral lipids by solubilization of ORO with isopropanol, plotted in Figure 5B, confirmed that lipid accumulation in POE + CQ cells increased by approximately 30% (102 ± 6%) compared to cells treated with POE alone (78 ± 7.7%).

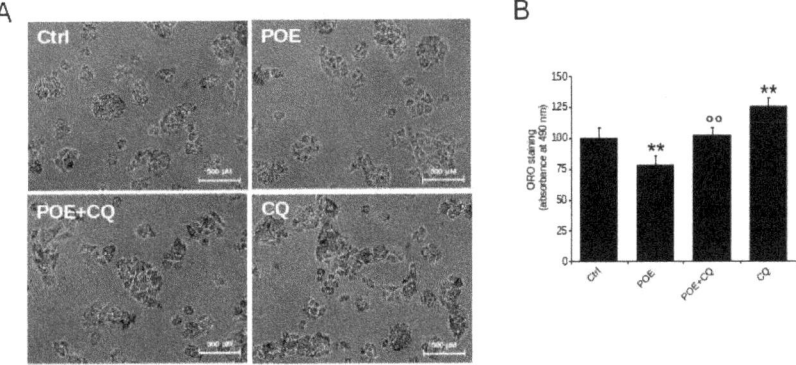

Figure 5. POE reduces lipid accumulation in HepG2 cells through autophagy activation. (**A**) Representative image of ORO-stained HepG2 cells treated with POE (7.2 µg/mL), CQ (10 µM), or POE added with CQ at 7 h (POE + CQ) until 24 h. (**B**) Changes in intracellular lipid content assessed by measuring ORO absorbance at 490 nm. Data were reported as the mean ± SD of at least three independent experiments. ** $p < 0.01$ vs. untreated control cells (Ctrl); °° $p < 0.01$ vs. POE-treated cells. Tukey's HSD test.

Recently, it has become known that autophagy mediates the elimination of stored lipid droplets [39]. Our data indicate that in the presence of CQ, the ability of autophagosomes to fuse with lysosomes is reduced, resulting in the accumulation of intracellular lipids; the altered autophagy flux provides a possible reason for the restoration of higher basal intracellular lipid levels in POE + CQ cells. This suggests that the effect of the POE phytocomplex on lipid accumulation is completely reversed by CQ-induced autophagy blockade.

Overall, this study provides evidence of the potential of POE to alleviate intracellular lipid accumulation through activation of autophagy. Thus, POE, which can control this process in liver cells, could have promising potential as an alternative medical strategy for a variety of disease conditions, including NAFLD [22,40].

3. Materials and Methods

3.1. Chemicals

Dulbecco's Modified Eagle's Medium (high-glucose DMEM-HG), fetal bovine serum (FBS), L-glutamine, penicillin and streptomycin, 1-(4,5-dimethylthiazol-2-yl)-3,5-diphenyl formazan (MTT), Oil red O (ORO), chloroquine (CQ), and rapamycin (Rapa) and all chemicals and solvents were purchased from Merck KGaA (Darmstadt, DA, Germany). Electrophoresis reagents were purchased from Bio-Rad Laboratories (Hercules, CA, USA). Primary antibodies were provided by Cell Signaling Technology (Beverly, MA, USA), Molecular Probes™ (Invitrogen, Carlsbad, CA, USA), and Abcam (Cambridge, UK) (Table 2). Anti-mouse IgG HRP-linked and anti-rabbit IgG HRP-linked secondary antibodies were obtained from Molecular Probes™ (Invitrogen, Carlsbad, CA, USA). Disposable plastics were from Sarstedt (Nümbrecht, Germany).

Table 2. Specifications of primary antibodies used in Western blotting experiments.

Primary Antibody	Target	Dilution	Host	Source	Lot
SQTSM1/p62	SQTSM1/p62 protein	1:1000	Rabbit	Abcam	#GR84445-1
LC3	Microtubule-associated protein light chain 3	1:1000	Rabbit	Invitrogen	#UD2753807C
Beclin-1	Beclin-1 protein	1:1000	Rabbit	Cell Signaling	#6
S6	Ribosomal protein S6	1:1000	Rabbit	Cell Signaling	#7
p-S6	Ribosomal protein S6 (Ser235/236)	1:2000	Rabbit	Cell Signaling	#16
α-Tubulin	α-Tubulin protein	1:1000	Mouse	Genetex	#43922

The leaves of *P. oceanica* were collected in July 2020 from the protected area of Meloria by personnel of the Interuniversity Center of Marine Biology and Applied Ecology G. Bacci (CIBM, Livorno, Tuscany, Italy) at a depth of about 15 m at the following geographical coordinates: 43° 35′ 13″ N and 010° 10′ 21″ E.

The CIBM was authorized for the collection of *P. oceanica* leaves by the Direction of Regional Parc of Migliarino, San Rossore, Massaciuccoli, formerly the managing institution of the Marine Protected Area (MPA) "Secche della Meloria." The following permission "Ente Parco Reg. M.S.R.M. Prot. 0012275 del 20-11-2019 partenza Cat. 7 Cl. 7 SCI.8" authorized the CIBM for institutional and research activities (including monitoring and sampling of both water and biota) inside all the MPA from 20 November 2018 to 31 December 2020.

3.2. Preparation of P. oceanica Extract

The collected leaves were removed from the epiphytes and carefully washed with bi-distilled water. The hydrophilic component was recovered according to the method previously described [5]. Briefly, 1 g of *P. oceanica* dried leaves were minced and suspended overnight in 10 mL of EtOH/H$_2$O (70:30 v/v) at 37 °C under stirring and subsequently at 65 °C for 3 h. The hydroalcoholic extract was then separated from the debris by centrifugation at 2000× g, and the recovered supernatant was mixed with n-hexane in a 1:1 ratio. The hydrophilic phase of the extract was recovered after vigorous agitation in a separating funnel, dispensed into 1 mL aliquots, and then dried using a Univapo™ vacuum concentrator. Each aliquot of *P. oceanica* leaf extract (1.8 mg of dry extract) was then dissolved in 0.5 mL of 70% (v/v) ethanol prior to use and hereafter referred to as POE.

3.3. Determination of Total Polyphenols and Carbohydrates

Total polyphenol (TP) and total carbohydrate (TC) content in POE was determined using the colorimetric Folin–Ciocalteau's method and phenol-sulfuric acid colorimetric methods, respectively [5]. Gallic acid (0.5 mg/mL) and D-glucose (1 mg/mL) were used as a reference in the range of 0–10 mg and 0–50 mg, respectively, to determine TP and TC values.

TP and TC were expressed as milligrams of gallic acid and D-glucose equivalents, respectively, per milliliter of extract after resuspension.

3.4. Antioxidant Assays

The antioxidant and radical-scavenging activities of POE were investigated using ferric-reducing/antioxidant power (FRAP) assay and α,α-diphenyl-β-picrylhydrazyl (DPPH) assay, respectively [5]. Ascorbic acid (0.1 mg/mL) was used as a reference in the range of 0–4 mg to evaluate both activities. The antioxidant and radical-scavenging activities of POE were expressed as milligrams of ascorbic acid equivalents per milliliter of extract after resuspension.

3.5. Cell Line and Culture Conditions

The human hepatoma cell line (HepG2), purchased from the American Type Culture Collection (ATCC®, HB-8065TM), was grown in a humidified atmosphere of 5% CO_2 at 37 °C in DMEM-HG supplemented with 10% FBS, 100 µg/mL streptomycin, 100 U/mL penicillin, and 2 mM L-glutamine (complete medium). At 90% confluence, cells were collected by scraping and seeded at an appropriate cell density.

3.6. Cell Viability Assay

Cell viability was determined by MTT assay. Cells were grown in 96-well plates (3×10^4 cells/well) for 24 h in complete medium. Next, cells were treated with 1:100, 1:250, and 1:500 dilutions of POE (corresponding to 36, 14, and 7.2 µg/mL dried weight of extract, respectively) for 24 h. Cells treated with the $EtOH/H_2O$ (70:30 v/v) vehicle and untreated cells were used as controls.

After cell treatments, 100 µL of MTT solution (0.5 mg/mL) was added to each well and cells were incubated in the dark at 37 °C for a further 1 h. After washing out the supernatant, the insoluble formazan product was dissolved in 100 µL/well of dimethyl sulfoxide (DMSO). Absorbance values were measured using a iMARK microplate reader (Bio-Rad Laboratories, USA) at 595 nm. Data were expressed in terms of percentages with respect to untreated control cells.

3.7. Western Blot Analysis

HepG2 cells (2×10^5 cells/well) were seeded in 35 mm dishes in complete medium and incubated overnight. To study the role of POE in the activation of an autophagic flux, cells were treated with POE (7.2 µg/mL) for different time points, from 3 h to 24 h. Cells treated with Rapa (0.5 µM) were used as an autophagy activation control. After treatments, cells were washed with PBS and then lysed in 80 µL of Laemmli buffer (62.5 mM Tris-HCl pH 6.8, 10% (w/v) SDS, 25% (w/v) glycerol) without bromophenol blue. Whole-cell lysates were collected and boiled at 95 °C for 5 min and centrifuged to remove cell debris ($12,000 \times g$ for 5 min at 4 °C). The BCA protein assay kit (Bio-Rad Laboratories, Hercules, CA, USA) was used to measure protein levels. Briefly, 25 µg of proteins from each sample, added with β-mercaptoethanol and bromophenol blue, were electrophoresed by 12% SDS-PAGE and transferred to PVDF membranes (0.45 µm). The membranes were incubated with blocking solution (5% (w/v) BSA in 0.1% (v/v) PBS-Tween®-20) for 1 h at room temperature. Membrane incubation with the desired primary antibody at appropriate dilution was conducted overnight at 4 °C (Table 1).

After three washes in 0.1% (v/v) PBS-Tween®-20 solution, the membranes were incubated for 1 h at room temperature with a specific secondary antibody (goat anti-rabbit IgG or goat anti-mouse IgG) diluted 1:10,000 in blocking solution. The membranes were finally washed three times in 0.5% (v/v) PBS-Tween®-20 before being stained with Clarity Western ECL solution. Signal of chemiluminescence were acquired with an Amersham™ 600 Imager imaging system (GE Healthcare Life Science, Pittsburgh, PA, USA). Quantity One software (Bio-Rad Laboratories) was used for densitometric analysis.

3.8. ORO Staining

HepG2 cells were seeded (6×10^4 cells/well) in 24-well plates overnight and then treated with POE (7.2 µg/mL) for 24 h. To test the impact of the autophagy process on lipid accumulation, cells were also exposed to CQ (10 µM) and Rapa (0.5 µM) treatment. Following this, the cells were washed with PBS and fixed for 10 min in 2% (v/v) paraformaldehyde. Subsequently, cells were washed twice with PBS and left to dry completely. Neutral lipids were stained for 30 min at 37 °C with 200 µL/well of Oil red O working solution (60% in distilled water). Excess dye was washed away with distilled water until the water no longer had a visible pink color. After the wells had completely dried, the stained lipid droplets in cells were examined and photographed under a Nikon TS-100 microscope equipped with a digital acquisition system (Nikon Digital Sight DS Fi-1; Nikon, Minato-ku, Tokyo, Japan). Finally, cellular lipid accumulation was measured by adding 200 µL/well of isopropanol. Absorption was measured at 490 nm using an iMARK microplate reader (Bio-Rad Laboratories, USA).

3.9. Statistical Analysis

Where not otherwise specified, data are expressed as the mean ± SD of at least three independent experiments.

For ORO and MTT experiments, signals acquired from independent experiments were normalized by mean centering (i.e., each replicate measurement was divided by the mean of the replicates in order to compensate for batch experimental fluctuations) and differences were assessed by one-way ANOVA followed by Tukey's HSD test after normality check with the Shapiro–Wilk test.

For Western blotting, difference between house-keeping-normalized intensity signals were assessed by the Kruskall–Wallis test, followed by the Conover post hoc test.

Statistical differences were called at $p \leq 0.05$.

4. Conclusions

In summary, this study revealed that POE protects against lipid accumulation in HepG2 cells by promoting autophagy through inhibition of the mTOR pathway.

P. oceanica is a marine plant with several bioactive properties, including antidiabetic and anti-inflammatory effects [41]. Thus, the possibility that *P. oceanica* may hit multiple pathogenic liver disease targets—lowering blood sugar, inhibiting the inflammatory state, and blocking the reduction in hepatic lipid accumulation—makes this traditional herbal remedy a potential effective weapon against the prevention and/or treatment of steatosis and related disease conditions. Indeed, NAFLD is a metabolic condition commonly associated with type 2 diabetes mellitus and often combined with a chronic inflammatory state. Given the lack of approved and recognized drug therapies for NAFLD, this study offers new insights into the mechanisms of action of *P. oceanica* that are a first step for further in vitro and in vivo studies in order to identify alternative and complementary strategies for disease management.

However, because this study was performed on the HepG2 cell line, it is essential that the data also be validated on primary hepatocytes in future studies. In addition, studies in in vivo models are absolutely necessary to test the applicability of *P. oceanica* in the management of NAFLD.

Supplementary Materials: The following are available online at https://www.mdpi.com/article/10.3390/ph14100969/s1, Figure S1. The effect of EtOH/H_2O vehicle (70:30 v/v) on the viability of HepG2 cells. MTT assay on untreated cells (-) or exposed to different dilutions of EtOH/H_2O (70:30 v/v) for 24 h. The amount of EtOH/H_2O (70:30 v/v) applied corresponds exactly to that used in POE cell treatment. Data were reported as mean ± SD of three independent experiments.

Author Contributions: Conceptualization, D.D.; formal analysis, M.V. and E.B.; investigation, M.V.; data curation, M.V. and E.B.; writing—original draft preparation, M.V. and D.D.; writing—review and editing, M.V., E.B., and D.D.; supervision, D.D.; project administration, D.D.; funding acquisition, D.D. All authors have read and agreed to the published version of the manuscript.

Funding: This research was funded by University of Florence, Fondi di Ateneo 2021, to D.D.

Institutional Review Board Statement: Not applicable.

Informed Consent Statement: Not applicable.

Data Availability Statement: All data has been present in main text and supplementary materials.

Conflicts of Interest: The authors declare no conflict of interest.

References

1. Gobert, S.; Cambridge, M.T.; Velimirov, B.; Pergent, G.; Lepoint, G.; Bouquegneau, J.M.; Dauby, P.; Pergent-Martini, C.; Walker, D.I. Biology of Posidonia. In *Seagrasses: Biology, Ecology and Conservation*; Larkum, A.W., Orth, R.J., Duarte, C., Eds.; Springer: Dordrecht, The Netherlands, 2006; pp. 387–408.
2. Batanouny, K.H. *Wild Medicinal Plants in Egypt. Academy of Scientific Research and Technology, Egypt*; The World Conservation Union (IUCN): Gland, Switzerland, 1999; pp. 166–167.
3. El-Mokasabi, F.M. Floristic composition and traditional uses of plant species at Wadi Alkuf, Al-Jabal Al-Akhder, Libya. *Am. Eur. J. Agric. Environ. Sci.* **2014**, *14*, 685–697. [CrossRef]
4. Gokce, G.; Haznedaroglu, M.Z. Evaluation of antidiabetic, antioxidant and vasoprotective effects of Posidonia oceanica extract. *J. Ethnopharmacol.* **2008**, *115*, 122–130. [CrossRef]
5. Barletta, E.; Ramazzotti, M.; Fratianni, F.; Pessani, D.; Degl'Innocenti, D. Hydrophilic extract from Posidonia oceanica inhibits activity and expression of gelatinases and prevents HT1080 human fibrosarcoma cell line invasion. *Cell. Adh. Migr.* **2015**, *9*, 422–431. [CrossRef] [PubMed]
6. Leri, M.; Ramazzotti, M.; Vasarri, M.; Peri, S.; Barletta, E.; Pretti, C.; Degl'Innocenti, D. Bioactive Compounds from Posidonia oceanica (L.) Delile Impair Malignant Cell Migration through Autophagy Modulation. *Mar. Drugs.* **2018**, *16*, 137. [CrossRef]
7. Piazzini, V.; Vasarri, M.; Degl'Innocenti, D.; Guastini, A.; Barletta, E.; Salvatici, M.C.; Bergonzi, M.C. Comparison of Chitosan Nanoparticles and Soluplus Micelles to Optimize the Bioactivity of Posidonia oceanica Extract on Human Neuroblastoma Cell Migration. *Pharmaceutics* **2019**, *11*, 655. [CrossRef] [PubMed]
8. Vasarri, M.; Leri, M.; Barletta, E.; Ramazzotti, M.; Marzocchini, R.; Degl'Innocenti, D. Anti-inflammatory properties of the marine plant Posidonia oceanica (L.) Delile. *J. Ethnopharmacol.* **2020**, *247*, 112252. [CrossRef] [PubMed]
9. Micheli, L.; Vasarri, M.; Barletta, E.; Lucarini, E.; Ghelardini, C.; Degl'Innocenti, D.; Di Cesare Mannelli, L. Efficacy of Posidonia oceanica Extract against Inflammatory Pain: In Vivo Studies in Mice. *Mar. Drugs.* **2021**, *19*, 48. [CrossRef]
10. Vasarri, M.; Barletta, E.; Ramazzotti, M.; Degl'Innocenti, D. In vitro anti-glycation activity of the marine plant Posidonia oceanica (L.) Delile. *J. Ethnopharmacol.* **2020**, *259*, 112960. [CrossRef] [PubMed]
11. Glick, D.; Barth, S.; Macleod, K.F. Autophagy: Cellular and molecular mechanisms. *J. Pathol.* **2010**, *221*, 3–12. [CrossRef]
12. Levine, B.; Kroemer, G. Autophagy in the pathogenesis of disease. *Cell* **2008**, *132*, 27–42. [CrossRef]
13. Ramos, V.M.; Kowaltowski, A.J.; Kakimoto, P.A. Autophagy in Hepatic Steatosis: A Structured Review. *Front. Cell Dev. Biol.* **2021**, *9*, 657389. [CrossRef]
14. Godoy-Matos, A.F.; Silva Júnior, W.S.; Valerio, C.M. NAFLD as a continuum: From obesity to metabolic syndrome and diabetes. *Diabetol. Metab. Syndr.* **2020**, *12*, 60. [CrossRef]
15. Gluchowski, N.L.; Becuwe, M.; Walther, T.C.; Farese, R.V., Jr. Lipid droplets and liver disease: From basic biology to clinical implications. *Nat. Rev. Gastroenterol. Hepatol.* **2017**, *14*, 343–355. [CrossRef]
16. Dong, H.; Czaja, M.J. Regulation of lipid droplets by autophagy. *Trends Endocrinol. Metab.* **2011**, *22*, 234–240. [CrossRef]
17. Czaja, M.J. Function of Autophagy in Nonalcoholic Fatty Liver Disease. *Dig. Dis. Sci.* **2016**, *61*, 1304–1313. [CrossRef]
18. Grefhorst, A.; van de Peppel, I.P.; Larsen, L.E.; Jonker, J.W.; Holleboom, A.G. The Role of Lipophagy in the Development and Treatment of Non-Alcoholic Fatty Liver Disease. *Front. Endocrinol. (Lausanne)* **2021**, *11*, 601627. [CrossRef]
19. Niture, S.; Lin, M.; Rios-Colon, L.; Qi, Q.; Moore, J.T.; Kumar, D. Emerging Roles of Impaired Autophagy in Fatty Liver Disease and Hepatocellular Carcinoma. *Int. J. Hepatol.* **2021**, *2021*, 6675762. [CrossRef] [PubMed]
20. Zhang, Y.; Li, K.; Kong, A.; Zhou, Y.; Chen, D.; Gu, J.; Shi, H. Dysregulation of autophagy acts as a pathogenic mechanism of non-alcoholic fatty liver disease (NAFLD) induced by common environmental pollutants. *Ecotoxicol. Environ. Saf.* **2021**, *217*, 112256. [CrossRef] [PubMed]
21. Mao, Y.; Yu, F.; Wang, J.; Guo, C.; Fan, X. Autophagy: A new target for nonalcoholic fatty liver disease therapy. *Hepat. Med.* **2016**, *8*, 27–37. [CrossRef] [PubMed]
22. Zhang, L.; Yao, Z.; Ji, G. Herbal Extracts and Natural Products in Alleviating Non-alcoholic Fatty Liver Disease via Activating Autophagy. *Front Pharmacol.* **2018**, *9*, 1459. [CrossRef]
23. Huang, Q.; Wang, T.; Yang, L.; Wang, H.Y. Ginsenoside Rb2 Alleviates Hepatic Lipid Accumulation by Restoring Autophagy via Induction of Sirt1 and Activation of AMPK. *Int. J. Mol. Sci.* **2017**, *18*, 1063. [CrossRef]

24. Zhang, Y.; Chen, M.L.; Zhou, Y.; Yi, L.; Gao, Y.X.; Ran, L.; Chen, S.H.; Zhang, T.; Zhou, X.; Zou, D.; et al. Resveratrol improves hepatic steatosis by inducing autophagy through the cAMP signaling pathway. *Mol. Nutr. Food Res.* **2015**, *59*, 1443–1457. [CrossRef]
25. Ding, S.; Jiang, J.; Zhang, G.; Bu, Y.; Zhang, G.; Zhao, X. Resveratrol and caloric restriction prevent hepatic steatosis by regulating SIRT1-autophagy pathway and alleviating endoplasmic reticulum stress in high-fat diet-fed rats. *PLoS ONE* **2017**, *12*, e0183541. [CrossRef]
26. Ji, G.; Wang, Y.; Deng, Y.; Li, X.; Jiang, Z. Resveratrol ameliorates hepatic steatosis and inflammation in methionine/choline-deficient diet-induced steatohepatitis through regulating autophagy. *Lipids Health Dis.* **2015**, *14*, 134. [CrossRef]
27. Parafati, M.; Lascala, A.; Morittu, V.M.; Trimboli, F.; Rizzuto, A.; Brunelli, E.; Coscarelli, F.; Costa, N.; Britti, D.; Ehrlich, J.; et al. Bergamot polyphenol fraction prevents nonalcoholic fatty liver disease via stimulation of lipophagy in cafeteria diet-induced rat model of metabolic syndrome. *J. Nutr. Biochem.* **2015**, *26*, 938–948. [CrossRef] [PubMed]
28. Li, Q.; Li, L.; Wang, F.; Chen, J.; Zhao, Y.; Wang, P.; Nilius, B.; Liu, D.; Zhu, Z. Dietary capsaicin prevents nonalcoholic fatty liver disease through transient receptor potential vanilloid 1-mediated peroxisome proliferator-activated receptor δ activation. *Pflugers Arch.* **2013**, *465*, 1303–1316. [CrossRef] [PubMed]
29. Pan, J.; Wang, M.; Song, H.; Wang, L.; Ji, G. The efficacy and safety of traditional chinese medicine (jiang zhi granule) for nonalcoholic Fatty liver: A multicenter, randomized, placebo-controlled study. *Evid. Based Complement. Alternat. Med.* **2013**, *2013*, 965723. [CrossRef]
30. Yan, H.M.; Xia, M.F.; Wang, Y.; Chang, X.X.; Yao, X.Z.; Rao, S.X.; Zeng, M.S.; Tu, Y.F.; Feng, R.; Jia, W.P.; et al. Efficacy of Berberine in Patients with Non-Alcoholic Fatty Liver Disease. *PLoS ONE* **2015**, *10*, e0134172. [CrossRef] [PubMed]
31. Chen, S.; Zhao, X.; Ran, L.; Wan, J.; Wang, X.; Qin, Y.; Shu, F.; Gao, Y.; Yuan, L.; Zhang, Q.; et al. Resveratrol improves insulin resistance, glucose and lipid metabolism in patients with non-alcoholic fatty liver disease: A randomized controlled trial. *Dig. Liver Dis.* **2015**, *47*, 226–232. [CrossRef]
32. Panahi, Y.; Kianpour, P.; Mohtashami, R.; Jafari, R.; Simental-Mendía, L.E.; Sahebkar, A. Efficacy and Safety of Phytosomal Curcumin in Non-Alcoholic Fatty Liver Disease: A Randomized Controlled Trial. *Drug Res.* **2017**, *67*, 244–251. [CrossRef] [PubMed]
33. Menon, M.B.; Dhamija, S. Beclin 1 Phosphorylation—At the Center of Autophagy Regulation. *Front. Cell. Dev. Biol.* **2018**, *6*, 137. [CrossRef] [PubMed]
34. Yoshii, S.R.; Mizushima, N. Monitoring and Measuring Autophagy. *Int. J. Mol. Sci.* **2017**, *18*, 1865. [CrossRef] [PubMed]
35. Pankiv, S.; Clausen, T.H.; Lamark, T.; Brech, A.; Bruun, J.A.; Outzen, H.; Øvervatn, A.; Bjørkøy, G.; Johansen, T. p62/SQSTM1 binds directly to Atg8/LC3 to facilitate degradation of ubiquitinated protein aggregates by autophagy. *J. Biol. Chem.* **2007**, *282*, 24131–24145. [CrossRef]
36. Zhang, Z.; Yao, Z.; Chen, Y.; Qian, L.; Jiang, S.; Zhou, J.; Shao, J.; Chen, A.; Zhang, F.; Zheng, S. Lipophagy and liver disease: New perspectives to better understanding and therapy. *Biomed. Pharmacother.* **2018**, *97*, 339–348. [CrossRef] [PubMed]
37. Takahashi, S.S.; Sou, Y.S.; Saito, T.; Kuma, A.; Yabe, T.; Sugiura, Y.; Lee, H.C.; Suematsu, M.; Yokomizo, T.; Koike, M.; et al. Loss of autophagy impairs physiological steatosis by accumulation of NCoR1. *Life Sci. Alliance* **2019**, *3*, e201900513. [CrossRef]
38. Czaja, M.J.; Ding, W.X.; Donohue, T.M.; Friedman, S.L., Jr.; Kim, J.S.; Komatsu, M.; Lemasters, J.J.; Lemoine, A.; Lin, J.D.; Ou, J.H.; et al. Functions of autophagy in normal and diseased liver. *Autophagy* **2013**, *9*, 1131–1158. [CrossRef]
39. Schulze, R.J.; Krueger, E.W.; Weller, S.G.; Johnson, K.M.; Casey, C.A.; Schott, M.B.; McNiven, M.A. Direct lysosome-based autophagy of lipid droplets in hepatocytes. *Proc. Natl. Acad. Sci. USA* **2020**, *117*, 32443–32452. [CrossRef] [PubMed]
40. Dyshlovoy, S.A. Blue-Print Autophagy in 2020: A Critical Review. *Mar. Drugs.* **2020**, *18*, 482. [CrossRef] [PubMed]
41. Vasarri, M.; De Biasi, A.M.; Barletta, E.; Pretti, C.; Degl'Innocenti, D. An Overview of New Insights into the Benefits of the Seagrass Posidonia oceanica for Human Health. *Mar. Drugs.* **2021**, *19*, 476. [CrossRef]

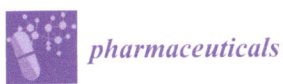

Article

Preliminary Biological Activity Screening of *Plectranthus* spp. Extracts for the Search of Anticancer Lead Molecules

Epole Ntungwe [1,2], Eva María Domínguez-Martín [1,2], Catarina Teodósio [1], Silvia Teixidó-Trujillo [3], Natalia Armas Capote [3], Lucilia Saraiva [4], Ana María Díaz-Lanza [2], Noélia Duarte [5] and Patrícia Rijo [1,5,*]

1. CBIOS—Universidade Lusófona Research Center for Biosciences & Health Technologies, Universidade Lusófona de Humanidades e Tecnologias, Campo Grande 376, 1749-024 Lisboa, Portugal; ntungweepolengolle@yahoo.com (E.N.); evam.dominguez@uah.es (E.M.D.-M.); catarina.teodosio@gmail.com (C.T.)
2. Department of Biomedical Sciences, Faculty of Pharmacy, University of Alcalá de Henares, Ctra. A2, Km 33.100—Campus Universitario, 28805 Alcalá de Henares, Spain; ana.diaz@uah.es
3. Centro Atlántico del Medicamento S.A., Avenida Trinidad 61, 7ª Planta, Torre Agustín Arévalo, 38204 La Laguna, Tenerife, Spain; teixido.silvia@gmail.com (S.T.-T.); nataliaarmas@ceamedsa.com (N.A.C.)
4. LAQV/REQUIMTE, Laboratório de Microbiologia, Departamento de Ciências Biológicas, Faculdade de Farmácia, Universidade do Porto, Rua de Jorge Viterbo Ferreira n.º 228, 4050-313 Porto, Portugal; lucilia.saraiva@ff.up.pt
5. Instituto de Investigação do Medicamento (iMed.ULisboa), Faculdade de Farmácia, Universidade de Lisboa, 1649-003 Lisboa, Portugal; mduarte@ff.ulisboa.pt
* Correspondence: patricia.rijo@ulusofona.pt

Citation: Ntungwe, E.; Domínguez-Martín, E.M.; Teodósio, C.; Teixidó-Trujillo, S.; Armas Capote, N.; Saraiva, L.; Díaz-Lanza, A.M.; Duarte, N.; Rijo, P. Preliminary Biological Activity Screening of *Plectranthus* spp. Extracts for the Search of Anticancer Lead Molecules. *Pharmaceuticals* **2021**, *14*, 402. https://doi.org/10.3390/ph14050402

Academic Editor: Maria Matilde Soares Duarte Marques

Received: 6 April 2021
Accepted: 20 April 2021
Published: 23 April 2021

Publisher's Note: MDPI stays neutral with regard to jurisdictional claims in published maps and institutional affiliations.

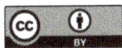

Copyright: © 2021 by the authors. Licensee MDPI, Basel, Switzerland. This article is an open access article distributed under the terms and conditions of the Creative Commons Attribution (CC BY) license (https:// creativecommons.org/licenses/by/ 4.0/).

Abstract: *Plectranthus* species (Lamiaceae) have been employed in traditional medicine and this is now validated by the presence of bioactive abietane-type diterpenoids. Herein, sixteen *Plectranthus* acetonic extracts were prepared by ultrasound-assisted extraction and their biological activity was screened. The antimicrobial activity of each extract was screened against yeasts, and Gram-positive and Gram-negative bacteria. The *P. hadiensis* and *P. mutabilis* extracts possessed significant activity against *Staphylococcus aureus* and *Candida albicans* (microdilution method). Moreover, all extracts showed antioxidant activity using the DPPH method, with *P. hadiensis* and *P. mutabilis* extracts having the highest scavenging activities. Selected by the *Artemia salina* model, *P. hadiensis* and *P.ciliatus* possessed low micromolar anti-proliferative activities in human colon, breast, and lung cancer cell lines. Furthermore, the most bioactive extract of *P. hadiensis* leaves and the known abietane diterpene, 7α-acetoxy-6β-hydroxyroyleanone isolated from this plant, were tested against the aggressive type triple negative breast cancer (MDA-MB-231S). *P. hadiensis* extract reduced the viability of MDA-MB-231S cancer cell line cells, showing an IC_{50} value of 25.6 µg/mL. The IC_{50} value of 7α-acetoxy-6β-hydroxyroyleanone was 5.5 µM (2.15 µg/mL), suggesting that this lead molecule is a potential starting tool for the development of anti-cancer drugs.

Keywords: *Plectranthus*; royleanone; 7α-acetoxy-6β-hydroxyroyleanone; *ent*-abietane; antitumoral activity; antimicrobial activity; antioxidant

1. Introduction

Over the centuries, plants and natural products derived from plants have been the basis of traditional medicine. Nowadays, plant-based medicines have been playing an important role in drug discovery and development. They are also widely employed in various public health practices as they are safe, cost-effective, and possess unique chemical diversity [1,2]. Cancer remains one of the leading causes of death globally, with approximately 18.1 million new cases and 9.6 million cancer-related deaths in 2018, according to the World Health Organization [3]. Furthermore, several types of chemotherapies used are ineffective and generate unwanted adverse side effects [4,5]. Similarly, there is an increasing number of cases of bacterial infections that are resistant to current antibiotics and are difficult or impossible to treat [6]. Currently, there is an emerging interest in developing drugs that overcome the problems stated above by using natural compounds.

Plectranthus L' Herit. is a major genus of the Lamiaceae family comprising about 300 species mainly distributed in the summer-rainfall savannahs and forested regions of tropical Africa, Asia, and Australia [7,8]. Most of the *Plectranthus* species are soft trailing semi-succulent to succulent herbs or shrubs and their stems, leaves, roots, and tubers are frequently used as traditional medicines for the treatment of various illnesses, including respiratory, digestive, and liver ailments [9]. Phytochemical studies on some species of *Plectranthus* revealed the presence of a large number of diterpenes and triterpenes [10,11]. Isolated terpenes from *Plectranthus* species are reported to possess antibacterial [12–14], antitumoral [15–18], antifungal [12,19], insecticidal [20], and antiplasmodial [20] activities. Moreover, our group has been focused on the phytochemical study of *Plectranthus* species and we have reported abietane diterpenoids with diverse bioactivity [16,17,21–25]. Therefore, the screening of other *Plectranthus* spp. extracts aiming at finding new sources of biologically active natural products is warranted.

Herein, sixteen *Plectranthus* species were screened for their bioactivity (antioxidant, antimicrobial activities, and general toxicity) and the main compound of the most bioactive extract was identified. To the best of our knowledge, the scientific literature concerning these species is scarce or even non-existent. *P. hadiensis* was earlier reported to have ethnopharmacological activity and to be a rich source of ent-abietane diterpenes [11]. This work aims to screen the antimicrobial, antioxidant, and cytotoxic properties of several *Plectranthus* spp. extracts and identifying the component in the most bioactive extract that may be responsible for its bioactivity.

2. Results and Discussion

All sixteen *Plectranthus* spp. extracts were prepared using ultrasound-assisted extraction in acetone. Previous studies of *Plectranthus* species showed that acetonic extracts are rich in diterpenoids, and high extraction yields are obtained when the ultrasound extraction method is carried out [21]. Therefore, using this extraction method, sixteen acetonic extracts of *Plectranthus* spp. were prepared. The extraction of all extracts was done in triplicate under the same conditions. All extracts were solubilized in DMSO (10 mg/mL) and stored at $-20\ °C$ until further analysis for their biological assays. *P. mutabilis* had the highest extraction yield (30.00% w/w) (Table 1).

The antioxidant activity of the extracts was quantitatively determined using the DPPH (2,2-diphenyl-1-picrylhydrazyl) scavenging radical assay. The antioxidant activity of the extracts was compared with quercetin, a well-known pure compound used as a positive control to understand the potential antioxidant activity of the extracts screen. The antioxidant activity indicates the capacity to quench reactive oxygen species (ROS), leading to decreased oxidative stress [26]. The results of the free radical scavenging capacity of extracts at a concentration of 10 µg/mL are shown in Table 1. *P. mutabilis* and *P. hadiensis* had the highest scavenging activity of 46.14% and 36.24%, respectively. These results are also in agreement with other studies with *Plectranthus* extracts, in which *P. madagascarensis P. neochilus*, *P. barbatus* and *P. verticillatus* extracts showed free radical scavenging abilities [27]. This could be due to the presence of abietane diterpenes known for their antioxidant activity. Recently, findings concerning the antioxidant activity of abietane diterpenes isolated from *Plectranthus* spp. suggest that the quinone moiety present in these compounds is probably responsible for their biological activity [28]. The presence of the 12-OH group and the carbonyl group at position C-7 (*p*-position) could serve as hydrogen- and/or electron-donating moieties, resulting in the formation of stable quinone derivatives [29].

To evaluate the antimicrobial activity, the extracts were screened against Gram-positive (*Staphylococcus aureus*, *Enterococcus faecalis*) and Gram-negative (*Pseudomonas aeruginosa* and *Escherichia coli*) bacteria and yeasts (*Candida albicans* and *Saccharomyces cerevisiae*) using the well diffusion assay. The antimicrobial activity of each acetonic extract was first screened by the well diffusion method at a concentration of 1 mg/mL. Only *P. hadiensis* and *P. mutabilis* extracts showed antimicrobial activity against *S. aureus* with inhibition zones of 16 mm and 15 mm, respectively. None of the extracts showed significant antibacterial activity against *E. faecalis* and Gram-negative bacteria. These results are in agreement with previous works on *Plectranthus* spp. [17,30] showing that only Gram-positive bacteria are sensitive to *Plectranthus* acetonic extracts [27,31]. When the zone of inhibition of the extracts was compared with the negative control, it was found that nine extracts (*P. ciliatus, P. welshii, P. mzumbulensis, P. inflexus, P. lucidus, P. xerophylus, P. lippio, P. hadiensis,* and *P. mutabilis.*) exhibited antimicrobial activity against *C. albicans* (10–11 mm). The remaining did not display any antimicrobial effects, showing inhibition zones similar to the negative control (data not shown).

Table 1. Extraction yields (dry weight % w/w), antioxidant activity, and general toxicity of sixteen *Plectranthus* spp. acetonic extracts.

Scientific Name	Yield (% w/w) [a]	Antioxidant Activity [b] (%)	General Toxicity	
			* Mortality (%)	LC_{50} (µg/mL) **
P. swynnertonii S. Moore †	3.89	20.24 ± 0.01	65.88 ± 5	0.036 ± 1.69
P. ciliatus E. Mey †	11.86	13.21 ± 0.01	60.14 ± 0.44	0.504 ± 1.13
P. mutabilis Codd. †	30.03	46.14 ± 0.02	51.50 ± 0.07	0.984 ± 2.92
P. hadiensis (Forssk.) Schweinf. Ex Sprenger †	13.49	36.24 ± 0.04	43.65 ± 3.04	0.88 ± 4.87
P. cylindraceus Hochst, ex Benth †	9.68	19.19 ± 0.07	43.50 ± 5.66	0.55 ± 1.96
P. lucidus (Benth.) Van Jaarsv. and T.J. Edwards †	6.29	23.96 ± 0.09	38.81 ± 3.75	1.053 ± 4.61
P. inflexus (Thunb.) Vahl ex Benth †	10.97	0.16 ± 0.05	38.70 ± 3.35	0.986 ± 2.87
P. lippio. Druce	2.09	30.5 ± 0.14	24.70 ± 6.22	N/A
P. crassus N.E.Br. †	7.77	27.27 ± 0.01	31.16 ± 1.29	N/A
P. mzimvubuensis Van Jaarsv. †	7.79	22.47 ± 0.05	33.95 ± 1.63	N/A
P. xerophylus Codd	10.16	20.15 ± 0.02	30.48 ± 3.24	N/A
P. welshii	2.15	15.06 ± 0.03	23.71 ± 0.60	N/A
P. petiolaris E. Mey ex Benth.	11.07	14.45 ± 0.01	23.42 ± 4.15	N/A
P. woodii Gürke	8.51	13.04 ± 0.01	29.95 ± 6.01	N/A
P. welwitschii (Briq. Codd)	3.59	12.63 ± 0.03	25.17 ± 5.54	N/A
P. spicatus E. Mey	4.75	10.57 ± 0.02	27 ± 0.28	N/A
Positive control	N/A	99.47 ± 0.10	98.89 ± 2.48	N/A
DMSO	N/A	N/A	21.87 ± 0.44	N/A

[a] (mg of extracts/g of the dried plant). [b] Antioxidant activity (%): Quercetin a potent free radical scavenging capacity was used as a positive control. Data are mean ± SD. * Screening of the *Plectranthus* spp. extracts for general toxicity at a concentration of 10 µg/mL using the *Artemia salina* test (24 h). ** LC_{50} values (µg/mL) for the most active extracts. Positive control = Potassium dichromate (10 µg/mL). Data are mean ± SD was calculated from three independent experiments and compared to DMSO († $p < 0.001$). Lethal concentration (%) = (Total *A.salina* − Alive *A.salina*)/(Total *A.salina*) × 100 was used to calculate the lethal concentration of all extracts. N/A—not applicable.

As the initial screening using the well diffusion assay identified *P. hadiensis* and *P. mutabilis* extracts as possessing the most promising antimicrobial activities, further studies were carried out to evaluate the minimum inhibitory concentration (MIC) and minimum bactericidal concentration (MBC) or minimum fungicidal concentration (MFC) against the susceptible strains (Table 2). The MIC values ranged from 3.91 µg/mL to 125 µg/mL. *P. hadiensis* was the most active extract, exhibiting a MIC value of 3.91 µg/mL against the methicillin-resistant *S. aureus* strain (MRSA), similar to that observed for the positive control (1.95 µg/mL). The MBC/MFC values ranged from 62.5 to 250 µg/mL. It is possible to conclude that the extracts are mainly bacteriostatic rather than bactericidal [32].

To identify the most promising extracts with cytotoxic activity, the screening of general toxicity using the *Artemia salina* model was carried out. This assay was employed to screen the sixteen extracts because it is low-cost, rapid, convenient, and requires only a relatively small amount of sample [31,33]. All of the acetonic extracts were tested at 10 µg/mL with values ranging from 23.42 to 65.88% mortality (see Table 1). The most active extracts were further studied to obtain the LC_{50} values at concentrations of 0.1, 0.5, and 1 mg/mL, after 24 h of exposure. The most toxic extracts (*P. mutabilis, P. swynnertonii, P. hadiensis, P. ciliatus,* and *P. cylindraceus*) with $LC_{50} \leq 1$ μg/mL (see Table 1) were then evaluated on human-derived cancer cell lines.

Table 2. MIC and MBC/MFC (μg/mL) values of the most active acetonic extracts.

Extracts	MIC (μg/mL)			MBC/MFC (μg/mL)		
	S. aureus	MRSA	*C. albicans*	*S. aureus*	MRSA	*C. albicans*
Positive Control	3.91	1.95	<0.48	-	-	-
P. mutabilis	31.25	31.25	125	250	250	125
P. hadiensis	15.62	3.91	62.5	250	250	62.5

Positive controls (1 mg/mL): Gram-positive = vancomycin, Gram-negative = norfloxacin, yeast = nystatin, Negative control = DMSO, methicillin-resistant *Staphylococcus aureus* = MRSA.

The cytotoxic activity was determined by the sulforhodamine B (SRB) assay in three different cancer cell lines: colon colorectal carcinoma (HCT116), human breast adenocarcinoma (MCF-7), and lung cancer carcinoma (NCI-H460). The IC_{50} values in all the cell lines tested ranged from 2.25 μg/mL to 36 μg/mL (Table 3). According to the National Cancer Institute (NCI), crude extracts that possess $IC_{50} \leq 500$ μg/mL are of potential interest for further studies [34] and a possible candidate for further development of cancer therapeutic agents. Thus, most of the selected extracts showed potential values, and *P. hadiensis* and *P. ciliatus* seem to be potential sources of lead anticancer molecules. *P. ciliatus* extract was most active against the colon cell line (HCT116), whereas the *P. hadiensis* extract was the most active against the breast (MCF-7) and lung (NCI-H460) cell lines with the lowest IC_{50} value in the MCF-7 cell lines. For this reason, this extract was further tested against the aggressive type triple-negative breast cancer (MDA-MB-231S). MCF-7 hormone receptors expressing breast cancers have a more favorable prognosis as opposed to triple-negative breast cancer (TNBC), which is characterized by a poor treatment outcome [35]. This cell line is a highly metastatic triple-negative breast cancer cell line that does not display estrogenic receptors (ER), progesterone receptors (PR), or human epidermal growth factor receptor 2 (HER2), and is thus difficult to treat [21]. *P. hadiensis* acetonic extract had a growth inhibition effect on MDA-MB-231 cancer cells (IC_{50} value of 25.6 μg/mL, Table 3). Many studies have attributed the cytotoxicity of *Plectranthus* extracts to the presence of royleanone-type abietane diterpenoids with known anticancer activities [18,36]. The abietane-type diterpenoid royleanones are a highly bioactive group of lead molecules, important for the development of new anticancer drugs [22] Given the good levels of bioactivity of *P. hadiensis* extract in all the cell lines tested, it was selected to identify its main bioactive component.

Table 3. IC_{50} (μg/mL) values for five selected acetonic extracts in HCT116, MCF-7, H460 and MDA-MB231S cell lines.

	HCT116 *	H460 *	MCF-7 *	MDA-MB231S **
P. hadiensis	3.45 ± 0.35	3.00 ± 0.10	2.90 ± 0.10	25.6
P. ciliatus	2.25 ± 0.75	6.45 ± 0.05	6.70 ± 0.30	N/A
P. swynnertonii	7.95 ± 0.35	13.50 ± 0.50	15.05 ± 0.02	N/A
P. cylindraceus	10.25 ± 0.75	12.50 ± 0.50	12.00 ± 1.00	N/A
P. mutabilis	28.00 ± 2.00	36.00 ± 2.00	35.00 ± 1.00	N/A
Doxorubicin	0.05 ± 3.24	0.29 ± 2.32	0.08 ± 4.10	0.07 ± 0.01

* The concentration that reduces growth by 50% (IC_{50}) was determined by sulforhodamine B assay after 48 h treatment. Data are mean ± SEM of 4–5 independent experiments. ** IC_{50} (μg/mL) of the most bioactive *P. hadiensis* acetonic extract in MDA-MB231S cancer cell lines. DMSO was used as the negative control. N/A—not applicable.

To unveil the chemical profile of the most bioactive *P. hadiensis* acetonic extract, and to identify the main compound responsible for the tested bioactivity, an HPLC–DAD study was carried out. The chromatogram revealed that the known *ent*-abietane diterpene,

7α-acetoxy-6β-hydroxyroyleanone, Roy (Figure 1) was the major compound in the extract (Supplementary Material). To isolate this diterpene, a bio-guided column and the preparative chromatographic procedure were carried out. Its structure was confirmed through comparison of its spectroscopic data (Supplementary Material) to those described in the literature [12,29,37].

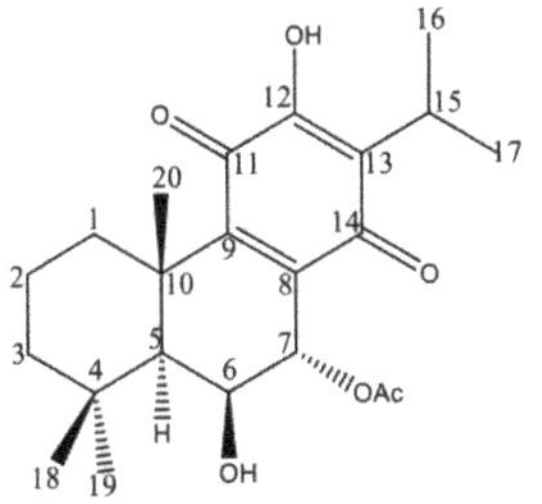

Figure 1. Chemical structure of 7α-acetoxy-6β-hydroxyroyleanone.

In previous studies, 7α-acetoxy-6β-hydroxyroyleanone showed cytotoxic activity against three human cell lines, namely, sensitive non-small cell lung carcinoma, NCI-H460 cell line (IC_{50} 2.7 ± 0.4), multidrug-resistant non-small cell lung carcinoma cell line with P-glycoprotein overexpression. NCI-H460/R (IC_{50} 3.1 ± 0.4), and human embryonal bronchial epithelial (MCR-5) cells (IC_{50} 8.6 ± 0.4) [21,38]. Given its cytotoxic properties, the presence of this compound in *P. hadiensis* acetonic extract may partially explain, the foreseen properties of the extract. To further explore its cytotoxicity, additional studies were performed.

The preliminary toxicity of the isolated 7α-acetoxy-6β-hydroxyroyleanone (Roy) was evaluated using the Brine shrimp lethality bioassay, which gave a percentage mortality of 30.95%. The cytotoxicity of 7α-acetoxy-6β-hydroxyroyleanone was further tested in the TNBC, MDA-MB231S cell line using the MTT assay. It had an IC_{50} value of 5.5 µM = 2.15 µg/mL (Supplementary Information Figure S4), being approximately 12-fold more active than the corresponding extract (MDA-MB231S IC_{50} value = 25.6 µg/mL). This diterpene has also exhibited cytotoxic activity against breast, renal, melanoma, and central nervous system cancer cell lines [24,29,30]. It was also found to induce apoptosis in the H7PX glioma cell line, through the G2/M cell cycle arrest and DSBs (double-strand breaks) [39]. The cytotoxicity of 7α-acetoxy-6β-hydroxyroyleanone could be due to its royleanone-type scaffold and by its high lipophilicity, which facilitates penetration into the interior of the cell membrane [21,22,29,39]. Moreover, 7α-acetoxy-6β-hydroxyroyleanone was found to exhibit better activity against Gram-positive bacteria, and more importantly, against MRSA strains than some of the existing antibiotics [37]. Roy is found in many other *Plectranthus* species like *P. madagascariensis*, *P. grandidentatus*, *P. actites*, *P. amboinicus*, *P. sanguineus*, *P. argentatus*, and thus can be considered as a chemomarker of the *Plectranthus* genus [21,22].

3. Materials and Methods

3.1. Plant Material

All *Plectranthus* spp. studied in this work (Table 1) were grown in the "Parque Botânico da Tapada da Ajuda", Lisbon-Portugal from cuttings provided by the Kirstenbosch National Botanical Gardens, South Africa. Plants were collected between 2007 and 2008, always in June and September. Voucher specimens were deposited in the Herbarium "João de Carvalho e Vasconcellos" of the Instituto Superior de Agronomia, Lisboa (LISI), Portugal. The plant names were verified with the Plant List [40].

Extraction Procedure

Plant extracts were obtained by the ultra-sonication method, adding 30 mL of acetone to 3 g of ground dry plants (*P. hadiensis* leaves and the whole plant for the remaining *Plectranthus* spp.), sonicated for 1 h, and filtered (Whatman No 5 paper, Inc., Clifton, NJ, USA). The extraction procedure was repeated three times until complete extraction [41]. The liquid samples were evaporated at 40–50 °C using a rotary evaporator (Sigma-Aldrich, IKA HBR 4 basic heating bath, Essen, Germany). All extracts were solubilized in DMSO (10 mg/mL, except for the exceptions that are mentioned) and stored at −20 °C until further analysis.

3.2. Phytochemical Study of P. Hadiensis

3.2.1. HPLC-DAD Fingerprint Analysis

Extract profiling was performed with an Agilent Technologies 1260 Infinity II Series system with diode array detector (DAD; Agilent, Santa Clara, CA, USA), equipped with an Eclipse XDB-C18, (250 × 4.0 mm i.d., 5 µm) column, from Merck and ChemStation Software (Hewlett-Packard, Alto Palo, CA, USA). Four detection wavelengths were selected: 254, 270, 280, and 360 nm. The mobile phase consisted of a mixture of methanol (A), acetonitrile (B), and 0.3% (w/v) trifluoroacetic acid in ultrapure water (C). The employed method was modified from the one previously published Matías et al. [21] as follows: 0 min, 15% A, 5% B, and 80% C; 10 min, 70% A, 30% B, and 0% C; 25 min, 70% A, 30% B, and 0% C; and 28 min, 15% A, 5% B, and 80% C. The flow rate was set at 1 mL/min at room temperature and the injection volume was 20 µL. Solvents were previously filtered and degassed through a 0.22 µm membrane filter. The major peak from the *P. hadiensis* leaves extract was identified by co-elution, comparing the retention time and UV-vis spectrum overlayed with an authentic standard (Supplementary Materials Figures S2 and S3).

3.2.2. Isolation and Structural Characterization of 7α-Acetoxy-6β-Hydroxyroyleanone

The *P. hadiensis* extract was fractionated by normal phase column chromatography over silica gel using mixtures of n-hexane: EtOAc (8: 2) as eluents to give 3 fractions (A, B, and C) in order of increasing polarity. Fraction B was further studied using preparative thin-layer chromatography (n-hexane/AcOEt 7:3) on pre-coated TLC sheets (Merck 7747, Darmstadt, Germany) giving 4 fractions B1 to B4. Visualization of spots was performed under visible light and UV light (λ 254 and 366 nm) followed by spraying with a mixture of H_2SO_4: AcOH: H_2O (4:80:16) and heating. Fraction B2 was further purified by preparative chromatography affording its major compound, 7α-acetoxy-6β-hydroxyroyleanone. The NMR spectra were collected on a Bruker Fourier 300 spectrometer (^{1}H 300 MHz, ^{13}C 75 MHz) using $CDCl_3$ as the solvent. ^{1}H and ^{13}C chemical shifts are expressed in δ (ppm) and the proton coupling constants (J) in hertz (Hz) Supplementary Materials Table S1.

3.3. DPPH Radical Scavenging Assay

The free radical scavenging activity was measured by the DPPH method, as described by Rijo et al. [26]. Briefly, 10 µL of each extracted sample (1 mg of dry plant extract/mL) were added to a 990 µL solution of DPPH (0.002% in methanol). The mixture was incubated for 30 minutes in the dark, at room temperature. The absorbance (Abs) was measured at 517 nm (U-1500 Hitachi Instruments, Inc; USA). The positive control used was quercetin (10 mg/mL in methanol). An absorbance control ($Abs_{control}$) containing 10 µL of methanol and 990 µL of DPPH was also prepared. Assays were carried out in triplicate and the free radical scavenging activity was calculated using Equation (1):

$$\text{Scavenging activity } (\%) = \frac{Abs_{control} - Abs_{sample}}{Abs_{control}} \times 100 \tag{1}$$

3.4. Antimicrobial Screening Assays

3.4.1. Microorganism Used

The microorganisms used in this study were obtained from the American Type Culture Collection (ATCC). They included five strains *Enterococcus faecalis* ATCC 29212, *Escherichia coli* ATCC 25922, *Pseudomonas aeruginosa* ATCC 27853, *Staphylococcus aureus* ATCC 25923, *Saccharomyces cerevisiae* ATCC 2601, *Staphylococcus aureus*. CIP were obtained from the CIP 106760, and the yeast strain *Candida albicans* ATCC 10231.

3.4.2. Well Diffusion Method

The antimicrobial activity of each obtained extract was evaluated against two Gram-positive bacteria (*E. faecalis* and *S. aureus*), two Gram-negative bacteria (*E. coli* and *P. aeruginosa*), and two yeasts (*S. cerevisiae* and *C. albicans*), according to Rijo et al. [41]. The extracts were diluted in DMSO from 10 mg/mL to a final concentration of 1 mg/mL. Stock solutions of reference antibiotics (vancomycin, norfloxacin, and nystatin) were also prepared at 1 mg/mL in DMSO.

In aseptic conditions, Petri dishes containing 20 mL of solid Mueller–Hinton for bacteria, or *Sabouraud* Dextrose Agar culture medium (from Biokar Diagnostics), for yeasts, were inoculated with 0.1 mL of bacterial suspension matching a 0.5 McFarland standard solution and uniformly spread on the medium surface using a sterile swab. Wells of approximately 5 mm in diameter were made in the medium, using a sterile glass Pasteur pipette, and 50 µL of each extract were added into the wells. A positive control of vancomycin for Gram-positive bacteria, norfloxacin for Gram-negative bacteria, and nystatin for yeasts, and a negative control of DMSO, were used in the assay. Plates were incubated at 37 °C for 24 h. The antimicrobial activity was evaluated by measuring the diameter (mm) of the inhibition zone formed around the wells and compared to controls.

3.4.3. Minimum Inhibitory Concentration (MIC) and Minimum Bactericidal Concentration (MBC)/ Minimum Fungicidal Concentration (MFC)

The MIC and MBC/MFC were determined using the microdilution technique proposed by National Committee for Clinical Laboratory Standards (NCCLS) [42]. Briefly, 100 mL of Mueller–Hilton broth for bacteria and *Sabouraud* for yeasts was placed into each well of a 96 microplate, under aseptic conditions. Each extracted sample (100 µL), the appropriate positive control of each microorganism, and negative controls at a concentration of 1 mg/mL, were added to the first well. Using a multichannel micropipette, a 1:2 microdilution series was made. A standardized bacterial suspension (10 µL), corresponding to 0.5 McFarland of each microorganism, was then placed in all wells. Finally, the plates were incubated at 37 °C for 24 h. The MIC was determined when no growth was detected in the well of the microplate. Each measurement was performed in triplicate using 96 well microtiter plates with enrichment. A total of 10 µL was withdrawn from the microplate and sown in a Petri dish to verify the MBC/MFC, which was determined when there was no visible microbial growth on the plates [43].

3.5. Evaluation of General Toxicity on Artemia salina Model

To evaluate the general toxicity of the different extracts and *ent*-abietane diterpene 7α-acetoxy-6β-hydroxyroyleanone, a test of lethality to *Artemia salina* (brine shrimp) was performed as described by Ntungwe et al. [31]. *A. salina* eggs, dry cyst (JBL GmbH and Co. KG, D-67141 Neuhofen Germany), were hatched in artificial seawater at 25–30 °C under aeration with a concentration of 35 g/L. A handmade container with two connected chambers was used for brine shrimp hatching. The eggs were placed in one of two compartments of a container separated by a boundary plate. The cysts were then incubated (in thermostat cabinet AQUA LYTIC®, Camberley, Surrey, United Kingdom) for 48 h at 24 °C. The compartment with the eggs was covered to maintain a dark ambiance. The other compartment was illuminated to attract the phototropic newly hatched nauplii through perforations on the boundary plate. The brine shrimps that had moved to the illuminated compartment were collected and used in the lethality assay. Ten to fifteen nauplii were transferred into 24-well plates containing artificial seawater, and 100 µL of each sample was added to the wells (final volume per well: 1 mL). After 24 h exposure to the samples (24 °C), the number of dead nauplii (mortality rate (%)) was determined (Equation (2)). In addition, LC_{50} (Lethal Concentration, 50%) values (µg/mL) were calculated for the most toxic extracts. DMSO was used as the solvent and was kept at 10% (v/v) in all samples tested. Potassium dichromate was used as the positive control. All samples were tested in triplicates-at a concentration of 10 ppm for each sample.

$$()\text{Lethal concentration } (\%) = \frac{\text{Total A. salina} - \text{Alive A. salina}}{\text{Total A. salina}} \times 100 \quad (2)$$

3.6. Cytotoxicity Screening Assays

3.6.1. Cells and Cell Culture

Human colon (HCT116), breast adenocarcinoma (MCF-7), lung carcinoma (H460), and triple-negative breast cancer, MDA-MB-231S, cell lines were purchased from ATCC (Rockville, MD, USA). Cell lines were routinely cultured in 293 RPMI-1640 with ultra-glutamine or DMEM (MDA-MB-231 cells) medium from Lonza (VWR, 294 Carnaxide, Portugal) supplemented with 10% fetal bovine serum from Gibco (Alfagene, Carcavelos, Portugal) and maintained in a humidified atmosphere at 37 °C with 5% CO_2.

3.6.2. Sulphorhodamine Assay

The cytotoxicity of five of the most toxic extracts on the brine shrimp lethality bioassay was carried out using the sulforhodamine B (SRB) assay as previously described [17,44,45]. Briefly, the extracts were tested in different cancer cell lines: colon colorectal carcinoma (HCT116), human breast adenocarcinoma (MCF-7), and lung cancer carcinoma (H460). Cells were plated in 96-well plates at a final density of 5.0×10^3 cells/well and incubated for 24 h. Cells were then exposed to serial dilutions of each extract (from 1.56 to 50 µg/mL). The effect of the extracts was analyzed following 48 h incubation, using the sulforhodamine B (SRB) assay. Briefly, following fixation with 10% trichloroacetic acid from Scharlau (Sigma–Aldrich, Sintra, Portugal), plates were stained with 0.4% SRB from Sigma–Aldrich (Sintra, Portugal) and washed with 1% acetic acid. The bound dye was then solubilized with 10 mM Tris Base and the absorbance was measured at 510 nm in a microplate reader (Biotek Instruments Inc., Synergy, MX, USA). The solvent of the extracts (DMSO) corresponding to the maximum concentration used in these assays (0.25%) was included as a control. The concentration of extract that causes a 50% reduction in the net protein increase in cells (IC_{50}) was determined for all tested extracts. Data are mean ± SEM of 4–5 independent experiments.

3.6.3. MTT Assay

MDA-MB231S cell line was grown in DMEM L050-500 culture medium Biowest supplemented with 10% fetal bovine serum, L-glutamine, and penicillin-streptomycin at 37 °C and 5% CO_2. For the MTT assay, 1000 cells/well were placed in a 96-well plate and the compound to be tested was added 24 h after sowing.

The extract and compound were prepared as stock solutions in DMSO (Scrharlau; SU01531000) at a concentration of 20 mg/mL in the case of the extract (which allowed us to use a reduced DMSO percentage at higher concentrations) and 10 mM in the case of the compound. They were stored at 4 °C. The extract and compound were prepared at different concentrations. For the extract, the following dilutions were made: 80 µg/mL, 40 µg/mL, 20 µg/mL, 10 µg/mL, and 2 µg/mL in culture medium. For the compound, the following dilutions were prepared: 10 µM, 3 µM, 1 µM, 0.3 µM, and 0.1 µM. Each concentration was assayed in triplicate in a 96-well plate.

After 48 h of treatment with the compound or extract, the cells were incubated for 2 h with MTT. After this time, the culture medium was removed, and the formazan crystals were dissolved by adding 200 µL of DMSO. The absorbance of each well was measured at 595 nm.

3.7. Statistical Analysis

The results were expressed as the mean value ± SD. Comparisons were performed within groups by the analysis of variance, using the ANOVA with Dunnett's post-test. Significant differences between control and experimental groups were assessed using GraphPad Prism version 5.00 for Windows, GraphPad Software, San Diego, CA, USA, www.graphpad.com, accessed on 5 February 2021. A probability level $p < 0.05$ was considered to indicate statistical significance.

4. Conclusions

Natural products are known to be an important source of new anticancer agents. This study investigated the diverse biological activity of sixteen *Plectranthus* extracts. Among the studied extracts, *P. hadiensis* leaves and *P. mutabilis* had the highest percentage extraction yield, antimicrobial and antioxidant activities. *P. hadiensis* and *P. ciliatus* were the most cytotoxic extract against HCT116, MCF-7, and H460 cancer cell lines. 7α-acetoxy-6β-hydroxyroyleanone was isolated from the most cytotoxic extract (*P. hadiensis*) and was found to be 12 times more bioactive than the extract in the MDA-MB-231S cell line (triple-negative breast cancer). Therefore, it is noteworthy that 7α-acetoxy-6β-hydroxyroyleanone present in the most cytotoxic extract has interesting antitumoral activities in different cancer cell lines and might thus be responsible for the biological activity of this extract. However further phytochemical studies should be done to find out more compounds that could contribute to the cytotoxicity of *P. hadiensis*.

Supplementary Materials: The following are available online at https://www.mdpi.com/article/10.3390/ph14050402/s1, Figure S1: 1H-NMR data information for 7α-acetoxy-6β-hydroxyroyleanone, Figure S2: HPLC chromatograms (270 nm) of *P. hadiensis* leaves showing the major compound, 7α-acetoxy-6β-hydroxyroyleanone, Figure S3: UV spectrum of 7α-acetoxy-6β-hydroxyroyleanone, Figure S4: Concentration-response curves (IC_{50} µM) for 7α-acetoxy-6β-hydroxyroyleanone; Table S1: NMR spectroscopy data characterization, ^{1}H NMR (300 MHz, CDCl$_3$), ^{13}C (75 MHz, CDCl$_3$.

Author Contributions: Conceptualization, P.R.; methodology, E.N., L.S., C.T., S.T.-T. and N.A.C.; validation, L.S., A.M.D.-L. and P.R.; investigation, E.N., L.S., C.T., S.T.-T. and N.A.C.; writing—original draft preparation, E.N.; writing—review and editing, E.M.D.-M., L.S, A.M.D.-L., P.R. and N.D.; supervision, N.D. and P.R. All authors have read and agreed to the published version of the manuscript.

Funding: This research was funded by Fundação para a Ciência e Tecnologia (FCT) projects UIDP/04567/2020, UIDB/04567/2020, CBIOS/COFAC/FIPID/1/2019 and COFAC/ILIND/CBIOS/1/2020. The authors gratefully acknowledge Fundação para a Ciência e Tecnologia (FCT) for the financial support under the reference CBIOS/COFAC/FIPID/1/2019, UIDB/50006/2020, UID/MULTI/04378/2013 and the project (3599-PPCDT) PTDC/DTP-FTO/1981/2014–POCI-01-0145-FEDER-016581 and the predoctoral FPU 2019 fellowship from the University of Alcalá awarded to E.M.D-M.

Data Availability Statement: Not applicable.

Acknowledgments: This work was supported by PADDIC 2019 (ALIES-COFAC) as part of the PhD Program in Health Sciences from Universidad de Alcalá and Universidade Lusófona de Humanidades e Tecnologias.

Conflicts of Interest: The authors declare no conflict of interest. The funders had no role in the design of the study; in the collection, analyses, or interpretation of data; in the writing of the manuscript, or in the decision to publish the results.

References

1. Wu, C.; Lee, S.L.; Taylor, C.; Li, J.; Chan, Y.M.; Agarwal, R.; Temple, R.; Throckmorton, D.; Tyner, K. Scientific and Regulatory Approach to Botanical Drug Development: A U.S. FDA Perspective. *J. Nat. Prod.* **2020**, *83*, 552–562. [CrossRef] [PubMed]
2. Newman, D.J.; Cragg, G.M. Natural Products as Sources of New Drugs over the Nearly Four Decades from 01/1981 to 09/2019. *J. Nat. Prod.* **2020**, *83*, 770–803. [CrossRef]
3. World Health Organization (WHO). Fact Sheet on Cancer. Available online: https://www.who.int/news-room/fact-sheets/detail/cancer (accessed on 5 February 2021).
4. Zhang, X.; Zhang, S.; Yang, Y.; Wang, D.; Gao, H. Natural barrigenol–like triterpenoids: A comprehensive review of their contributions to medicinal chemistry. *Phytochemistry* **2019**, *161*, 41–74. [CrossRef] [PubMed]
5. Alam, A.; Jaiswal, V.; Akhtar, S.; Jayashree, B.S.; Dhar, K.L. Isolation of isoflavones from Iris kashmiriana Baker as potential anti proliferative agents targeting NF-kappaB. *Phytochemistry* **2017**, *136*, 70–80. [CrossRef] [PubMed]
6. Saksham Garg, A.R. A Current Perspective of Plants as an Antibacterial Agent: A Review. *Curr. Pharm. Biotechnol.* **2020**, *21*, 1588. [CrossRef] [PubMed]
7. Arumugam, G.; Swamy, M.K.; Sinniah, U.R. Plectranthus amboinicus (Lour.) Spreng: Botanical, Phytochemical, Pharmacological and Nutritional Significance. *Molecules* **2016**, *21*, 369. [CrossRef] [PubMed]
8. Al Musayeib, N.M.; Amina, M.; Al-Hamoud, G.A.; Mohamed, G.A.; Ibrahim, S.R.M.; Shabana, S. Plectrabarbene, a new abietane diterpene from plectranthus barbatus aerial parts. *Molecules* **2020**, *25*, 2365. [CrossRef] [PubMed]
9. Garcia, C.; Silva, C.O.; Monteiro, C.M.; Nicolai, M.; Gonz, I.; Ana, M.D. Anticancer properties of the abietane diterpene 6,7-dehydroroyleanone obtained by optimized extraction. *Future Med. Chem.* **2018**, *10*. [CrossRef] [PubMed]
10. Pereira, M.; Matias, D.; Pereira, F.; Reis, C.; Simões, M.F.; Rijo, P. Antimicrobial screening of Plectranthus madagascariensis and P. neochilus extracts. *Biomed. Biopharm. Res.* **2015**, *12*, 127–138. [CrossRef]
11. Garcia, C.; Teodósio, C.; Oliveira, C.; Oliveira, A.; Reis, C.; Duarte, N.; Rijo, P. Naturally Occurring Plectranthus-derived Diterpenes with Antitumoral Activities. *Curr. Pharm. Des.* **2019**, *24*, 4207–4236. [CrossRef]
12. Abdissa, N.; Frese, M.; Sewald, N. Antimicrobial abietane-type diterpenoids from plectranthus punctatus. *Molecules* **2017**, *22*, 1919. [CrossRef]
13. Pirttimaa, M.; Nasereddin, A.; Kopelyanskiy, D.; Kaiser, M.; Yli-Kauhaluoma, J.; Oksman-Caldentey, K.M.; Brun, R.; Jaffe, C.L.; Moreira, V.M.; Alakurtti, S. Abietane-Type Diterpenoid Amides with Highly Potent and Selective Activity against Leishmania donovani and Trypanosoma cruzi. *J. Nat. Prod.* **2016**, *79*, 362–368. [CrossRef]
14. Isca, V.M.S.; Andrade, J.; Fernandes, A.S.; Paix, P.; Uriel, C.; Mar, A. In Vitro Antimicrobial Activity of Isopimarane-Type Diterpenoids. *Molecules* **2020**, *25*, 4250. [CrossRef]
15. Mesquita, L.S.F.; Matos, T.S.; Do Nascimento Ávila, F.; Da Silva Batista, A.; Moura, A.F.; De Moraes, M.O.; Da Silva, M.C.M.; Ferreira, T.L.A.; Nascimento, N.R.F.; Monteiro, N.K.V.; et al. Diterpenoids from Leaves of cultivated Plectranthus ornatus. *Planta Med.* **2020**. [CrossRef]
16. Śliwiński, T.; Sitarek, P.; Skała, E.; Isca, V.M.S.; Synowiec, E.; Kowalczyk, T.; Bijak, M.; Rijo, P. Diterpenoids from Plectranthus spp. As potential chemotherapeutic agents via apoptosis. *Pharmaceuticals* **2020**, *13*, 123. [CrossRef]
17. Garcia, C.; Ntungwe, E.; Rebelo, A.; Bessa, C.; Stankovic, T.; Dinic, J.; Díaz-Lanza, A.; Reis, C.P.; Roberto, A.; Pereira, P.; et al. Parvifloron D from Plectranthus strigosus: Cytotoxicity screening of Plectranthus spp. extracts. *Biomolecules* **2019**, *9*, 616. [CrossRef]
18. Cretton, S.; Saraux, N.; Monteillier, A.; Righi, D.; Marcourt, L.; Genta-Jouve, G.; Wolfender, J.L.; Cuendet, M.; Christen, P. Anti-inflammatory and antiproliferative diterpenoids from Plectranthus scutellarioides. *Phytochemistry* **2018**, *154*, 39–46. [CrossRef]
19. Simões, M.F.; Rijo, P.; Duarte, A.; Barbosa, D.; Matias, D.; Delgado, J.; Cirilo, N.; Rodríguez, B. Two new diterpenoids from Plectranthus species. *Phytochem. Lett.* **2010**, *3*, 221–225. [CrossRef]
20. Mothana, R.A.; Al-Said, M.S.; Al-Musayeib, N.M.; El Gamal, A.A.; Al-Massarani, S.M.; Al-Rehaily, A.J.; Abdulkader, M.; Maes, L. In vitro antiprotozoal activity of abietane diterpenoids isolated from Plectranthus barbatus andr. *Int. J. Mol. Sci.* **2014**, *15*, 8360–8371. [CrossRef]
21. Matias, D.; Nicolai, M.; Saraiva, L.; Pinheiro, R.; Faustino, C.; Diaz Lanza, A.; Pinto Reis, C.; Stankovic, T.; Dinic, J.; Pesic, M.; et al. Cytotoxic Activity of Royleanone Diterpenes from Plectranthus madagascariensis Benth. *ACS Omega* **2019**, *4*, 8094–8103. [CrossRef]
22. Garcia, C.; Isca, V.M.S.; Pereira, F.; Monteiro, C.M.; Ntungwe, E.; Sousa, F.; Dinic, J.; Holmstedt, S.; Roberto, A.; Díaz-Lanza, A.; et al. Royleanone Derivatives from Plectranthus spp. as a Novel Class of P-Glycoprotein Inhibitors. *Front. Pharmacol.* **2020**, *11*, 1711. [CrossRef]
23. Isca, V.M.S.; Ferreira, R.J.; Garcia, C.; Monteiro, C.M.; Dinic, J.; Holmstedt, S.; André, V.; Pesic, M.; Dos Santos, D.J.V.A.; Candeias, N.R.; et al. Molecular Docking Studies of Royleanone Diterpenoids from Plectranthus spp. as P-Glycoprotein Inhibitors. *ACS Med. Chem. Lett.* **2020**, *11*, 839–845. [CrossRef]
24. Isca, V.M.S.; Sencanski, M.; Filipovic, N.; Dos Santos, D.J.V.A.; Gašparović, A.Č.; Saraíva, L.; Afonso, C.A.M.; Rijo, P.; García-Sosa, A.T. Activity to breast cancer cell lines of different malignancy and predicted interaction with protein kinase C isoforms of royleanones. *Int. J. Mol. Sci.* **2020**, *21*, 3671. [CrossRef]
25. Saraiva, N.; Costa, J.G.; Reis, C.; Almeida, N.; Rijo, P.; Fernandes, A.S. Anti-migratory and pro-apoptotic properties of parvifloron d on triple-negative breast cancer cells. *Biomolecules* **2020**, *10*, 158. [CrossRef]
26. Padmapriya, R.; Ashwini, S.; Raveendran, R. In vitro antioxidant and cytotoxic potential of different parts of Tephrosia purpurea. *Res. Pharm. Sci.* **2017**, *12*, 31–37. [CrossRef]

27. Rijo, P.; Batista, M.; Matos, M.; Rocha, H.; Jesus, S.; Simões, M.F. Screening of antioxidant and antimicrobial activities on *Plectranthus* spp. extracts. *Biomed. Biopharm. Res.* **2012**, *9*, 225–235. [CrossRef]
28. Andrade, J.M.; Domínguez-Martín, E.M.; Nicolai, M.; Faustino, C.; Rodrigues, L.M.; Rijo, P. Screening the dermatological potential of plectranthus species components: Antioxidant and inhibitory capacities over elastase, collagenase and tyrosinase. *J. Enzym. Inhib. Med. Chem.* **2021**, *36*, 257–269. [CrossRef]
29. Ndjoubi, K.O.; Sharma, R.; Badmus, J.A.; Jacobs, A.; Jordaan, A.; Marnewick, J.; Warner, D.F.; Hussein, A.A. Antimycobacterial, Cytotoxic, and Antioxidant Activities of Abietane Diterpenoids Isolated from *Plectranthus madagascariensis*. *Plants* **2021**, *10*, 175. [CrossRef]
30. Matias, D.; Nicolai, M.; Fernandes, A.S.; Saraiva, N.; Almeida, J.; Saraiva, L.; Faustino, C.; Díaz-Lanza, A.M.; Reis, C.P.; Rijo, P. Comparison study of different extracts of *Plectranthus madagascariensis*, *P. neochilus* and the rare *P. porcatus* (lamiaceae): Chemical characterization, antioxidant, antimicrobial and cytotoxic activities. *Biomolecules* **2019**, *9*, 179. [CrossRef]
31. Ntungwe, N.E.; Marçalo, J.; Garcia, C.; Reis, C.; Teodósio, C.; Oliveira, C.; Oliveira, C.; Roberto, A. Biological activity screening of seven *Plectranthus* species. *J. Biomed. Biopharm. Res.* **2017**, *14*, 95–108. [CrossRef]
32. Mogana, R.; Adhikari, A.; Tzar, M.N.; Ramliza, R.; Wiart, C. Antibacterial activities of the extracts, fractions and isolated compounds from *Canarium patentinervium* miq. Against bacterial clinical isolates. *BMC Complement. Med. Ther.* **2020**, *20*, 55. [CrossRef] [PubMed]
33. Ntungwe, N.E.; Domínguez-Martín, E.M.; Roberto, A.; Tavares, J.; Isca, V.M.S.; Pereira, P.; Cebola, M.-J.; Rijo, P. *Artemia* species: An Important Tool to Screen General Toxicity Samples. *Curr. Pharm. Des.* **2020**, *26*, 2892–2908. [CrossRef] [PubMed]
34. Srisawat, T.; Chumkaew, P.; Heed-Chim, W.; Sukpondma, Y.; Kanokwiroon, K. Phytochemical screening and cytotoxicity of crude extracts of vatica diospyroides Symington type LS. *Trop. J. Pharm. Res.* **2013**, *12*, 71–76. [CrossRef]
35. Kathryn, J.; Sireesha, V.; Stanley, L. Triple Negative Breast Cancer Cell Lines: One Tool in the Search for Better Treatment of Triple Negative Breast Cancer. *Breast Dis.* **2012**, *32*, 35–48. [CrossRef]
36. Burmistrova, O.; Simões, M.F.; Rijo, P.; Quintana, J.; Bermejo, J.; Estévez, F. Antiproliferative activity of abietane diterpenoids against human tumor cells. *J. Nat. Prod.* **2013**, *76*, 1413–1423. [CrossRef]
37. Bernardes, C.E.S.; Garcia, C.; Pereira, F.; Mota, J.; Pereira, P.; Cebola, M.J.; Reis, C.P.; Correia, I.; Piedade, M.F.M.; Minas Da Piedade, M.E.; et al. Extraction Optimization and Structural and Thermal Characterization of the Antimicrobial Abietane 7α-Acetoxy-6β-hydroxyroyleanone. *Mol. Pharm.* **2018**, *15*, 1412–1419. [CrossRef]
38. Abdel-Mogib, M.; Albar, H.A.; Batterjee, S.M. Chemistry of the genus *Plectranthus*. *Molecules* **2002**, *7*, 271–301. [CrossRef]
39. Sitarek, P.; Toma, M.; Ntungwe, E.; Kowalczyk, T.; Skała, E.; Wieczfinska, J.; Śliwiński, T.; Rijo, P. Insight the biological activities of selected abietane diterpenes isolated from *Plectranthus* spp. *Biomolecules* **2020**, *10*, 194. [CrossRef]
40. The Plant List. Version 1.1. 2013. Available online: http://www.theplantlist.org/ (accessed on 1 January 2021).
41. Rijo, P.; Matias, D.; Fernandes, A.S.; Simões, M.F.; Nicolai, M.; Reis, C.P. Antimicrobial plant extracts encapsulated into polymeric beads for potential application on the skin. *Polymers* **2014**, *6*, 479–490. [CrossRef]
42. CLSI Padronização dos Testes de Sensibilidade a Antimicrobianos por Disco-difusão. In *Norma Aprovada—Oitava Edição*; NCCLS: Wayne, PA, USA, 2003; Volume 23, ISBN 1-56238-485-6.
43. Brandão, F.; Isabel, M.; Ramos, L.; Miyagusku, L. Antimicrobial activity of hydroalcoholic extracts from genipap, baru and taruma. *Cienc. Rural* **2017**, *47*, 6–11. [CrossRef]
44. Leão, M.; Soares, J.; Gomes, S.; Raimundo, L.; Ramos, H.; Bessa, C.; Queiroz, G.; Domingos, S.; Pinto, M.; Inga, A.; et al. Enhanced cytotoxicity of prenylated chalcone against tumour cells via disruption of the p53-MDM2 interaction. *Life Sci.* **2015**, *142*, 60–65. [CrossRef]
45. Soares, J.; Pereira, N.A.; Monteiro, Â.; Leão, M.; Bessa, C.; Dos Santos, D.J.; Raimundo, L.; Queiroz, G.; Bisio, A.; Inga, A.; et al. Oxazoloisoindolinones with in vitro antitumor activity selectively activate a p53-pathway through potential inhibition of the p53–MDM2 interaction. *Eur. J. Pharm. Sci.* **2015**, *66*, 138–147. [CrossRef]

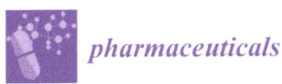

Article

Effects of Essential Oils and Some Constituents from Ingredients of Anti-Cellulite Herbal Compress on 3T3-L1 Adipocytes and Rat Aortae

Ngamrayu Ngamdokmai [1], Tamkeen Urooj Paracha [2], Neti Waranuch [3], Krongkarn Chootip [4], Wudtichai Wisuitiprot [5], Nungruthai Suphrom [6], Kamonlak Insumrong [6] and Kornkanok Ingkaninan [1,*]

[1] Centre of Excellence in Cannabis Research, Department of Pharmaceutical Chemistry and Pharmacognosy, Faculty of Pharmaceutical Sciences and Center of Excellence for Innovation in Chemistry, Naresuan University, Phitsanulok 65000, Thailand; ngamrayun59@nu.ac.th

[2] Department of Pharmacology, Faculty of Pharmacy, Hamdard University, Main Campus, Karachi 74600, Pakistan; tamkeen.urooj@hamdard.edu

[3] Cosmetics and Natural Products Research Center and Center of Excellence for Innovation in Chemistry, Department of Pharmaceutical Technology, Faculty of Pharmaceutical Sciences, Naresuan University, Phitsanulok 65000, Thailand; netiw@nu.ac.th

[4] Department of Physiology, Faculty of Medical Sciences, Naresuan University, Phitsanulok 65000, Thailand; krongkarnc@nu.ac.th

[5] Department of Thai Traditional Medicine, Sirindhorn College of Public Health, Phitsanulok 65130, Thailand; wudtichai@scphpl.ac.th

[6] Department of Chemistry, Faculty of Science and Center of Excellence for Innovation in Chemistry, Naresuan University, Phitsanulok 65000, Thailand; nungruthais@nu.ac.th (N.S.); kamonlaki59@nu.ac.th (K.I.)

* Correspondence: k_ingkaninan@yahoo.com or kornkanoki@nu.ac.th; Tel.: +66-5596-1860 or +66-8148-17350; Fax: +66-5596-3731

Abstract: Cellulite is associated with a complex array of adipocytes under the skin and vascular system. A herbal compress that was previously developed was proven to have an anti-cellulite effect in healthy volunteers within 2 weeks of treatment. However, its mechanism and ingredients responsible for reducing cellulite were not known. The purpose of this study was to investigate the activity of eight essential oils in, and two water extracts from, the ingredients of the herbal compress together with nine monoterpenoid constituents on the 3T3-L1 adipocytes. The vasodilatory effect on rat aortae was also studied. The adipocytes were induced by dexamethasone, 3-isobutyl-1-methylxanthine and insulin. At all concentrations tested, all essential oils, water extracts and their monoterpenoid constituents significantly inhibited lipid accumulation activity ($p < 0.05$) and decreased the amount of triglycerides when compared to untreated cells ($p < 0.01$). In addition, our results showed that the mixed oil distilled from the herbal compress mixed ingredients could relax the isolated rat aorta ($EC_{50} = 14.74 \pm 2.65$ µg/mL). In conclusion, all essential oils, extracts and chemical constituents tested showed effects on adipogenesis inhibition and lipolysis induction on the cultured adipocytes with the mixed oil demonstrating vasorelaxation activity, all of which might be the mechanisms of the anti-cellulite effects of the herbal compress.

Keywords: cellulite; essential oil; monoterpenes; Thai herbal compress; adipogenesis; lipolysis; vasorelaxation

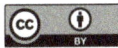

1. Introduction

Cellulite is associated with excessive fat accumulation and increases in size and number of adipocytes under the skin, which is caused by genetic, dietary, behavior and hormones. Cellulite is usually found around the thighs and buttocks of post-pubescent females. The increase in these cellulite deposits causes them to invade the dermis which disrupts the tissue architecture, microcirculation, skin elasticity and dermal thickness, resulting in the orange peel-like appearance of the skin [1,2].

There are basically two pathways which can be targeted to achieve cellulite reduction. First, the inhibition of lipogenesis to prevent fat storage in the adipocytes, and, second, the induction of lipolysis which is the metabolic pathway through which lipid triglycerides are hydrolyzed into a glycerol and three fatty acids. Essentially, this is the process of the decomposition of the chemical that causes fat to be released from the adipose tissue by the hydrolysis of the ester bonds in the triglycerides of the fatty tissue under the skin. In addition, the enlarged fat cells, evident as cellulite, lead to the alteration in the microvascular network of the fat tissue, resulting in water retention, which results in the compression of the vascular vessels and in cellular changes [3,4]. There are known compounds, such as retinol, that improve the appearance of cellulite by increasing the microcirculation [5]. The mixture of retinol, caffeine and ruscogenin could increase microcirculation on the thigh of 46 women who showed moderate degrees of cellulite [6].

The use of herbal compresses is popular in traditional Thai therapies, such as in traditional message and spa. These compresses contain herbs bundled within a cloth to form a ball which is warmed and applied to relieve muscle pains, stress and strains. In previous studies [7,8], we modified a Thai traditional herbal compress to use as an anti-cellulite product. The formulation contained *Zingiber officinale* Roscoe rhizomes (ginger), *Piper nigrum* L. fruit (black pepper), *Piper retrofractum* Vahl. Fruit (java long pepper), *Camellia sinensis* (L.) Kuntze leaf (tea) and *Coffea arabica* L. seed (coffee) as the principal ingredients together with some auxiliary herbs i.e., *Zingiber montanum* (J. Koenig) Link ex A.Dietr. rhizomes (Cassumunar ginger or plai), *Curcuma longa* L. rhizomes (turmeric), *Cymbopogon citratus* DC. Stapf. leaves (lemon grass), *Citrus hystrix* DC. fruit peels (kaffir lime), with camphor and salts added for both scent and skin penetration. In those prior studies, the anti-cellulite effects of the herbal compress were determined via a double-blinded, randomized placebo-controlled trial conducted on 21 female volunteers aged 20 to 55 over an 8-week test period. The results showed that the herbal compress could significantly reduce thigh circumference, skin fold thickness and the severity of cellulite within 2 weeks. However, the mechanisms of this action and the bioactive constituents responsible for such an action were not identified.

In our current study, we distilled the essential oils of the herbal compress and each ingredient, with the tea leaves and coffee beans being extracted by water. All samples were tested, together with their major monoterpenoid constituents (camphor, camphene, citral, 3-carene, limonene, myrcene, alpha-pinene, beta-pinene and terpinene-4-ol), for their anti-cellulite effects. The effects of these samples on lipid accumulation were demonstrated, in vitro, on the mouse adipocyte cell 3T3L1 model and the inhibiting of adipogenesis and stimulation of lipolysis was observed and measured. Further, the vasorelaxant effect of the mixture of the essential oil, distilled from the powdered form of all ingredients, was tested on the aortae isolated from rats.

2. Results and Discussion

2.1. Cell Viability

Notably, 3T3-L1 adipocytes are widely used in assays of adipogenesis because they can tolerate an increased number of passages and homogeneously respond to treatments [9,10]. Prior to our study of the effects of essential oils/extracts and their major monoterpenoid constituents on adipogenesis and lipolysis of 3T3-L1 adipocytes, we tested the viability of the various concentrations (1–500 µg/mL) of the samples on the preadipocytes and adipocytes.

In addition, the viability of the samples on keratinocyte, fibroblast was studied to provide safety information. The highest dilution that resulted in more than 80% cells being viable was considered to be the non-toxic concentration to be used in our further studies on adipogenesis and lipolysis of 3T3-L1 adipocytes. Table 1 illustrates the non-toxic levels of the tested concentrations.

Table 1. Non-toxic concentrations of 7 essential oils, mixed oil, tea and coffee extracts, and their major constituents in anti-cellulite herbal compress selected from 3-(4,5-dimethylthiazol-2-yl)-2,5-diphenyl-tetrazolium bromide (MTT) assay.

Samples	Concentrations (µg/mL)			
	KR [1]	FB [2]	PA [3]	A [4]
1. Lemon grass oil	31.25	31.25	31.25	62.5
2. Ginger oil	62.5	125	62.5	125
3. Black pepper oil	125	125	125	125
4. Long pepper oil	125	250	125	250
5. Tea water extract	125	250	125	250
6. Turmeric oil	125	250	125	250
7. Cassumunar ginger oil	250	250	250	250
8. Coffee water extract	250	250	250	250
9. Kaffir lime oil	250	250	250	250
10. Mixed oil	250	250	250	250
11. Camphor	ND	ND	200	200
12. Camphene	ND	ND	200	200
13. Citral	ND	ND	200	200
14. 3-carene	ND	ND	200	200
15. D-limonene	ND	ND	200	200
16. β-myrcene	ND	ND	200	200
17. α-pinene	ND	ND	200	200
18. β-pinene	ND	ND	200	200
19. Terpinene-4-ol	ND	ND	200	200
20. Caffeine		1 mM (194.2 µg/mL)		
21. Adrenaline		0.1 mM (18.3 µg/mL)		

[1] Keratinocyte; [2] Fibroblast; [3] 3T3-L1 preadipocyte; and [4] adipocyte cells. (ND = not determined).

2.2. Preventive and Treatment Effects of Essential Oils/Extracts and Their Major Monoterpenoid Constituents on Adipogenesis of 3T3-L1 Cells

Adipogenesis is a complex process by which pre-adipocytes transform into adipocytes. Oil red O staining is the most commonly used method for distinguishing adipocytes from other cells and has recently been used as a quantitative method to assess different degrees of adipocyte differentiation [11]. In our study, the pre-adipocytes were treated with dexamethasone, 3-isobutyl-1-methyl xanthine (IBMX) and insulin to induce the differentiation. After nine days, the formation of adipocytes was evaluated. The preventive and treatment effects of the essential oils distilled from the ingredients of the herbal compress and the aqueous extracts of tea and coffee on adipogenesis were studied at the concentrations that were non-toxic to the cells. To investigate the preventive effect, the samples were added to the media on day 3, 5 and 7 after the initiation. Their effects on 3T3-L1 adipocyte differentiation were observed via lipid accumulation oil red O staining on day 9. To evaluate the treatment effect, the samples were incubated with the mature adipocyte on day 9 after the initiation and their effects were measured on day 10.

The results showed that all samples had preventive effects on adipogenesis in a dose-dependent manner. Of the samples tested, lemon grass oil demonstrated inhibition of lipid accumulations at a concentration of 12.5 µg/mL that was 23 ± 6%, which was the lowest effective concentration of all samples tested (Figure 1A). As well as lemon grass, another promising sample was ginger oil, which gave 33 ± 5% inhibition at the concentration of 50 µg/mL. The remaining essential oils and extracts tested showed around 30% inhibition at the concentration of 100–200 µg/mL, whereas the positive controls i.e., 18 µg/mL adrenaline and 194 µg/mL caffeine expressed 24 ± 5% and 25 ± 2% inhibition, respectively. Manaharan et al. 2016 reported that ginger oil at various concentrations (50 to 800 µg/mL) significantly decreased lipid content in mature adipocytes in a dose-dependent fashion [12]. Coffee and tea have shown anti-obesity and anti-adiposity activities in adipocytes in some previous studies [13,14]. Both coffee extracts and their major constituents, namely caffeine, caffeic acid, chlorogenic acid and trigonelline, increased glycerol release while also reducing the accumulation in the 3T3-L1 cells during adipocytic differentiation. Also, the expression of the peroxisome proliferator-activated receptor γ (PPARγ), a transcription factor that controls the differentiation of adipocytes, is inhibited by the consumption of coffee. Also, as reported by [15,16], the main theaflavin of tea, polyphenols and theaflavin-3,3′-digallate (TF3), demonstrated an anti-adiposity effect in mature adipocytes through the activation of the AMPK pathway. Further, Goto et al. [17] showed that several bioactive terpenoids, which are derived from herbal and dietary plants, function as PPAR modulators as regulators of carbohydrate and lipid metabolism. However, the anti-adipogenic effects of the essential oils distilled from lemongrass, black pepper, long pepper, turmeric and cassumunar ginger, as well as the mixed oil from herbal compresses, are reported here for the first time.

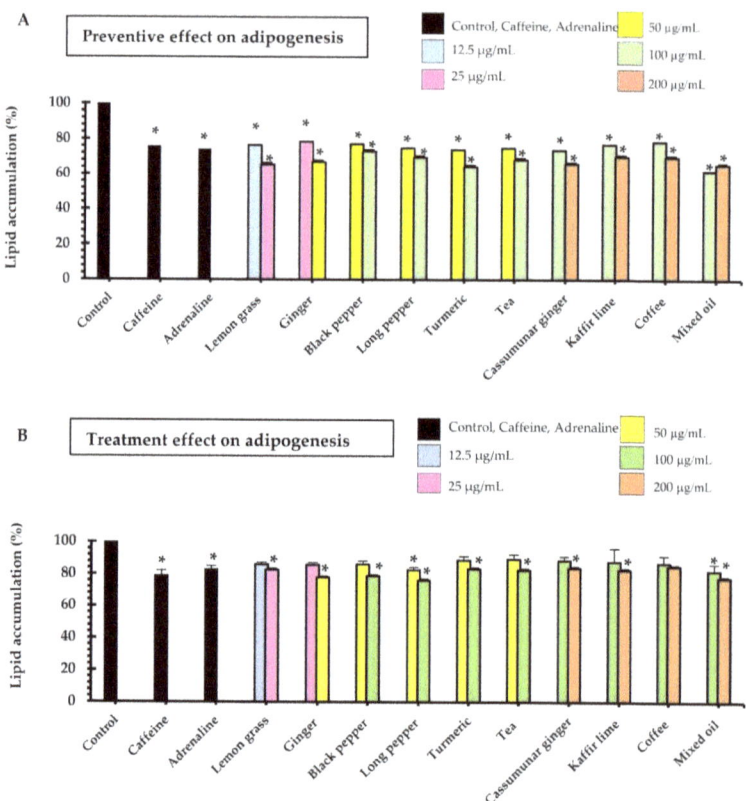

Figure 1. Lipid accumulation in 3T3-L1 adipocytes after treated with essential oil, extracts and positive controls (adrenaline 0.1 mM or 18.3 µg/mL and caffeine 1 mM or 194.2 µg/mL); (**A**) in the preventive experiments where the pre-adipocytes were treated with the samples during the differentiation on days 3, 5 and 7, and (**B**) in the treatment experiments where the samples were added after the pre-adipocytes were differentiated to adipocytes (on day 9) and incubated for one day. The lipid accumulation was measured by Oil Red O assay, and the results are expressed as the mean ± SEM of triplicate tests. Data expressed in percentage in comparison with control. One-way ANOVA showed significant value, * $p < 0.05$ as compared to control.

The lipid accumulation, after the mature adipocytes had been treated with samples of the essential oils and tea and coffee extract, was evaluated to ascertain the effect of the treatment. Figure 1B shows that lemon grass (25 µg/mL), ginger (50 µg/mL), black pepper (100 µg/mL), long pepper (50, 100 µg/mL) and mixed oil (100, 200 µg/mL) significantly inhibited lipid accumulation in the range of 12–24%. Interestingly, the positive controls i.e., 18 µg/mL adrenaline and 194 µg/mL caffeine showed the same range of % lipid accumulation inhibition (21% and 17%, respectively). All samples tended to decrease intracellular lipids in a concentration-dependent manner. The maximum inhibition of lipid accumulation (24%) was observed from 100 µg/mL long pepper oil. It is noted that the positive controls as well as all test samples could reduce lipid accumulations on 3T3-L1 adipocytes in both preventive and treatment experiments where the degree of reduction was greater in the preventive experiments. The samples that clearly showed significantly higher % lipid accumulation in the preventive experiments when compared to the treatment experiments were turmeric, cassumunar ginger, tea and mixed oil ($p < 0.05$).

Nine monoterpenoid constituents of the herbal compress ingredients were tested for their preventive and treatment effects on adipogenesis of 3T3-L1 adipocytes (Figure 2). The results showed that all samples significantly inhibited lipid accumulation as compared to the control cells in both preventive and treatment ways, although most samples tended to have a higher preventive effect than the treatmentive effect. The significant difference between preventive effects and treatment effects are shown in citral (50, and 100 µg/mL, $p < 0.001$), and 3-carene (100 µg/mL, $p < 0.05$). For the effective effect, the highest inhibition of lipid accumulation was observed in limonene at the concentration of 100 µg/mL, with 47 ± 2% inhibition. The limonene compound significantly decreased lipid accumulation more than the caffeine (194.2 µg/mL, 38 ± 1% inhibition) and adrenaline (18.3 µg/mL, 34 ± 3% inhibition). For the treatment effect of the intracellular lipid accumulation, these results indicated that the nine major monoterpenoid constituents inhibited lipid accumulation (Figure 2B). These data also show that camphor, camphene, citral, 3-carene, alpha-pinene in the concentration of 100 µg/mL as well as limonene, myrcene, beta-pinene and terpinene-4-ol in the concentrations of 50 and 100 µg/mL significantly inhibited lipid accumulation by 20–33% where caffeine (18 µg/mL) showed 18 ± 1% inhibition and adrenaline (194 µg/mL) showed 21 ± 3% inhibition. The highest % inhibition of lipid accumulation was observed in limonene at 100 µg/mL (38 ± 4%), which was significantly higher than caffeine and adrenaline ($p < 0.05$). A previous animal study [18] showed the preventive effects of limonene on hyperglycemia and dyslipidemia in high-fat diet-induced obesity mice. In addition, limonene was reported to be effective in regulating the peroxisome proliferator-activated receptor (PPAR)-α signaling and liver X receptor (LXR)-β signaling. The microscopic pictures of 3T3-L1 adipocytes after stained with Oil Red O in preventive and treatment experiments are shown in Figure 3.

2.3. Effects of Essential Oils/Extracts and Their Major Monoterpenoid Constituents on Triglyceride Accumulation of Adipogenesis of 3T3-L1 Cells

In addition to inhibition of adipocyte differentiation and mature adipocyte, we also determined the effect of the test samples on triglyceride accumulation of 3T3-L1 adipocytes causing the in vitro lipolysis effect. Excessive amounts of triglyceride accumulation in the adipocyte is related to an increased risk of a variety metabolic disease. In our study, treatment of cells with seven essential oils, mixed oil and tea and coffee extracts decreased triglyceride accumulation in differentiated 3T3-L1 cells. The amount of intracellular triglyceride accumulated in adipocytes was significantly decreased at all concentration levels tested (Figure 4A,B) when compared to the effect in the untreated control cells.

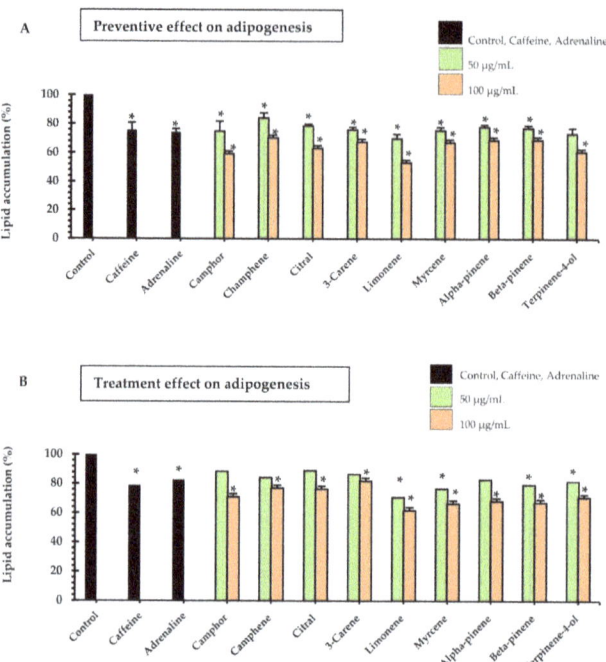

Figure 2. Lipid accumulation in 3T3-L1 adipocytes after treated with monoterpenoid constituents of the herbal compress ingredients and positive controls (adrenaline 0.1 mM or 18.3 μg/mL and caffeine 1 mM or 194.2 μg/mL); (**A**) in the preventive experiments where the pre-adipocytes were treated with the samples during the differentiation on days 3, 5 and 7, and (**B**) in the treatment experiments where the samples were added after the pre-adipocytes were differentiated to adipocytes (on day 9) and incubated for one day. The lipid accumulation was measured by Oil Red O assay, and the results expressed as the mean ± SEM of triplicate tests. Data expressed in percentage in comparison with control. One-way ANOVA showed significant value, * $p < 0.05$ as compared to control.

The lowest concentration that significantly decreased triglyceride content was observed in lemon grass oil (25 μg/mL, 53 ± 3% triglyceride content). Five essential oils that demonstrated the most prominent decrease for the triglyceride content were long pepper oil (100 μg/mL, 42 ± 6% triglyceride content), black pepper (100 μg/mL, 47 ± 5% triglyceride content), coffee (200 μg/mL, 47 ± 7% triglyceride content), kaffir lime (200 μg/mL, 50 ± 5% triglyceride content) and mixed oil (200 μg/mL, 50 ± 2% triglyceride content). A total of 1 mM of Caffeine decreased the triglyceride contents by 41 ± 2% and 0.1 mM adrenaline decreased triglyceride accumulation by 67 ± 4% (relative to the control).

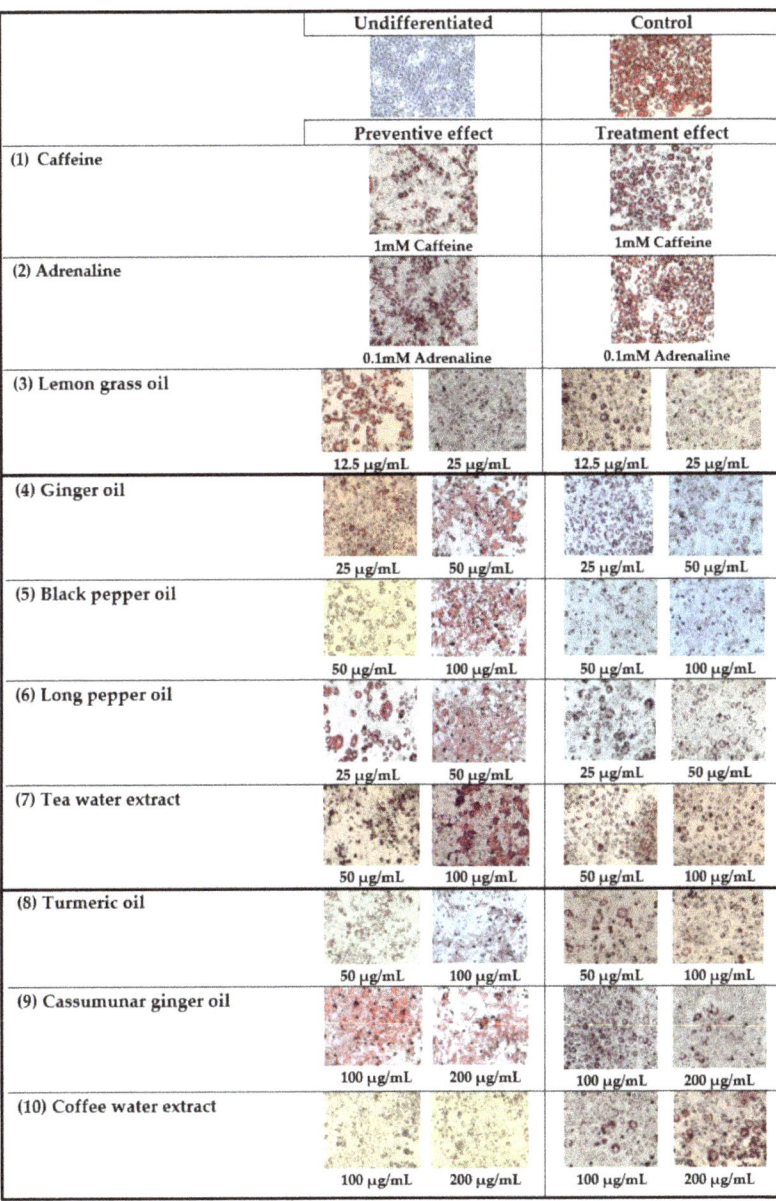

Figure 3. Cont.

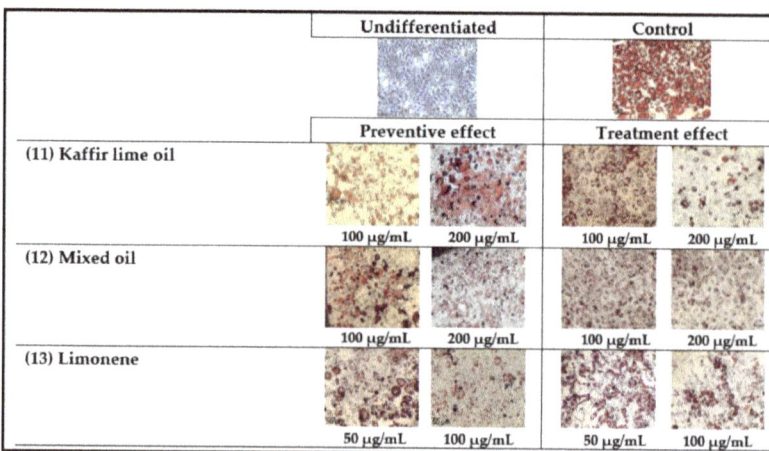

Figure 3. Representative photographs (20×) of 3T3-L1 adipocytes stained with Oil Red O after treatment with the essential oils, extracts and limonene in comparison with undifferentiated and control cells. To study the preventive effect, the mature adipocytes were treated with samples (1–13) on days 3, 5 and 7 after the initiation and the oil red O staining was conducted on day 9. For treatment effect, the samples were incubated with the mature adipocyte on day 9 and their effects were measured on day 10. Notably, 1 mM (18.3 µg/mL) caffeine and 0.1 mM (194.2 µg/mL) adrenaline were used as positive controls.

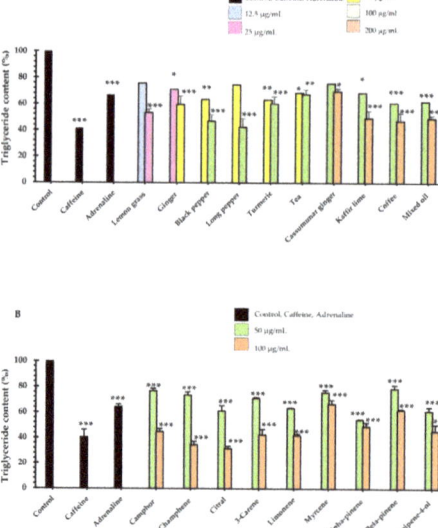

Figure 4. The effects of (**A**) the essential oils/extracts, and (**B**) monoterpenoid constituents on triglyceride content of 3T3-L1 adipocytes after treatment for 24 h. Intracellular triacylglycerol content was determined using enzymatic colorimetric methods. We used 1 mM (18.2 µg/mL) caffeine and 0.1 mM (194.3 µg/mL) as positive controls. Values are expressed as mean ± SE of three independent experiments. One-way ANOVA showed significant value, * $p < 0.05$, ** $p < 0.01$, and *** $p < 0.001$ vs. control cells (untreated).

For nine monoterpenoid constituents on lipolysis of lipid accumulation in adipocytes, at day 10, were measured using intracellular triglyceride content, as shown in Figure 4B. The maximum significant decrease of triglyceride content was identified in the presence of citral (100 µg/mL concentration, 32 ± 1% triglyceride content) and camphene (100 µg/mL, 35 ± 2% triglyceride content), relative to the control. In addition, two constituents: camphene and citral at 100 µg/mL concentrations, decreased triglyceride content more than caffeine ($p < 0.01$). We also found that nine constituents had decreased triglyceride content more than adrenaline. These were camphor, camphene, citral, 3-carene, limonene, myrcene, alpha-pinene, beta-pinene and terpinene-4-ol at 100 µg/mL concentration. Interestingly, triglyceride determination of camphene, citral and limonene showed similar decreases in total lipid accumulation in mature adipocytes as compared to the 1% dimethyl sulfoxide (DMSO) control. Our results concur with the animal study reported in [19], which showed that there was a significant inhibition of differentiation of preadipocytes to mature adipocytes was observed, and it was evident from reduced lipid accumulation in the cells. Cellular lipid content was decreased by 18% by camphene at 10 µM, by 29% at 50 µM and by 37% at 100 µM, when compared with the control cells treated with DMSO. Previous work has also found that 30 µM citral exhibits significant inhibition of total triglyceride accumulation using the triglyceride determination kit by 30%, while 40 µM showed a 50% inhibition, and 50 µM showed 80% inhibition [20]. In another study [21], a quick screening on the lipolytic effect of monoterpenes in 3T3-L1 adipocyte was conducted with the result that 1µM of limonene stimulated lipolysis by 17%. Caffeine and adrenaline were used as a positive control in this study. Figure 4A,B show that caffeine at the concentration of 1 mM or 194 µg/mL increased lipolysis with a triglyceride accumulation reduction of 41 ± 2% triglyceride content. Adrenaline at the concentration of 0.1 mM or 18 µg/mL also decreased triglyceride accumulation (67 ± 4% triglyceride content). These results are supported by a previous report that showed that caffeine inhibited triglyceride content by 11%, 22% and 34% at the concentration of 1, 5 and 10 µg/mL [22]. In addition, adrenaline (1 µM) stimulated lipolysis for about a 30% glycerol release. Total glycerol content in the medium indicates the lipolytic effect of adrenaline in 3T3-L1 adipocytes [21]. Previous studies demonstrated that lemon grass oils are rich in citral [23,24], and also that citral inhibited the formation of intracellular lipid accumulation in a concentration-dependent manner (10–50 µM) for 30, 40 and 50 µM concentrations of citral [20]. It should be noted that the present research has shown the potent impact on the lipolytic effect of nine essential oils, mixed oil and their major constituents, which are monoterpenes, The potential anti-cellulite activity of the seven essential oils, mixed oil and tea and coffee water extracts, and their nine major monoterpenoid constituents, extracted from the anti-cellulite herbal compress that we had developed, were assayed on the 3T3-L1 cell lines of preadipocyte, a commonly used cell model for adipose cell biology research. Furthermore, anti-cellulite effects can be exerted by reducing the size and number of intracellular lipid accumulations in adipocytes and assayed triglyceride accumulations. It is suggested that further work be undertaken to study the molecular mechanisms and to substantiate the effectiveness of bioactive compounds as anti-lipogenesis or lipolysis substances, and the beneficial anti-cellulite activities that we have shown to be demonstrated by the herbal compress.

2.4. Vasorelaxant Effects Of Mixed Oil on Rat Aortae

Our previous clinical study showed that the anti-cellulite herbal compress improved cellulite appearance, as assessed by measurement of thigh circumferences, skin thickness and severity of cellulite [7]. Blood flow enhancement via vasodilation could be one of the mechanisms activated by the anti-cellulite herbal compress. Therefore, the mixed oil derived from hydrodistillation of the herbal compress was tested on isolated rat aortae. This test revealed a concentration-dependent (1–300 µg/mL) vasorelaxant effect of mixed oil on the phenylephrine pre-contracted endothelium-intact vessel (EC_{50} = 14.74 ± 2.65 µg/mL and E_{max} = 99.51 ± 0.49%, Figure 5). The vascular action of the herbal compress could be attributed to some of the major constituents of mixed oil, in particular monoterpenes i.e., α-pinene, camphene, β-pinene, β-myrcene, 3-carene, D-limonene, camphor, terpinene-4-ol β-citral and α-citral, which were displayed on chromatographic profiles shown in a GC-MS chromatogram (Figure 6). The mechanism of vasorelaxant actions of the mixed oil could involve the endothelium dependent pathway i.e., nitric oxide release, as reported by several studies evaluating vascular actions of the volatile oils and plants containing similar monoterpene profiles [7,25,26].

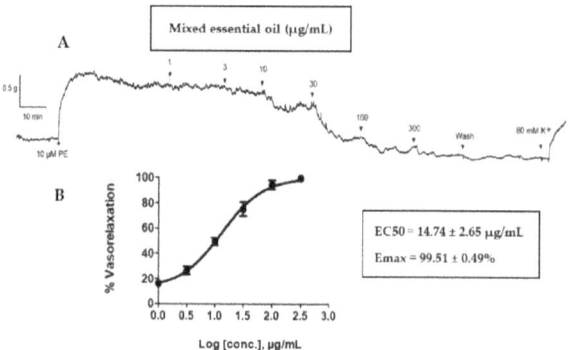

Figure 5. (**A**) A typical trace of the vasorelaxant effect of the mixed oil distilled from the herbal compress mixed ingredients (0–300 μg/mL) on endothelium-intact aortae. (**B**) Concentration-relaxation curves for mixed oil from anti-cellulite herbal compress (1–300 μg/mL) on endothelium-intact aortic rings. All data points are means ± SEMs (n = 5).

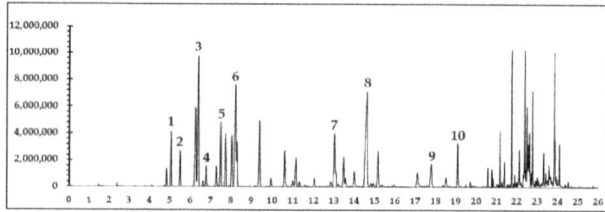

Figure 6. GC-MS total ion chromatogram of the mixed oil distilled from the herbal compress mixed ingredients. The peaks of the main constituents were identified by comparing the molecular mass from mass spectra data of each compound with the NIST library (Version 2.2) as (1) α-pinene, (2) camphene, (3) β-pinene, (4) β-myrcene, (5) 3-carene (6) D-limonene, (7) camphor, (8) terpinene-4-ol, (9) β-citral and (10) α-citral.

3. Materials and Methods

3.1. Chemicals and Plant Materials

Keratinocyte serum-free medium (KSFM) and supplements (2.5 μg of recombinant human epidermal growth factor and 25 mg of bovine pituitary extract), high glucose Dulbecco's Modified Eagle's Medium (DMEM), bovine calf serum (BCS), fetal bovine serum (FBS), phosphate buffered saline (PBS) and antibiotics were purchased from GIBCO (Grand Island, NY, USA), while 3-(4,5-dimethylthiazol-2-yl)-2,5-diphenyl-tetrazolium bromide (MTT), DMSO, Oil Red O reagent and human recombinant insulin were purchased from Sigma-Aldrich (St. Louis, MO, USA. Dexamethasone and IBMX were purchased from Merck (Kenilworth, NJ, USA). Caffeine, camphene, camphor, 3-carene, α-citral, β-citral, limonene, β-myrcene, α-pinene, β-pinene and terpinene-4-ol were purchased from Sigma-Aldrich (Buchs, Switzerland). Adrenaline was purchased from MARCH (Bangkok, Thailand).

The ingredients of the herbal compress i.e., ginger (rhizome), black pepper (fruit), java long pepper (fruit), turmeric (rhizome), plai (rhizome), lemongrass (stalk) and kaffir lime (fruit peel) were purchased in Phitsanulok, Thailand. Specimens of all nine herbs were collected and authenticated by comparing with voucher lots available in the Biological Sciences Herbarium, Naresuan University, Phitsanulok or comparing with botanical illustrations. Roasted coffee beans (Arabica100% Coffman®) were produced by Coffman International. Co., Ltd., Bangkok, Thailand and the tea (Three Horses®) was purchased from Three Horses Tea Co., Ltd., Bangkok, Thailand.

3.2. Extraction

Essential oil extraction: The essential oil of each seven plant ingredients as well as the mixed oil were extracted using hydro-distillation. The plant materials were cut into small pieces, dried at 45–50 °C and ground into powder. The powder of each plant (50 g) was placed in a round-bottomed flask with 500 mL of distilled water. For the mixed oil, the 150 g of mixture of seven plant herbal compress ingredients in the ratio that reported in previous study [7] was placed in a round-bottomed flask with 1500 mL of distilled water. The distillation apparatus was set to 100 °C for 3 to 5 h of distillation [27,28]. Tea and coffee water extraction: Tea and coffee (100 g) were boiled in 400 mL of distilled water for 3 times, and filtered through a filter cloth, followed by 5 min of centrifuging, then the supernatant was lyophilized and stored at -20 °C in screw cap bottles.

3.3. Cell Culture

The protocol was approved by Naresuan University Institutional Review Board for human keratinocyte and fibroblast cells (Approval number 608/59), and for 3T3-L1 preadipocytes and adipocytes (Approval number 0044/61). 3T3-L1 preadipocyte cell line was obtained from ATCC (Manassas, VA, USA). Keratinocyte cells were cultured in KFSM supplemented with 5 µg/mL epidermal growth factor human recombinant, 50 µg/mL bovine pituitary extract and 1% P/S solution [29]. Fibroblast and 3T3-L1 preadipocyte cells were cultured in DMEM, 10% FBS (fibroblast), or 10% BCS (3T3-L1), 3.7 g/L sodium bicarbonate and 1% P/S solution. The cells culture condition was maintained at 37 °C, and humidified in an atmosphere of 5% CO_2.

3.4. Adipocyte Differentiation (Adipogenesis Assay)

For adipocyte differentiation, the 3T3-L1 pre-adipocytes were plated in 96 well plates at a density of 2×10^3/well and cultured in DMEM supplemented with 10% BCS and 1% P/S solution. Two days after confluence; day 0, the media was removed and the fresh differentiation media i.e., DMEM with 10% FBS, 1 µM dexamethasone, 0.5 mM IBMX and 5 µg/mL insulin was added and maintained for 2 days at 37 °C in an atmosphere of 5% CO_2. The media was replaced with fresh DMEM containing insulin every second day. By day 9, more than 90% of the cells had differentiated into lipid droplets [30,31].

3.5. Cell Viability

Human keratinocyte and fibroblast cells were separated from human foreskins. The keratinocytes were seeded at 2×10^4 cells/well and the fibroblast cells were seeded at 2×10^4 cells/well. The 3T3-L1 pre-adipocytes were seeded at 1×10^4 cells/well and 3T3-L1 pre-adipocytes, for differentiation to the adipocytes, were seeded at 2×10^3 cells/well in a 96-well plate. The essential oils and extracts and their major compounds were dissolved in 100% DMSO and the culture medium was then replaced with 100 µL serial dilutions (0.97, 1.95, 3.90, 7.81, 15.62, 31.25, 62.5, 125, 250 and 500 µg/mL) of the extracts for keratinocytes, fibroblast and pre-adipocytes, and 12.5, 25, 50, 100, 200 and 500 µg/mL for the adipocytes. The cells were then incubated with the essential oils/extracts at 37 °C, and 5% CO_2, for 24 h. The viability of the differentiated cells adipocyte and post-confluent adipocytes was ascertained by treating them with a sample solution in differentiation medium every 2 days for 9 days, after which the viability was assayed. Where the final concentration of DMSO was less than 1% v/v in the cell culture medium, the cells were added to each well with 50 µL of MTT working solution (1 mg/mL) in PBS (pH = 7.4) and incubated for a further three hours. The solution was measured at a test wavelength of 595 nm by microplate reader [32–34].

3.6. Quantification of Lipid Content by Lipid Accumulation

The accumulation of lipids in the cells was quantified by Oil-Red-O assay. The inhibition of essential oils and extracts, and their major monoterpenoids, were evaluated for their preventive and treatment effects against adipogenesis. Various concentrations of the essential oils and extracts (12.5 to 200 µg/mL) were added to the differentiation media (with insulin) on days 3, 5 and 7. After day 7, the lipid droplets in the mature adipocytes were stained then visualized through Oil Red O staining and photographed. To evaluate the treatment effect, the samples were incubated with the mature adipocyte on day 9 for 24 h and their effects were stained with Oil Red O on day 10 [12,20].

3.7. Oil-Red-O Staining

After the lipid droplets were stained and showed through the Oil Red O staining of 3T3-L1, the adipocytes were treated with different concentrations of the extracts, as described above. The cells were washed twice with PBS, fixed with 10% formalin for 8 min and left for 1 h at room temperature when they were washed again with 60% Isopropanol and stained with freshly prepared Oil Red O solution diluted with 3 parts of 0.5% Oil Red O in 2 parts of distilled water, for 45 min at room temperature. The cells were again washed twice with distilled water to remove the excess stain and then were dried. The cells were then examined under a microscope. After 10 min, the Oil Red O staining was extracted by isopropanol. The absorbance was measured using a microplate reader at 500 nm [31,35] and examined under a microscope (Nikon) and the images were captured.

3.8. Determination of Triglyceride (TG) Content

Next, 3T3-L1 adipocytes were induced for differentiation in the same fashion as stated in session 3.5. At day 9, they were treated with samples of essential oils, extracts and monoterpenoids, or positive controls of caffeine and adrenaline, and incubated at 37 °C, and 5% CO_2 for 24 h. The cells were then collected and lysed using sonication. The total triglyceride contents in the cells were determined using the Triglyceride Assay Kit (Cayman Chemical Company, Ann Arbor, MI, USA) [20,35,36].

3.9. Vasorelaxant Effects of Mixed Oil

This study was approved and conducted in accordance with the guidelines of the Naresuan University Animal Care and Use Committee (NUACUC; Animal Ethics Approval Number: NU-AE601021). After anesthetizing the male Wistar rats, using intraperitoneal injection of thiopental sodium (100 mg/kg), the rats' aortae were excised and kept in cold physiological Krebs' solution (mM): NaCl 122 mM; KCl 5 mM; [N-(2-hydroxyethyl) piperazine N'-(2-ethanesulfonic acid)] HEPES 10 mM; KH_2PO_4 0.5 mM; NaH_2PO_4 0.5 mM; $MgCl_2$ 1 mM; glucose 11 mM; and $CaCl_2$ 1.8 mM (pH = 7.4). After removal of the superficial connective tissues, each aorta was cut into ring segments, 3–4 mm in length, which were then mounted in standard 10 mL organ baths continuously aerated (95% O_2:5% CO_2) and filled with Krebs-Hensleit (KH) buffer (pH = 7.4) at 37 °C. A Mac Lab A/D converter (Chart V5, A.D. Instruments, Castle Hill, NSW, Australia) was used to measure the isometric tension of the force transducers which were connected with intra-luminal wires. The resting tension of the aortic rings was maintained at 1 g and the rings were equilibrated for 60 min to ensure a stable contraction with 10 µM phenylephrine (PE). Presence of the endothelial lining was evaluated by observing >70% relaxation with 10 µM acetylcholine (Ach) after stable contraction with PE [37].

The experiment was conducted on endothelium intact rat aortae equilibrated at 1 g initially and pre contracted with 10 µM PE. A stable contraction plateau was observed which was then followed by the cumulative addition of mixed oil from 1 µg/mL, 3 µg/mL, 10 µg/mL, 30 µg/mL, 100 µg/mL and 300 µg/mL. Each concentration was incubated until the relaxation was stable. Identical concentrations of DMSO alone were added to serve as the negative control group at the same time interval as the addition of the mixed oil, in order to ensure that the relaxation was rendered by the mixed oil rather than the DMSO. The vessel was washed with physiological Kreb's solution after complete relaxation had been observed at the highest concentration of the mixed oil. To evaluate the vessels' integrity, 80 mM K^+ solution was added. The immediate contraction plateau of each vessel was observed, signifying the vessel's viability throughout the experimental protocol. The % relaxation was calculated as % contraction in response to PE.

3.10. Gas Chromatography-Mass Spectrometry Analysis of Monoterpenoid Constituents in Mixed Oil

GC-MS analysis used an Agilent 7890B, Gas Chromatography System-5977B coupled to an Agilent 5977B MSD model mass spectrometer (Agilent Technologies, Singapore). Mixed oil was prepared by dissolving 5 mg into 1 mL of methanol and injected into a capillary column HP-5 5% Phenyl Methyl Silox (30 m × 250 μm × 0.25 μm; Agilent 19091S-433) with a constant flow rate of Helium 1.0 mL/min. The injector was set at 250 °C and performed by split mode with a split ratio of 100:1 (in 1.0 μL). The GC oven temperature was initially set at 70 °C for 5 min, then increased to 100 °C at a rate of 3 °C/min and held for 3 min, then increased to 250 °C at a rate of 20 °C/min and held for another 1 min, with a total run time of 26.5 min (Figure 6).

Monoterpenoid constituents of the mixed oil were identified by mass spectrometry in full scan mode using mass analyzer and confirmed by comparing their spectra to those of the NIST MS search 2.2 library. The mass spectrometer was operated in the electron impact ionization mode (70 eV), with a scan range of 50 to 550 amu. The interested constituents of mixed oil from the anti-cellulite herbal compress and their relative peak areas were listed in Table 2.

Table 2. The GC-MS retention times and the relative peak areas of the interested monoterpenoid constituents of mixed oil from the anti-cellulite herbal compress.

Monoterpenes Constituents [1]	Retention Time (min)	Relative Area (%) [2]
α-pinene (1)	5.044	6.13
Camphene (2)	5.478	3.73
β-Pinene (3)	6.383	20.99
β-myrcene (4)	6.774	2.63
3-carene (5)	7.495	8.34
D-limonene (6)	8.221	20.70
Camphor (7)	13.036	8.38
Terpinene-4-ol (8)	14.630	20.93
β-citral (9)	17.791	3.84
α-citral (10)	19.108	4.33

[1] Relative area (%) obtained by area of the interested peak/total area of 10 interested peaks × 100. [2] The number in the brackets of represent the peak in Figure 6.

3.11. Statistical Analysis

All adipogenesis experiments, each with a set of 3 wells, were carried out in triplicate. Data were statistically evaluated by a one-way analysis of variance (ANOVA). Determination of significant differences ($p < 0.05$) between means was supported by Tukey's multiple comparison test (GraphPad Prism software version 8.0, San Diego, CA, USA). Values are given as mean ± standard error of the sample animals. The EC_{50} values and Emax values to achieve maximum relaxation were obtained by concentration-response curve fitting using GraphPad Prism software version 8.0, San Diego, CA, USA.

4. Conclusions

This study presents the preclinical effects, on cellular lipid accumulation, triglyceride content and the vasodilatation effect of on rat aortae, of the essential oils and extracts obtained from Thai traditional herbal compresses and their constituents. These findings demonstrate the abilities of the test samples to decrease lipid accumulation resulting in the inhibition of adipocyte differentiation and increasing lipolysis on 3T3-L1 adipocyte cells. The mixed oils showed vasodilatory effects on rat aortae via endothelium-dependent release of vasodilators. Our study is the first to report on the anti-cellulite mechanisms of Thai traditional herbal compresses, including prevention of lipid accumulation and increasing blood flow. Our findings allow us to confidently suggest that the anti-cellulite activity of volatile oils and their monoterpenes constituents, or combinations of them, are useful in the treatment for cellulite.

Author Contributions: Conceptualization, N.N., N.W., K.C. and K.I. (Kornkanok Ingkaninan); methodology and experimental design, N.N., T.U.P., W.W., K.C. and K.I. (Kornkanok Ingkaninan); software, N.N.; validation, N.N., N.S., K.I. (Kamonlak Insumrong) and K.I. (Kornkanok Ingkaninan); formal analysis, N.N., T.U.P., K.C. and K.I. (Kornkanok Ingkaninan); investigation, N.N.; resources, N.W., K.C. and K.I. (Kornkanok Ingkaninan); data curation and interpretation, N.N. and K.I. (Kornkanok Ingkaninan); writing original draft preparation, N.N., K.C. and K.I. (Kornkanok Ingkaninan); writing review and editing, N.N., T.U.P., K.I. (Kornkanok Ingkaninan) and K.C.; visualization, N.N., N.W., K.C. and K.I. (Kornkanok Ingkaninan); supervision N.W., K.C. and K.I. (Kornkanok Ingkaninan); project administration, K.I. (Kornkanok Ingkaninan); funding acquisition, N.W. and K.I. (Kornkanok Ingkaninan). All authors have read and agreed to the published version of the manuscript.

Funding: This research was funded by Royal Golden Jubilee Program (RGJ-PhD) [0008/2560], Thailand Center of Excellence for Life Sciences (TCEL) [TC-A2/62], National Research Council of Thailand [DBG6080005, IRN61W0005], and the Center of Excellence for Innovation in Chemistry (PERCH-CIC), the Ministry of Higher Education, Science, Research and Innovation Neither funding agency influenced or restricted any part of the trial, its data or publication.

Institutional Review Board Statement: The study was conducted according to the guidelines of the Declaration of Helsinki, and approved by the Institutional Review Board of Naresuan University for human keratinocyte and fibroblast cells (Approval number 608/59), and for 3T3-L1 pre-adipocytes and adipocytes (Approval number 0044/61) and Institutional Animal Care and Use Committee at the Naresuan University for animal (Approval Number: NU-AE601021).

Informed Consent Statement: Not applicable.

Data Availability Statement: The data presented in this study are available on request from the corresponding author.

Acknowledgments: We would like to acknowledge the Center of Excellence for Innovation in Chemistry (PERCH-CIC) and Cosmetics and Natural Products Research Center (COSNAT), Naresuan University on research facility support. We also wish to thank Roy I. Morien of the Naresuan University Graduate School for his efforts in editing the English grammar and expressions in this paper.

Conflicts of Interest: The authors declare no conflict of interest.

References

1. De la Casa Almeida, M.; Suarez Serrano, C.; Rebollo Roldán, J.; Jiménez Rejano, J. Cellulite's aetiology: A review. *J. Eur. Acad. Dermatol.* **2013**, *27*, 273–278. [CrossRef] [PubMed]
2. Terranova, F.; Berardesca, E.; Maibach, H. Cellulite: Nature and aetiopathogenesis. *Int. J. Cosmet. Sci.* **2006**, *28*, 157–167. [CrossRef]
3. Khan, M.H.; Victor, F.; Rao, B.; Sadick, N.S. Treatment of cellulite: Part I. Pathophysiology. *J. Am. Acad. Dermatol.* **2010**, *62*, 361–370. [CrossRef]
4. Khan, M.H.; Victor, F.; Rao, B.; Sadick, N.S. Treatment of cellulite: Part II. Advances and controversies. *J. Am. Acad. Dermatol.* **2010**, *62*, 373–384. [CrossRef] [PubMed]
5. Kligman, A.; Pagnoni, A.; Stoudemayer, T. Topical retinol improves cellulite. *J. Dermatol. Treat.* **1999**, *10*, 119–125. [CrossRef]
6. Bertin, C.; Zunino, H.; Pittet, J.-C.; Beau, P.; Pineau, P.; Massonneau, M.; Robert, C.; Hopkins, J. A double-blind evaluation of the activity of an anti-cellulite product containing retinol, caffeine, and ruscogenine by a combination of several non-invasive methods. *J. Cosmet. Sci.* **2001**, *52*, 199–210. [PubMed]
7. Ngamdokmai, N.; Waranuch, N.; Chootip, K.; Jampachaisri, K.; Scholfield, C.N.; Ingkaninan, K. Cellulite Reduction by Modified Thai Herbal Compresses; A Randomized Double-Blind Trial. *JEBIM* **2018**, *23*. [CrossRef] [PubMed]
8. Ngamdokmai, N.; Waranuch, N.; Chootip, K.; Neungchamnong, N.; Ingkaninan, K. HPLC-QTOF-MS method for quantitative determination of active compounds in an anti-cellulite herbal compress. *Songklanakarin J. Sci. Technol.* **2017**, *39*, 463–470.

9. Green, H.; Meuth, M. An established pre-adipose cell line and its differentiation in culture. *Cell* **1974**, *3*, 127–133. [CrossRef]
10. Poulos, S.P.; Dodson, M.V.; Hausman, G.J. Cell line models for differentiation: Preadipocytes and adipocytes. *Exp. Biol. Med.* **2010**, *235*, 1185–1193. [CrossRef]
11. Kraus, N.A.; Ehebauer, F.; Zapp, B.; Rudolphi, B.; Kraus, B.J.; Kraus, D. Quantitative assessment of adipocyte differentiation in cell culture. *Adipocyte* **2016**, *5*, 351–358. [CrossRef]
12. Manaharan, T.; Kanthimathi, M. Ginger oil-mediated down-regulation of adipocyte specific genes inhibits adipogenesis and induces apoptosis in 3T3-L1 adipocytes. *Biochem. Biotechnol. Res.* **2016**, *4*, 38–47.
13. Aoyagi, R.; Funakoshi-Tago, M.; Fujiwara, Y.; Tamura, H. Coffee inhibits adipocyte differentiation via inactivation of PPARγ. *Biol. Pharm. Bull.* **2014**, *37*, 1820–1825. [CrossRef] [PubMed]
14. Duangjai, A.; Nuengchamnong, N.; Suphrom, N.; Trisat, K.; Limpeanchob, N.; Saokaew, S. Potential of coffee fruit extract and quinic acid on adipogenesis and lipolysis in 3T3-L1 adipocytes. *Kobe J. Med. Sci.* **2018**, *64*, E84. [PubMed]
15. Ko, H.-J.; Lo, C.-Y.; Wang, B.-J.; Chiou, R.Y.-Y.; Lin, S.-M. Theaflavin-3,3′-digallate, a black tea polyphenol, stimulates lipolysis associated with the induction of mitochondrial uncoupling proteins and AMPK–FoxO3A–MnSOD pathway in 3T3-L1 adipocytes. *J. Funct. Foods* **2015**, *17*, 271–282. [CrossRef]
16. Lin, J.K.; Lin-Shiau, S.Y. Mechanisms of hypolipidemic and anti-obesity effects of tea and tea polyphenols. *Mol. Nutr. Food Res.* **2006**, *50*, 211–217. [CrossRef]
17. Goto, T.; Takahashi, N.; Hirai, S.; Kawada, T. Various terpenoids derived from herbal and dietary plants function as PPAR modulators and regulate carbohydrate and lipid metabolism. *PPAR Res.* **2010**, *2010*, 483958. [CrossRef]
18. Jing, L.; Zhang, Y.; Fan, S.; Gu, M.; Guan, Y.; Lu, X.; Huang, C.; Zhou, Z. Preventive and ameliorating effects of citrus D-limonene on dyslipidemia and hyperglycemia in mice with high-fat diet-induced obesity. *Eur. J. Pharmacol.* **2013**, *715*, 46–55. [CrossRef]
19. Kim, Y.; Choi, Y.; Choi, S.; Choi, Y.; Park, T. Dietary camphene attenuates hepatic steatosis and insulin resistance in mice. *Obesity* **2014**, *22*, 408–417. [CrossRef]
20. Devi, S.S.; Ashokkumar, N. Citral, a Monoterpene Inhibits Adipogenesis through Modulation of Adipogenic Transcription Factors in 3T3-L1 Cells. *Indian J. Clin. Biochem.* **2018**, *33*, 414–421. [CrossRef]
21. Tan, X.C.; Chua, K.H.; Ravishankar Ram, M.; Kuppusamy, U.R. Monoterpenes: Novel insights into their biological effects and roles on glucose uptake and lipid metabolism in 3T3-L1 adipocytes. *Food Chem.* **2016**, *196*, 242–250. [CrossRef]
22. Saraphanchotiwitthaya, A.; Sripalakit, P. Inhibition of lipid accumulation in 3T3-L1 adipocytes by *Morinda citrifolia* Linn. Leaf extracts and commercial herbal formulas for weight control. *Int. J. Pharm. Pharm. Sci.* **2016**, *8*, 199–204. [CrossRef]
23. Piaru, S.P.; Perumal, S.; Cai, L.W.; Mahmud, R.; Majid, A.M.S.A.; Ismail, S.; Man, C.N. Chemical composition, anti-angiogenic and cytotoxicity activities of the essential oils of *Cymbopogan citratus* (lemon grass) against colorectal and breast carcinoma cell lines. *J. Essent. Oil Res.* **2012**, *24*, 453–459. [CrossRef]
24. Shah, G.; Shri, R.; Panchal, V.; Sharma, N.; Singh, B.; Mann, A. Scientific basis for the therapeutic use of *Cymbopogon citratus*, stapf (Lemon grass). *J. Adv. Pharm. Technol.* **2011**, *2*, 3–8. [CrossRef]
25. Cunha, G.; Fechine, F.; Frota Bezerra, F.; Moraes, M.; Silveira, E.; Canuto, K.; Moraes, M. Comparative study of the antihypertensive effects of hexane, chloroform and methanol fractions of essential oil of *Alpinia zerumbet* in rats Wistar. *Rev. Bras. Plantas Med.* **2016**, *18*, 113–124. [CrossRef]
26. Buddhakala, N. Physiological Study of the Effects of Ginger Oil on Rat Uterine Contraction. Ph.D. Thesis, Suranaree Suranaree University of Technology Intellectual Respository of Technology, Korat, Thailand, 2007.
27. Department of Medical Sciences, Ministry of Public Health. *Thai Herbal Pharmacopoeia*, 2nd ed.; Office of National Buddishm Press: Bangkok, Thailand, 2000; pp. 9–15.
28. Department of Medical Sciences, Ministry of Public Health. *Thai Herbal Pharmacopoeia*, 1st ed.; Office of National Buddishm Press: Bangkok, Thailand, 2009; pp. 18–20.
29. Wongwad, E.; Pingyod, C.; Saesong, T.; Waranuch, N.; Wisuitiprot, W.; Sritularak, B.; Temkitthawon, P.; Ingkaninan, K. Assessment of the bioactive components, antioxidant, antiglycation and anti-inflammatory properties of *Aquilaria crassna* Pierre ex Lecomte leaves. *Ind. Crop. Prod.* **2019**, *138*, 111448. [CrossRef]
30. Sadick, N. Treatment for cellulite. *Int. J. Womens Dermatol.* **2019**, *5*, 68–72. [CrossRef]
31. Chang, W.-T.; Wu, C.-H.; Hsu, C.-L. Diallyl trisulphide inhibits adipogenesis in 3T3-L1 adipocytes through lipogenesis, fatty acid transport, and fatty acid oxidation pathways. *J. Funct. Foods* **2015**, *16*, 414–422. [CrossRef]
32. Saravanan, M.; Ignacimuthu, S. Effect of *Ichnocarpus frutescens* (L.) R. Br. hexane extract on preadipocytes viability and lipid accumulation in 3T3-L1 cells. *Asian Pac. J. Trop. Med.* **2013**, *6*, 360–365. [CrossRef]
33. Cetin, Y.; Bullerman, L.B. Cytotoxicity of Fusarium mycotoxins to mammalian cell cultures as determined by the MTT bioassay. *Food Chem. Toxicol.* **2005**, *43*, 755–764. [CrossRef]
34. Arechabala, B.; Coiffard, C.; Rivalland, P.; Coiffard, L.J.M.; Roeck-Holtzhauer, Y.D. Comparison of cytotoxicity of various surfactants tested on normal human fibroblast cultures using the neutral red test, MTT assay and LDH release. *J. Appl. Toxicol.* **1999**, *19*, 163–165. [CrossRef]
35. Khattak, M.M.A.K.; Taher, M.; Ichwan, S.J.A.; Azahari, N. Selected Herbal Extracts Improve Diabetes Associated Factors in 3T3-L1 Adipocytes. *Procedia Soc. Behav. Sci.* **2013**, *91*, 357–375. [CrossRef]

36. Wu, M.; Liu, D.; Zeng, R.; Xian, T.; Lu, Y.; Zeng, G.; Sun, Z.; Huang, B.; Huang, Q. Epigallocatechin-3-gallate inhibits adipogenesis through down-regulation of PPARγ and FAS expression mediated by PI3K-AKT signaling in 3T3-L1 cells. *Eur. J. Pharmacol.* **2017**, *795*, 134–142. [CrossRef]
37. Kamkaew, N.; Paracha, T.U.; Ingkaninan, K.; Waranuch, N.; Chootip, K. Vasodilatory Effects and Mechanisms of Action of *Bacopa monnieri* Active Compounds on Rat Mesenteric Arteries. *Molecules* **2019**, *24*, 2243. [CrossRef] [PubMed]

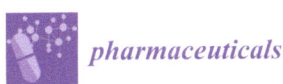

Article

Melatonin Improves Endoplasmic Reticulum Stress-Mediated IRE1α Pathway in Zücker Diabetic Fatty Rat

Samira Aouichat [1,2], Miguel Navarro-Alarcon [3], Pablo Alarcón-Guijo [1], Diego Salagre [1], Marwa Ncir [4], Lazhar Zourgui [4] and Ahmad Agil [1,5,*]

1. Department of Pharmacology, Bioheath Institute and Neurosciences Institute, School of Medicine, University of Granada, 18016 Granada, Spain; samira_aouichat@outlook.fr (S.A.); pabloang30@correo.ugr.es (P.A.-G.); dsalagres@correo.ugr.es (D.S.)
2. Team of Cellular and Molecular Physiopathology, Faculty of Biological Sciences, University of Sciences and Technology Houari Boumediene, El Alia, Algiers 16111, Algeria
3. Department of Nutrition and Bromatology, School of Pharmacy, University of Granada, 18071 Granada, Spain; nalarcon@ugr.es
4. Bioactive Molecule Valorization Research Unit, Higher Institute of Applied Biology of Medenine, University of Gabes, Gabes 4119, Tunisia; nsirrmarwaa@yahoo.fr (M.N.); lazhar.zourgui@gmail.com (L.Z.)
5. Biosanitary Research Institute of Granada (ibs. GRANADA), University Hospital of Granada, 18016 Granada, Spain
* Correspondence: aagil@ugr.es; Tel.: +34-958-24-35

Abstract: Obesity and diabetes are linked to an increased prevalence of kidney disease. Endoplasmic reticulum stress has recently gained growing importance in the pathogenesis of obesity and diabetes-related kidney disease. Melatonin, is an important anti-obesogenic natural bioactive compound. Previously, our research group showed that the renoprotective effect of melatonin administration was associated with restoring mitochondrial fission/fusion balance and function in a rat model of diabesity-induced kidney injury. This study was carried out to further investigate whether melatonin could suppress renal endoplasmic reticulum (ER) stress response and the downstream unfolded protein response activation under obese and diabetic conditions. Zücker diabetic fatty (ZDF) rats and lean littermates (ZL) were orally supplemented either with melatonin (10 mg/kg body weight (BW)/day) (M–ZDF and M–ZL) or vehicle (C–ZDF and C–ZL) for 17 weeks. Western blot analysis of ER stress-related markers and renal morphology were assessed. Compared to C–ZL rats, higher ER stress response associated with impaired renal morphology was observed in C–ZDF rats. Melatonin supplementation alleviated renal ER stress response in ZDF rats, by decreasing glucose-regulated protein 78 (GRP78), phosphoinositol-requiring enzyme1α (IRE1α), and ATF6 levels but had no effect on phospho–protein kinase RNA–like endoplasmic reticulum kinase (PERK) level. In addition, melatonin supplementation also restrained the ER stress-mediated apoptotic pathway, as indicated by decreased pro-apoptotic proteins phospho–c–jun amino terminal kinase (JNK), Bax, and cleaved caspase-3, as well as by upregulation of B cell lymphoma (Bcl)-2 protein. These improvements were associated with renal structural recovery. Taken together, our findings revealed that melatonin play a renoprotective role, at least in part, by suppressing ER stress and related pro-apoptotic IRE1α/JNK signaling pathway.

Keywords: melatonin; endoplasmic reticulum stress; diabesity; kidney

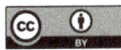

Citation: Aouichat, S.; Navarro-Alarcon, M.; Alarcón-Guijo, P.; Salagre, D.; Ncir, M.; Zourgui, L.; Agil, A. Melatonin Improves Endoplasmic Reticulum Stress-Mediated IRE1α Pathway in Zücker Diabetic Fatty Rat. *Pharmaceuticals* **2021**, *14*, 232. https://doi.org/10.3390/ph14030232

Academic Editor: Noelia Duarte

Received: 15 February 2021
Accepted: 4 March 2021
Published: 8 March 2021

Publisher's Note: MDPI stays neutral with regard to jurisdictional claims in published maps and institutional affiliations.

Copyright: © 2021 by the authors. Licensee MDPI, Basel, Switzerland. This article is an open access article distributed under the terms and conditions of the Creative Commons Attribution (CC BY) license (https://creativecommons.org/licenses/by/4.0/).

1. Introduction

Chronic metabolic diseases, particularly obesity and type 2 diabetes mellitus (T2DM), are a major health problem worldwide, and kidney disease associated to them is an important complication that is emerging as a major cause of morbidity and mortality [1]. Despite great progress in the control of obesity and T2DM, effective clinical therapy of obesity and diabetes-related kidney injury is still limited, emphasizing the urgent necessity for the development of new therapeutic strategies that target novel signaling pathways.

It is well accepted that obese and diabetic kidney microenvironments play a pivotal role in the pathogenesis of chronic kidney disease, through a mechanism involving the endoplasmic reticulum (ER), the intracellular organelle responsible for synthesis, folding, and maturation of protein, and for Ca^{+2} homeostasis modulation and lipids or steroids synthesis [2–4]. Pathophysiological states that increase the demand for protein folding or that disrupt normal folding processes result in accumulation of misfolded proteins in the ER and cause ER stress [3]. At the initial stage of ER stress, a protective process termed unfolded protein response (UPR) is initiated in the ER, which is mediated by three transmembrane sensors, including protein kinase RNA–like endoplasmic reticulum kinase (PERK), activated transcription factor 6 (ATF–6) and inositol-requiring enzyme1α (IRE1α) [5]. Under non-stress conditions, the proteins are bound to the ER chaperone protein glucose-regulated protein 78 kDa (GRP78), and thus remain inactive. Upon accumulation of unfolded proteins in the ER, GRP78 becomes dissociated from these transducers proteins, and UPR cascade is activated after dimerization and autophosphorylation of PERK and IRE1α, and regulated intramembrane proteolysis of ATF6. This response induced by UPR triggers the reduction in global protein synthesis, the degradation of misfolded or unfolded proteins, and the increase of protein chaperones synthesis, especially GRP78. When the adaptive ER stress fails to restore cell homeostasis, this response can also trigger an apoptotic pathway to remove the damaged cells [2]. One or more pro-apoptotic signaling pathways are known to contribute to cell death under prolonged or chronic activation of the three UPR pathways. According to the literature, UPR-mediated pro-apoptotic signaling is divided between that mediated by IRE1α and that mediated by CCAAT/enhancer-binding protein homologous protein (CHOP). Although CHOP can be induced by all three ER stress sensors, it is most strongly induced by activation of PERK. IRE1α initiates ER stress-associated apoptosis by recruiting tumor necrosis factor receptor-associated factor 2 (TRAF2), leading to the activation of the c–jun amino terminal kinase (JNK) pathway of apoptosis, which suppresses the expression of B cell lymphoma (Bcl-2) and induces that of Bcl–2-associated x–protein (Bax). Another mechanism of ER stress-associated apoptosis is via upregulation of Ca^{2+}-mediated signaling, where ER stress leads to the release of Ca^{2+} from ER to mitochondria, resulting in the activation of the caspase family for apoptosis [6].

Accumulating evidence indicates that ER stress is pathogenic in various kidney diseases [7]. The link between chronic ER stress and renal damage was established by the presence of ER stress markers in both renal glomeruli and tubular interstitium of animal models of both obesity and diabetes [8–12] and in diabetic patients [13]. Obese and diabetic kidney microenvironment (e.g., lipotoxicity, glucotoxicity, and proteinuria) has been postulated to induce several conditions that impose an ER stress response and UPR pathway activation, leading to renal cells death [9,13–15]. Hence, therapeutic strategies targeting ER stress and its downstream signaling might have the potential to provide a powerful tool in an attempt to prevent renal injury in obesity and diabetes.

Melatonin (N-acetyl-5-methoxytryptamine) is a highly lipophilic molecule that can easily cross the cell membrane in many organs and organelles [16]. It is an indoleamine synthesized and secreted from the pineal gland and is mainly responsible for controlling the circadian cycle [17]. Melatonin is also produced extrapineally by many peripheral tissues, including kidney, owing to the expression of the two key enzymes involved in its synthesis (arylalkylamine-N-acetyltransferase (AA-NAT) and hydroxyindole-O-methyltransferase (HIOMT)) [18,19]. Exogenous melatonin is widely used to remedy sleep disorders and jet-lag, either as a dietary supplement or as a drug, in many countries in Europe and USA [20,21]. Apart from this, melatonin was shown to possess remarkable anti-obesity and metabolic effects, as well as robust cell-protective properties, including anti-inflammatory and anti-apoptotic properties [22–24]. The effectiveness of melatonin to reduce kidney injury and dysfunction caused by various pathological conditions, such as obesity and diabetes, has been widely investigated, and various mechanisms have been reported to underlie its beneficial effects, including anti-oxidative stress, anti-inflammatory, and anti-apoptotic mechanisms [16,25–35]. Our group has recently shown that melatonin improved outcomes of renal dysfunction through the modulation of mitochondrial dynamics and function in an animal model of diabesity-induced kidney injury [36]. This mechanism could not rule out the possibility that melatonin may also depend on ER stress response and its downstream signaling mechanism to limit kidney damage under conditions of obesity and associated diabetes, given that melatonin has been shown to be effective in modulating ER stress response and UPR activation in different pathological situations [37–39]. With respect to kidney diseases, so far, there has been only two studies, in which melatonin was able to reduce renal ER stress in human in–vivo kidney stones model [40] and in a rat model of renal warm ischemia–reperfusion [41]. However, whether melatonin can mitigate renal ER stress in a rat model of obesity and diabetes-associated kidney injury has not yet been investigated. The present study was undertaken to investigate whether melatonin is effective against ER stress-induced renal damage in ZDF rat, and whether its renoprotective effect implicates the inactivation of UPR signaling pathway. ZDF is an excellent animal model of human obesity-induced type 2 diabetes, recapitulating pathological features similar to that seen in human, including progressive insulin resistance, glucose intolerance, hyperglycemia, hyperinsulinemia, hyperlipidemia, moderate hypertension, and progressive renal injury. The ZDF rats spontaneously develop proteinuria and focal segmental glomerulosclerosis (FSGS) by 14 to 20 weeks, which ultimately lead to renal insufficiency by 22 weeks of age [36,42–46]. Our findings provide new insight into the beneficial effect of melatonin supplementation on ER stress-induced kidney damage under diabesity conditions.

2. Results

2.1. Effects of Melatonin on Kidney ER Stress Response

ER stress plays an important role in the development of diabesity-related kidney disease [7]. To study ER stress in the kidney of ZDF rats and the possible effect of melatonin supplementation on this situation, we assayed the expression level of the main ER stress markers (GRP78, phospho–PERK, phospho–IRE1α, and ATF6) using Western blot analysis.

The upregulated expression of GRP78 is considered a major hallmark of ER stress. The protein expression of GRP78 was significantly higher in the C–ZDF group compared with the C–ZL group (2.2-fold; $p < 0.001$; Figure 1a) and was found to be significantly decreased after melatonin supplementation in both ZDF (2.2-fold) and ZL (1.3-fold) groups, as compared to their control counterparts without supplementation ($p < 0.01$ and $p < 0.05$, respectively; Figure 1a).

In this study phospho–PERK, phospho–IRE1α, and ATF6 were investigated as markers of ER stress. Notably, although, the relative protein level of phospho–PERK was significantly increased in C–ZFD group compared with C–ZL group (2.1-fold; $p < 0.01$; Figure 1b), the extent of this change was not attenuated in either ZDF or ZL groups with melatonin supplementation, as compared to their corresponding without supplementation ($p > 0.05$; Figure 1b). The relative protein amount of phospho–IRE1α and ATF6 were found to be significantly increased in the C–ZDF group compared with the C–ZL group (3.1-fold and 3.0-fold, respectively; $p < 0.001$; Figure 1c,d), and melatonin supplementation lowered their expression in ZDF group (4.5-fold and 4.1-fold, respectively) but not in ZL group, as compared with the respective control ZDF ($p < 0.001$ and $p < 0.001$, respectively) and ZL ($p > 0.05$ and $p > 0.05$, respectively) without supplementation (Figure 1c,d). Interestingly, the expressed amount of phospho–IRE1α and ATF6 in M-ZDF group was restored to that of C–ZL group.

2.2. Effects of Melatonin on Kidney ER Stress-Related Apopotosis Markers

Apoptosis could be stimulated with the activation of prolonged UPR. To investigate whether the relieve effect of melatonin for the ER stress can be accompanied by the subsequent repression of the ER stress-induced apoptosis, we choose to evaluate the IRE1α branch of ER stress-associated apoptosis pathway.

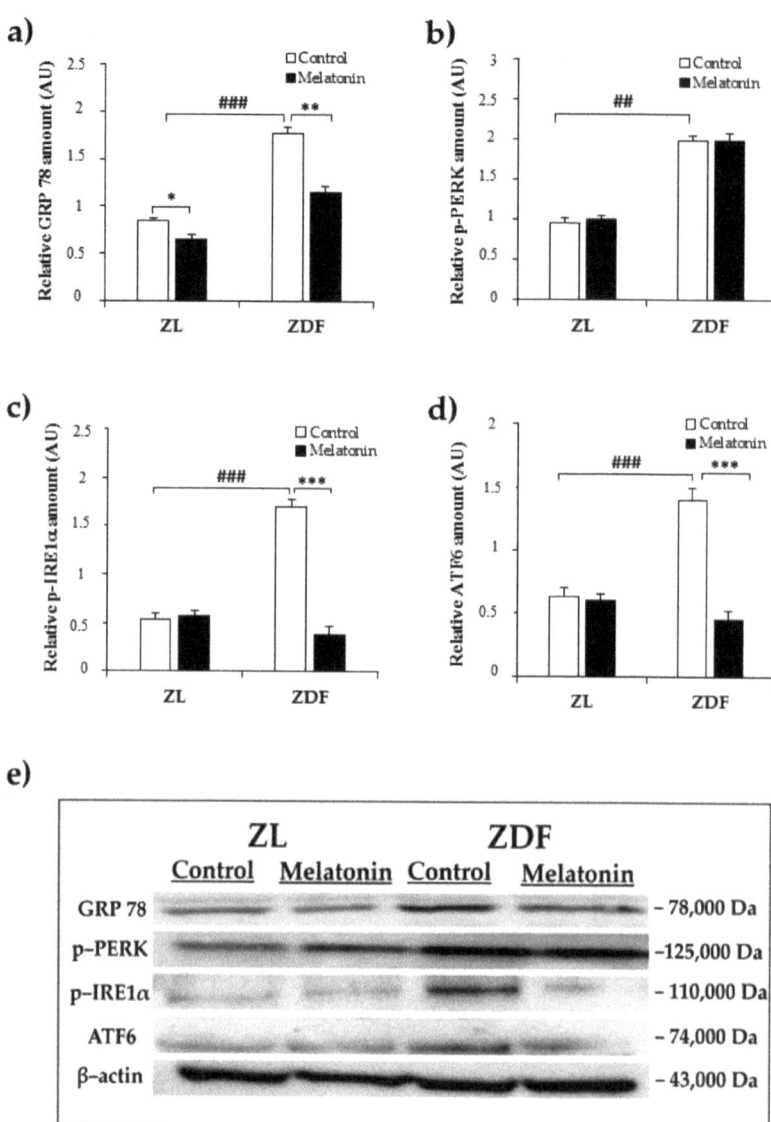

Figure 1. Effects of melatonin supplementation on endoplasmic reticulum (ER) stress markers in the kidney of Zücker lean and diabetic fatty rats as measured by Western blot. (**a–d**) Densitometry quantification of glucose-regulated protein 78 (GRP78) p–protein kinase RNA–like endoplasmic reticulum kinase (PERK), p–inositol-requiring enzyme1α (IRE1α), and ATF6 protein levels. (**e**) Representative blot of GRP78, phospho–PERK, phospho–IRE1α, and ATF6. C–ZL: control lean rats without melatonin; M–ZL: lean rats with melatonin; C–ZDF: control diabetic fatty rats without melatonin; M–ZDF: diabetic fatty rats with melatonin; ZL: Zücker lean rats; ZDF: Zücker diabetic fatty rats. Values are means ± S.E.M ($n = 3$) of ratios of specific protein levels to β–actin (Loading protein). ## $p < 0.01$, ### $p < 0.001$ C-ZDF vs. C-ZL; * $p < 0.05$ M-ZL vs. C-ZL; ** $p < 0.01$, *** $p < 0.001$ M-ZDF vs. C-ZDF (Tukey post hoc test).

The IRE1α contributes to the ER stress-induced apoptosis through phosphorylation of JNK, which has been proposed to be a pro-apoptotic event through down–regulation of the anti-apoptotic protein Bcl-2 and upregulation of mitochondrial-associated pro-apoptotic factors, including Bax, leading to cleavage of caspase-3, as the terminal apoptotic effector [47].

We first examined the expression of the activated form of JNK (phospho-JNK). As shown in Figure 2a, western blot analysis revealed higher relative content in renal tissue from C–ZDF in comparison with C–ZL group (2.4-fold; $p < 0.01$; Figure 2a). Melatonin supplementation resulted in a significant loss of JNK phosphorylation in the ZDF group (1.7-fold) but had no effect on JNK phosphorylation in ZL group, as compared to the respective control group without supplementation ($p < 0.01$ and $p > 0.05$, respectively; Figure 2a). In line with this, we also evaluated the expression of mitochondria-associated pro-apoptotic Bax and anti-apoptotic Bcl-2 factors. The analysis showed that protein expression of Bax significantly increased in C–ZDF group when compared to C–ZL group (1.6-fold; $p < 0.05$; Figure 2b). This was concomitant with a significant decrease in the protein level of Bcl-2 in the C–ZDF group, as compared to C–ZL group (1.9-fold; $p < 0.01$; Figure 2c). These protein changes resulted in a significant increase in Bax/Bcl-2 ratio, as compared to C–ZL group (3.1-fold; $p < 0.001$; Figure 2d). After melatonin supplementation, the protein level of Bax significantly reduced, whereas that of Bcl-2 increased, resulting in a reduced Bax/Bcl-2 ratio expression in both ZDF (1.5-fold, 2.9-fold, and 4.2-fold, respectively) and ZL (1.3-fold, 1.3-fold, and 1.5-fold) groups, as compared to the corresponding control ZDF ($p < 0.05$, $p < 0.05$, and $p < 0.001$, respectively) and ZL ($p < 0.05$, $p < 0.05$, and $p < 0.05$, respectively) groups without supplementation (Figure 2b–d). To finally explore the relevance of melatonin on ER stress-mediated apoptosis, we detected the protein level of the activated form of caspase-3. We found that the level of activated caspase-3 (cleaved caspase-3) was significantly higher in C–ZDF group than in C–ZL group (1.4-fold; $p < 0.05$; Figure 2e), and that melatonin supplementation significantly reduced its cleavage in both ZDF (1.8-fold) and ZL (1.7-fold) groups compared to their control counterparts without supplementation ($p < 0.05$ and $p < 0.01$, respectively; Figure 2e). Interestingly, the expression levels of all the aforementioned ER stress-related apoptotic markers (phospho-JNK, Bax, Bcl-2, and cleaved caspase-3) in M–ZDF group were restored to those of the C–ZL group.

2.3. Effects of Melatonin on Renal Tissue Morphology

Given our previous findings of improved renal dysfunction outcomes with melatonin supplementation [36], we next examined whether melatonin can prevent renal structural damage. Compared with renal tissues from C–ZL rats, C–ZDF rats exhibited an early FSGS with glomerular hypertrophy, mesangial expansion, segmental mesangial hypercellularity, and capillary collapse (endocapillary) (Figure 3c). Furthermore, tubulointerstitial damage, such as interstitial fibrosis and dilated tubules with atrophic epithelial cells and destructed brush borders were also observed in C–ZDF rats (Figure 3c). The semi-quantitative histopathological analysis indicated that both glomerulosclerosis index and tubular scarring index scores were significantly higher in C–ZDF rats compared with C–ZL rats (0.67 ± 0.03 vs. $0.04 \pm 0.05/100$ glomeruli and 65.42 ± 3.12 vs. $7.12 \pm 4.11/100$ glomeruli, respectively; $p < 0.001$; Figure 3e,f). Melatonin supplementation prevented FSGS and tubular degeneration (Figure 3d) and significantly lowered the glomerulosclerosis index and tubular index scores in ZDF rats ($0.23 \pm 0.04/100$ glomeruli and $11.78 \pm 3.71/100$ glomeruli, respectively), as compared to their control counterparts without supplementation ($p < 0.001$; Figure 3e,f). The renal tissue from M–ZL rats exhibited a similar histological aspect to that from C–ZL rats (Figure 3a,b), and no significant difference in either glomerulosclerosis index or tubular scarring index was observed in them ($0.06 \pm 0.03/100$ glomeruli and $6.23 \pm 3.89/100$ glomeruli, respectively), when compared to their respective control rats without supplementation ($p < 0.001$; Figure 3e,f).

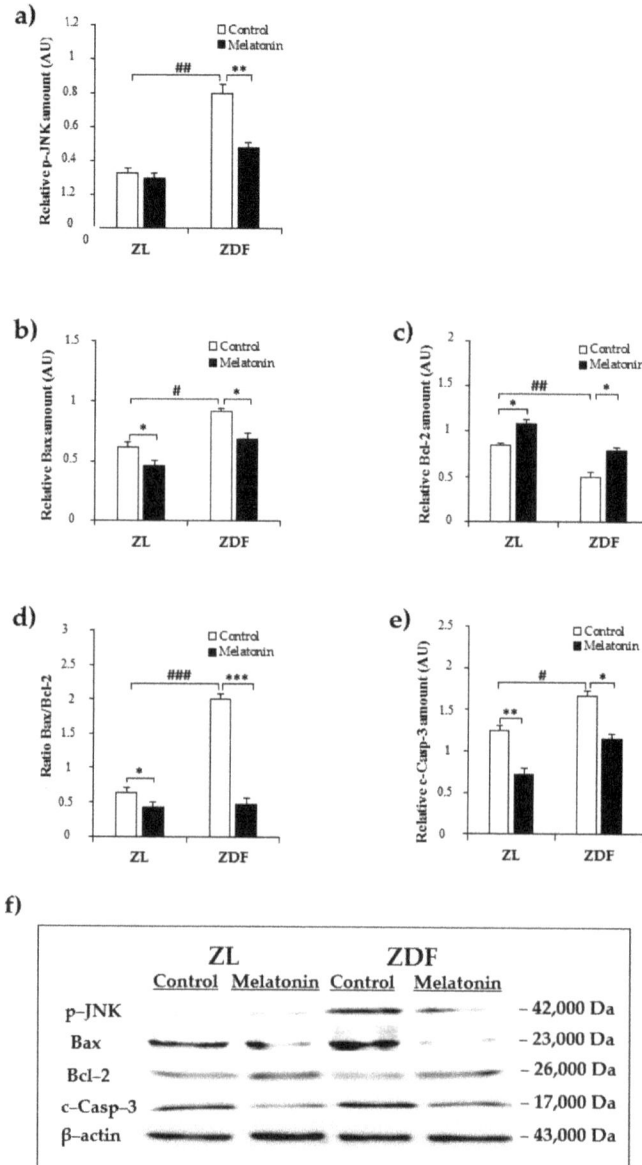

Figure 2. Effects of melatonin supplementation on ER stress-related apoptotic markers in the kidney of Zücker lean and diabetic fatty rats as measured by Western blot. (**a–c,e**) Densitometry quantification of p–c–jun amino terminal kinase (JNK), Bax, B cell lymphoma (Bcl)-2, and cleaved caspase-3 protein levels. (**d**) Bax/Bcl-2 ratio expression. (**f**) Representative blot of phospho–JNK, Bax, Bcl-2, and cleaved caspase-3. C–ZL: control lean rats without melatonin; M–ZL: lean rats with melatonin; C–ZDF: control diabetic fatty rats without melatonin; M–ZDF: diabetic fatty rats with melatonin; ZL: Zücker lean rats; ZDF: Zücker diabetic fatty rats. Values are means ± S.E.M (n = 3) of ratios of specific protein levels to β–actin (Loading protein). # $p < 0.05$, ## $p < 0.01$, ### $p < 0.001$ C–ZDF vs. C–ZL; * $p < 0.05$, ** $p < 0.01$ M–ZL vs. C–ZL; *** $p < 0.001$ M–ZL vs. C–ZL; * $p < 0.05$, *** $p < 0.001$ M–ZDF vs. C–ZDF (Tukey post hoc test).

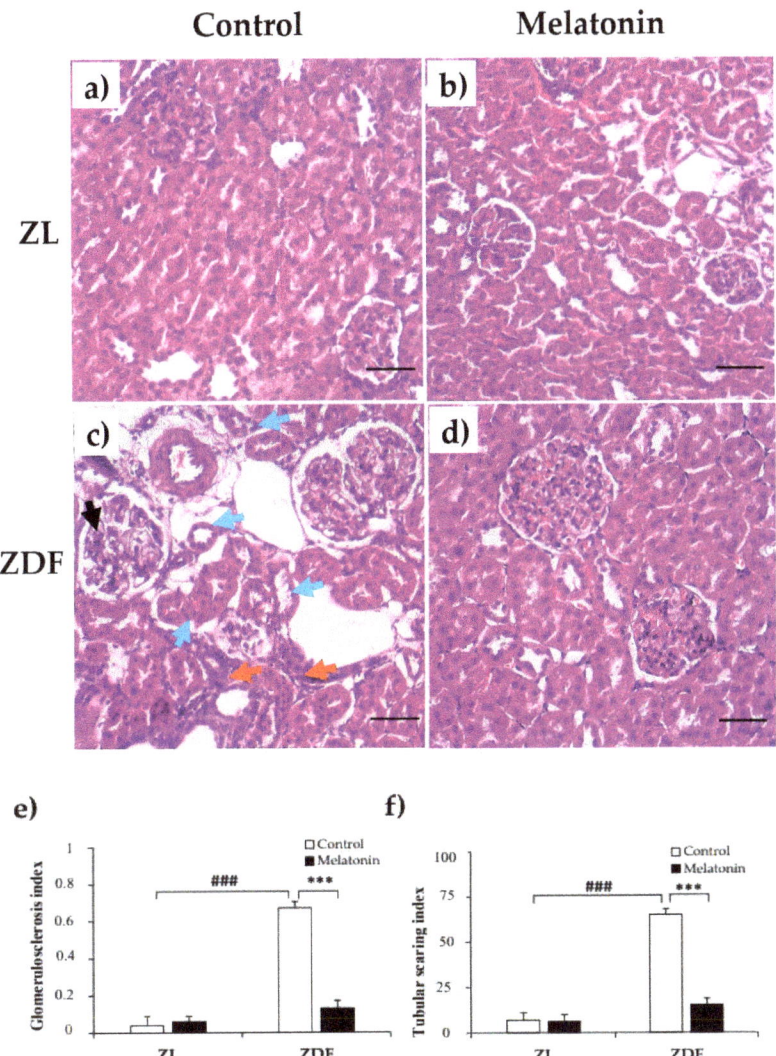

Figure 3. Effects of melatonin on renal tissue morphology of Zücker lean and diabetic fatty rats. (a,b) Representative photomicrographs showing normal appearance of the glomerulus and tubules in C–ZL (left panel) and M–ZL rats (right panel). (c) Early focal segmental glomerulosclerosis (FSGS) and tubulointerstitial damage were noted in C–ZDF rats, with a left glomerulus showing segmental mesangial hypercellularity and mild segmental endocapillary (black arrow) and on the right showing hypertrophy, associated with interstitial fibrosis (red arrows) and mild tubular degeneration as shown with epithelial cells atrophy and loss of brush borders and cell polarity (blue arrows). (d) Normal structure of renal tissue was observed in M–ZDF rats, with lower severity of FSGS and normal renal tubules, and no signs of fibrosis. (H&E stain; original magnification at ×100). (e,f) Semi-quantitative analysis of glomerulosclerosis index (left panel) and tubular index (right panel) scores in ZL and ZDF rats. C–ZL: control lean rats without melatonin; M–ZL: lean rats with melatonin; C–ZDF: control diabetic fatty rats without melatonin; M–ZDF: diabetic fatty rats with melatonin; ZL: Zücker lean rats; ZDF: Zücker diabetic fatty rats. Values are means ± S.E.M ($n = 6$). ### $p < 0.001$ C–ZDF vs. C–ZL; *** $p < 0.001$ M–ZDF vs. C–ZDF (Tukey post hoc test). Scale bar: 200 µm.

3. Discussion

Results from this study revealed for the first time that melatonin supplementation alleviated renal ER stress response and subsequent pro-apoptotic IRE1α–JNK signaling pathway in a rat model of diabesity-induced kidney injury. This was associated with the restoration of normal renal morphology. Based on these findings, we suggest that the therapeutic benefit of melatonin in the obese and diabetic kidney could be attributed, at least in part, to the modulation of ER stress-mediated cell death pathway. The present study also stresses the role of renal ER stress in the pathogenesis of diabesity-related kidney injury.

ER stress has been reported to be activated in renal tissue under conditions of obesity and associated diabetes, contributing to the development and progression of kidney disease [48]. In the present study, we proved that ER stress was induced in the renal tissue from control diabetic obese rats, as evidenced by amplified levels of GRP78, phospho–PERK phospho–IRE1α, and ATF6 stress markers. The precise trigger of ER stress cannot be deduced from this study. However, we postulate that it is likely to be a combination of increased reactive oxygen species, hyperglycemia, lipid accumulation, and excessive protein load in the ER, known to occur under obese and diabetic conditions [3]. Interestingly, the current study showed that melatonin supplementation usefully restored the levels of GRP78, phospho–IRE1α, and ATF6 proteins in diabetic obese rats. Meanwhile, melatonin supplementation had no effect on the protein level of phospho–PERK. These data clearly indicate that melatonin may exert a protective effect on obese diabetic kidneys by inhibiting the IRE1α and ATF6 pathways. Our results are in keeping with recent findings demonstrating that melatonin reduced ER stress in different models of kidney injury. For instance, melatonin attenuated the ER stress response markers in–vitro kidney stones model [40]. Similar effects were also observed in rat model of renal ischemia/reperfusion injury [41]. In lean rats, melatonin supplementation reduced the levels of GRP78 but had no effect on the three ER stress sensors, suggesting reduced acute ER stress level, which possibly reflects the fact that melatonin minimizes oxidative stress that is known to cause accumulation of unfolded proteins; bearing additionally in mind that myriad of studies, including ours, highlighted melatonin as a powerful antioxidant [16,49]. To our knowledge, this study provides the first evidence that melatonin might exert its protective effects on obese diabetic kidneys through inhibiting ER stress.

Based on the above finding showing that melatonin preferentially suppressed the IRE1α and ATF6 pathways among the three major arms of the ER stress response, we investigated the effect of melatonin on the protein expression of some IRE1α-downstream targets. It is known that IRE1α branch played a vital role in ER stress related to apoptosis [47]. This branch is highly regulated and could be the link between the survival role of ER stress and the apoptotic features related to UPR [50]. During prolonged ER stress, enhanced IRE1α kinase activity can phosphorylate the downstream JNK target to induce cell death. The induction of JNK is regarded as an important element of the switch from pro-survival to pro-apoptotic signaling cascades [47]. This study clearly shows that renal tissue from control diabetic obese rats contain a high amount of phosphorylated JNK, which indicates the activation of the apoptotic signaling. The activation of JNK signaling is critical in the development of various forms of human kidney injury [51]. JNK activation was also been evident in wide array of animal models of glomerular diseases and in the aging kidney [52–57]. ER stress-associated apoptosis is a complex process controlled by many factors, such as Bax and Bcl-2. Bcl-2 is an anti-apoptotic factor that reduces the permeability of the mitochondria membrane and regulates the mitochondrial apoptosis, while Bax is a pro-apoptotic factor that promotes the activation of caspase-3 [47]. It has been reported that the phosphorylation of IRE1α/JNK activates both pro-apoptotic Bax and concomitantly inhibited Bcl-2 factor [47]. Consistent with the activated IRE1α pro-apoptotic pathway in control diabetic obese rats, we logically found an increased level of apoptotic cell markers (Bax and cleaved caspase-3) and decreased level of anti-apoptotic Bcl-2 protein in the control diabetic obese rats compared with control lean rats. The ratio of

Bax/Bcl-2 is regarded as a key factor in determining whether cells can enter the apoptosis process [58]. Our data showed an elevated Bax/Bcl-2 ratio, which confirms the activation of the apoptotic pathway. Apoptosis is considered to be closely associated with the pathogenesis of diabetic and obesity-related kidney disease [59]. It has also been reported that diabetic and obesity-related kidney disease undergoes apoptosis in response to diabetic hyperglycemia and proteinuria [6].

In the current study, melatonin supplementation attenuates the upregulation of JNK and Bax expressions, the cleavage of caspase-3, the downregulation of Bcl-2 expression, and the Bax/Bcl-2 ratio expression in renal tissue from diabetic obese rats. Based on these data, we speculate that melatonin protects against kidney damage occurred under obese and diabetic state, by activating the pro–survival mechanisms and preventing the excessive upregulation of pro-apoptotic pathways. Moreover, because melatonin completely eliminated the induction of JNK signaling effectors and restored them to those of the control lean rats, we hypothesize that melatonin intervened with the downstream components of the JNK signaling pathway rather than it controls upstream of the ER stress signaling. Results from lean rats are a further argument in support of this hypothesis, according to which melatonin enhanced the level of Bcl-2 and reduced that of Bax and cleaved-caspase-3 but had no effect on the level of either JNK or IRE1α, which would, on the one hand, be in a favor of adaptive capacity enhancement and, on the other, be explained by the fact that melatonin target components of the Bcl-2 signaling in order to suppress the IRE1α/JNK pro-apoptotic pathway, which remains to be verified. In support with this suggestion, melatonin was shown to interfere with the intrinsic pathway of apoptosis by inducing the mitochondrial re–localization of Bcl-2 [60] and directly inhibiting Bax and caspase-3 activation [61]. Previously, other examples of melatonin reducing the ER stress-associated apoptotic conditions have been reported. For instance, melatonin protected the heart by ameliorating cardiac ER stress-induced apoptosis in rat with diabetic cardiomyopathy [62]. Additionally, melatonin protected the brain against ischemia–reperfusion injury by attenuating ER stress trigged autophagy through both PERK and IRE1α pathways [63]. Inhibition of the JNK pathway by genetic or pharmacologic approaches has also been demonstrated to be effective at preventing and suppressing glomerulosclerosis and tubulointerstitial fibrosis [51]. The current data demonstrated that in addition to suppression of the IRE1α branch of JNK signaling, melatonin supplementation prevented glomerulosclerosis, glomerular hypertrophy, and tubulointerstitial damage, which are common features seen in patients with obesity and T2DM [64,65]. Of note, a positive correlation between elevated JNK activation and increased glomerulosclerosis was observed in human renal biopsies from patients with hypertension and diabetic nephropathy [66]. Taken together, the present data suggest that melatonin might exert its renoprotective effect by targeting components of the pro-apoptotic IRE1α/JNK pathway.

Even though our current and previous data suggest that the renoprotective mechanism of melatonin under conditions of obesity and diabetes may be due, partially, to the suppression of ER stress and related IRE1α branch of JNK signaling and modulation of the mitochondrial fission/fusion balance and function, it could not rule out the possibility that the protective effect of melatonin on kidney may also be attributed to the improvement of the metabolic complications of obesity, such as dyslipidemia, insulin resistance, hyperglycemia, hypertension, and oxidative stress, which are well accepted as risk factors for the development of kidney disease [67], given that several studies, including ours, showed a beneficial effect of melatonin to counteract these risk factors [49,68,69].

4. Materials and Methods

4.1. Reagents

All reagents used were of the highest purity available. Melatonin was purchased from Sigma-Aldrich (Madrid, Spain).

4.2. Animals and Experimental Protocol

Male Zücker diabetic fatty rats (ZDF; *fa/fa*) and their male lean littermates (ZL; *fa/−*) were purchased at 5 weeks of age from Charles River Laboratory (Charles River Laboratories, SA, Barcelona, Spain). This study was conducted in compliance with the European Union guidelines for animal care and protection. Rats were housed 2 per clear plastic cage under a 12-h light/dark cycle (lights on at 07:00 a.m.) in a temperature-controlled room (25–28 °C). Tap water and Purina 5008 rat chow (protein 23%, fat 6.5%, carbohydrates 58.5%, fiber 4%, and ash 8%; Charles River Laboratories, SA, Barcelona, Spain) were provided *ad libitum*. All animals were acclimatized for 1 week before starting the experiments.

At the age of 6 weeks, the animals were randomly divided into four groups ($n = 6$ per group): the non-supplemented control groups (C–ZDF and C–ZL) and the melatonin-supplemented groups (M–ZDF and M–ZL). Melatonin was dissolved in a minimum volume of absolute ethanol and then diluted to the final solution of 0.066% (*w/v*) in the drinking water to yield a dose of 10 mg/kg body weight and was received daily for 17 weeks. The animals in the non-supplemented control groups received the vehicle in the drinking water at a comparable dose and supplementation duration. Fresh melatonin and vehicle solutions were prepared twice a week, and the melatonin dose was adjusted for body weight over the entire period of the study. Water bottles were covered with aluminum foil to protect from light, and the drinking fluid was changed twice weekly.

At the end of the experiment, the animals were sacrificed under sodium thiobarbital (thiopental) anesthesia, and the kidney of each rat was immediately removed and frozen at −80 °C until further use.

4.3. Protein Extraction and Western Blotting

Western blot analysis was performed according to the instructions previously described by our research group [70]. Briefly, about 200 mg of kidney tissue was homogenized in lysis buffer (150 mM NaCl, 5 mM ethylene diamine tetra-acetic acid EDTA, 50 mM Tris–HCl; pH 7.4) without Triton X–100 and homogenized with a Teflon pestle, maintaining the temperature at 4 °C throughout all procedures. Homogenates were centrifuged ($3000 \times g \times 15$ min; 4 °C), and the fat cake was removed from the top of the tube. Then, Triton X–100 was added to a final concentration of 1%. After incubating at 4 °C for 30 min, extracts were cleared by centrifugation at $15,000 \times g$ for 15 min at 4 °C. The supernatant fraction was stored at 80 °C in aliquots until use. Protein concentration was measured by the Bradford method using the bovine–serum albumin (BSA) as a standard. Equal amounts of protein extracts were resolved on SDS–PAGE (sodium dodecylsulfate polyacrylamide gel electrophoresis). The gels for immunoblot analyses were transferred to a nitrocellulose membrane (Bio-Rad Trans-Blot SD, Bio-Rad Laboratories). The membranes were then blocked with 5% non-fat dry milk in tris-buffered saline (TBS) containing 0.05% Tween-20 (TBS-T) for 1 h at 37 °C and incubated overnight at 4 °C with primary antibodies against GRP78 (cat#G–8918), phospho–PERK (cat#SAB–5700521), phospho–IRE1α (cat#I–6785), ATF6 (cat#SAB–2100170), phospho–JNK (cat#07–175), Bax (cat#SAB–4502546), Bcl-2 (cat#SAB–4500003), and cleaved caspase-3 (cat#AB–3623). All antibodies were obtained from Sigma-Aldrich (Sigma-Aldrich, Madrid, Spain) at 1:200–1:2000 dilution with TBS–T containing 2.5% non-fat dry milk. Equal loading of protein was demonstrated by incubating the membranes with mouse β–actin antibody (cat#SC–81178) (Santa Cruz Biotechnology, Santa Cruz, CA, USA) at 0:1000 dilution. After the incubation, the membranes were washed three times for 20 min in TBS-T and incubated for 1 h at room temperature with respective horseradish peroxidase–conjugated secondary antibodies (Sigma-Aldrich, Madrid, Spain) at 1:1000 dilution. The membrane was washed three times for 20 min in the TBS-T, and then a chemiluminescence assay system (ECL kit, GE Healthcare Life Sciences, Buckinghamshire, UK) was used to develop the immunoreactive bands. Finally, the protein band densities were quantitatively analyzed using Image J 1.33 software (National Institutes of Health, Bethesda, MD, USA). The results were normalized to β-actin as a loading control. All experiments were performed in triplicate.

4.4. Microscopic Analysis

Kidney tissues were cut into sections and fixed with 4% paraformaldehyde for 24 h, dehydrated, and embedded in paraffin following routine protocols. After embedding in paraffin, 4-μm-thick sections were stained with hematoxylin and eosin (H&E) and finally inspected under a light microscope (Olympus, Germany) equipped with a digital camera system (Carl Zeiss camera, model Axiocam ERc 5s. Göttingen, Germany). The glomerular lesions and tubular degeneration were evaluated semiquantitatively. The glomerular lesion was defined as glomerular hypertrophy, mesangial expansion, glomerulosclerosis, and capillary occlusion, and semiquantitatively scored from 0 to 3 + on the basis of severity of the lesion for each glomerulus (0 = none, 1 < 25%, 2 = up to 50%, and 3 > 50%). The glomerulosclerosis index was then calculated as described [45]. Briefly, 100 glomeruli were randomly chosen from each rat kidney and carefully scored for glomerular lesion and then adding all the scores and divided by 100. This was done in a sequential manner to ensure that the same glomerulus was not graded twice. To evaluate tubular degeneration, tubular scarring index was evaluated by counting the total number of atrophic or atrophying tubular in the same area that contained these 100 glomeruli in each section [45].

4.5. Statistical Analysis

Statistical Package of Social Science (IBM SPSS Software, version 15, Michigan, IL, USA) was used for statistical analysis. All results are expressed as mean ± standard error of the mean (S.E.M) values. Comparisons between experimental groups were analyzed using one-way ANOVA followed by Tukey post hoc test. Differences between group means were considered statistically significant if $p < 0.05$. A $p < 0.05$ was considered statistically significant, and levels of significance were labeled on the figures as follows: *** $p < 0.001$; ** $p < 0.01$; * $p < 0.05$, and ### $p < 0.001$; ## $p < 0.01$; # $p < 0.05$.

5. Conclusions

This study is the first to demonstrate that chronic melatonin supplementation in obese and diabetic-induced kidney injury rat model acts as a renal ER stress suppressor, and the mechanism is possibly through targeting IRE1α signaling pathway. This, in concert with our previously reported effect via mitochondria in the same strain animal model, showing that melatonin supplementation improves kidney function under conditions of obesity and diabetes [34]. Data from our unpublished studies showed that melatonin doses ranged between 1–10 mg/kg body weight (BW) reduces body weight and improves metabolic outcomes in diabetic obese rats. Based on human equivalent dose calculation [71], we estimated that a clinically effective dose of 0.16–1.6 mg/Kg BW might have potential therapeutic implications, especially among the obese diabetic population with a high risk of kidney disease. Hence, clinical trials should be promoted to investigate the optimal effective dose in humans. Further in–vitro studies are required to fully elaborate on the effect of melatonin on ER stress-induced kidney injury and decipher the precise underlying related molecular mechanism.

Author Contributions: Conceptualization, A.A.; Formal analysis, A.A., P.A.-G., and L.Z.; Funding acquisition, A.A.; Methodology, S.A., M.N., and D.S.; Project administration, A.A.; Software, M.N.-A.; Supervision, A.A.; Writing-original draft, S.A. All authors have read and agreed to the published version of the manuscript.

Funding: This work was supported by grant SAF2016-79794-R from the Ministerio de Ciencia e Innovación (Spain) and European Regional Development Fund (ERDF).

Institutional Review Board Statement: The study was conducted according to the guidelines of the Declaration of Helsinki, and approved by the Ethical Committee of the University of Granada (Granada, Spain) according to the European Union guidelines. The protocol code is 4 09-2016-CEEA.

Informed Consent Statement: Not applicable.

Data Availability Statement: Not applicable.

Acknowledgments: The authors thank Mohamed Tassi for his histology preparation and analysis of morphology assistance (Service of Microscopy, CIBM, University of Granada). Samira Aouichat was a visiting researcher from University of Sciences and Technology Houari Boumediene, Algiers, Algeria and Lazahar Zourgui from University of Gabes, Gabes, Tunisia. Zourgui and Aouichat were supported by Erasmus + Mobility Program Dimensión Internacional (grant number KA 107) from "European Commission".

Conflicts of Interest: No conflict of interest.

References

1. Cao, Z.; Cooper, M.E. Pathogenesis of diabetic nephropathy. *J. Diabetes Investig.* **2011**, *2*, 243–247. [CrossRef] [PubMed]
2. Ghemrawi, R.; Battaglia-Hsu, S.-F.; Arnold, C. Endoplasmic reticulum stress in metabolic disorders. *Cells* **2018**, *7*, 63. [CrossRef]
3. Hotamisligil, G.S. Endoplasmic reticulum stress and the inflammatory basis of metabolic disease. *Cell* **2010**, *140*, 900–917. [CrossRef] [PubMed]
4. Cybulsky, A.V. Endoplasmic reticulum stress, the unfolded protein response and autophagy in kidney diseases. *Nat. Rev. Nephrol.* **2017**, *13*, 681–696. [CrossRef] [PubMed]
5. Cnop, M.; Foufelle, F.; Velloso, L.A. Endoplasmic reticulum stress, obesity and diabetes. *Trends Mol. Med.* **2012**, *18*, 59–68. [CrossRef] [PubMed]
6. Yan, M.; Shu, S.; Guo, C.; Tang, C.; Dong, Z. Endoplasmic reticulum stress in ischemic and nephrotoxic acute kidney injury. *Ann. Med.* **2018**, *50*, 381–390. [CrossRef]
7. Cunard, R. Endoplasmic reticulum stress in the diabetic kidney, the good, the bad and the ugly. *J. Clin. Med.* **2015**, *4*, 715–740. [CrossRef]
8. Wang, C.; Wu, M.; Arvapalli, R.; Dai, X.; Mahmood, M.; Driscoll, H.; Rice, K.M.; Blough, E. Acetaminophen attenuates obesity-related renal injury through ER-mediated stress mechanisms. *Cell. Physiol. Biochem.* **2014**, *33*, 1139–1148. [CrossRef]
9. Li, B.; Leung, J.C.K.; Chan, L.Y.Y.; Yiu, W.H.; Li, Y.; Lok, S.W.Y.; Liu, W.H.; Chan, K.W.; Tse, H.F.; Lai, K.N.; et al. Amelioration of Endoplasmic reticulum Stress by Mesenchymal Stem Cells via Hepatocyte Growth Factor/c-Met Signaling in Obesity-Associated Kidney Injury. *Stem Cells Transl. Med.* **2019**, *8*, 898–910. [CrossRef] [PubMed]
10. Liu, G.; Sun, Y.; Li, Z.; Song, T.; Wang, H.; Zhang, Y.; Ge, Z. Apoptosis induced by endoplasmic reticulum stress involved in diabetic kidney disease. *Biochem. Biophys. Res. Commun.* **2008**, *370*, 651–656. [CrossRef] [PubMed]
11. Morse, E.; Schroth, J.; You, N.H.; Pizzo, D.P.; Okada, S.; RamachandraRao, S.; Vallon, V.; Sharma, K.; Cunard, R. TRB3 is stimulated in diabetic kidneys, regulated by the ER stress marker CHOP, and is a suppressor of podocyte MCP-1. *Am. J. Physiol. Ren. Physiol.* **2010**, *299*. [CrossRef]
12. Chen, J.; Guo, Y.; Zeng, W.; Huang, L.; Pang, Q.; Nie, L.; Mu, J.; Yuan, F.; Feng, B. ER stress triggers MCP-1 expression through SET7/9-induced histone methylation in the kidneys of db/db mice. *Am. J. Physiol. Ren. Physiol.* **2014**, *306*. [CrossRef] [PubMed]
13. Lindenmeyer, M.T.; Rastaldi, M.P.; Ikehata, M.; Neusser, M.A.; Kretzler, M.; Cohen, C.D.; Schlöndorff, D. Proteinuria and hyperglycemia induce endoplasmic reticulum stress. *J. Am. Soc. Nephrol.* **2008**, *19*, 2225–2236. [CrossRef] [PubMed]
14. Cheng, D.W.; Jiang, Y.; Shalev, A.; Kowluru, R.; Crook, E.D.; Singh, L.P. An analysis of high glucose and glucosamine-induced gene expression and oxidative stress in renal mesangial cells. *Arch. Physiol. Biochem.* **2006**, *112*, 189–218. [CrossRef]
15. Ohse, T.; Inagi, R.; Tanaka, T.; Ota, T.; Miyata, T.; Kojima, I.; Ingelfinger, J.R.; Ogawa, S.; Fujita, T.; Nangaku, M. Albumin induces endoplasmic reticulum stress and apoptosis in renal proximal tubular cells. *Kidney Int.* **2006**, *70*, 1447–1455. [CrossRef] [PubMed]
16. Promsan, S.; Lungkaphin, A. The roles of melatonin on kidney injury in obese and diabetic conditions. *BioFactors* **2020**, *46*, 531–549. [CrossRef]
17. Navarro-Alarcón, M.; Ruiz-Ojeda, F.J.; Blanca-Herrera, R.M.; A-Serrano, M.M.; Acuña-Castroviejo, D.; Fernández-Vázquez, G.; Agil, A. Melatonin and metabolic regulation: A review. *Food Funct.* **2014**, *5*, 2806–2832. [CrossRef]
18. Acuña-Castroviejo, D.; Escames, G.; Venegas, C.; Díaz-Casado, M.E.; Lima-Cabello, E.; López, L.C.; Rosales-Corral, S.; Tan, D.X.; Reiter, R.J. Extrapineal melatonin: Sources, regulation, and potential functions. *Cell. Mol. Life Sci.* **2014**, *71*, 2997–3025. [CrossRef]
19. Sanchez-Hidalgo, M.; de la Lastra, C.A.; Carrascosa-Salmoral, M.P.; Naranjo, M.C.; Gomez-Corvera, A.; Caballero, B.; Guerrero, J.M. Age-related changes in melatonin synthesis in rat extrapineal tissues. *Exp. Gerontol.* **2009**, *44*, 328–334. [CrossRef]
20. Karamitri, A.; Jockers, R. Melatonin in type 2 diabetes mellitus and obesity. *Nat. Rev. Endocrinol.* **2019**, *15*, 105–125. [CrossRef] [PubMed]
21. Meng, X.; Li, Y.; Li, S.; Zhou, Y.; Gan, R.Y.; Xu, D.P.; Li, H. Bin Dietary sources and bioactivities of melatonin. *Nutrients* **2017**, *9*, 367. [CrossRef] [PubMed]
22. Cipolla-Neto, J.; Amaral, F.G.; Afeche, S.C.; Tan, D.X.; Reiter, R.J. Melatonin, energy metabolism, and obesity: A review. *J. Pineal Res.* **2014**, *56*, 371–381. [CrossRef] [PubMed]
23. Mauriz, J.L.; Collado, P.S.; Veneroso, C.; Reiter, R.J.; González-Gallego, J. A review of the molecular aspects of melatonin's anti-inflammatory actions: Recent insights and new perspectives. *J. Pineal Res.* **2013**, *54*, 1–14. [CrossRef]
24. Galano, A.; Tan, D.X.; Reiter, R.J. Melatonin as a natural ally against oxidative stress: A physicochemical examination. *J. Pineal Res.* **2011**, *51*, 1–16. [CrossRef]
25. Ebaid, H.; Bashandy, S.A.E.; Abdel-Mageed, A.M.; Al-Tamimi, J.; Hassan, I.; Alhazza, I.M. Folic acid and melatonin mitigate diabetic nephropathy in rats via inhibition of oxidative stress. *Nutr. Metab.* **2020**, *17*. [CrossRef]

26. Ko, J.W.; Shin, N.R.; Jung, T.Y.; Shin, I.S.; Moon, C.; Kim, S.H.; Lee, I.C.; Kim, S.H.; Yun, W.K.; Kim, H.C.; et al. Melatonin attenuates cisplatin-induced acute kidney injury in rats via induction of anti-aging protein, Klotho. *Food Chem. Toxicol.* **2019**, *129*, 201–210. [CrossRef] [PubMed]
27. Leibowitz, A.; Volkov, A.; Voloshin, K.; Shemesh, C.; Barshack, I.; Grossman, E. Melatonin prevents kidney injury in a high salt diet-induced hypertension model by decreasing oxidative stress. *J. Pineal Res.* **2016**, *60*, 48–54. [CrossRef]
28. Wang, W.; Zhang, J.; Wang, X.; Wang, H.; Ren, Q.; Li, Y. Effects of melatonin on diabetic nephropathy rats via Wnt/β-catenin signaling pathway and TGF-β-Smad signaling pathway. *Int. J. Clin. Exp. Pathol.* **2018**, *11*, 2488–2496. [PubMed]
29. Kim, J.Y.; Leem, J.; Jeon, E.J. Protective effects of melatonin against aristolochic acid-induced nephropathy in mice. *Biomolecules* **2020**, *10*, 11. [CrossRef]
30. Dutta, S.; Saha, S.; Mahalanobish, S.; Sadhukhan, P.; Sil, P.C. Melatonin attenuates arsenic induced nephropathy via the regulation of oxidative stress and inflammatory signaling cascades in mice. *Food Chem. Toxicol.* **2018**, *118*, 303–316. [CrossRef] [PubMed]
31. Motawi, T.K.; Ahmed, S.A.; Hamed, M.A.; El-Maraghy, S.A.; Aziz, W.M. Combination of melatonin and certain drugs for treatment of diabetic nephropathy in streptozotocin-induced diabetes in rats. *Diabetol. Int.* **2016**, *7*, 413–424. [CrossRef]
32. Shi, S.; Lei, S.; Tang, C.; Wang, K.; Xia, Z. Melatonin attenuates acute kidney ischemia/reperfusion injury in diabetic rats by activation of the SIRT1/Nrf2/HO-1 signaling pathway. *Biosci. Rep.* **2019**, *39*. [CrossRef]
33. Kim, J.W.; Jo, J.; Kim, J.Y.; Choe, M.; Leem, J.; Park, J.H. Melatonin attenuates cisplatin-induced acute kidney injury through dual suppression of apoptosis and necroptosis. *Biology* **2019**, *8*. [CrossRef] [PubMed]
34. Potić, M.; Ignjatović, I.; Nićković, V.P.; Živković, J.B.; Krdžić, J.D.; Mitić, J.S.; Popović, D.; Ilić, I.R.; Stojanović, N.M.; Sokolović, D.T. Two different melatonin treatment regimens prevent an increase in kidney injury marker-1 induced by carbon tetrachloride in rat kidneys. *Can. J. Physiol. Pharmacol.* **2019**, *97*, 422–428. [CrossRef] [PubMed]
35. Bai, X.Z.; He, T.; Gao, J.X.; Liu, Y.; Liu, J.Q.; Han, S.C.; Li, Y.; Shi, J.H.; Han, J.T.; Tao, K.; et al. Melatonin prevents acute kidney injury in severely burned rats via the activation of SIRT1. *Sci. Rep.* **2016**, *6*. [CrossRef]
36. Agil, A.; Chayah, M.; Visiedo, L.; Navarro-Alarcon, M.; Rodríguez Ferrer, J.M.; Tassi, M.; Reiter, R.J.; Fernández-Vázquez, G. Melatonin improves mitochondrial dynamics and function in the kidney of zücker diabetic fatty rats. *J. Clin. Med.* **2020**, *9*, 2916. [CrossRef]
37. de Luxán-Delgado, B.; Potes, Y.; Rubio-González, A.; Caballero, B.; Solano, J.J.; Fernández-Fernández, M.; Bermúdez, M.; Rodrigues Moreira Guimarães, M.; Vega-Naredo, I.; Boga, J.A.; et al. Melatonin reduces endoplasmic reticulum stress and autophagy in liver of leptin-deficient mice. *J. Pineal Res.* **2016**, *61*, 108–123. [CrossRef]
38. Kim, S.J.; Kang, H.S.; Lee, J.H.; Park, J.H.; Jung, C.H.; Bae, J.H.; Oh, B.C.; Song, D.K.; Baek, W.K.; Im, S.S. Melatonin ameliorates ER stress-mediated hepatic steatosis through miR-23a in the liver. *Biochem. Biophys. Res. Commun.* **2015**, *458*, 462–469. [CrossRef]
39. Fernández, A.; Ordóñez, R.; Reiter, R.J.; González-Gallego, J.; Mauriz, J.L. Melatonin and endoplasmic reticulum stress: Relation to autophagy and apoptosis. *J. Pineal Res.* **2015**, *59*, 292–307. [CrossRef] [PubMed]
40. Song, Q.; He, Z.; Li, B.; Liu, J.; Liu, L.; Liao, W.; Xiong, Y.; Song, C.; Yang, S.; Liu, Y. Melatonin inhibits oxalate-induced endoplasmic reticulum stress and apoptosis in HK-2 cells by activating the AMPK pathway. *Cell Cycle* **2020**, *19*, 2600–2610. [CrossRef] [PubMed]
41. Hadj Ayed Tka, K.; Mahfoudh Boussaid, A.; Zaouali, M.A.; Kammoun, R.; Bejaoui, M.; Ghoul Mazgar, S.; Rosello Catafau, J.; Ben Abdennebi, H. Melatonin Modulates Endoplasmic Reticulum Stress and Akt/GSK3-Beta Signaling Pathway in a Rat Model of Renal Warm Ischemia Reperfusion. *Anal. Cell. Pathol.* **2015**, *72*, 6351. [CrossRef]
42. Peterson, R.G.; Shaw, W.N.; Neel, M.-A.; Little, L.A.; Eichberg, J. Zucker diabetic fatty rat as a model for non-insulin-dependent diabetes mellitus. *ILAR J.* **1990**, *32*, 16–19. [CrossRef]
43. Kasiske, B.L.; O'Donnell, M.P.; Keane, W.F. The zucker rat model of obesity, insulin resistance, hyperlipidemia, and renal injury. *Hypertension* **1992**, *19*, I-110–I-115. [CrossRef]
44. Chander, P.N.; Gealekman, O.; Brodsky, S.V.; Elitok, S.; Tojo, A.; Crabtree, M.; Gross, S.S.; Goligorsky, M.S. Nephropathy in Zucker diabetic fat rat is associated with oxidative and nitrosative stress: Prevention by chronic therapy with a peroxynitrite scavenger ebselen. *J. Am. Soc. Nephrol.* **2004**, *15*, 2391–2403. [CrossRef]
45. Ionescu, E.; Sauter, J.F.; Jeanrenaud, B. Abnormal oral glucose tolerance in genetically obese (fa/fa) rats. *Am. J. Physiol. Endocrinol. Metab.* **1985**, *248*, E500–E506. [CrossRef]
46. Coimbra, T.M.; Janssen, U.; Gröne, H.J.; Ostendorf, T.; Kunter, U.; Schmidt, H.; Brabant, G.; Floege, J. Early events leading to renal injury in obese Zucker (fatty) rats with type II diabetes. *Kidney Int.* **2000**, *57*, 167–182. [CrossRef]
47. Binukumar, B.K. Crosstalk Between the unfolded protein response, micrornas, and insulin signaling pathways: In search of biomarkers for the diagnosis and treatment of type 2 diabetes. *Front. Endocrinol.* **2018**, *9*. [CrossRef]
48. Sankrityayan, H.; Oza, M.J.; Kulkarni, Y.A.; Mulay, S.R.; Gaikwad, A.B. ER stress response mediates diabetic microvascular complications. *Drug Discov. Today* **2019**, *24*, 2247–2257. [CrossRef] [PubMed]
49. Agil, A.; Reiter, R.J.; Jiménez-Aranda, A.; Ibán-Arias, R.; Navarro-Alarcón, M.; Marchal, J.A.; Adem, A.; Fernández-Vázquez, G. Melatonin ameliorates low-grade inflammation and oxidative stress in young Zucker diabetic fatty rats. *J. Pineal Res.* **2013**, *54*, 381–388. [CrossRef] [PubMed]
50. Bhattarai, K.R.; Chaudhary, M.; Kim, H.; Chae, H. Endoplasmic reticulum (ER) stress response failure in diseases trends in cell biology. *Trends Cell Biol.* **2020**, *30*, 672–675. [CrossRef]
51. Grynberg, K.; Ma, F.Y.; Nikolic-Paterson, D.J. The JNK signaling pathway in renal fibrosis. *Front. Physiol.* **2017**, *8*, 829. [CrossRef]

52. Nishiyama, A.; Yoshizumi, M.; Hitomi, H.; Kagami, S.; Kondo, S.; Miyatake, A.; Fukunaga, M.; Tamaki, T.; Kiyomoto, H.; Kohno, M.; et al. The SOD mimetic tempol ameliorates glomerular injury and reduces mitogen-activated protein kinase activity in dahl salt-sensitive rats. *J. Am. Soc. Nephrol.* **2004**, *15*, 306–315. [CrossRef] [PubMed]
53. Park, S.J.; Jeong, K.S. Cell-type-specific activation of mitogen-activated protein kinases in PAN-induced progressive renal disease in rats. *Biochem. Biophys. Res. Commun.* **2004**, *323*, 1–8. [CrossRef] [PubMed]
54. Flanc, R.S.; Ma, F.Y.; Tesch, G.H.; Han, Y.; Atkins, R.C.; Bennett, B.L.; Friedman, G.C.; Fan, J.H.; Nikolic-Paterson, D.J. A pathogenic role for JNK signaling in experimental anti-GBM glomerulonephritis. *Kidney Int.* **2007**, *72*, 698–708. [CrossRef] [PubMed]
55. Lim, A.K.H.; Ma, F.Y.; Nikolic-Paterson, D.J.; Ozols, E.; Young, M.J.; Bennet, B.L.; Friedman, G.C.; Tesh, G.H. Evaluation of JNK blockade as an early intervention treatment for type 1 diabetic nephropathy in hypertensive rats. *Am. J. Nephrol.* **2011**, *34*, 337–346. [CrossRef]
56. Nakagawa, N.; Barron, L.; Gomez, I.G.; Johnson, B.G.; Roach, A.M.; Kameoka, S.; Jack, R.M.; Lupher, M.L.; Gharib, S.A.; Duffield, J.S. Pentraxin-2 suppresses c-Jun/AP-1 signaling to inhibit progressive fibrotic disease. *JCI Insight* **2016**, *1*, e87446. [CrossRef] [PubMed]
57. Kim, H.J.; Jung, K.J.; Yu, B.P.; Cho, C.G.; Chung, H.Y. Influence of aging and calorie restriction on MAPKs activity in rat kidney. *Exp. Gerontol.* **2002**, *37*, 1041–1053. [CrossRef]
58. Bilbault, P.; Lavaux, T.; Launoy, A.; Gaub, M.P.; Meyer, N.; Oudet, P.; Pottecher, T.; Jaeger, A.; Schneider, F. Influence of drotrecogin alpha (activated) infusion on the variation of Bax/Bcl-2 and Bax/Bcl-xl ratios in circulating mononuclear cells: A cohort study in septic shock patients. *Crit. Care Med.* **2007**, *35*, 69–75. [CrossRef]
59. Manucha, W.; Vallés, P.G. Apoptosis modulated by oxidative stress and inflammation during obstructive nephropathy. *Inflamm. Allergy Drug Targets* **2012**, *11*, 303–312. [CrossRef]
60. Radogna, F.; Cristofanon, S.; Paternoster, L.; D'Alessio, M.; De Nicola, M.; Cerella, C.; Dicato, M.; Diederich, M.; Ghibelli, L. Melatonin antagonizes the intrinsic pathway of apoptosis via mitochondrial targeting of Bcl-2. *J. Pineal Res.* **2008**, *44*, 316–325. [CrossRef]
61. Juknat, A.A.; del Valle Armanino Méndez, M.; Quaglino, A.; Fameli, C.I.; Mena, M.; Kotler, M.L. Melatonin prevents hydrogen peroxide-induced Bax expression in cultured rat astrocytes. *J. Pineal Res.* **2005**, *38*, 84–92. [CrossRef] [PubMed]
62. Xiong, F.Y.; Tang, S.T.; Su, H.; Tang, H.Q.; Jiang, P.; Zhou, Q.; Wang, Y.; Zhu, H.Q. Melatonin ameliorates myocardial apoptosis by suppressing endoplasmic reticulum stress in rats with long-term diabetic cardiomyopathy. *Mol. Med. Rep.* **2018**, *17*, 374–381. [CrossRef] [PubMed]
63. Feng, D.; Wang, B.; Wang, L.; Abraham, N.; Tao, K.; Huang, L.; Shi, W.; Dong, Y.; Qu, Y. Pre-ischemia melatonin treatment alleviated acute neuronal injury after ischemic stroke by inhibiting endoplasmic reticulum stress-dependent autophagy via PERK and IRE1 signalings. *J. Pineal Res.* **2017**, *62*, e12395. [CrossRef]
64. Lehmann, R.; Schleicher, E.D. Molecular mechanism of diabetic nephropathy. *Clin. Chim. Acta* **2000**, *297*, 135–144. [CrossRef]
65. Raptis, A.E.; Viberti, G. Pathogenesis of diabetic nephropathy. *Exp. Clin. Endocrinol. Diabetes* **2001**, *109*, S424–S437. [CrossRef]
66. De Borst, M.H.; Prakash, J.; Melenhorst, W.B.W.H.; Van Den Heuvel, M.C.; Kok, R.J.; Navis, G.; Van Goor, H. Glomerular and tubular induction of the transcription factor c-Jun in human renal disease. *J. Pathol.* **2007**, *213*, 219–228. [CrossRef]
67. Maric-Bilkan, C. Obesity and Diabetic Kidney Disease. *Med. Clin.* **2013**, *97*, 59–74. [CrossRef]
68. Agil, A.; Navarro-Alarcón, M.; Ruiz, R.; Abuhamadah, S.; El-Mir, M.Y.; Vázquez, G.F. Beneficial effects of melatonin on obesity and lipid profile in young Zucker diabetic fatty rats. *J. Pineal Res.* **2011**, *50*, 207–212. [CrossRef]
69. Agil, A.; Rosado, I.; Ruiz, R.; Figueroa, A.; Zen, N.; Fernández-Vázquez, G. Melatonin improves glucose homeostasis in young Zucker diabetic fatty rats. *J. Pineal Res.* **2012**, *52*, 203–210. [CrossRef]
70. Jiménez-Aranda, A.; Fernández-Vázquez, G.; Campos, D.; Tassi, M.; Velasco-Perez, L.; Tan, D.X.; Reiter, R.J.; Agil, A. Melatonin induces browning of inguinal white adipose tissue in Zucker diabetic fatty rats. *J. Pineal Res.* **2013**, *55*, 416–423. [CrossRef]
71. Reagan-Shaw, S.; Nihal, M.; Ahmad, N. Dose translation from animal to human studies revisited. *FASEB J.* **2008**, *22*, 659–661. [CrossRef]

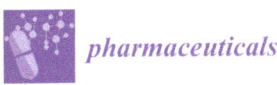

Article

Analytical Characterization of an Inulin-Type Fructooligosaccharide from Root-Tubers of *Asphodelus ramosus* L

Valentina Noemi Madia [1,†], Daniela De Vita [2,†], Antonella Messore [1,*], Chiara Toniolo [2], Valeria Tudino [1], Alessandro De Leo [1], Ivano Pindinello [1], Davide Ialongo [1], Francesco Saccoliti [3], Anna Maria D'Ursi [4], Manuela Grimaldi [4], Pietro Ceccobelli [5], Luigi Scipione [1], Roberto Di Santo [1] and Roberta Costi [1]

1. Istituto Pasteur-Fondazione Cenci Bolognetti, Dipartimento di Chimica e Tecnologie del Farmaco, "Sapienza" Università di Roma, p.le Aldo Moro 5, 00185 Rome, Italy; valentinanoemi.madia@gmail.com (V.N.M.); valeria.tudino@uniroma1.it (V.T.); alessandro.deleo@uniroma1.it (A.D.L.); ivano.pindinello@uniroma1.it (I.P.); ialongo.1679357@studenti.uniroma1.it (D.I.); luigi.scipione@uniroma1.it (L.S.); roberto.disanto@uniroma1.it (R.D.S.); roberta.costi@uniroma1.it (R.C.)
2. Department of Environmental Biology, "Sapienza" University of Rome, p.le Aldo Moro 5, 00185 Rome, Italy; daniela.devita@uniroma1.it (D.D.V.); chiara.toniolo@uniroma1.it (C.T.)
3. D3 PharmaChemistry, Italian Institute of Technology, Via Morego 30, 16163 Genova, Italy; francesco.saccoliti@iit.it
4. Department of Pharmacy, University of Salerno, Via Giovanni Paolo II, Fisciano, 84084 Salerno, Italy; dursi@unisa.it (A.M.D.); magrimaldi@unisa.it (M.G.)
5. Local Health Authority (ASL)/rm202, 00157 Rome, Italy; pietro.ceccobelli@libero.it
* Correspondence: antonella.messore@uniroma1.it; Tel.: +39-06-4991-3965
† These authors contributed equally.

Abstract: Plant-based systems continue to play a pivotal role in healthcare, and their use has been extensively documented. *Asphodelus* L. is a genus comprising various herbaceous species, known by the trivial name Asphodelus. These plants have been known since antiquity for both food and therapeutic uses, especially for treating several diseases associated with inflammatory and infectious skin disorders. Phytochemical studies revealed the presence of different constituents, mainly anthraquinones, triterpenoids, phenolic acids, and flavonoids. Although extensive literature has been published on these constituents, a paucity of information has been reported regarding the carbohydrate composition, such as fructans and fructan-like derivatives. The extraction of water-soluble neutral polysaccharides is commonly performed using water extraction, at times assisted by microwaves and ultrasounds. Herein, we reported the investigation of the alkaline extraction of root-tubers of *Asphodelus ramosus* L., analyzing the water-soluble polysaccharides obtained by precipitation from the alkaline extract and its subsequent purification by chromatography. A polysaccharide was isolated by alkaline extraction; the HPTLC study to determine its composition showed fructose as the main monosaccharide. FT-IR analysis showed the presence of an inulin-type structure, and NMR analyses allowed us to conclude that *A. ramosus* roots contain polysaccharide with an inulin-type fructooligosaccharide with a degree of polymerization of 7–8.

Keywords: *Asphodelus ramosus*; root-tubers; inulin; fructans; fructooligosaccharide; alkaline extraction; high-performance thin layer chromatography; NMR spectroscopy; 2D NMR analyses; infrared spectroscopy

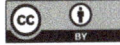

1. Introduction

The genus *Asphodelus* L. belongs to the Liliaceae [1] or Asphodelaceae family according to APG IV classification of 2016 [2]. It is native to South Europe, Africa, the Middle East, and the Indian Subcontinent, which is where it is mainly distributed [3], and reaches its maximum diversity in the west of the Mediterranean, particularly in the Iberian Peninsula and in northwest Africa [4]. Plants of genus *Asphodelus* have been known since antiquity for their both therapeutic and food uses. Indeed, root-tubers are used as daily food, after being moistened and fried beforehand to eliminate the astringent compounds [5], and also the young stem, the leaves, and the roasted seeds [6]. Additionally, various ethnomedical uses were described for *Asphodelus* species, including the treatment of skin eczema or solar erythema, alopecia, paralysis, rheumatism, or earache [3]. *Asphodelus ramosus* L. is a species abundant in Mediterranean areas [5,7,8]. Its phytochemical studies revealed the presence of different constituents, mostly depending on the part of the plant. The roots mostly exhibit the presence of anthraquinones [9–11], while the aerial parts are mainly reported to have flavonoids and phenolic acids [12,13]. A paucity of information has been reported regarding carbohydrate composition [14,15], even though the members of *Asphodelus* genus are known to contain fructans [16], water-soluble carbohydrates consisting of repeating fructose. Here, we analyzed the water-soluble polysaccharide isolated from the alkaline extract of *A. ramosus*, resulting in an inulin-type fructan. The most common inulin-type fructans (ITFs) are inulin and fructooligosaccharides (FOSs), consisting of linear chains of fructose units linked by beta (2 → 1) fructosyl-fructose glycosidic bonds bound to a terminal glucose unit and a residue of glucose [17]. From a chemical point of view, FOS and inulin differ only in the degree of polymerization (DP): FOSs have a short chain with a DP between 2 and 9, while inulin can reach 60 units [18]. Inulin is widely used in industry because it improves the taste and mouthfeel of food and can replace fats in dairy and baked products [19]. Together with FOS, inulin is classified as a dietary fiber included in the class of nondigestible carbohydrates, since they cannot be hydrolyzed by intestinal enzyme; on the contrary, the microbiome can digest FOS and inulin giving several metabolites (i.e., short-chain fatty acids) [20] that gut microbiota and the host can utilize to improve gastrointestinal physiology with benefits on lipid metabolism, with decreased levels of serum cholesterol, triacylglycerols and phospholipids [21], and levels of glucose and insulin [22], immune function, and mineral absorption [23]. Other beneficial effects include host metabolism, and even in the development and homeostasis of the CNS [24]. Currently, FOS are increasingly included in food products and infant formulas due to their prebiotic effect, stimulating the growth of nonpathogenic intestinal microflora [21]. Inulin is used as a prebiotic, fat replacer, sugar replacer, texture modifier, and for the development of functional foods in order to improve health due to its beneficial role in gastric health. Indeed, inulin plays a preventive role against gastrointestinal complications such as constipation and many diseases of the intestinal tract, particularly irritable bowel diseases and colon cancer. Moreover, inulin consumption enhances the absorption of calcium, magnesium, and iron, and stimulates the immune system [25]. Interestingly, in vitro studies showed that inulin has radical scavenging activity and ferric reducing power, although they are weaker than vitamin C. Additionally, in vivo studies of laying hens showed that dietary supplementation with inulin significantly improved the antioxidant status of these animals [26].

Therefore, natural sources of inulin and FOS have great value, possessing health benefits for humans.

2. Results and Discussion

2.1. Extraction and Purification of Water-Soluble Polysaccharides from Root-Tubers of A. ramosus

Usually, the extraction of water-soluble polysaccharides is performed using hot water, at times assisted by microwaves [27] and ultrasound [28] to overcome some disadvantages, including the long time and low efficiency of extraction. The cooking processes were reported as a method to increase the efficiency of polysaccharide extraction from plant material, breaking hydrogen and hydrophobic bonds without the degradation of the covalent ones [29]. Therefore, we performed an extraction under high-pressure cooking treatment giving the solid called AR3. Nevertheless, since hot water extraction is associated with high extraction temperature, more time consumption, and low efficiency [30], an alternative way to increase extraction yield is alkaline extraction [31]. Therefore, we also performed an alkaline extraction of *A. ramosus* root-tubers, followed by the precipitation by ethanol of a brown solid (AR1).

A fast comparison by TLC of AR1 and AR3, using commercial inulin as a standard, allowed us to conclude that only AR1 contained water-soluble polysaccharide, as preliminarily confirmed by HPTLC analysis. Then, AR1 was purified by column chromatography on silica gel using an aqueous binary mobile phase (isopropanol:water), giving AR2.

2.2. High-Performance Thin-Layer Chromatography (HPTLC) Analysis

Commonly, the polysaccharides are subjected to hydrolysis followed by the determination of their monosaccharides by cleaving a glycosidic bond in a strong acid medium. Therefore, due to the instability of sugar monomers with strong mineral acids [32], milder hydrolysis is preferred. Here, we used an aqueous solution of trifluoroacetic acid (TFA) that seemed more advantageous than other ones reported in the literature, such as oxalic acid [33], because of the possibility to remove the residual TFA at the end of the hydrolysis process. Indeed, in our hands, the co-presence of residual oxalic acid influenced the retention factor (Rf) values of the monosaccharides (data not shown). The hydrolysis with TFA was previously investigated by Li et al. [29], giving the best conditions of temperature, time, and acid concentration to cleave the glycosidic bond and preserve the stability of the corresponding monomers. For the HPTLC analysis, in addition to fructose, the aldoses (glucose, galactose and arabinose) were used as references as, in a previous work [34], these monosaccharides were found to compose the mucilage isolated from tubers of *A. microcarpus* Salzm. and Viv. As the mobile phase, we chose a binary mixture (acetonitrile/water) where water is necessary to avoid diffused spots on the silica plate. Moreover, a sample of commercial inulin underwent hydrolysis with TFA in the same condition of AR2. After acidic hydrolysis of *A. ramosus* extract by TFA, the presence in the chromatogram of fructose is very evident from both AR1 (data not shown) and AR2 (Figure 1), evidenced as a brown spot visualized by derivatization with a solution of sulfuric acid in methanol. On the contrary, other monosaccharides were not found. This allowed us to conclude that AR2 is a fructose polymer.

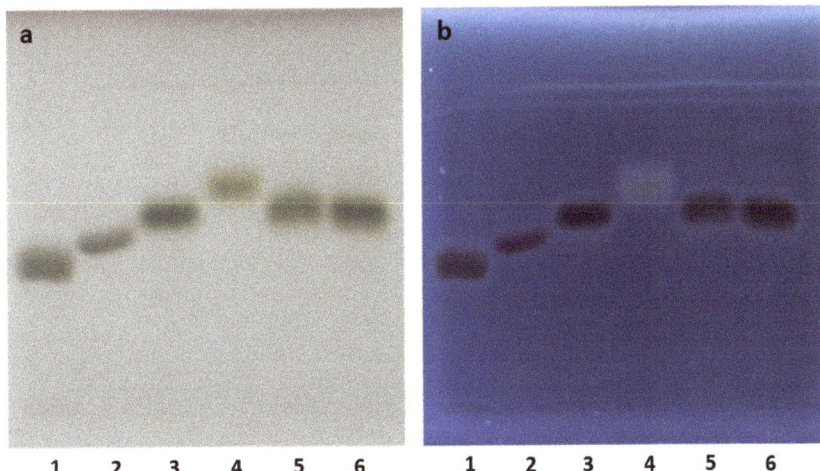

Figure 1. HPTLC analysis of the hydrolysate of the water-soluble polysaccharides from *A. ramosus* roots. Mobile phase: acetonitrile:water (85:15 v/v). (**a**) Visualization, WRT light, derivatization with a solution of sulfuric acid in methanol. (**b**) Visualization, UV 366 nm, derivatization with a solution of sulfuric acid in methanol. Tracks: 1. galactose (1 mg/mL; 8 µL); 2. glucose (1 mg/mL; 8 µL); 3 fructose (1 mg/mL; 8 µL); 4. arabinose (1 mg/mL; 8 µL); 5. hydrolyzed AR2 (1 mg/mL; 8 µL); 6. hydrolyzed inulin (1 mg/mL; 8 µL).

2.3. Fourier-Transform Infrared Spectroscopy (FTIR) Analysis

The FT-IR spectrum (Figure S4) of AR2 shows a broad band due to the vibrations of hydroxyl groups (OH stretching) at 3275 cm^{-1} [35,36], while, in the region 1500-900 cm^{-1}, the strongest bands at 1114 and 1020 cm^{-1} can be assigned to the stretching vibrations of C-OC- groups in furanosyl residues [35]. Lastly, the so-called "finger-print" region (1300-900 cm^{-1}) can be useful for the characterization of a molecule since it is characteristic of every compound. The superposition of the inulin spectrum with that of AR2 (Figure S5) shows no significant differences in FT-IR spectra of commercial inulin and the saccharide extracted from A. ramosus.

2.4. Nuclear Magnetic Resonance (NMR) Studies

Data of ^{1}H and ^{13}C NMR, heteronuclear single quantum coherence (HSQC), and heteronuclear multiple bond correlation (HMBC) are compatible with inulin structure (Figure S2) and in accordance with the literature [35,37–39]. The ^{1}H NMR spectrum (Figure S1) of AR2 showed the characteristic signals of polysaccharides in the region δ 3.40–5.40 ppm, with a higher magnitude below δ 4.20 ppm and a lower doublet in the anomeric region at 5.35 ppm (J = 3.8 Hz) related to H-1 proton of the α-Glc unit present. Intense signals were observed at more shielded fields: a doublet at 4.18 ppm (J = 8.8 Hz) and a triplet at 4.04 ppm (J = 8.8 Hz) related to H-3 and H-4 fructose, respectively, are present. The presence of fructosyl residues is also highlighted by ^{13}C NMR and DEPT-135 spectra, whose signals are in agreement with literature data [35].

^{1}H-^{13}C multiplicity-edited HSQC NMR spectrum of AR2 (Figure 2 and Figure S3) confirmed the assignments (Table 1). In details, the signals $δ_H$ 4.18/$δ_C$ 78.48, $δ_H$ 4.04/$δ_C$ 75.48, and $δ_H$ 3.80/$δ_C$ 82.20 can be assigned to C3, C4, and C5 of fructose, respectively, in agreement with literature data [35,39]. Moreover, the cross-peak $δ_H$ 5.35/$δ_C$ 93.38 belongs to the anomeric signal of glucose with an α-configuration, while the signal $δ_H$ 3.75/$δ_C$ 61.42 confirmed that glucose residue is in a terminal position of the chain.

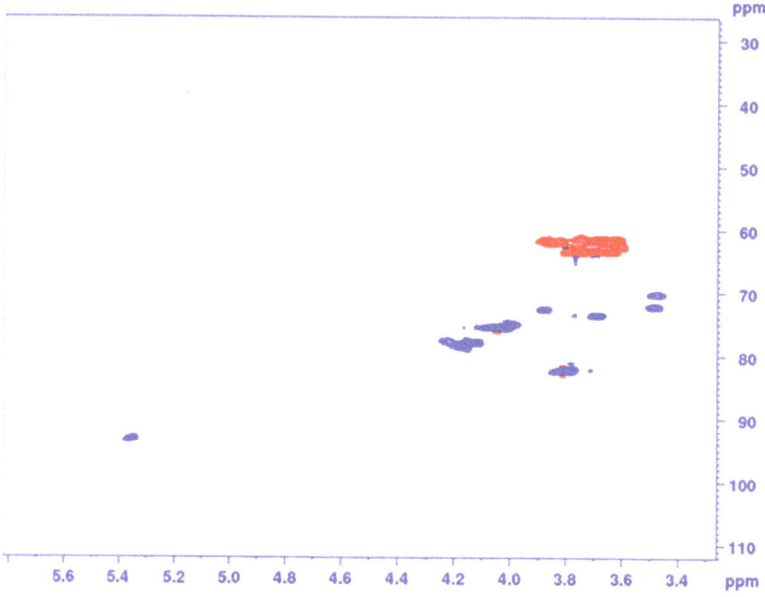

Figure 2. ^{1}H-^{13}C multiplicity-edited HSQC spectrum of AR2.

Table 1. ¹H and ¹³C NMR chemical shifts of AR2.

Residue	H-1/C-1 (ppm)	H-2/C-2 (ppm)	H-3/C-3 (ppm)	H-4/C-4 (ppm)	H-5/C-5 (ppm)	H-6/C-6 (ppm)
→1)-β-D-Fru$f$-(2→	3.85/3.66 61.94	- 104.10	4.18 78.48	4.04 75.48	3.80 82.20	3.78/3.70 63.32
α-D-Glc$p$-(1→	5.35 93.38	3.49 72.26	3.69 73.49	3.48 70.31	3.88 72.66	3.75 61.42

HMBC spectrum of AR2 showed the correlation between the H-1 of the glucosyl residue and C-2 fructosyl residue (Figure 3). Indeed, because of the cross-peak between H-1 of glucose and C-2 of fructose residue, glucose was confirmed to be terminally linked to a fructose chain with a non-reducing end [38].

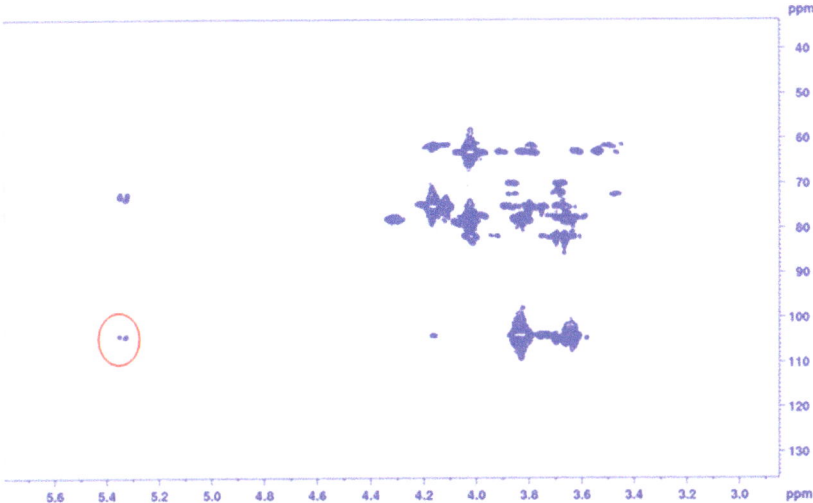

Figure 3. ¹H-¹³C 2D heteronuclear multiple bond correlation (HMBC) spectrum of AR2, correlation between the H-1 of the glucosyl residue and C-2 fructosyl residue is highlighted.

Lastly, 2D NMR studies confirmed the (2 → 1) glycosidic bonds of fructosyl residue in the chain, in line with an inulin-type structure and in agreement with previous literature data [35,37,39].

To calculate the degree of polymerization (DP) of inulin, we followed the procedure previously described [40]. According to their experimental procedure, the degree of polymerization (DP) or the number of repeating units of a polymer can be calculated by comparing the ¹H NMR signal intensity of a known moiety (typically, end-group(s) with a known number of protons) to that of the repeating chain unit of interest. By applying our data to the equation reported in the Material and Methods section, the DP of the polymer under scrutiny is found to be 7–8.

3. Materials and Methods

3.1. Materials

Roots of *A. ramosus* were collected in Vallecorsa (Lazio, Italy). Inulin, fructose, glucose, galactose, arabinose, trifluoroacetic acid, and deuterium oxide were purchased from Sigma-Aldrich (Milan, Italy). All chemical standards were of analytical grade. Concentrated sulfuric acid was obtained from Carlo Erba (Milan, Italy). Silica gel high-purity grade (pore size 60 Å, 220–440 mesh particle size, 35–75 µm particle size) were obtained from Sigma-

Aldrich (Milan, Italy). Thin layer chromatography (TLC) was performed on Kieselgel GF254 plates and the plates were heated at 150–200 °C by spraying with $KMnO_4$ solution until yellow coloration took place. The high-performance thin-layer chromatography (HPTLC) plates 10 × 10 cm with glass-backed layers silica gel 60 F_{254} (2 μm thickness) were purchased from Merck (Darmstadt, Germany) and prewashed by methanol. HPLC grade solvents were purchased from Sigma-Aldrich (Milan, Italy) and VWR (Milan, Italy). HPLC-grade water was prepared with a Milli-Q gradient (Millipore, Vimodrone, Italy) water purification system.

3.2. Extraction and Purification of the Water-Soluble Polysaccharides from Root-Tubers of A. ramosus

The alkaline solution was obtained as previously reported by us [41] by treating the fresh roots (1 kg) of *A. ramosus* with NaOH in pellets (100 g). Water-soluble polysaccharides were precipitated from the alkaline solutions by the addition of absolute ethanol as follows: 1 mL of alkaline solution was diluted with distilled water (1 mL). From the resulting solution, polysaccharides were precipitated by slow addition of absolute ethanol (ca. 5 mL). The solid was collected and dissolved with water; from the resulting solution, the solid was then precipitated with ethanol and dried under vacuum over P_2O_5 to constant weight. Fifty milligrams of a brown solid, called AR1, were obtained. Purification of AR1 was carried out on a gravity column using silica for flash chromatography as a stationary phase (weight ratio stationary phase: AR1 1:100). The mobile phase was a mixture of isopropanol:water 11:9 (*v/v*). The spot with the Rf equal to inulin was isolated and dried at low pressure to give a brownish solid, referred to as AR2, that was analyzed to elucidate its composition.

The aqueous extraction was performed with 10 g of dried root-tubers and hot water (1 L) under high-pressure cooking treatment, autoclaved for 10 min and left to rest for 24 h. An aliquot of the filtrate was concentrated under vacuum until the volume is reduced by 10 times and then added with 10-fold volume of ethanol. The precipitate was collected by centrifugation at 4000× g for 10 min, washed with ethanol 3 times, and dried until gaining a constant weight, obtaining the brownish solid AR3 (5% yield).

3.3. High-Performance Thin-Layer Chromatography Analysis

The samples (8 μL each) were applied with nitrogen flow by Linomat 5 sample applicator (CAMAG, Muttenz, Switzerland). The operating conditions were: syringe delivery speed, 10 s μL^{-1} (100 nL s^{-1}); injection volume, 8 μL; band width, 6 mm; distance from bottom, 15 mm. The HPTLC plates were developed in the Automatic Developing Chamber 2 (ADC 2), the automatic and reproducibly developing chamber (CAMAG, Muttenz, Switzerland), saturated with the same mobile phase, acetonitrile:water (85:15 *v/v*), for 20 min at room temperature. The developed solvents (i.e., type of solvents and ratios) were carefully optimized before the analyses. The length of the chromatogram run was 70 mm from the point of application. The developed layers were allowed to dry on TLC Plate Heater III (CAMAG, Muttenz, Switzerland) for 5 min at 120 °C and then derivatized with sulfuric acid. Lastly, the plates were warmed for 5 min at 120 °C before inspection. All treated plates were then inspected under a UV light at 254 or 366 nm or under reflectance and transmission white light (WRT), respectively, at a Camag TLC visualizer (CAMAG, Muttenz, Switzerland), before and after derivatization. Aqueous solutions of AR1 and AR2 (4.5 mg/mL) were analyzed before and after hydrolysis with 3 mL of TFA (1 mg/mL) for 60 min at 90 °C, according to the procedure reported in the literature [29]. The hydrolyzed sample was evaporated to remove all the volatile components, taken up with water to obtain a final concentration of 1 mg/mL. Inulin, used as a reference, was subjected to the same acidic hydrolysis and reconstituted to the final concentration of 1 mg/mL. Aqueous solutions (1 mg/mL) of galactose, glucose, fructose, and arabinose were used as a reference.

3.4. FR-IR Analysis

FT-IR spectra of sample powders were collected using a FT-IR Perkin-Elmer Spectrometer One equipped with ATR (Attenuated Total Reflection) sampling device. Spectra were recorded over the spectral range of 400–4000 cm^{-1} at a 4 cm^{-1} resolution, coadding 32 scans. Before performing the analysis, the sample was dried under vacuum with P_2O_5 until gaining a constant weight.

3.5. NMR Experiments

For monodimensional experiments, 3 mg of AR2 were dissolved in 500 µL in 99.95% D_2O. NMR spectra were recorded at 298 K and 400 MHz for ^1H and 100 MHz for ^{13}C on Bruker (Billerica, MA, USA) Avance 400 (Milano, Italy) spectrometer. Two-dimensional heteronuclear experiments were performed on 500 MHz Bruker DRX-500 spectrometer equipped with 5 mm BBI ^1H-BB/^2H Z-GRD probe, at 298 K. Two-dimensional ^1H-^{13}C heteronuclear multiple bond correlation (HMBC) and ^1H-^{13}C heteronuclear single quantum coherence (HSQC) spectra were acquired using hmbcgplpndqf (dummy scans 16, number of scans 92, time domain 256) and hsqcedetgpsp.3 (dummy scans 32, number of scans 80, time domain 256) pulse sequences available on Bruker software (Bruker, Wissembourg, France). ^1H NMR and ^{13}C resonances were assigned from the ^1H-^{13}C correlations observed in the. Chemical shifts were expressed in ppm and *J* values are shown in Hz. Quantitative measurements of signal intensity performed on both 1D and 2D experiments led to the DP calculation. In the 1D spectrum, we chose the isolated glucose unit signal at 5.35 ppm, and the fructose unit signal at 4.18 ppm.

The DP was calculated using the following equation:

$$n_x = (a_x\, m_y\, n_y) : (a_y\, m_x) \qquad (1)$$

where a_x is the area or intensity of the ^1H NMR peak of moiety x; n_x is the number of repeating units of moiety x; m_x is the number of protons of moiety x; a_y is the area or intensity of the ^1H NMR peak of moiety y; n_y is the number of repeating units of moiety y; and m_y is the number of protons of moiety y. By applying our data to this equation, the DP of the polymer under scrutiny was found to be 7–8.

4. Conclusions

A polysaccharide was isolated from the root-tubers of *A. ramosus* by alkaline extraction and purified by column chromatography. HPTLC study was performed in order to determine the monosaccharide composition of the polysaccharide after acid hydrolysis. The results show fructose as the main monosaccharide into the polymer. The identity of the fructan was further confirmed by FT-IR analysis, where comparison of AR2 and inulin spectra showed the presence of the inulin-type structure. Furthermore, 1D and 2D NMR analyses allowed us to conclude that the water-soluble polysaccharide isolated from *A. ramosus* roots is an inulin-type fructan. Lastly, the degree of polymerization was calculated by ^1H NMR, giving a DP of 7–8.

Supplementary Materials: The following are available online at https://www.mdpi.com/1424-8247/14/3/278/s1, Figure S1: ^1H spectrum of AR sample in D_2O, Figure S2: inulin structure, Figure S3: 2D ^1H-^{13}C-HSQC spectrum of AR sample in D_2O, Figure S4: FT-IR spectrum of AR2 (neat), Figure S5: FT-IR spectra (neat) of AR2 (red) and standard inulin (black) in the region 1600–600 cm^{-1}.

Author Contributions: Conceptualization, D.D.V., L.S., R.C., R.D.S., P.C. and A.M.D.; methodology, A.M., D.D.V. and M.G.; validation, A.M., A.D.L., V.T., I.P., V.N.M., C.T. and M.G.; formal analysis, M.G. and A.M.D.; investigation, A.M., D.D.V., V.N.M., C.T., A.D.L., V.T., D.I. and M.G.; resources and project administration, L.S., R.C., R.D.S. and A.M.D.; writing—original draft preparation, V.N.M., D.D.V., and M.G.; writing—review and editing, V.N.M., D.D.V., A.M., F.S., I.P., P.C. and A.M.D.; visualization, A.M., V.N.M., D.D.V., and M.G.; supervision, D.D.V., L.S., R.C., R.D.S. and A.M.D.; funding acquisition, R.C. and A.M.D. All authors have read and agreed to the published version of the manuscript.

Funding: Not applicable.

Institutional Review Board Statement: Not applicable.

Informed Consent Statement: Not applicable.

Data Availability Statement: Data are contained within the article.

Conflicts of Interest: The authors declare no conflict of interest.

Sample Availability: Samples of roots of *Asphodelus ramosus* L. are available from the authors.

References

1. El-Seedi, H.R. Antimicrobial arylcoumarins from *Asphodelus microcarpus*. *J. Nat. Prod.* **2007**, *70*, 118–120. [CrossRef] [PubMed]
2. Chase, M.W.; Christenhusz, M.J.M.; Fay, M.F.; Byng, J.W.; Judd, W.S.; Soltis, D.E.; Mabberley, D.J.; Sennikov, A.N.; Soltis, P.S.; Stevens, P.F. An update of the Angiosperm Phylogeny Group classification for the orders and families of flowering plants: APG IV. *Bot. J. Linn. Soc.* **2016**, *181*, 1–20.
3. Malmir, M.; Serrano, R.; Caniça, M.; Silva-Lima, B.; Silva, O. A comprehensive review on the medicinal plants from the genus *Asphodelus*. *Plants* **2018**, *7*, 20. [CrossRef] [PubMed]
4. Díaz Linfante, Z. *Asphodelus* L. In *Flora Iberica*, 1st ed.; Liliaceae-Agavaceae, Talavera, S., Andrés, C., Arista, M., Piedra, M.P.F., Rico, E., Crespo, M.B., Quintanar, A., Herrero, A., Aedo, C., Eds.; Real Jardin Botánico, Consejo Superior de Investigaciones Científicas (CSIC): Madrid, Spain, 2013; Volume 20, pp. 1–33.
5. Geraci, A.; Amato, F.; Di Noto, G.; Bazan, G.; Schicchi, R. The wild taxa utilized as vegetables in Sicily (Italy): A traditional component of the Mediterranean diet. *J. Ethnobiol. Ethnomed.* **2018**, *14*, 14. [CrossRef]
6. Peksel, A.; Imamoglu, S.; Altas Kiymaz, N.; Orhan, N. Antioxidant and radical scavenging activities of *Asphodelus aestivus* Brot. extracts. *Int. J. Food Prop.* **2013**, *16*, 1339–1350. [CrossRef]
7. Crosti, R.; Ladd, P.G.; Dixon, K.W.; Piotto, B. Post-fire germination: The effect of smoke on seeds of selected species from the central Mediterranean basin. *For. Ecol. Manag.* **2006**, *221*, 306–312. [CrossRef]
8. Perrino, E.V.; Signorile, G.; Marvulli, M. A first checklist of the vascular flora of the Polignano a Mare coast (Apulia, southern Italy). *Nat. Croat.* **2013**, *22*, 295–318.
9. Adinolfi, M.; Corsaro, M.M.; Lanzetta, R.; Parrilli, M.; Scopa, A.A. Bianthrone C glycoside from *Asphodelus ramosus* tubers. *Phytochemistry* **1989**, *28*, 284–288. [CrossRef]
10. Adinolfi, M.; Lanzelta, R.; Marciano, C.E.; Parrilli, M.; Giulio, A.D.E. A new class of anthraquinone-anthrone-C-glycosides from *Asphodelus ramosus* tubers. *Tetrahedron* **1991**, *47*, 4435–4440. [CrossRef]
11. Lanzetta, R.; Parrilli, M.; Adinolfi, M.; Aquila, T.; Corsaro, M.M. Bianthrone C-glycosides. 2. Three new compounds from *Asphodelus ramosus* tubers. *Tetrahedron* **1990**, *46*, 1287–1294. [CrossRef]
12. Reynaud, J.; Lussignol, M.; Flament, M.M.; Becchi, M. Flavonoid content of *Asphodelus ramosus* (Liliaceae). *Can. J. Bot.* **1997**, *75*, 2105–2107. [CrossRef]
13. Chimona, C.; Karioti, A.; Skaltsa, H.; Rhizopoulou, S. Occurrence of secondary metabolites in tepals of *Asphodelus ramosus* L. *Plant Biosyst.* **2014**, *148*, 31–34. [CrossRef]
14. Incoll, L.D.; Bonnett, G.D. The occurrence of fructan in food plants. In *Studies in Plant Science*, 1st ed.; Fuchs, A., Ed.; Elsevier: Amsterdam, The Netherlands, 1993; Volume 3, pp. 309–322.
15. Meier, H.; Reid, J.S.G. Reserve polysaccharides other than starch in higher plants. In *Plant Carbohydrates I. Encyclopedia of Plant Physiology*; New Series; Loewus, F.A., Tanner, W., Eds.; Springer: Berlin/Heidelberg, Germany, 1982; Volume 13, pp. 418–471.
16. Loewus, F.A.; Tanner, W. *Plant Carbohydrates I: Intracellular Carbohydrates*; New Series; Springer: Berlin/Heidelberg, Germany, 2012.
17. Franco-Robles, E.; López, M.G. Implication of fructans in health: Immunomodulatory and antioxidant mechanisms. *Sci. World J.* **2015**, *2015*, 289267.
18. Brites, M.L.; Noreña, C.P.Z. Obtaining fructooligosaccharides from yacon (*Smallanthus sonchifolius*) by an ultrafiltration process. *Braz. J. Chem. Eng.* **2016**, *33*, 1011–1020. [CrossRef]
19. Franck, A. Technological functionality of inulin and oligofructose. *Br. J. Nutr.* **2002**, *87*, S287–S291. [CrossRef]
20. Kumar, J.; Rani, K.; Datt, C. Molecular link between dietary fibre, gut microbiota and health. *Mol. Biol. Rep.* **2020**, *47*, 6229–6237. [CrossRef] [PubMed]
21. Sabater-Molina, M.; Larqué, E.; Torrella, F.; Zamora, S. Dietary fructooligosaccharides and potential benefits on health. *J. Physiol. Biochem.* **2009**, *65*, 315–328. [CrossRef]
22. Ahmed, W.; Rashid, S. Functional and therapeutic potential of inulin: A comprehensive review. *Crit. Rev. Food Sci. Nutr.* **2019**, *59*, 1–13. [CrossRef]
23. Saeed, F.; Pasha, I.; Arshad, M.U.; Anjum, F.M.; Hussain, S.; Rasheed, R.; Nasir, M.A.; Shafique, B. Physiological and nutraceutical perspectives of fructan. *Int. J. Food Prop.* **2015**, *18*, 1895–1904. [CrossRef]
24. Silva, Y.P.; Bernardi, A.; Frozza, R.L. The role of short-chain fatty acids from gut microbiota in gut-brain communication. *Front. Endocrinol.* **2020**, *11*, 25. [CrossRef] [PubMed]
25. Shoaib, M.; Shehzad, A.; Omar, M.; Rakha, A.; Raza, H.; Sharif, H.R.; Shakeel, A.; Ansari, A.; Niazi, S. Inulin: Properties, health benefits and food applications. *Carbohydr. Polym.* **2016**, *147*, 444–454. [CrossRef]
26. Shang, H.M.; Zhou, H.Z.; Yang, J.Y.; Li, R.; Song, H.; Wu, H.X. In vitro and in vivo antioxidant activities of inulin. *PLoS ONE* **2018**, *13*, e0192273. [CrossRef] [PubMed]

27. Zhao, J.L.; Zhang, M.; Zhou, H.L. Microwave-assisted extraction, purification, partial characterization, and bioactivity of polysaccharides from *Panax ginseng*. *Molecules* **2019**, *24*, 1605. [CrossRef] [PubMed]
28. Wang, J.; Lu, H.D.; Muḥammad, U.; Han, J.Z.; Wei, Z.H.; Lu, Z.X.; Bie, X.M.; Lu, F.X. Ultrasound-assisted extraction of polysaccharides from *Artemisia selengensis* Turcz and its antioxidant and anticancer activities. *Int. J. Food Sci.* **2016**, *53*, 1025–1034. [CrossRef] [PubMed]
29. Li, S.; Wu, Q.; Yin, F.; Zhu, Z.; He, J.; Barba, F.J. Development of a combined trifluoroacetic acid hydrolysis and HPLC-ELSD method to identify and quantify inulin recovered from *Jerusalem artichoke* assisted by ultrasound extraction. *Appl. Sci.* **2018**, *8*, 710. [CrossRef]
30. Huang, S.Q.; Li, J.W.; Wang, Z.; Pan, H.X.; Chen, J.X.; Ning, Z.X. Optimization of alkaline extraction of polysaccharides from *Ganoderma lucidum* and their effect on immune function in mice. *Molecules* **2010**, *15*, 3694–3708. [CrossRef] [PubMed]
31. Chen, Y.; Yin, L.; Zhang, X.; Wang, Y.; Chen, Q.; Jin, C.; Hu, Y.; Wang, J. Optimization of alkaline extraction and bioactivities of polysaccharides from rhizome of *Polygonatum odoratum*. *Biomed. Res. Int.* **2014**, *2014*, 504896.
32. Antal, M.J., Jr.; Mok, W.S.; Richards, G.N. Mechanism of formation of 5-(hydroxymethyl)-2-furaldehyde from D-fructose and sucrose. *Carbohydr. Res.* **1990**, *199*, 91–109. [CrossRef]
33. Simonovska, B. Determination of inulin in foods. *J. Assoc. Off. Anal. Chem.* **2000**, *83*, 675–678. [CrossRef]
34. Rizk, A.M.; Hammouda, F.M. Phytochemical Studies of Asphodelus microcarpus (Lipids and Carbohydrates). *Planta Med.* **1970**, *18*, 168–172. [CrossRef]
35. Sun, Q.; Zhu, L.; Li, Y.; Cui, Y.; Jiang, S.; Tao, N.; Chen, H.; Zhao, Z.; Xu, J.; Dong, C. A novel inulin-type fructan from *Asparagus cochinchinensis* and its beneficial impact on human intestinal microbiota. *Carbohydr. Polym.* **2020**, *247*, 116761. [CrossRef] [PubMed]
36. Chen, J.; Cheong, K.; Song, Z.; Shi, Y.; Huang, X. Structure and protective effect on UVB-induced keratinocyte damage of fructan from white garlic. *Carbohydr. Polym.* **2013**, *92*, 200–205. [CrossRef] [PubMed]
37. Meng, Y.; Xu, Y.; Chang, C.; Qiu, Z.; Hu, J.; Wu, Y.; Zhang, B.; Zheng, G. Extraction, characterization and anti-inflammatory activities of an inulin-type fructan from *Codonopsis pilosula*. *Int. J. Biol. Macromol.* **2020**, *163*, 1677–1686. [CrossRef]
38. Zhang, X.; Hu, P.; Zhang, X.; Li, X. Chemical structure elucidation of an inulin-type fructan isolated from *Lobelia chinensis* lour with anti-obesity activity on diet-induced mice. *Carbohydr. Polym.* **2020**, *240*, 116357. [CrossRef]
39. Cerantola, S.; Kervarec, N.; Pichon, R.; Magné, C.; Bessieres, M.A.; Deslandes, E. NMR characterization of inulin-type fructooligosaccharides as the major water-soluble carbohydrates from *Matricaria maritima* (L.). *Carbohydr. Res.* **2004**, *339*, 2445–2449. [CrossRef] [PubMed]
40. Josephat, U.I.; Higginbotham, C.L. Polymer molecular weight analysis by ^{1}H NMR spectroscopy. *J. Chem. Educ.* **2011**, *88*, 1098–1104.
41. Ceccobelli, P.; Mirabella, C. WO-Composition of Asphodelus root extracts. PCT International Patent Application 2017/137887, 17 August 2017.

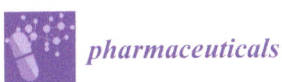

Article

A Newfangled Collagenase Inhibitor Topical Formulation Based on Ethosomes with *Sambucus nigra* L. Extract

Ana Henriques Mota [1], Inês Prazeres [2,3], Henrique Mestre [1], Andreia Bento-Silva [1], Maria João Rodrigues [4], Noélia Duarte [1], Ana Teresa Serra [2,3], Maria Rosário Bronze [1,2,3], Patrícia Rijo [1,5], Maria Manuela Gaspar [1], Ana Silveira Viana [6], Lia Ascensão [7], Pedro Pinto [8], Pradeep Kumar [9], António José Almeida [1] and Catarina Pinto Reis [1,10,*]

[1] iMED.Ulisboa, Research Institute for Medicines, Faculdade de Farmácia, Universidade de Lisboa, Av. Prof. Gama Pinto, 1649-003 Lisboa, Portugal; ana.luisa.mota@campus.ul.pt (A.H.M.); henriquemestre@campus.ul.pt (H.M.); abentosilva@ff.ulisboa.pt (A.B.-S.); mduarte@ff.ulisboa.pt (N.D.); mrbronze@ff.ulisboa.pt (M.R.B.); patricia.rijo@ulusofona.pt (P.R.); mgaspar@ff.ulisboa.pt (M.M.G.); aalmeida@ff.ulisboa.pt (A.J.A.)

[2] IBET, Instituto de Biologia Experimental e Tecnológica, Av. da República, Estação Agronómica, Apartado 12, 2780-901 Oeiras, Portugal; ines.prazeres@ibet.pt (I.P.); tserra@ibet.pt (A.T.S.)

[3] Instituto de Tecnologia Química e Biológica António Xavier, Universidade Nova de Lisboa (ITQB NOVA), Av. da República, 2780-157 Oeiras, Portugal

[4] Centre of Marine Sciences, Faculty of Sciences and Technology, University of Algarve, Ed. 7, Campus of Gambelas, 8005-139 Faro, Portugal; mary_p@sapo.pt

[5] CBiOS—Research Center for Biosciences & Health Technologies, Universidade Lusófona de Humanidades e Tecnologias, Campo Grande 376, 1749-024 Lisboa, Portugal

[6] Centro de Química Estrutural, Faculdade de Ciências, Universidade de Lisboa, Campo Grande, 1749-016 Lisboa, Portugal; apsemedo@fc.ul.pt

[7] Centro de Estudos do Ambiente e do Mar (CESAM), Faculdade de Ciências, Universidade de Lisboa, Campo Grande, 1749-016 Lisboa, Portugal; lmpsousa@fc.ul.pt

[8] PhDTrials—International Contract Research Organization, Av. Maria Helena Vieira da Silva n° 24 A, 1750-182 Lisboa, Portugal; pcontreiras@sapo.pt

[9] Wits Advanced Drug Delivery Platform Research Unit, Department of Pharmacy and Pharmacology, School of Therapeutic Sciences, Faculty of Health Sciences, University of the Witwatersrand, Johannesburg 2193, South Africa; pradeep.kumar@wits.ac.za

[10] IBEB, Biophysics and Biomedical Engineering, Faculdade de Ciências, Universidade de Lisboa, 1749-016 Lisboa, Portugal

* Correspondence: catarinareis@ff.ulisboa.pt; Tel.: +351-21-794-6400

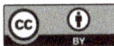

Abstract: *Sambucus nigra* L. (*S. nigra*) is a shrub widespread in Europe and western Asia, traditionally used in medicine, that has become popular in recent years as a potential source of a wide range of interesting bioactive compounds. The aim of the present work was to develop a topical *S. nigra* extract formulation based on ethosomes and thus to support its health claims with scientific evidence. *S. nigra* extract was prepared by an ultrasound-assisted method and then included in ethosomes. The ethosomes were analyzed in terms of their size, stability over time, morphology, entrapment capacity (EC), extract release profile, stability over time and several biological activities. The prepared ethosomes were indicated to be well defined, presenting sizes around 600 nm. The extract entrapment capacity in ethosomes was 73.9 ± 24.8%, with an interesting slow extract release profile over 24 h. The extract-loaded ethosomes presented collagenase inhibition activity and a very good skin compatibility after human application. This study demonstrates the potential use of *S. nigra* extract incorporated in ethosomes as a potential cosmeceutical ingredient and on further studies should be performed to better understand the impact of *S. nigra* compounds on skin care over the time.

Keywords: *Sambucus nigra* L.; ethosomes; collagenase inhibition; skin compatibility

1. Introduction

The skin constitutes the interface between the organism and the external environment, acting as an epidermal barrier, protecting and supporting the life that it encloses. It presents three different layers (epidermis, dermis and hypodermis). The epidermis in turn can be divided in distinct layers: stratum corneum, lucidum, granulosum, spinosum and basale [1–3].

Over the years, skin disorders have been emerging, affecting millions of people particularly in developing countries. Several factors can disturb this barrier function by damaging the stratum corneum (SC). These factors are associated with ultrastructural anomalies in the upper granular layer [1], related to a change of integrity of the skin layers and respective structures. These disorders can appear due to many factors, underlying medical conditions and other pathologies, such as inflamed skin, infections, chronic inflammatory skin disorders (e.g., psoriasis), sensitive skin (e.g., allergic contact dermatitis, atopic dermatitis, seborrhea dermatitis or rosacea), among others [1]. Inflamed skin is generally characterized by redness, swelling, itching, heat and pain [2]. The cause or trigger for skin inflammation may be acute or chronic. Most cases are curable, and the treatment depends on what is causing the inflammation. On the other hand, skin infections occur when bacteria, virus, fungus or other foreign substances enter the skin through a wound or cut. These can lead to several diseases like cellulitis, impetigo, staphylococcal infections, shingles, warts, yeast infections, among others. Symptoms include swelling, redness, pain, irritation, itching and burning sensation. Finally, sensitive skin is described as a discomfort situation with stinging, burning or tingling sensations and sometimes it can be very painful and itch [2]. Thus, finding new protective bioactive ingredients that can help in skin care is crucial.

S. nigra has been used in traditional medicine for several purposes [4,5]. One of them is related to its microbiological properties. Recent studies reported that a flower extract of *S. nigra* has several important biological activities, such as anti-inflammatory properties and collagenase (Coll)-inhibitory activity [4,5]. Coll is a matrix metalloprotease (MMP) enzyme responsible for the degradation of collagen [5,6]. In general, this enzyme is produced by fibroblasts like synoviocytes [6], and the degradation of the extracellular matrix by Coll has an important part in the invasion of tumor cells [7]. Collagen can be classified in different types, being collagen type I, the most abundant protein of the skin [8] and collagen I and III fibrils, responsible for the strength and resiliency of the skin. The skin aging is associated with an overexpression of Coll activity [9], as well as a reduced production of type I and III collagen as well as an abundance of degraded and disorganized collagen fibrils [8,10]. Furthermore, tumor cells may induce host cells to produce Coll [7]. In this sense, like many other species, elderflower extracts might have some potential and interesting properties against skin aging, although, its direct skin application can be compromised by thermal degradation [11], or by photodegradation which might affect its phenolic content [12]. Thus, the encapsulation or entrapment of extracts using protective carriers may present several advantages [4,13]. The characterization of the extract was already performed by our research group [4,5]. It was possible to identify malic acid, rutin, isoquercetin, isorhamnetin-3-O-glucoside, naringenin, quercetin-4-O-glucoside, isorhamnetin-3-rutinoside and luteolin-7-O-glucoside (see Supplementary Material Figure S1).

Nanotechnology has been used in the delivery of therapeutic agents or active ingredients through the skin. Among nanocarriers, vesicular systems are frequently used, since they present many advantages as enhancer agents of the stability of loaded agents, preventing its degradation and improving its penetration across the skin. These advantages are a consequence of their size, elasticity and lipid content, which allows to interact with the SC [2]. Among vesicles, ethosomes represent the third generation of elastic lipid carriers. They are phospholipid nanovesicles with ability to overcome the natural dermal barrier and capacity to delivery drugs through the skin layers. Ethosomes are constituted by phospholipids (20–45%), water and high concentrations of short chain alcohols (in general between 20–45% ethanol) and isopropyl alcohol or propylene glycol (up to 15%). A contributing factor that could explain the enhanced delivery when compared with other vesicles, such as liposomes, is the presence of ethanol, a known permeation enhancer, which provides ultradeformability. Ethanol is interspersed in the intercellular lipids, enhancing the lipid fluidity and decreasing the density of the lipid multilayer, event that is known as "ethanol effect". Afterwards, the "ethosomes effect" occurs, consisting of the interlipid penetration and permeation by the opening of new pathways due to the malleability and fusion of these nanovesicles with skin lipids. Thus resulting in the release of bioactive compounds into the deep layers of the skin [14].

This study aimed to develop a possible ultradeformable skin carrier for *Sambucus* extract, to protect the bioactive compounds from degradation and to obtain a slow bioactive compound release [1–3,15,16].

2. Results and Discussion

2.1. Physical Characterization of Ethosomes

Empty and extract-loaded ethosomes were successfully produced and then characterized in terms of size, polidispersity index (PdI) and pH. This characterization was also performed for stored particles at three different temperatures: refrigerated conditions (RC), room temperature (RT) and accelerated conditions (AC) for 12 months as depicted in Figure 1.

It is noteworthy that an increase of the size was observed after the extract encapsulation. The temperature of storage had influence on particle size. After loading the particle size of extract-loaded ethosomes was 630.1 ± 113.8 nm at RC (0 months) and 573.3 ± 192.3 nm (0 months) at AC, but a slight decrease was observed after 12 months in storage. The final particle size was 580.7 ± 57.1 nm and 549.8 ± 147.4 nm for RC and AC, respectively. However, at RT, the extract-loaded ethosomes presented an increase of the particle size from 601.6 ± 103.6 nm to 726.4 ± 133.6 nm (12 months). But, in all cases, those changes were very small in particular at AC. The particle size has influence in many properties of particulate materials, being a crucial key factor for quality and performance of the formulation [4,17]. It is very important to maintain this parameter over the time and to control the tendency of creating agglomerates.

In terms of the PdI, at RC, the extract-loaded ethosomes presented a slight increase of PdI from 0.725 ± 0.086 (0 months) to 0.784 ± 0.111 (12 months). While, at RT and AC there was a reduction of the PdI, from 0.731 ± 0.116 (0 months) to 0.707 ± 0.194 (12 months) and 0.755 ± 0.111 (0 months) to 0.569 ± 0.210 (12 months), respectively.

In terms of pH, after the extract encapsulation, a decrease of the pH was verified. Concerning the pH values, the extract-loaded ethosomes suspension revealed differences ($p < 0.001$) over time at RC and at AC. Less evident differences were observed at RT with a $p < 0.01$ (0–12 months). This data is in accordance with previous studies where the pH values were 4.11 ± 0.04 and 3.90 ± 0.03, for empty and rutin-loaded ethosomes, respectively [18].

Finally, the zeta potential analysis showed that the empty and extract-loaded ethosomes presented negative charge. When comparing both, i.e., empty and loaded ethosomes, the results suggest that the extract encapsulation led to an increase of the negative charge of the ethosomes.

As section summary, the extract-loaded ethosomes were stable over time in terms of size and pH. The temperature of storage had influence on the tested parameters especially on PdI. The extract-loaded ethosomes showed a better stability at RT in terms of size, PdI, pH and zeta potential when compared with other temperatures.

2.2. Lipid Quantification of Ethosomes

Considering the nature of these carriers, lipid composition was determined to correctly assess the amount of ethosomes for the next studies. The calibration curve was established between 10 and 80 nmol/tube ($y = 0.013x + 0.0033$ with a R^2 of 0.9996). The theoretical concentration for this formulation was of 25.95 µmol/mL. However, the obtained result suggested a concentration of 28.33 µmol/mL. Thus, the result was near the empiric concentration.

2.3. Histochemical Characterization of Ethosomes Lipidic Constitution and of Their Morphology

In light microscopy, the empty ethosomes in suspension state had the appearance of small spherical granules (Figure 2a). After staining with Nile blue A (a stain for in situ detection of all the major classes of cellular lipids), they stained blue, indicating the presence of acidic lipids (Figure 2b). Neutral lipids generally stain red with this histochemical test. When Nile Blue A was used as a fluorochrome, an intense bright red fluorescence was observed under green light (Figure 2c) which confirms the lipidic constitution of ethosomes.

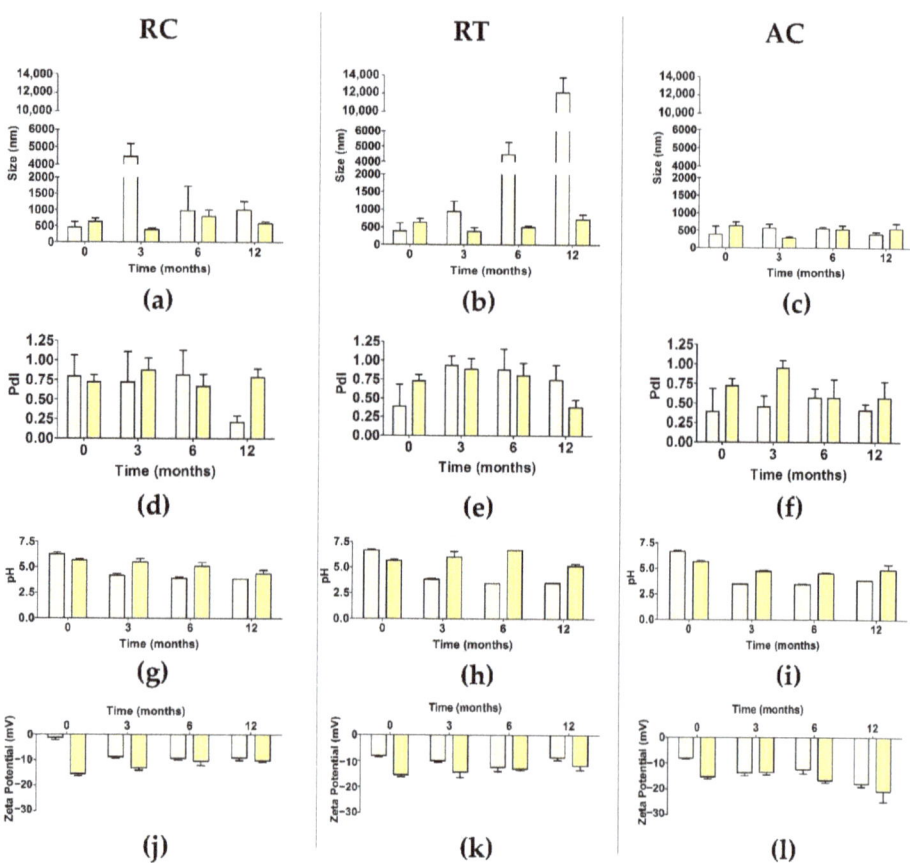

Figure 1. (a–l) Variation of mean size, PdI, pH and zeta potential over the time (0, 3, 6 and 12 months) of empty ethosomes (light yellow columns) and extract-loaded ethosomes (dark yellow columns) using different temperature of storage, namely, RC, RT and AC (mean ± S.D., n = 9).

The micrographs obtained with Nile blue support the quantification of lipids determined previously, where the same tendency was observed. In Figure 2c, the amount of red points was significant, revealing an important amount of lipids into the formulation, which corresponds to the phosphatidylcholine (SPC) used.

Furthermore, empty and extract-loaded ethosomes were observed by scanning and transmission electron microscopy (SEM and TEM), as well as by atomic force microscopy (AFM). By SEM, all ethosomes presented a spherical or a very near-spherical-shape and a smooth surface (Figure 3a,b). The morphology of ethosomes does not seem to change after entrapment of the extract. TEM observations also showed spherical shaped unilamellar vesicles (Figure 3c,d), confirming the results obtained by Dynamic Light Scattering (DLS).

By AFM (Figure 4), another technique and sample treatment, sizes between ca 140 and 350 nm were observed for empty ethosomes, whereas extract-loaded ones exhibited approximately 300 nm, as represented in the cross-section profiles of Figure 4b,d. Overall, the sizes observed by AFM were lower than the ones determined by DLS. AFM generally delivers a high contrast images and signal to noise ratio. However, it can be very sensitive to cleanliness of the samples [19]. In case of DLS, this technique measures Brownian motion and relates to the hydrodynamic diameter. This value refers to how a particle diffused within a fluid and it strongly depends on the particle "core", particle surface as well the concentration and type of the ions in that medium that forms a double layer. These ions can influence the thickness of the electric double layer. All techniques showed that empty and extract-loaded ethosomes exhibited a spherical or near-spherical-shape, which is a good indicator for the potential topical use, since the surface area versus volume should be high in principle [20].

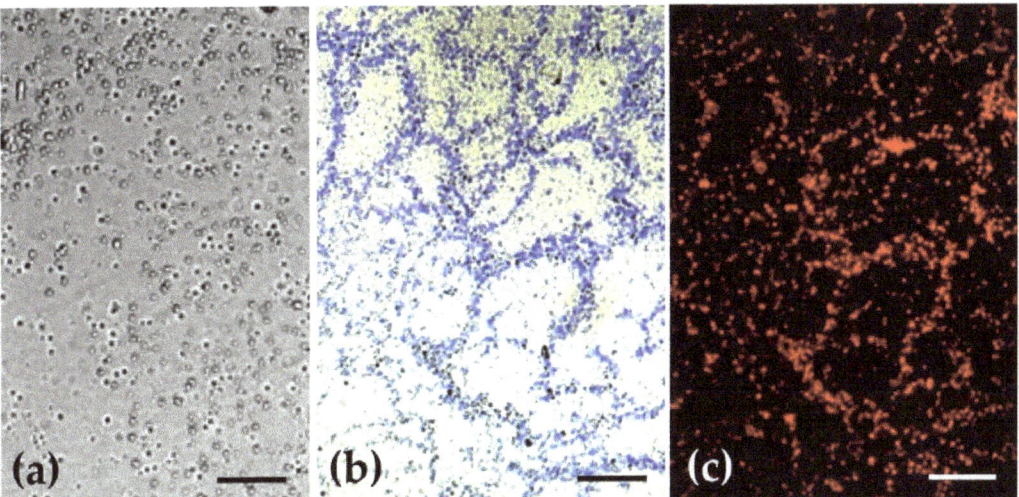

Figure 2. Light micrographs of empty ethosomes. (**a**) Unstained and observed with Nomarsky optics; (**b**) Stained with Nile blue A and observed under bright field illumination; (**c**) Stained with Nile blue A and observed under green light. Note the bright red secondary fluorescence of lipids. Scale bars = 5 µm.

2.4. Entrapment Capacity of Extract in Ethosomes

The entrapment capacity (EC) was determined for extract-loaded ethosomes using rutin as reference (Figure 5). Rutin is the major phenolic compound of this extract (74.93 ± 17.00 mg/g of extract). This observed value is in accordance with the values found in literature [21–23]. In the current study, the ethosomes presented an EC of 73.91 ± 24.80% (n = 20) which might be a good indicator of the presence of stable interactions between extract and SPC. Besides other factors, the EC is generally dependent on the composition of ethosomes [24–26]. In previous works with similar composition of ethosomes, the value ranged between 65% and 71% of rutin [26–28], similar to our value.

2.5. Characterization of Rutin and Ethosomes Complexes

Table 1 displays the inherent molecular energy attributes for various biomolecular complexes (SPC-rutin), while Figure 6 presents the corresponding geometrical positions. Here, the target was the major compound of the extract, rutin. In terms of the overall energy, the SPC-rutin complex was stabilized by the Van der Waals energy and it was accompanied by dihedral and electrostatic destabilizations. Interestingly, this comparatively destabilization of SPC-rutin molecular complex ($\Delta E \approx -6$ kcal/mol) may provide enhanced diffusivity of rutin across the lipidic matrix, in comparison to the polymer-rutin complexes in a previous study performed by our group, where poly-glycolic-lactic acid-rutin and poly-caprolactone-rutin revealed higher molecular complex ($\Delta E \approx -20$ kcal/mol and -18 kcal/mol, respectively) [4]. These chemical interactions might somehow justify the extract entrapment of around 70%, i.e., the interactions are not too strong in terms of energy.

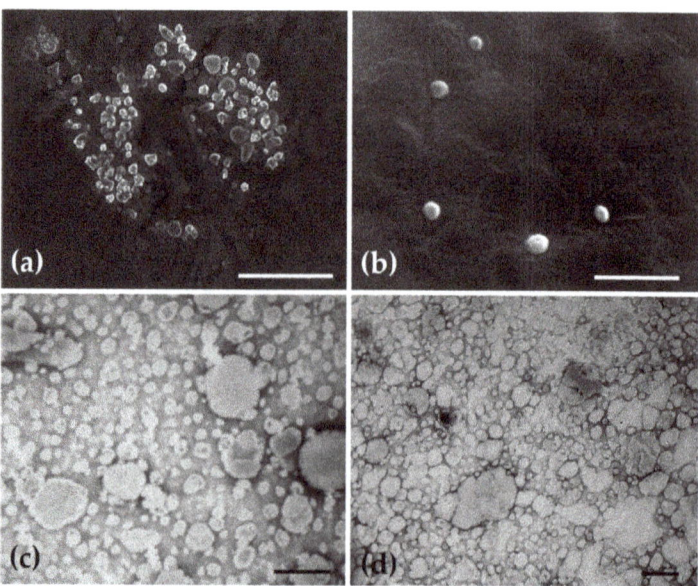

Figure 3. Representative SEM and TEM micrographs showing the morphology of ethosomes. (a,b) SEM images of empty and extract-loaded ethosomes, respectively. (c,d), TEM images of empty and extract-loaded ethosomes, respectively. Scale bars = 5 µm (a); 3 µm (b); 2 µm (c,d).

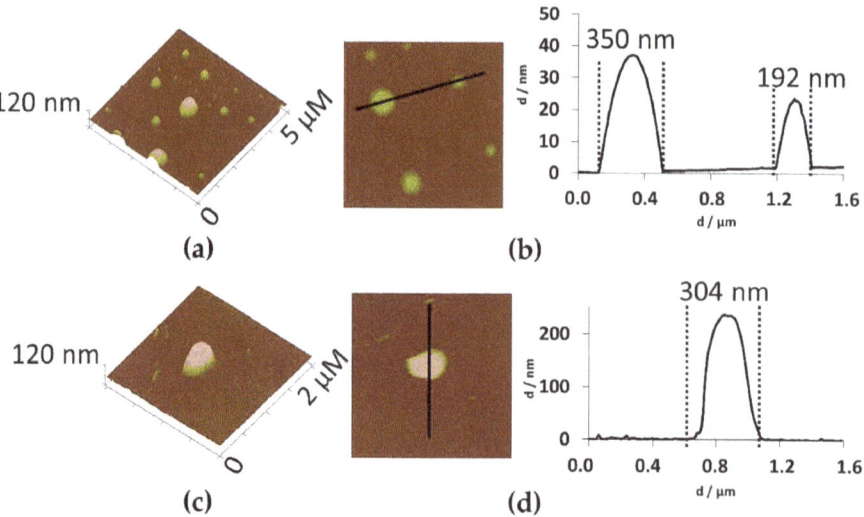

Figure 4. AFM topographic images of ethosomes. (a,b) empty and (c,d) extract-loaded. 3D images (a,c) and cross section analysis (b,d).

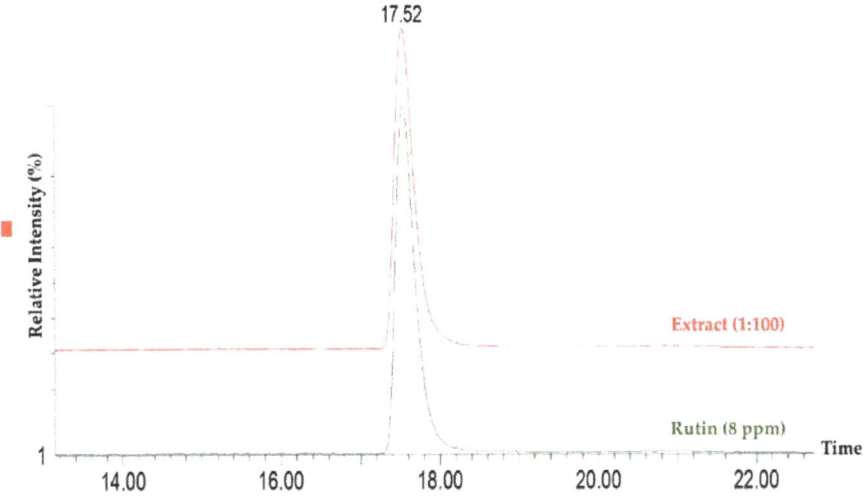

Figure 5. MRM overlay chromatograms of rutin in the extract with a standard solution.

Table 1. Inherent energy attributes of SPC-rutin complexes calculated using static-lattice atomistic simulations (SLAS) in vacuum.

Energy	Rutin	SPC	SPC-Rutin	ΔE [1]
Total [2]	23.09	1.10	18.61	−5.58 [8]
Bond [3]	1.16	1.39	2.49	−0.05 [8]
Angle [4]	7.57	35.69	42.85	−0.41 [8]
Dihed [5]	14.32	10.28	27.60	3.00 [9]
vdW [6]	0.04	−4.25	−14.35	−10.15 [8]
Elec [7]	0.00	−42.01	−39.97	2.04 [9]

[1] ΔE(A/B) = E(A/B) − [E(A) + E(B)]; [2] total steric energy for an optimized structure; [3] bond stretching contributions; [4] bond angle contributions; [5] torsional contribution arising from deviations from optimum dihedral angles; [6] Van der Waals interactions; [7] electrostatic interactions; [8] values represent the structure stabilizing contribution; and [9] values represent the structure destabilizing contribution.

2.6. In Vitro Release Studies of Extract from Ethosomes

The release profile of extract from ethosomes was performed using PBS at two different pHs, at pH 5.5 which is similar to the pH of the skin [2], and at pH 7.4 which corresponds to the biological pH of blood [29]. The assays were performed at controlled room temperature (RT ≈ 25 °C). The obtained results are displayed in Figure 7. The release studies showed that the extract-loaded ethosomes presented the same release profiles, independently of pH, achieving 83.8 ± 8.3% and 82.8 ± 6.4%, for PBS pH 5.5 and pH 7.4, respectively. This behavior was quite different from the free extract where its complete solubilization instantaneously occurred after 5 min. Here, the extract encapsulation into ethosomes led to a slight delay, which can favor the extract release in the target area. This retention time can be additionally modulated after inclusion in Carbopol gel as it was already reported in literature [30,31]. This effect is still controversial; some studies showed a slower release of the encapsulant but other described the same profile after inclusion in a semi-solid dosage form [32]. As a representative example, a very recent work described the preparation of ethosomes with *Achillea millefolium* L. extract. In the permeation study, ethosomes alone or after inclusion of Carbopol had the same behavior. Thus, further studies should be done with aim to verify this hypothesis.

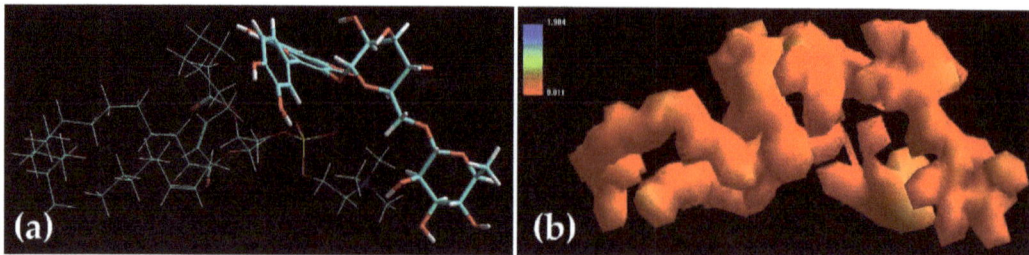

Figure 6. Representation of (**a**) geometrical preferences (**b**) electrostatic molecular graph after molecular mechanics simulations in vacuum (**a,b**) SPC-Rutin [Colour code for elements: C = cyan; H = white; O = red; N = blue]. Rutin: tube rendering; SPC: stick rendering.

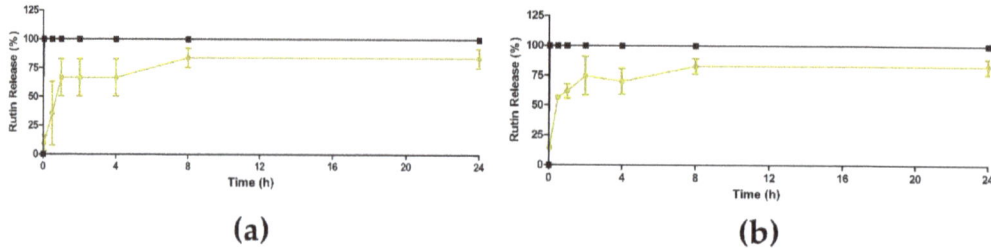

Figure 7. Percentage of rutin release free extract (black line) and extract-loaded ethosomes (yellow line), (**a**) in PBS pH 5.5, (**b**) in PBS pH 7.4.

2.7. In Vitro Collagenase Inhibition Activity of Extract after Encapsulation

The results obtained for the in vitro collagenase inhibition activity are showed in Figure 8. The free extract (93.57 ± 0.61%) presented higher Coll inhibition activity the positive control (84.36 ± 0.91%). At equivalent concentration of the extract, extract-loaded ethosomes had the highest Coll inhibition activity (99.67 ± 0.09%).

This enzyme is generally involved in some skin diseases or disorders, being associated with the degradation of the collagen-rich extracellular matrix (ECM). Furthermore, there is a relationship between Coll-assisted ECM breakdown and tumor invasion [5]. The inhibition of this enzyme can prevent skin disorders or contribute for the treatment of these diseases. Among the phytocompounds previously identified in this extract, this inhibition can be related to the presence of naringenin [33]. This value was higher than some values described in previous studies. As an example, Zofia et al. tested different extracts in terms of Coll inhibition. Inhibition ranged between 10–40% to *Meum athamanticum* L., less than 30% to *Centella asiatica* L. and varied between 20–75% to *Aegopodium podagraria* L. [34].

2.8. Preliminary In Vitro Safety Assessment of Extract in Ethosomes

One important parameter in any formulation development is the safety [4]. Cell viability of HaCaT cells was performed for free extract as well as empty and extract-loaded ethosomes. The tested concentrations ranged from 8.13 to 130.00 µg of rutin/mL, and results are depicted in Figure 9. A dose-dependent effect for free extract and loaded ethosomes was observed but this tendency was not observed for empty ethosomes. This reduction of cell viability observed in the ethosomes (empty or loaded) is possibly due to the presence of ethanol, which was not present in the extract. Besides the presence of ethanol, the ethosomes sizes by itself can be another possible reason, since they can act as physical barriers and thus interfere with cell growth. This observation is already well documented in several previous studies.

A wide number of published works have stated that ethosomes are safe to be applied in humans and animals, presenting an excellent skin tolerability [35]. In fact, SPC presents a very high tolerability and biocompatibility [36]. In terms of in vitro scenario, keratinocyte (HaCat) cells represent 95% of epidermal cells [4,37], being more sensible than skin by itself in a real scenario [4,38]. Thus, in principle, there should be no concerns in terms of its application in humans as further section confirmed it.

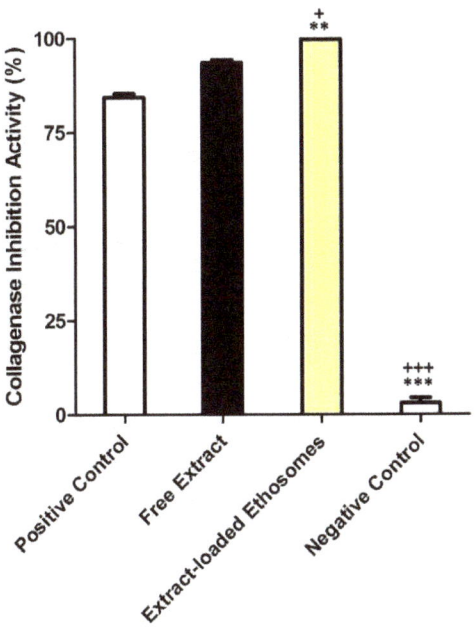

Figure 8. Coll inhibition activity of samples (1 mg of sample/mL, mean ± S.D., $n = 3$, ** $p < 0.01$ and *** $p < 0.001$, when compared to epigallocatechin gallate (EGCG, positive control—250 µM) and + $p < 0.05$ and +++ $p < 0.001$, when compared to free extract).

2.9. Preliminary Stability Test of Semi-Solid Formulation with Free Extract and Ethosomes
2.9.1. Heating and Cooling Testing

The organoleptic characteristics, pH and viscosity of each sample were evaluated over one week for heating and cooling tests, with analyses in four different times (immediately after the incorporation of the ethosomes into the gels, on the second, fourth and last day). Samples of gel with extract (Gel + E), gel with empty ethosomes (Gel + Etho) and extract-loaded ethosomes (Gel + E-Etho) were compared to the gel (Carbopol® 940 as control). This study reports for the first time that all these combinations were studied by diverse parameters and for different assays over time.

Concerning the Carbopol® 940, no phase separation (PS) was observed over time, after inclusion of extract, empty ethosomes and loaded ethosomes. The organoleptic characteristics did not change over time, with maintenance of similar colour for each sample. The pH values were registered for each sample, and a stable pH was verified for all samples, with slight variations (1.04 maximum) over time. These small changes of pH did not have any impact on the consistency of the gel, which is in conformity with the results reported by Islam et al. [39]. Viscosity is another main parameter of a potential semi-solid formulation for topical use. This parameter was measured for all samples over the time and the values are registered in Table 2. A decrease of viscosity over time was noticed. The comparison between the gel (control) and the Gel + E revealed a statistical difference of $p < 0.001$ on day 0 and 4, but for the other time-points no difference was observed. The data suggested that the addition of extract led to an initial increase of viscosity, but after the second day, a decrease of the value of this parameter was registered, and this tendency was maintained over time. Concerning the samples of empty and extract-loaded ethosomes, it was verified a decrease of viscosity, which was maintained over time. This event can be a consequence of the addition of ethosomes in a solution. Regarding the free extract, it was included in gel in powder.

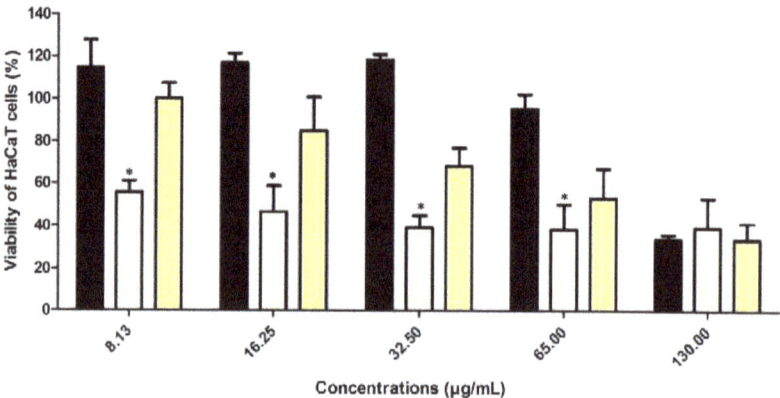

Figure 9. Cell viability (%) of HaCaT following 48 h incubation of free extract (black columns), empty (light yellow columns) and extract-loaded ethosomes (dark yellow columns). Tested concentration ranged from 8–130 µg of rutin/mL (%, mean ± S.D.; $n = 6$; * $p < 0.05$, when compared with free extract). Empty ethosomes were used at equivalent concentration of loaded ethosomes.

2.9.2. Centrifugation Stress of Semi-Solid Formulation with Free Extract and Ethosomes

The results of the organoleptic characteristics showed a normal appearance before and after centrifugation for all the samples. The pH values after the centrifugation ranged between 5.39–7.00, for Carbopol gel. In general, the samples presented similar pH before and after the centrifugation. Concerning viscosity, it was observed a decrease after centrifugation as can be seen in Table 2. Results suggested that for all samples, the addition of extract and ethosomes (empty or loaded) decreased the viscosity of the gel after centrifugation.

2.10. Accelerated Stability of Semi-Solid Formulation with Free Extract and Ethosomes
2.10.1. Tests Cycles of Heating and Cooling

Organoleptic characteristics observations revealed a normal appearance over time for all samples. The addition of extract into the gel decreases the pH of the gel and this behavior was maintained over the assay. On the other hand, the Gel + E-Etho led to an increase of pH value in the first moment and that was maintain until the end of assay. In terms of viscosity, samples of gel (control) and Gel + E presented a decrease at the end of the study. On the contrary, the sample of Gel + E-Etho presented a slight increase of viscosity over time and with the cycles of heating and cooling. Thus, concerning to viscosity this assay suggests that these samples present some vulnerability with the exposition to different temperature exposition.

Table 2. Stability data of the tested samples (Gel; Gel + E; Gel + Etho and Gel + E-Etho) at different testing conditions (mean ± SD, $n = 3$). OC means organoleptic characteristics, E means extract, Etho means ethosomes and E-Etho means extract-loaded ethosomes (N—normal, AC* at 40 ± 2 °C).

Time (Days)	Gel			Gel + E			Gel + Etho			Gel + E-Etho		
	OC	pH	Viscosity	OC	pH	Viscosity	OC	pH	Viscosity	OC	pH	Viscosity
Preliminary Stability Testing (Heating and Cooling)												
0	N	7.68 ± 0.01	134,050 ± 14,453	N	6.39 ± 0.03	159,800 ± 200	N	7.39 ± 0.02	183,933 ± 14,609	N	8.77 ± 0.01	155,533 ± 1922
2	N	7.65 ± 0.01	128,333 ± 1246	N	6.35 ± 0.21	123,933 ± 306	N	7.37 ± 0.02	129,667 ± 874	N	8.55 ± 0.04	28,200 ± 200
4	N	7.59 ± 0.02	124,867 ± 566	N	6.33 ± 0.12	107,333 ± 416	N	7.21 ± 0.03	100,067 ± 2055	N	8.50 ± 0.01	53,400 ± 872
7	N	7.45 ± 0.01	111,717 ± 58	N	6.13 ± 0.03	108,333 ± 643	N	7.27 ± 0.01	122,700 ± 200	N	8.45 ± 0.02	29,800 ± 200
Preliminary Stability Testing (Centrifugation Stress)												
Before	N	6.89 ± 0.01	192622 ± 518	N	6.60 ± 0.03	162,533 ± 306	N	5.38 ± 0.02	28,000 ± 200	N	7.11 ± 0.04	53,600 ± 529
After	N	6.96 ± 0.02	190933 ± 115	N	6.63 ± 0.01	150,733 ± 306	N	5.39 ± 0.03	27,867 ± 115	N	7.00 ± 0.01	49,000 ± 200
Accelerated Stability Testing (Heating and Cooling)												
0	N	7.58 ± 0.18	158,267 ± 2203	N	6.19 ± 0.02	156,933 ± 3252				N	7.50 ± 0.02	20,800 ± 529
2	N	6.72 ± 0.02	175,467 ± 25015	N	6.16 ± 0.08	133,800 ± 200				N	7.63 ± 0.04	38,733 ± 306
4	N	6.78 ± 0.02	193,800 ± 200	N	6.10 ± 0.02	98,600 ± 200				N	7.59 ± 0.02	31,200 ± 200
6	N	6.72 ± 0.02	133,400 ± 200	N	6.11 ± 0.01	128,933 ± 1890				N	7.61 ± 0.02	30,200 ± 200
8	N	6.73 ± 0.01	194,867 ± 5601	N	6.07 ± 0.04	62,600 ± 721				N	7.64 ± 0.01	40,867 ± 306
10	N	6.70 ± 0.01	114,600 ± 529	N	6.09 ± 0.17	57,800 ± 200				N	7.67 ± 0.04	25,000 ± 200
12	N	6.66 ± 0.02	96,467 ± 416	N	6.43 ± 0.16	73,467 ± 306				N	7.62 ± 0.02	28,533 ± 115

Time (days)	Gel			Gel + E			Gel + Etho			Gel + E-Etho		
	OC	pH	Viscosity	OC	pH	Viscosity	OC	pH	Viscosity	OC	pH	Viscosity
Accelerated Stability Testing (14 Days)—RC												
0	N	8.88 ± 0.14	168,333 ± 306	N	6.34 ± 0.01	104,000 ± 200				N	6.77 ± 0.03	33,467 ± 306
3	N	9.17 ± 0.08	66,533 ± 306	N	6.33 ± 0.02	151,200 ± 200				N	6.72 ± 0.01	42,200 ± 200
7	N	9.01 ± 0.06	68,000 ± 200	N	6.18 ± 0.01	118,333 ± 306				N	6.73 ± 0.03	41,333 ± 987
14	N	8.89 ± 0.02	50,200 ± 200	N	6.26 ± 0.17	99,933 ± 306				N	6.70 ± 0.02	64,733 ± 503
Accelerated Stability Testing (14 Days)—RT												
0	N	6.31 ± 0.06	194,533 ± 503	N	6.78 ± 0.02	167,200 ± 400				N	8.50 ± 0.01	21,800 ± 200
3	N	6.61 ± 0.02	185,467 ± 306	N	6.68 ± 0.03	138,200 ± 200				N	8.44 ± 0.02	29,400 ± 200
7	N	6.50 ± 0.03	121,200 ± 200	N	6.60 ± 0.04	109,600 ± 800				N	8.34 ± 0.01	129,400 ± 3470
14	N	6.54 ± 0.03	138,867 ± 416	N	6.55 ± 0.02	101,133 ± 306				N	8.03 ± 0.05	81,600 ± 4386

Table 2. *Cont.*

Time (Days)	Gel			Gel + E			Gel + Etho			Gel + E-Etho		
	OC	pH	Viscosity	OC	pH	Viscosity	OC	pH	Viscosity	OC	pH	Viscosity
Accelerated Stability Testing (14 Days)—AC												
0	N	5.89 ± 0.04	159,267 ± 2444	N	7.42 ± 0.02	145,200 ± 200				N	8.02 ± 0.02	127,333 ± 503
3	N	6.15 ± 0.03	181,200 ± 200	N	7.35 ± 0.02	118,200 ± 200				N	7.79 ± 0.01	27,600 ± 200
7	N	6.21 ± 0.01	136,933 ± 306	N	7.08 ± 0.01	103,533 ± 611				N	7.78 ± 0.01	33,200 ± 200
14	N	6.27 ± 0.02	121,800 ± 200	N	7.01 ± 0.02	105,200 ± 200				N	7.67 ± 0.01	35,933 ± 306
Accelerated Stability Testing (14 Days)—AC *												
0	N	6.57 ± 0.01	158,667 ± 1617	N	6.74 ± 0.01	163,000 ± 1929				N	7.40 ± 0.01	71,533 ± 2759
3	N	6.60 ± 0.02	190,800 ± 721	N	6.77 ± 0.01	109,600 ± 917				N	7.11 ± 0.01	92,867 ± 643
7	N	6.60 ± 0.03	119,867 ± 306	N	6.77 ± 0.03	87,800 ± 200				N	7.09 ± 0.02	32,667 ± 306
14	N	6.58 ± 0.02	113,867 ± 115	N	6.80 ± 0.01	102,800 ± 600				N	7.09 ± 0.01	33,400 ± 200
Accelerated Stability Testing (14 Days)—Temperature Cycles												
Before	N	6.60 ± 0.32	161,000 ± 1217	N	6.56 ± 0.01	180,733 ± 22,689				N	6.55 ± 0.09	108,333 ± 416
After	N	7.21 ± 0.04	171,200 ± 20101	N	6.61 ± 0.03	156,533 ± 306				N	6.48 ± 0.01	38,467 ± 306
Accelerated Stability Testing (3 Months)—RC												
0	N	8.88 ± 0.14	168,333 ± 306	N	6.34 ± 0.01	104,000 ± 200				N	6.77 ± 0.03	33,467 ± 306
30	N	8.79 ± 0.01	44,733 ± 416	N	6.09 ± 0.01	70,067 ± 611				N	6.62 ± 0.04	40,600 ± 200
60	N	8.77 ± 0.03	45,667 ± 757	N	6.20 ± 0.01	53,000 ± 1058				N	6.73 ± 0.04	36,533 ± 1332
90	N	8.80 ± 0.01	186,467 ± 8612	N	6.30 ± 0.01	126,000 ± 9035				N	6.90 ± 0.01	113,133 ± 1553
Accelerated Stability Testing (3 Months)—RT												
0	N	6.31 ± 0.06	194,533 ± 503	N	6.78 ± 0.02	167,200 ± 400				N	8.50 ± 0.01	21,800 ± 200
30	N	6.56 ± 0.03	42,933 ± 416	N	6.51 ± 0.01	50,533 ± 115				N	7.94 ± 0.01	97,800 ± 529
60	N	6.50 ± 0.02	105,000 ± 6630	N	6.58 ± 0.04	109,133 ± 3775				N	7.44 ± 0.02	95,267 ± 8425
90	N	6.51 ± 0.01	132,600 ± 1929	N	6.67 ± 0.01	186,933 ± 2023				N	7.17 ± 0.03	56,400 ± 200
Accelerated Stability Testing (3 Months)—AC												
0	N	5.89 ± 0.04	159,267 ± 2444	N	7.42 ± 0.02	145,200 ± 200				N	8.02 ± 0.02	127,333 ± 503
30	N	6.33 ± 0.03	60,867 ± 416	N	6.87 ± 0.06	54,400 ± 200				N	7.52 ± 0.01	30,467 ± 833
60	N	6.36 ± 0.03	55,800 ± 2163	N	6.80 ± 0.01	72,467 ± 5623				N	7.37 ± 0.01	27,867 ± 702
90	N	6.47 ± 0.02	145,733 ± 1026	N	6.96 ± 0.02	168,733 ± 16,931				N	6.95 ± 0.04	100,600 ± 1562

2.10.2. Stability Test over 14 Days

Organoleptic characteristics observations revealed a normal appearance over time for all samples under the different exposition temperatures. The addition of extract and extract-loaded ethosomes led to a slight decrease of the pH value that was kept over the assay, which suggest a stability of the samples under RC. Concerning the RT, the addition of extract or extract-loaded ethosomes increased the pH value and this difference was maintained over time. At AC, the addition of extract and extract-loaded ethosomes increased the pH value and this difference was also kept over time. The influence of temperature in the pH of the gel was evident, like previous study demonstrated [40]. The viscosity was measured for all samples in Carbopol® 940 gel; it was observed an increase of viscosity over time at RC and RT for Gel + E-Etho but a decrease when exposed to AC and AC*, suggesting a direct correlation with the temperature to the Gel + E. Nevertheless, no correlation was noticed to the Gel (control) and to Gel + E-Etho.

2.10.3. Temperature Cycles

The temperature cycles have no interference with organoleptic parameters and pH values, but regarding the viscosity, it was verified a decrease of values at the end of assay, that was more evident for the Gel + E-Etho. With the increase of temperature, the molecular vibrations might have also increase, changing polymer entanglement [32]. The change can be also due to the syneresis of the sample by itself, presence of ethanol and other compounds from the loaded ethosomes. This behavior was already reported in previous studies described in the literature [41,42].

2.11. Stability over Three Months

Organoleptic characteristics observations were registered over three months, every month, under three different temperatures (RC, RT and AC). The results did not reveal any change. The results for pH showed a decrease of difference over time with the increase of temperature for some of the samples, probably due to the release of some phytocompounds of the extract entrapped into the ethosomes. Regarding the viscosity, this parameter changed in the presence of extract, ethosomes, the presence of both and with temperature. This variation was already observed in previous studies. As an example, Dave et al. developed several ethosomes with gel formulations, but the most similar formula with this study revealed a viscosity of 7063 ± 2.8 cP [43]. Another example revealed that the addition of ethosomes in Carbopol gel affects its flow and viscoelastic behavior [44]. These authors suggested that the increase of temperature led to a decrease of viscosity, a consequence of the loosing of polymer entanglement at higher temperatures.

2.12. Rheology of Semi-Solid Formulation with Free Extract and Ethosomes

The rheology is important to characterize the stability of samples as well as to develop consumer acceptable final products [45]. This parameter allows to understand the rheological nature of the formulation, to perform studies of quality control of the effect of parameters like formulation, storage time and temperature on the quality of the formulation and to assess a product with regard to actual usage, such as spreading and adherence to the skin and removal from a tube or a jar. Profiles of all samples are presented in Figure 10. The results suggest that these samples present a shear thinning pseudoplastic behavior, which is according to the literature [46]. All tested samples consisted of hydrogels that are classified as non-Newtonian systems, exhibiting a non-linear relationship between stress and shear rate.

2.13. Texture of Semi-Solid Formulation with Free Extract and Ethosomes

It is generally accepted that the ideal characteristics of a fine semi-solid formulation for a better consumer acceptance are a good skin spread ability, an easy removal of product from the package and a good skin adhesion [47]. So, the aim of this study was to evaluate the textural properties of the different formulations concerning the physical gel structure [48]. The samples were analyzed in triplicate and the maximum peak force of displacement, also named hardness (F_{max}, N) and area of the peak (AUC, N/s) are displayed in Figure 11. It was observed that the Gel + E seems to be more adhesive than the Gel + E-Etho, probably due to the presence of ethanol and dilution after ethosomes inclusion.

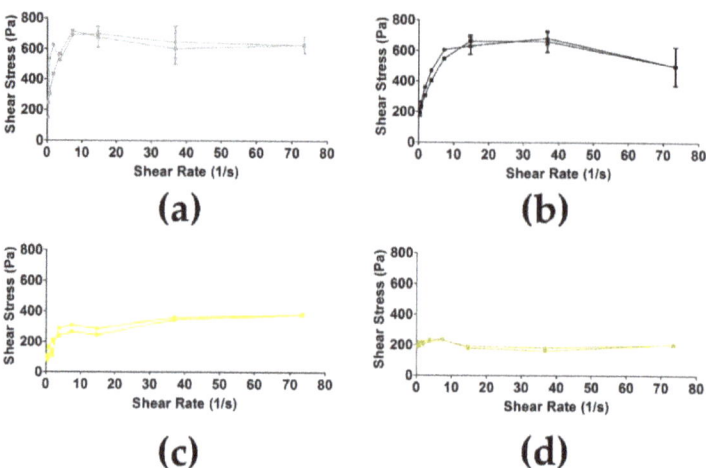

Figure 10. Rheology profile of samples (•) when increase the speed and (■) when decrease the speed (**a**) Gel (control), (**b**) Gel + E, (**c**) Gel + Etho, and (**d**) Gel + E-Etho (mean ± S.D.; n = 3).

2.14. Skin Compatibility Test of Semi-Solid Formulation with Free Extract and Ethosomes

The obtained results are presented in Table 3. Both samples showed very good skin compatibility. No reaction was detected for both samples in all the volunteers, confirming the safety of this formulation. The decrease of adhesion of the Gel + E-Etho observed in the texture analysis suggests that this change did not have any impact after topically delivered. Other properties are also important to achieve a suitable and effective topical delivery, such as the thixotropic properties and spreadability of the gel.

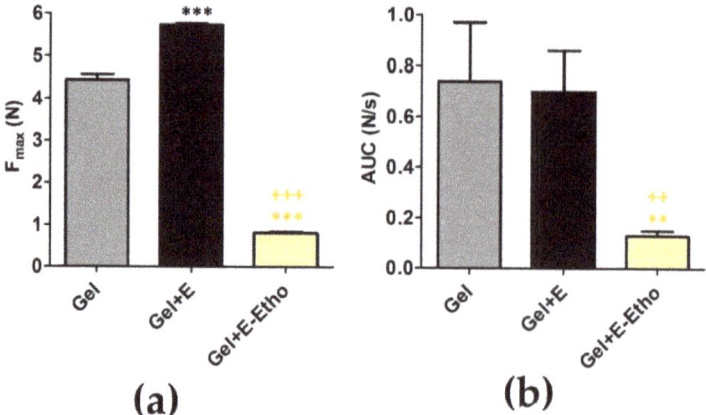

Figure 11. The (**a**) peak force of displacement (F_{max}, N) and the (**b**) area of the peak (AUC, N/s) obtained from the force versus time curves. The results are presented regarding the mean ± S.D.; n = 3 (** $p < 0.01$ and *** $p < 0.001$ when compared with gel (control); ++ $p < 0.01$ and +++ $p < 0.001$, when compared with Gel + E).

Table 3. Skin compatibility test for Gel + E and Gel + E-Etho (n = 6 each group, mean ± S.D.).

Samples	Control Time after Patch Removal	Reactive Subjects (n)	Types of Reaction	Mean Daily Irritation Score (Mdis)
Gel + E	15 min	0	None	0 ± 0
	24 h	0	None	0 ± 0
	48 h	0	None	0 ± 0
Gel + E-Etho	15 min	0	None	0 ± 0
	24 h	0	None	0 ± 0
	48 h	0	None	0 ± 0

3. Materials and Methods

3.1. Materials

3.1.1. Plant Material

S. nigra L. flowers (elderflowers) were supplied by *Régiefrutas—Cooperativa Agrícola de Interesse Público Távora-Varosa*, CIPRL, collected from commercial crops at Tarouca, Beira Alta, Portugal (lat. 40° 59′ 06″ N; long. 7° 37′ 03″ W; 695 m alt.) in May 2019.

3.1.2. Chemicals

Phosphatidylcholine (L-α-Phosphatidylcholine, also named soybean hosphatidylcholine, SPC) was supplied by Sigma Aldrich (St. Louis, MO, USA). Oleic Acid was acquired by Fluka Chemika (Buchs, Switzerland). Coll from Clostridium histolyticum type IA, Dulbecco's Modified Eagle's Medium—high glucose (DMEM), quercetin, thiazolyl blue tetrazolium bromide (MTT), Span 20®, Nile Blue A and ascorbic acid were supplied by Sigma Aldrich (Steinheim, Germany). Fetal bovine serum (FBS) purchased from Biowest (Riverside, CA, USA). L-Glutamine was supplied by Lonza (Leuven, Belgium). Rutin was acquired from Extrasynthese (Genay, France). Methanol was purchased from António M. S. Cruz (Amadora, Portugal) and sodium chloride (NaCl) from José M. Vaz Pereira (Benavente, Portugal). Epigallocatechingallate (EGCG), *N*-[3-furyl-acryloyl]-Leu-Gly-Pro-Ala (FALGPA) were purchased from Panreac (Barcelona, Spain). Tricine buffer was acquired by VWR (Leuven, Belgium). Carbopol 940® was purchased from Fagron (Barcelona, Spain). Folin reagent was supplied by Merck (Darmstadt, Germany). High performance liquid chromatography (HPLC) grade acetonitrile and formic acid were obtained from Chem-Lab NV (Zedelgem, Belgium). Milli-Q water (18.2 MΩ cm^{-1} resistivity) was obtained from a Millipore-Direct Q3 UV system (Millipore®, Burlington, MA, USA). All other chemicals were of analytical grade.

3.1.3. Cell Lines

The HaCaT cell line was supplied by Cell-Line-Service (cat: 300493, Eppelheim, Germany).

3.2. Methods

3.2.1. Extraction

The extract was obtained from fresh elderflowers, using methanol as solvent through ultrasonication method (Sonorex Super RK 510 H; Bandelin, Berlin, Germany) for 1 h. The procedure was repeated three times until complete extraction [4,5,49]. The extract was then filtered, and the methanol was removed by rotary evaporation (VV2000 rotary evaporator from Heidolph, Apeldoorn, The Netherlands).

3.2.2. Ethosomes Preparation Method

To produce ethosomes, 2% of SPC (w/v), 40% of ethanol (v/v) and 58% of MilliQ water (v/v) were used. Ethosomes then were centrifuged at 10,460× g (Centrifuge, Sigma Laborzentrifugen, Osterode am Harz, Germany) for 10 min at room temperature (RT) and then resuspended in MilliQ water. For the extract-loaded ethosomes, the same method was performed, and the amount of extract used was according to the proportion 1:1, w/w, lipid:extract. Empty and extract-loaded ethosomes were stored at 4 ± 2 °C—refrigeration conditions (RC). The ethosomes stored at these conditions were further used in all the assays.

3.2.3. Lipid Quantification

The lipid content of vesicles was determined using the modified colorimetric method described by Rouser et al. [50,51]. Briefly, the samples (in triplicate) with an amount of phosphate between 20 and 80 nmol (sample volume below 100 µL) were cooled and after that 0.3 mL of perchloric acid (70–72%) was added. Furthermore, all tubes were heated at 180 °C for 45 min, in order to convert all the organic lipid phosphate to its inorganic form and the samples were cooled to RT. Subsequently, 1.0 mL of H_2O and 0.4 mL of hexa-ammonium heptamolybdate solution [1.25% (w/v)] followed by 0.4 mL of ascorbic acid solution [5% (w/v)] were added. It was obtained a blue color solution due to the reduction of ascorbic acid over the heating process. In the end of method, the absorbance of all samples was recorded at 797 nm) in a UV-mini 1240 spectrophotometer (Shimadzu, Kyoto, Japan) [51]. In parallel, a calibration curve was also prepared with amounts of phosphate ranging from 20 and 80 µmol/tube, also in triplicate. All tubes were heated (180 °C) in a heating block until dryness.

3.2.4. Physical Characterization of Ethosomes: Size, Surface Charge and pH

Mean size, PdI, zeta potential and pH of empty and extract-loaded ethosomes were evaluated for up to 12 months [52]. Zeta potential of the ethosomes was measured in diluted NaCl (0.1 M) solution (1:10, v/v). The size, PdI and zeta potential were measured in diluted samples (1:16, v/v) by DLS, using a Malvern Zetasizer Nano-S and Nano-Z (Malvern Instruments, Worcestershire, UK). Results were expressed as mean of measurements in triplicate ($n = 3$). Stability study at different temperature was performed using three different temperatures (4 ± 2 °C—RC, 25 ± 5 °C—RT and 40 ± 2 °C—AC). Results were expressed as the mean ± S.D. ($n = 3$). The pH of the obtained suspension of ethosomes was measured using a pH electrode meter (827 pH Lab, Metrohm, Herisau, Switzerland), calibrated every day of measurements, with buffer solutions pH 4.00 ± 0.02 and 7.00 ± 0.02 (20 °C) ST (Panreac).

3.2.5. Histochemical Characterization of the Lipidic Constitution of Ethosomes and Study of their Morphology

The lipidic constitution of ethosomes was histochemically demonstrated by Nile blue A, a stain used for detection of acidic and neutral lipids [53]. Microscope slides were prepared with a drop of the vesicular suspension, previously stained with an aqueous solution of 0.1% Nile blue A. Observations were carried out in bright field and in fluorescence with an BX51 light microscope (Olympus, Tokyo, Japan) equipped with a Nomarski and an epifluorescence condenser. For fluorescence, a filter set for green light with excitation at 535/30 nm and emission at 580 nm was used. Images were recorded digitally.

The morphological characteristics of the particles were investigated by scanning, transmission and atomic force microscopy techniques (SEM, TEM and AFM, respectively). For SEM, aliquots (20 µL) of the vesicular suspensions were carefully dispersed on round glass coverslips coated with poly L-lysine and previously attached to the microscope stubs. The samples, after dried in a desiccator, were sputter-coating with gold and observed with a 5200LV scanning electron microscope (JEOL Ltd., Tokyo, Japan) at an accelerating voltage of 20 kV. Images were recorded digitally. For TEM, aliquots (10 µL) of NPs suspensions were placed on Formvar/carbon coated grids and the excess solution was removed with a filter paper. Then, the material was negatively stained with 1% of uranyl acetate and left in room conditions for air-drying. Observations were carried out on a 1200EX transmission electron microscope (JEOL Ltd., Tokyo, Japan) operating at 80 kV and images were recorded digitally.

For the atomic force microscopy (AFM) analysis, the samples were centrifuged at 7378× g (Sigma Laborzentrifugen, Osterode am Harz, Germany) for 10 and 20 min, for empty and extract-loaded vesicles, respectively, followed by resuspension in water (in half of the previous volume) [54]. AFM uses a diluted sample, 1:2 without any pre-treatment. A freshly cleaved mica surface was used to place a drop (≈40 µL of sample), being allowed to adsorb for around 30 min [54]. After drying using a stream of N2, samples were analyzed in intermittent mode (Multimode 8 HR Microscope, produced by Bruker, Billerica, MA, USA) [54]. Images were acquired in ambient conditions (≈21 °C), through the use of etched silicon tips with a resonance frequency of around 320 kHz (NCHV, Bruker), at a scan rate near to 1.3 Hz [54]. All images were recorded digitally.

3.2.6. Entrapment Capacity of Extract in Ethosomes

To determine the EC of the elderflower extract, the samples were analyzed by HPLC-MS/MS aiming at quantifying rutin, the major compound of the methanolic extract. The Waters® Alliance 2695 HPLC system (Waters®, Dublin, Ireland) equipped with an autosampler, quaternary pumps, column furnace, and a diode-array detector (DAD) Waters 996 DAD (Waters®) was used to performer the assays. Chromatographic analyses were carried out using a LiChrospher® 100 RP-18, 5 µm (250 × 4 mm) column at 35 °C. A mixture of formic acid (0.5% v/v in ultrapure water) (eluent A) and 0.5% formic acid in acetonitrile (eluent B) at a flow rate of 0.3 mL/min, were used as a mobile phase. The initial conditions were maintained for 20 min as a re-equilibration step. The gradient was: 5% B (0–10 min), 15% B (10–30 min), 20% B (30–45 min), 20% B (45–65 min), 54% B (65–95 min), 63% B (65–110 min), and 5% B (110–115 min). The total running time was 135 min and the injection volume 20 µL. The HPLC system was coupled to a triple quadrupole mass spectrometer MicroMass Quattromicro® API (Waters®, Dublin, Ireland) equipped with an electrospray ionization source (ESI).

MS/MS conditions were optimized for the identification and quantification of rutin. The electrospray ion source (ESI) was set to operate at 120 °C in negative mode, using a capillary voltage of 2.5 kV, cone voltage of 45 V and collision energies of 32, and 34 eV. High purity nitrogen was used as drying and as a nebulizing gas. The collision gas used was the ultra-high purity argon. Analyses were performed in multiple reaction monitoring mode (MRM), selecting the one product ion with the highest signal as the monitored transitions for quantification (MRM1, 609.00 > 300.00) and confirmation (MRM2, 609.00 > 271.00) purposes. MassLynx Version 4.1 software (Waters) was used for instrument control, data acquisition, and data processing.

The *EC* was determined by analyzing the rutin present in the supernatant—indirect method). EC was determined by the Equation (1):

$$EC = \left(\frac{Total\ amount_{major\ bioactive\ compound} - Amount\ free_{major\ bioactive\ compound}}{Total\ amount_{major\ bioactive\ compound}} \right) \times 100 \quad (1)$$

3.2.7. Rutin and Ethosomes Complex Simulation

The reactional profile of extract and ethosomes system was assessed in silico via molecular mechanics simulations and the ensuing energetic-geometric stabilization provided an insight into the antioxidant potential of ethosomes. To analyze the mechanism governing the CoII potential of the ethosomes, energetic and geometrical stabilization of the drug-lipid molecular complexes were conducted using atomistic simulations (HyperChemLite Molecular Modelling Software, Hypercube Inc., Gainesville, FL, USA). The structures of SPC and rutin were generated as natural bond angles. The individual molecules and the biomolecular complexes (SPC-rutin) were energy minimized and optimized employing MM3 Force Field algorithm which was further accompanied by a Polak–Ribiere Conjugate Gradient method until an RMS gradient of 0.001 kcal/mol was achieved [55,56].

3.2.8. In Vitro Release Studies

Extract-loaded ethosomes were previously lyophilized over 24 h at −50 °C (freeze–dryer model, Edwards, Edwards, CO, USA). Afterwards, they were solubilized into phosphate buffer solution (PBS) (USP41) pH 5.5 (10 mL) to simulate human skin pH and stirred

(200 rpm) at 32 °C in a multiplate stirring plate. Sink conditions were assured over the whole assay. Aliquots of the release medium were collected at appropriate time intervals (5 and 30 min, 1, 2, 4, 8 and 24 h), and replaced immediately with fresh buffer. The same assay was performed in PBS at pH 7.4 (USP41). As reference, rutin was previously identified as the major flavonoid of the extract [5], therefore a standard calibration curve was performed with rutin solution in PBS buffer pH 5.5 or 7.4, depending on the assay. Extract concentration at each time point was determined using HPLC-DAD-MS/MS.

HPLC-DAD-MS/MS assays were carried out on a Waters® Alliance 2695 HPLC system (Waters®) coupled to a 2996 Photodiode Array Detector and a Micromass® Quattro Micro triple quadrupole (TQ) (Waters®). These analyses were performed at 35 °C on a LiChrospher® 100 RP-18 (250 × 4 mm, 5 μm) column. The mobile phase used was the same as described in Section 3.2.6. The elution program consisted of 20% B (0–5 min), with increase to 90% B in 10 min, 90% B (15–20 min), and with a decrease to 20% B in 1 min, and ultimately the initial conditions were maintained for 20 min as a re-equilibration step. Total run time was 40 min and the injection volume 10 μL. MS/MS conditions were already described in Section 3.2.6.

3.2.9. In Vitro Collagenase Inhibition Activity

The protocol used was already described in previous works [4,5,57]. This assay was performed in 50 mM tricine buffer (pH 7.5) enriched with 400 mM NaCl, and 10 mM $CaCl_2$. The FALGPA (substrate) was dissolved in tricine buffer (2 mM) whereas Coll from *Clostridium histolyticum* (EC.3.4.23.3) was dissolved in a buffer at an initial concentration of 0.8 Units/mL and according to the supplier's activity data. Negative controls were the respective sample solvent. The absorbance was measured at 405 nm after the substrate addition over 10 min using a microplate reader (Thermo Scientific Multiskan FC, Shanghai, China). The positive control (EGCG) was used at a concentration of 250 μM. This compound has been reported as being a strong inhibitor of collagen degradation [58]. The Coll inhibition (%) was determined using the Equations (2) and (3):

$$Velocity\ reaction\ of\ control\ or\ inhibitor = \frac{Corrected\ Abs}{time\ (min)} \quad (2)$$

$$Collagenase\ inhibition\ activity\ (\%) = 100 - \left(\frac{100 \times Velocity\ reaction\ of\ inhibitor}{Velocity\ reaction\ of\ control}\right) \quad (3)$$

For the Coll activity, the absorbance decrease was calculated using the Equation (2) for the velocity reaction of negative control (ΔAbs_{405nm}/min) and after to determine the Coll inhibitions activity, it was used the Equation (3) [4,5,57].

3.2.10. In Vitro Safety Assessment

The in vitro safety of the free extract, empty and extract-loaded ethosomes were evaluated using the MTT assay in the human keratinocyte cell line (HaCaT, cell line). These cells were seeded in 96-wells plate at a density of 5×10^4 cells/mL in DMEM with high-glucose (4500 mg/L), supplemented with 10% FBS, and 100 IU/mL of penicillin and 100 μg/mL streptomycin [(Pen/Strep, 1%, v/v)], and allowed to grow for 24 h in a humidified chamber at 37 °C in a 5% CO_2 atmosphere [59]. For this assay, the medium was removed and samples at concentrations ranging from 8.13–130.00 μg of rutin/mL (free extract and equivalent concentrations of extract into ethosomes, according to the results obtained for EC were prepared and added to HaCaT cells. After 48 h, the samples were removed, and the cell monolayers were washed with PBS. Then, 50 μL of MTT at 0.5 mg/mL was added to the cells and the plates were incubated for 4 h in a humidified chamber at 37 °C and 5% CO_2 atmosphere. After this incubation time, 100 μL of DMSO was added to each well to solubilize the formazan crystals. The absorbance (Abs) was measured, and cell viability was calculated using the same Equation (4):

$$Cell\ Viability\ (\%) = \frac{Abs_t}{Abs_c} \times 100 \qquad (4)$$

where Abs_t is the absorbance of the sample and Abs_c the absorbance of the control.

3.2.11. Inclusion of Extract-Loaded Ethosomes in a Semi-Solid Formulation

Carbopol® 940 gel was prepared based on previous literature with slight modifications [60]. Briefly, 500 mg of Carbopol® 940 was dispersed in water under stirring (400 rpm) until complete solubilization. Then, 0.2% of methyl 4-hydroxybenzoate and 0.02% of propyl-4-hydroxybenzoate were added under constant stirring. Finally, NaOH was added to Carbopol (0.4 g of NaOH per gram of Carbopol) under magnetic stirring. This last reagent was responsible for the gelling effect.

The resultant Carbopol® 940 gel was then characterized. A total of four different samples were tested: gel only (control); gel + Extract (Gel + E); gel + empty ethosomes (Gel + Etho) and gel + extract-loaded ethosomes (Gel + E-Etho), as schematic illustrated on the Figure 12. Incorporation of extract was performed according HPLC values (Section 3.2.6). Specifically, 1.5 mg of extract was mixed with 1 mL of Carbopol gel, followed by vortexing 5 s. Incorporation of ethosomes was performed by adding 2.34 mL of ethosomes suspension/mL of Gel to a tube, followed by same vortexing.

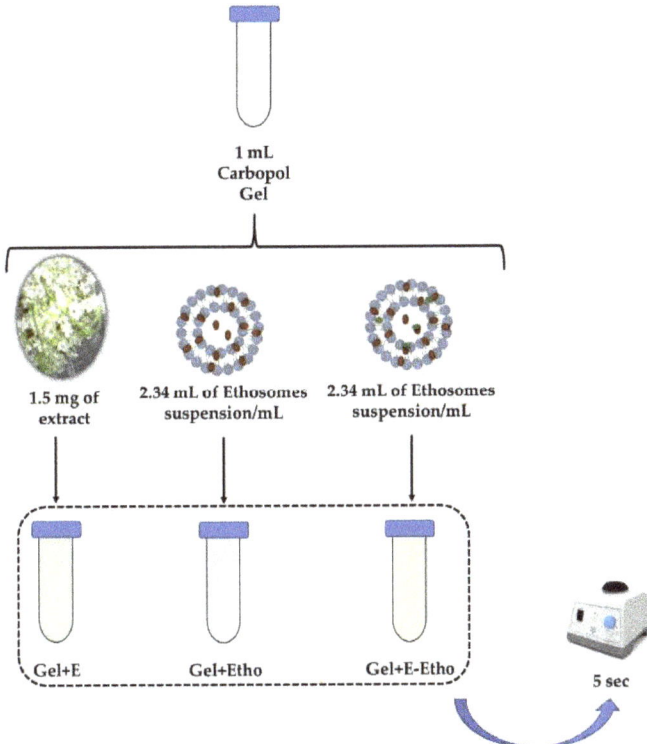

Figure 12. Schematic representation of inclusion of Extract-Loaded Ethosomes in a Semi-Solid Formulation.

3.2.12. Characterization of the Semi-Solid Formulation for Skin Delivery of *S. nigra* Extract

- Organoleptic Characteristics

The obtained gels with and without ethosomes were characterized in terms of aspect (colour and homogeneity) and odor. The organoleptic characteristics were evaluated by direct observation of samples. When the physical appearance was maintained, the samples were classified as normal whereas they were classified as PS when a phase separation was observed.

- pH Measurement

Measurement of the pH was performed at RT in triplicate using potentiometer (827 pH Lab, Metrohm, Herisau, Switzerland). This equipment was daily calibrated with buffer solutions pH 4.00 ± 0.02 and 7.00 ± 0.02 (20 °C) (Panreac).

- Viscosity Measurement

The viscosity was measured using a DV-I + Viscometer (Brookfield Engineering Labs. Inc., Middeborough, MA, USA) with the n° 4 needle and using a speed rate of 3 rpm.

- Preliminary Stability Assays of Semi-Solid Formulation with Free Extract and Ethosomes

The following tests were performed in all samples, i.e., with and without empty and extract-loaded ethosomes as previously reported by Reis et al. [61] and according to the International Guideline ICHQ1A (R2) [62]. The preliminary stability assays included the heating and cooling, as well as the centrifugation stress:

(1) Heating and Cooling

Samples were submitted to heat-freeze cycles [25 ± 2 °C in an oven (24 h), then cooled to -5 ± 2 °C in a freezer (24 h)], over one week. Frozen samples were allowed to melt and cool down to RT prior measurements. Samples were analyzed at 48, 96 and 168 h in terms of organoleptic characteristics, pH measurement and viscosity, as previously presented [61].

(2) Centrifugation Stress

This assay was adapted from Reis et al. (2015) [61]. Each sample (approximately 6 g) was exposed to a 50 °C water bath (Heidolph MR3001, Heidolph Instruments, Schwabach, Germany) and, subsequently, centrifuged at $1077 \times g$ for 30 min (Beckman Gpr Refrigerated Centrifuge Rotor, Indianapolis, IN, USA). The parameters of organoleptic characteristics, pH measurement and viscosity, were verified before and after centrifugation.

- Accelerated Stability Assays of Semi-Solid Formulation with Free Extract and Ethosomes

The following tests were performed in empty and extract-loaded ethosomes as previously reported [61] and under Guideline ICHQ1A (R2) [62].

(1) Tests Cycles of Heating and Cooling

Samples were incubated at 45 ± 2 °C in the oven and cooled in the freezer at -10 ± 2 °C (cycles of 24 h at each condition) for twelve days. Samples were analyzed every two days. This analysis included the evaluation of the parameters referred above (organoleptic characteristics, pH measurement and viscosity).

(2) Stability Test over 14 Days

Samples were exposed to three different settings: refrigerated conditions (RC, -5 ± 2 °C); RT (20 ± 5 °C), and accelerated conditions (AC, 50 ± 2 °C and AC*, 40 ± 2 °C) for 14 days. In this case, two different ovens were used to evaluate different conditions, one of them in regular or normal oven at 50 ± 2 °C, and the other one in a climatic chamber at 40 ± 2 °C. After 3, 7 and 14 days, formulations were analyzed and the parameters, already mentioned evaluated.

(3) Temperature Cycles

Samples were exposed to water bath at 40 °C, with a controlled heating rate of 10 °C/30 min of up to 80 °C. After returning to RT, the samples were analyzed in the same parameters than the previous tests.

- Stability over Three Months

Samples were exposed to three different settings: RC (-5 ± 2 °C); RT (20 ± 5 °C), and AC (50 ± 2 °C) for 3 months. After 1, 2 and 3 months, formulations were analyzed and organoleptic characteristics, pH measurement and viscosity determined.

- Rheological Properties

The procedure was based on the method of Braden [63], with slight modifications. The same needle was used and the values of viscosity for different speeds starting with the lowest (0.3 rpm) and gradually increasing the speed until 60 rpm.

- Texture Analysis

The texture of all samples was assessed by the TA.XT.plus (Texture Analyzer Stable Micro Systems, Surrey, UK). This assay was done using the following characteristics: pretest speed (0.50 mm/s); test speed (0.50 mm/s); post-test speed (10.00 mm/s); applied force (500.0 g); return distance (10.000 mm); contact time (10.00 s); trigger type (automatic) and trigger force (5.0 g). The estimated mean areas under the force-time curve were calculated for each sample, in triplicate analysis.

3.2.13. Human Skin's Compatibility Testing

The skin's compatibility was performed by occlusive patch Finn Chamber® standard [64] with some modifications made by Mazulli et al. [65]. A group of 12 subjects (n = 6 each group) with age between 18 to 70 years, female and male, with phototype (Fitzpatrick) I to IV and to all type of skin was randomized in two different groups: one group dosed with gel with extract and the other group dosed with gel with extract-loaded ethosomes. The goal of the present case was reached after a single application to the human skin. The tested samples were: the final formulation of Gel + E and Gel + E-Etho (20 µL each). The formulations were in contact with skin, under patch in the back, for 48 ± 5 h. The examination was carried out, visually under standard "daylight", before patching on first day and about 15 min (or more if some redness appeared after patch removal), then 24 and 48 h after patch removal. All the tests were made according to the Declaration of Helsinki and received the approval of the local Ethics Committee.

The mean daily irritation score (Mdis) was determined using Equation (5), where Idis represents the individual daily irritation score, which is obtained by the sum of the marks obtained for all the signs observed [66].

$$Mdis = \frac{\sum Idis}{number\ of\ valid\ cases} \tag{5}$$

3.2.14. Statistical Analysis

Results were expressed as mean ± standard deviation (S.D.). The results concerning the biological assays were expressed as mean ± standard error of the mean (S.E.M.). One-Way ANOVA for multiple comparisons was used to assess the significance of differences by Graph Prisma Version 5.03 (GraphPad Software, San Diego, CA, USA). Only it was considered the significant differences when $p < 0.05$. Two-Way ANOVA for multiple comparisons between all samples. Concerning to the results of incorporation of the extract-loaded ethosomes were expressed as mean ± S.D. Statistical analysis was performed using Two-Way ANOVA for multiple comparisons between control and different formulations by Bonferroni test, using GraphPad Prism 5.03. Results were considered significantly different when $p < 0.05$.

4. Conclusions

Ethosomes demonstrated to be a good nanocarrier for the *Sambucus nigra* L. flower extract, regarding the high EC. In addition, these nanocarriers showed a high value of Coll inhibition. After the incorporation in Carbopol gel, these results suggested to be a stable gel over the time, in terms of organoleptic characteristics, pH and viscosity at different temperatures of storage. This formulation was also safe for humans and thus it can be considered a promising topical formulation, attracting a wide interest from cosmetic industry.

Supplementary Materials: The following are available online at https://www.mdpi.com/article/10.3390/ph14050467/s1, Figure S1. Chromatogram of methanolic elderflowers extract at 280 nm.

Author Contributions: Conceptualization: C.P.R.; Formal analysis, A.H.M., I.P., H.M., A.B.-S., M.J.R., N.D., A.T.S., M.R.B., P.R., M.M.G., A.S.V., L.A., P.P., P.K., A.J.A. and C.P.R.; Funding acquisition, N.D., P.R., M.M.G., P.K., A.J.A. and C.P.R.; Investigation, A.H.M., I.P., H.M., A.B.-S., M.J.R., N.D., A.T.S., M.R.B., P.R., M.M.G., A.S.V., L.A., P.P., P.K., A.J.A. and C.P.R.; Methodology, C.P.R.; Project administration, C.P.R.; Supervision, A.J.A. and C.P.R.; Writing—original draft, A.H.M., I.P. and H.M.; Writing—review & editing, N.D., M.M.G., A.S.V., L.A., P.P., P.K., A.J.A. and C.P.R. All authors have read and agreed to the published version of the manuscript.

Funding: Authors also gratefully acknowledge the Régiefrutas, iMed and Fundação para a Ciência e a Tecnologia (FCT) (UIDB/04138/2020, UIDB/00100/2020, UIDP/50017/2020+UIDB/50017/2020, COFAC/ILIND/CBIOS/1/2020 and CCMAR/Multi/04326/2019 project), Portugal 2020, Portuguese Mass Spectrometry Network (LISBOA-01-0145-FEDER-402-022125), FCT/MCTES for the financial support to CESAM (UIDP/50017/2020, UIDB/50017/2020), INTERFACE Programme (Innovation, Technology and Circular Economy Fund (FITEC) and iNOVA4Health—UIDB/04462/2020, a program financially also supported by FCT. A.T.S. also acknowledge FCT/Ministério da Educação e Ciência for the Individual Grant CEECIND/04801/2017.

Institutional Review Board Statement: The study was conducted according to the guidelines of the Declaration of Helsinki and approved by the Institutional Review Board (or Ethics Committee) of PhD trials, protocol code 15860121.C and 15860121.D and approved on 27 January 2021.

Informed Consent Statement: Informed consent was obtained from all subjects involved in the study.

Data Availability Statement: The data presented in this study are available on request from the corresponding author.

Acknowledgments: The authors are also grateful to Jacinta Pinho from iMED.Ulisboa, Faculty of Pharmacy, University of Lisboa (Lisbon, Portugal) and João Mota from Faculty of Pharmacy, University of Lisboa (Lisbon, Portugal), as well as Sheila Alves from Instituto de Biologia Experimental e Tecnológica (Oeiras, Portugal) in conducting some experiments.

Conflicts of Interest: The authors declare no conflict of interest. The funders had no role in the design of the study; in the collection, analyses, or interpretation of data; in the writing of the manuscript, or in the decision to publish the results.

References

1. Mota, A.H.; Santos-Rebelo, A.; Almeida, A.J.; Reis, C.P. Therapeutic Implications of Nanopharmaceuticals in Skin Delivery. In *Nanopharmaceuticals: Principles and Applications*; Yata, V.K., Ranjan, S., Dasgupta, N., Lichtfouse, E., Eds.; Environmental Chemistry for a Sustainable World; Springer International Publishing: Cham, Switzerland, 2021; Volume 1, pp. 205–272. ISBN 9783030449247.
2. Mota, A.H.; Rijo, P.; Molpeceres, J.; Reis, C.P. Broad overview of engineering of functional nanosystems for skin delivery. *Int. J. Pharm.* **2017**, *532*, 710–728. [CrossRef]
3. Mota, A.H.; Sousa, A.; Figueira, M.; Amaral, M.; Sousa, B.; Rocha, J.; Fattal, E.; Almeida, A.J.; Reis, C.P. Natural-based consumer health nanoproducts: Medicines, cosmetics, and food supplements. In *Handbook of Functionalized Nanomaterials for Industrial Applications*; Hussain, C.M., Ed.; Micro and Nano Technologies; Elsevier: Amsterdam, The Netherlands, 2020; pp. 527–578, ISBN 9780128167885.
4. Mota, A.H.; Duarte, N.; Serra, A.T.; Ferreira, A.; Bronze, M.R.; Custódio, L.; Gaspar, M.M.; Simões, S.; Rijo, P.; Ascensão, L.; et al. Further Evidence of Possible Therapeutic Uses of Sambucus nigra L. Extracts by the Assessment of the In Vitro and In Vivo Anti-Inflammatory Properties of Its PLGA and PCL-Based Nanoformulations. *Pharmaceutics* **2020**, *12*, 1181. [CrossRef] [PubMed]

5. Mota, A.H.; Andrade, J.M.; Rodrigues, M.J.; Custódio, L.; Bronze, M.R.; Duarte, N.; Baby, A.; Rocha, J.; Gaspar, M.M.; Simões, S.; et al. Synchronous insight of in vitro and in vivo biological activities of *Sambucus nigra* L. extracts for industrial uses. *Ind. Crops Prod.* **2020**, *154*, 1–11. [CrossRef]
6. Leverett, J.C.; Chandra, A.; Rana, J.; Fast, D.J.; Missler, S.R.; Flower, D.M. Extracts of durian fruit for use in skin care compositions. U.S. Patent Application No. 11/655,015, 24 May 2007.
7. Liotta, A.; Unnur, P.; Universio, P. Role of collagenases in tumor cell invasion. *Cancer Metastasis Rev.* **1982**, *288*, 277–288. [CrossRef]
8. Fisher, G.J.; Kang, S.; Varani, J.; Bata-Csorgo, Z.; Wan, Y.; Datta, S.; Voorhees, J.J. Mechanisms of photoaging and chronological skin aging. *Arch. Dermatol.* **2002**, *138*, 1462–1470. [CrossRef]
9. Ricciarelli, R.; Maroni, P.; Özer, N.; Zingg, J.M.; Azzi, A. Age-dependent increase of collagenase expression can be reduced by α-tocopherol via protein kinase C inhibition. *Free Radic. Biol. Med.* **1999**, *27*, 729–737. [CrossRef]
10. Krutmann, J. Skin Aging. In *Nutrition Health Skin*; Springer: Berlin/Heidelberg, Germany, 2010; pp. 15–24. ISBN 9783642122637.
11. Oancea, A.M.; Onofrei, C.; Turturică, M.; Bahrim, G.; Râpeanu, G.; Stănciuc, N. The kinetics of thermal degradation of polyphenolic compounds from elderberry (*Sambucus nigra* L.) extract. *Food Sci. Technol. Int.* **2018**, *24*, 361–369. [CrossRef]
12. Carlsen, C.; Stapelfeldt, H. Light sensitivity of elderberry extract. Quantum yields for photodegradation in aqueous solution. *Food Chem.* **1997**, *60*, 383–387. [CrossRef]
13. Rijo, P.; Matias, D.; Fernandes, A.; Simões, M.; Nicolai, M.; Reis, C. Antimicrobial plant extracts encapsulated into polymeric beads for potential application on the skin. *Polymers* **2014**, *6*, 479–490. [CrossRef]
14. Sudhakar, C.K.; Upadhyay, N.; Jain, S.; Charyulu, R.N. Ethosomes as Non-invasive Loom for Transdermal Drug Delivery System. In *Nanomedicine and Drug Delivery-Adavnces in Nanoscience and Nanotechnology*; Sebastian, M., Ninan, N., Haghi, A.K., Eds.; CRC Press/Taylor & Francis: Oakville, ON, Canada, 2012; Volume 1, pp. 1–16. ISBN 9781466560079.
15. Kaul, S.; Gulati, N.; Verma, D.; Mukherjee, S.; Nagaich, U. Role of Nanotechnology in Cosmeceuticals: A Review of Recent Advances. *J. Pharm.* **2018**, *2018*, 1–19. [CrossRef]
16. Lohani, A.; Verma, A.; Joshi, H.; Yadav, N.; Karki, N. Nanotechnology-Based Cosmeceuticals. *ISRN Dermatol.* **2014**, *2014*, 1–14. [CrossRef]
17. *A Guidebook to Particle Size Analysis*; Horiba Scientific: Piscataway, NJ, USA, 2016; Available online: https://docplayer.net/18477598-A-guidebook-to-particle-size-analysis.html (accessed on 13 January 2017).
18. Cândido, T.M.; De Oliveira, C.A.; Ariede, M.B.; Velasco, M.V.R.; Rosado, C.; Baby, A.R. Safety and Antioxidant Efficacy Profiles of Rutin-Loaded Ethosomes for Topical Application. *AAPS PharmSciTech* **2018**, *19*, 1773–1780. [CrossRef]
19. Eaton, P.; Quaresma, P.; Soares, C.; Neves, C.; de Almeida, M.P.; Pereira, E.; West, P. A direct comparison of experimental methods to measure dimensions of synthetic nanoparticles. *Ultramicroscopy* **2017**, *182*, 179–190. [CrossRef] [PubMed]
20. Liu, Y.; Tan, J.; Thomas, A.; Ou-Yang, D.; Muzykantov, V.R. The shape of things to come: Importance of design in nanotechnology for drug delivery. *Ther. Deliv.* **2012**, *3*, 181–194. [CrossRef] [PubMed]
21. Scopel, M.; Mentz, L.A.; Henriques, A.T. Comparative analysis of sambucus nigra and sambucus australis flowers: Development and validation of an HPLC method for raw material quantification and preliminary stability study. *Planta Medica* **2010**, *76*, 1026–1031. [CrossRef] [PubMed]
22. Testoni, L.D.; De Souza, A.B.; De Krueger, C.M.A.; Quintão, N.L.M.; Couto, A.G.; Bresolin, T.M.B. Quantification of sambucus nigra (Adoxaceae) markers related to tincture stability. *Nat. Prod. Commun.* **2019**, *14*, 59–62. [CrossRef]
23. Oniszczuk, A.; Olech, M.; Oniszczuk, T.; Wojtunik-Kulesza, K.; Wójtowicz, A. Extraction methods, LC-ESI-MS/MS analysis of phenolic compounds and antiradical properties of functional food enriched with elderberry flowers or fruits. *Arab. J. Chem.* **2019**, *12*, 4719–4730. [CrossRef]
24. Barupal, A.K.; Gupta, V.; Ramteke, S. Preparation and Characterization of Ethosomes for Topical delivery of Aceclofenac. *Indian J. Pharm. Sci.* **2010**, *72*, 582–586.
25. Iizhar, S.A.; Syed, I.A.; Satar, R.; Ansari, S.A. In vitro assessment of pharmaceutical potential of ethosomes entrapped with terbinafine hydrochloride. *J. Adv. Res.* **2016**, *7*, 453–461. [CrossRef]
26. Dhiman, A.; Singh, D.; Fatima, K.; Zia, G. Development of Rutin Ethosomes for Enhanced Skin Permeation. *Int. J. Tradit. Med. Appl.* **2019**, *1*, 4–10. [CrossRef]
27. Jacob, M.; Agrawal, N.; Paul, D. Development, characterization & in vitro skin permeation of rutin ethosomes as a novel vesicular carrier. *Int. J. Biomed. Res.* **2017**, *8*, 559–566.
28. Park, S.N.; Lee, H.J.; Gu, H.A. Enhanced skin delivery and characterization of rutin-loaded ethosomes. *Korean J. Chem. Eng.* **2014**, *31*, 485–489. [CrossRef]
29. Proksch, E. pH in nature, humans and skin. *J. Dermatol.* **2018**, *45*, 1044–1052. [CrossRef] [PubMed]
30. Chandra, A.; Aggarwal, G.; Manchanda, S.; Narula, A. Development of Topical Gel of Methotrexate Incorporated Ethosomes and Salicylic Acid for the Treatment of Psoriasis. *Pharm. Nanotechnol.* **2019**, *7*, 362–374. [CrossRef]
31. Marto, J.; Baltazar, D.; Duarte, A.; Fernandes, A.; Gouveia, L.; Militão, M.; Salgado, A.; Simões, S.; Oliveira, E.; Ribeiro, H.M. Topical gels of etofenamate: In vitro and in vivo evaluation. *Pharm. Dev. Technol.* **2015**, *20*, 710–715. [CrossRef] [PubMed]
32. Andleeb, M.; Shoaib Khan, H.M.; Daniyal, M. Development, Characterization and Stability Evaluation of Topical Gel Loaded with Ethosomes Containing *Achillea millefolium* L. Extract. *Front. Pharmacol.* **2021**, *12*, 1–11. [CrossRef]

33. Pannu, A.; Goyal, R.K.; Ojha, S.; Nandave, M. Naringenin: A Promising Flavonoid for Herbal Treatment of Rheumatoid Arthritis and Associated Inflammatory Disorders. In *Bioactive Food as Dietary Interventions for Arthritis and Related Inflammatory Diseases*; Elsevier: Amsterdam, The Netherlands, 2019; pp. 343–354. ISBN 9780128138205.
34. Zofia, N.Ł.; Martyna, Z.D.; Aleksandra, Z.; Tomasz, B. Comparison of the Antiaging and Protective Properties of Plants from the Apiaceae Family. *Oxid. Med. Cell. Longev.* **2020**, *2020*. [CrossRef] [PubMed]
35. Karim, N.A. Ethosomal nanocarriers: The impact of constituents and formulation techniques on ethosomal properties, in vivo studies, and clinical trials. *Int. J. Nanomed.* **2016**, *11*, 2279–2304.
36. Van Hoogevest, P.; Wendel, A. Review Article The use of natural and synthetic phospholipids as pharmaceutical excipients Â. *Eur. J. Lipid Sci. Technol.* **2014**, *116*, 1088–1107. [CrossRef]
37. Colombo, I.; Sangiovanni, E.; Maggio, R.; Mattozzi, C.; Zava, S.; Corbett, Y.; Fumagalli, M.; Carlino, C.; Corsetto, P.A.; Scaccabarozzi, D.; et al. HaCaT Cells as a Reliable In Vitro Differentiation Model to Dissect the Inflammatory/Repair Response of Human Keratinocytes. *Mediat. Inflamm.* **2017**, *2017*, 1–12. [CrossRef]
38. Marques, P.; Marto, J.; Gonçalves, L.M.; Pacheco, R.; Fitas, M.; Pinto, P.; Serralheiro, M.L.M.; Ribeiro, H. *Cynara scolymus* L.: A promising Mediterranean extract for topical anti-aging prevention. *Ind. Crops Prod.* **2017**, *109*, 699–706. [CrossRef]
39. Islam, M.T.; Ciotti, S.; Ackermann, C. Rheological Characterization of Topical Carbomer Gels Neutralized to Different pH. *Pharm. Res.* **2004**, *21*, 1192–1199. [CrossRef]
40. Feil, H.; Bae, Y.H.; Feijen, J.; Kim, S.W. Mutual influence of pH and temperature on the swelling of ionizable and thermosensitive hydrogels. *Macromolecules* **1992**, *25*, 5528–5530. [CrossRef]
41. Barry, B.W.; Meyer, M.C. The rheological properties of carbopol gels I. Continuous shear and creep properties of carbopol gels. *Int. J. Pharm.* **1979**, *2*, 1–25. [CrossRef]
42. Kunitz, M. Syneresis and swelling of gelatin. *J. Gen. Physiol.* **1928**, *12*, 289–312. [CrossRef]
43. Dave, V.; Bhardwaj, N.; Gupta, N.; Tak, K. Herbal ethosomal gel containing luliconazole for productive relevance in the field of biomedicine. *3 Biotech* **2020**, *10*, 1–15. [CrossRef]
44. Jain, S.; Patel, N.; Madan, P.; Lin, S. Formulation and rheological evaluation of ethosome-loaded carbopol hydrogel for transdermal application. *Drug Dev. Ind. Pharm.* **2016**, *42*, 1315–1324. [CrossRef] [PubMed]
45. Walicka, A.; Falicki, J. Rheology of Drugs for Topical and Transdermal Delivery. *Int. J. Appl. Mech. Eng.* **2019**, *24*, 179–198. [CrossRef]
46. Ortan, A.; Parvu, C.D.; Ghica, M.V.; Popescu, L.M.; Ionita, L. Rheological study of a liposomal hydrogel based on carbopol. *Rom. Biotechnol. Lett.* **2011**, *16*, 47–54.
47. Pawar, J.; Narkhede, R.; Amin, P.; Tawde, V. Design and Evaluation of Topical Diclofenac Sodium Gel Using Hot Melt Extrusion Technology as a Continuous Manufacturing Process with Kolliphor® P407. *AAPS PharmSciTech* **2017**, *18*, 2303–2315. [CrossRef]
48. Bonacucina, G.; Cespi, M.; Misici-Falzi, M.; Palmieri, G.F. Rheological, adhesive and release characterisation of semisolid Carbopol/tetraglycol systems. *Int. J. Pharm.* **2006**, *307*, 129–140. [CrossRef]
49. Rijo, P.; Falé, P.L.; Serralheiro, M.L.; Simões, M.F.; Gomes, A.; Reis, C. Optimization of medicinal plant extraction methods and their encapsulation through extrusion technology. *Meas. J. Int. Meas. Confed.* **2014**, *58*, 249–255. [CrossRef]
50. Rouser, G.; Fleischer, S.; Yamamoto, A. Two dimensional thin layer chromatographic separation of polar lipids and determination of phospholipids by phosphorus analysis of spots. *Lipids* **1970**, *5*, 494–496. [CrossRef]
51. Gaspar, M.M.; Cruz, A.; Penha, A.F.; Reymão, J.; Sousa, A.C.; Eleutério, C.V.; Domingues, S.A.; Fraga, A.G.; Filho, A.L.; Cruz, M.E.M.; et al. Rifabutin encapsulated in liposomes exhibits increased therapeutic activity in a model of disseminated tuberculosis. *Int. J. Antimicrob. Agents* **2008**, *31*, 37–45. [CrossRef] [PubMed]
52. Silva, C.O.; Rijo, P.; Molpeceres, J.; Figueiredo, I.V.; Ascensão, L.; Fernandes, A.S.; Roberto, A.; Reis, C.P. Polymeric nanoparticles modified with fatty acids encapsulating betamethasone for anti-inflammatory treatment. *Int. J. Pharm.* **2015**, *493*, 271–284. [CrossRef] [PubMed]
53. Vijayalakshmi, S.; Karthika, T.N.; Mishra, A.K.; Chandra, T.S. Spectrofluorimetric method for the estimation of total lipids in Eremothecium ashbyii fungal filaments using Nile blue and avoiding interference of autofluorescent riboflavin. *J. Microbiol. Methods* **2003**, *55*, 99–103. [CrossRef]
54. Mota, A.H.; Direito, R.; Carrasco, M.P.; Rijo, P.; Ascensão, L.; Silveira Viana, A.; Rocha, J.; Eduardo-Figueira, M.; João Rodrigues, M.; Custódio, L.; et al. Combination of hyaluronic acid and PLGA particles as hybrid systems for viscosupplementation in osteoarthritis. *Int. J. Pharm.* **2019**, *559*, 13–22. [CrossRef] [PubMed]
55. Kumar, P.; Choonara, Y.E.; Pillay, V. In silico analytico-mathematical interpretation of biopolymeric assemblies: Quantification of energy surfaces and molecular attributes via atomistic simulations. *Bioeng. Transl. Med.* **2018**, *3*, 222–231. [CrossRef] [PubMed]
56. Santos-Rebelo, A.; Kumar, P.; Pillay, V.; Choonara, Y.E.; Eleutério, C.; Figueira, M.; Viana, A.S.; Ascensão, L.; Molpeceres, J.; Rijo, P.; et al. Development and mechanistic insight into the enhanced cytotoxic potential of parvifloron D albumin nanoparticles in EGFR-overexpressing pancreatic cancer cells. *Cancers* **2019**, *11*, 1733. [CrossRef]
57. Mota, A.H.; Andrade, J.M.; Ntungwe, E.N.; Pereira, P.; Cebola, M.J.; Bernardo-Gil, M.G.; Molpeceres, J.; Rijo, P.; Viana, A.S.; Ascensão, L.; et al. Green extraction of *Sambucus nigra* L. for potential application in skin nanocarriers. *Green Mater.* **2020**, *8*, 181–193. [CrossRef]

58. Jackson, J.K.; Zhao, J.; Wong, W.; Burt, H.M. The inhibition of collagenase induced degradation of collagen by the galloyl-containing polyphenols tannic acid, epigallocatechin gallate and epicatechin gallate. *J. Mater. Sci. Mater. Med.* **2010**, *21*, 1435–1443. [CrossRef] [PubMed]
59. Santos-Rebelo, A.; Garcia, C.; Eleutério, C.; Bastos, A.; Coelho, S.C.; Coelho, M.A.N.; Molpeceres, J.; Viana, A.S.; Ascensão, L.; Pinto, J.F.; et al. Development of parvifloron D-loaded smart nanoparticles to target pancreatic cancer. *Pharmaceutics* **2018**, *10*, 216. [CrossRef]
60. Delfim Fernando Gonçalves dos Santos Absorção percutânea-geles de carbopol contendo fentiazac, Faculdade de Farmacia do Porto. 1995. Available online: http://hdl.handle.net/10216/10158 (accessed on 31 October 2019).
61. Reis, C.; Antunes, A.F.; Rijo, P.; Baptista, M.; Mota, J.P.; Monteiro Rodrigues, L. A novel topical association with zinc oxide, chamomile and aloe vera extracts-stability and safety studies. *Biomed. Biopharm. Res.* **2015**, *12*, 251–264. [CrossRef]
62. EMA/CPMC/ICH/2736/99 ICH Topic Q1A (R2). 2003. Available online: https://www.ema.europa.eu/en/documents/scientific-guideline/ich-q-1-r2-stability-testing-new-drug-substances-products-step-5_en.pdf (accessed on 6 August 2020).
63. Braden, M. Tissue Conditioners: II. Rheologic Properties. *J. Dent. Res.* **1970**, *49*, 496–501. [CrossRef]
64. Reis, C.P.; Gomes, A.; Rijo, P.; Candeias, S.; Pinto, P. Evaluation of a New Topical Treatment for Acne with Azelaic Acid-Loaded Nanoparticles. *Microsc. Microanal.* **2013**, *19*, 1141–1150. [CrossRef] [PubMed]
65. Marzulli, F.N.; Maibach, H.I. Contact allergy: Predictive testing in man. *Contact Dermatitis* **1976**, *2*, 1–17. [CrossRef] [PubMed]
66. PhD Trials Patch Test study protocol n° PT.02.01/final03, RNEC n° 127504.

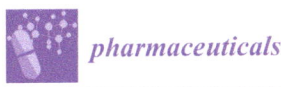

Article

Development of a Topical Amphotericin B and *Bursera graveolens* Essential Oil-Loaded Gel for the Treatment of Dermal Candidiasis

Lupe Carolina Espinoza [1,2], Lilian Sosa [3], Paulo C. Granda [2,4], Nuria Bozal [5], Natalia Díaz-Garrido [6,7], Brenda Chulca-Torres [1] and Ana Cristina Calpena [2,4,*]

1 Departamento de Química, Universidad Técnica Particular de Loja, Loja 1101608, Ecuador; lcespinoza@utpl.edu.ec (L.C.E.); bachulca@utpl.edu.ec (B.C.-T.)
2 Institute of Nanoscience and Nanotechnology (IN2UB), University of Barcelona, 08028 Barcelona, Spain; paulogranda92@gmail.com
3 Faculty of Chemical Sciences and Pharmacy, National Autonomous University of Honduras (UNAH), Tegucigalpa 11101, Honduras; lilian.sosa@unah.edu.hn
4 Department of Pharmacy, Pharmaceutical Technology and Physical Chemistry, Faculty of Pharmacy and Food Sciences, University of Barcelona, 08028 Barcelona, Spain
5 Department of Biology, Healthcare and the Environment, School of Pharmacy and Food Sciences, University of Barcelona, 08028 Barcelona, Spain; nuriabozaldefebrer@ub.edu
6 Department of Biochemistry and Physiology, Faculty of Pharmacy and Food Sciences, University of Barcelona, 08028 Barcelona, Spain; natalia.diaz.garrido@gmail.com
7 Institute of Biomedicine of the University of Barcelona-Sant Joan de Déu Research Institute (IBUB-IRSJD), 08028 Barcelona, Spain
* Correspondence: anacalpena@ub.edu

Abstract: The higher molecular weight and low solubility of amphotericin B (AmB) hinders its topical administration. The aim of this study was to incorporate *Bursera graveolens* essential oil into an AmB topical gel (AmB + BGEO gel) in order to promote the diffusion of the drug through the skin in the treatment of cutaneous candidiasis. AmB + BGEO gel formulation was determined using a factorial experiment. Physical and chemical parameters, stability, in vitro release profile and ex vivo permeation in human skin were evaluated. In vitro antimicrobial activity was studied using strains of *C. albicans*, *C. glabrata* and *C. parapsilosis*. The tolerability was evaluated using in vitro and in vivo models. AmB + BGEO gel presented appropriate characteristics for topical administration, including pH of 5.85, pseudoplastic behavior, optimal extensibility, as well as high stability and acceptable tolerability. In vitro release studies showed that the formulation releases the drug following a Boltzmann sigmoidal model. Finally, AmB + BGEO gel exhibited higher amount of drug retained inside the skin and lower Minimum Inhibitory Concentration than a formulation sans essential oil. Therefore, these results suggest that the incorporation of *B. graveolens* essential oil in the formulation could be used as strategy to promote a local effect in the treatment of cutaneous candidiasis.

Keywords: amphotericin B; candidiasis; gel; essential oil; *Bursera graveolens*; topical treatment

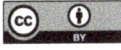

1. Introduction

Cutaneous candidiasis is a superficial mycosis caused by proliferation in the skin by fungal organisms belonging to the genus *Candida* [1]. *C. albicans* is responsible for approximately 70% of skin infections associated with *Candida* spp. [2,3]. This type of mycosis mainly affects intertriginous areas and produces dryness, erythema, edema, erosions and pustules [4]. Topical treatments for cutaneous candidiasis include the application of azoles and polyenes such as clotrimazole, miconazole, fluconazole, itraconazole and nystatin [5–7]. However, resistance mechanisms both intrinsic and acquired to these antifungal drugs have been reported. Intrinsic resistance is highly stable and is predictive of therapeutic failure whereas acquired resistance can be either stable or transient and is developed due to long exposure to antifungals [8–10]. Although polyene resistance is still uncommon compared to resistance to other antifungals, some mechanisms of resistance have been proposed, including: (1) alterations in the sterol composition of the fungal cell membrane due to several mutations in genes (ERG) of the ergosterol biosynthesis pathway, (2) oxidative stress, and (3) alterations of the fungal cell wall characterized by an increased glucan production [11].

AmB is a polyene macrolide antibiotic produced by *Streptomyces nodosus* that acts by binding with the sterols (ergosterol) present in the cell membrane of susceptible fungi, resulting in the creation of transmembrane channels that induce ion permeability, loss of protons and monovalent cations, and consequently depolarization and concentration-dependent cell killing [12,13]. AmB has been clinically used to treat *Candida*, *Cryptoccocus* and *Aspergillus* via intravenous infusion [14,15]. However, its systemic adverse effects are well-known, including symptoms from acute toxicity such as nausea, vomiting, rigors, fever, hypertension or hypotension, and hypoxia as well as chronic adverse effects such as nephrotoxicity [16]. A topically administered AmB formulation can bypass these disadvantages from invasive administration techniques and thus permit treatment of localized infections in skin or mucous membranes [17]. However, the higher molecular weight (926 Da) and low solubility in water of AmB could limit its passage through the skin [18]. These complications could be circumvented by incorporating excipients with permeation-enhancing properties that promote the penetration of drugs through the stratum corneum (SC) and its distribution to the epidermis and dermis [19].

Examples of commonly studied permeation enhancers for dermal drug delivery include azone, pyrrolidones, sulphoxides, fatty acids, and surfactants as well as essential oils and their components [20]. Ideally, these compounds induce a temporary and reversible reduction in the barrier function of the SC in order to facilitate the drug permeation across the skin [21,22].

Essential oils are natural products extracted from aromatic plant materials and contain complex mixtures of several volatile compounds such as terpenes, terpenoids and phenylpropanoids [22]. Essential oils are widely used in pharmaceutical, cosmetic, agricultural and food industries in several applications including improvement of drug permeation in addition to antibacterial, antifungal, antioxidant and anti-inflammatory activities [23]. As permeation enhancers, the active compounds derived from essential oils increase drug diffusion by changes in the SC structure and interaction with intercellular lipids in the SC [22,23]. In particular, the *Bursera graveolens* essential oil has been reported to inhibit the growth of breast tumor cells and amastigotes of *Leishmania amazonensis* while also having antioxidant, antifungal and anticarcinogenic properties [24,25]. *B. graveolens* is a deciduous tree found from western Mexico to northwestern Peru. Its wood exhibits a characteristic sweet, spicy and balsamic aroma that has traditionally been used as incense [26]. It is widely referred to as "palo santo" by local populations, which in Spanish means "holy wood" [27]. Essential oil obtained from the fruit of *B. graveolens* primarily contains D-limonene (49.89%), α-phellandrene (37.64%) and menthofuran (6.08%) [25,27].

The purpose of this study was to develop and characterize a topical gel of AmB and *B. graveolens* essential oil (AmB + BGEO gel) as strategy to promote drug permeation through the SC and its retention in human skin in order to achieve a local effect in the treatment of cutaneous candidiasis.

2. Results

2.1. Solubility Studies

The AmB solubility in different components are shown in Figure 1. DMSO (solubility 3.82 ± 0.05 mg/mL) exhibited greater ability to solubilize the drug and was, therefore, used as solvent in the formulation. Propylene glycol 400 (solubility 1.09 ± 0.04 mg/mL) and glycerin (solubility 1.02 ± 0.04 mg/mL) were evaluated by a 2^3 factorial experiment in order to determine the most appropriate cosolvent for the formulation.

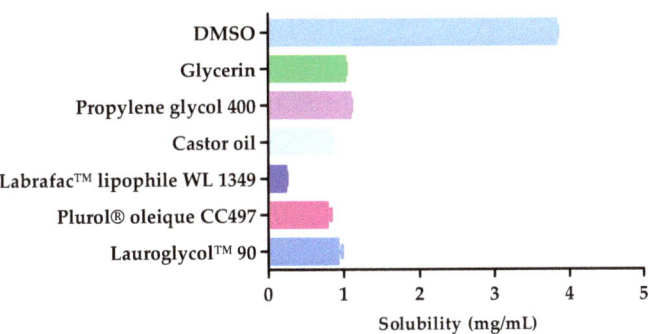

Figure 1. Amphotericin B (AmB) solubility in different excipients ($n = 3$).

2.2. Design and Preparation of AmB + BGEO Gel Formulation

Table 1 shows the physical and chemical characterization of the eight formulations obtained by 2^3 factorial experiment. After 60 days of storage at 30 °C, formulations 1, 4, 6 and 8 showed precipitates or formed lumps, whereas formulations 2 and 5 were homogeneous but showed significant changes in pH. These signs of instability were accompanied by a decrease in drug content. Finally, when comparing formulations 3 and 7, it was observed that formulation 3 was more stable, especially with regard to drug content, and was therefore selected as the final formulation for the AmB + BGEO gel.

Table 1. Physical and chemical characterization of the 8 formulations obtained by 2^3 factorial experiment after one and 60 days of preparation and storage at 30 °C.

	1 Day			60 Days		
Formulation	Appearance	pH	Drug Content (%)	Appearance	pH	Drug Content (%)
F1	Homogeneous	4.80 ± 0.03	99.68 ± 0.16	Precipitates	4.12 ± 0.09	96.78 ± 1.67
F2	Homogeneous	6.76 ± 0.05	99.73 ± 0.12	Homogeneous	4.98 ± 0.07	98.25 ± 0.82
F3	Homogeneous	5.85 ± 0.09	99.65 ± 0.08	Homogeneous	5.57 ± 0.04	99.18 ± 0.43
F4	Homogeneous	6.81 ± 0.07	99.66 ± 0.10	Lumps	6.02 ± 0.10	98.86 ± 1.35
F5	Homogeneous	5.28 ± 0.01	99.52 ± 0.09	Homogeneous	4.16 ± 0.15	98.16 ± 0.98
F6	Homogeneous	7.12 ± 0.08	99.59 ± 0.13	Precipitates	6.15 ± 0.09	97.63 ± 1.82
F7	Homogeneous	5.92 ± 0.04	99.81 ± 0.09	Homogeneous	5.05 ± 0.07	98.83 ± 0.66
F8	Homogeneous	6.70 ± 0.06	99.65 ± 0.11	Precipitates	5.72 ± 0.25	97.15 ± 1.68

AmB + BGEO gel (0.1%) was prepared by dissolving AmB in 5% DMSO, 20% Propylene glycol 400, and 2% *B. graveolens* essential oil. This mixture was then incorporated into a gel base composed of 3% CMC, 0.20% citric acid, 0.02% sodium benzoate, and 69.68% water (Table 2).

Table 2. Final formulation of AmB + BGEO gel.

Component (%)	
Amphotericin B (AmB)	0.1
B. graveolens essential oil (BGEO)	2
Carboxymethylcelullose (CMC)	3
Propylene glycol 400	20
Sodium benzoate	0.02
Citric acid	0.2
Dimethylsulfoxyde (DMSO)	5
Water	69.68

2.3. Characterization of AmB + BGEO Gel

AmB + BGEO gel showed a homogeneous appearance without signs of lumps or precipitates while also exhibiting a slightly yellowish color and a pleasant citrus scent characteristic of essential oil. The drug content in the formulation was of 99.65 ± 0.08% and with a pH value of 5.85 ± 0.09, which is biocompatible with the natural acidity of the skin.

Rheological studies (Figure 2) confirmed pseudoplastic behavior of the formulation (Cross model $r^2 = 0.999$) with a mean viscosity at 50 s^{-1} of 5036 ± 45.71 mPa·s. A hysteresis loop with an area of 4269 Pa/s was observed.

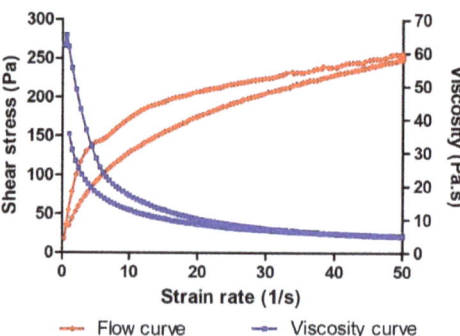

Figure 2. Rheological behavior of AmB + BGEO gel showing a hysteresis loop.

The extensibility profile of AmB + BGEO gel at 25 °C described in Figure 3 showed that the extensibility values increased proportionally to loading weight until reaching a maximum extensibility of 27.81 cm^2 following a one-phase association mathematical model.

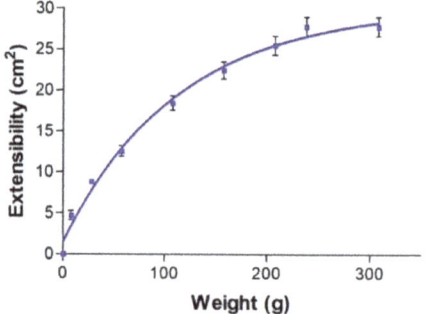

Figure 3. Extensibility profile of AmB + BGEO gel at 25 °C.

2.4. Stability Studies

The short-term stability evaluation of AmB + BGEO gel (Table 3) confirmed that after 120 days of storage at 30 °C and 40 °C, the formulation maintained a homogeneous aspect and suitable pH values for its application on skin (5.48 ± 0.12 to 5.85 ± 0.09 and 5.12 ± 0.07 to 5.83 ± 0.07, respectively). In the same way, the content of AmB present in the formulation remained without significant changes during the time of the stability study with a decrease of 0.86% at 30 °C and 1.1% at 40 °C.

Table 3. Stability studies of AmB + BGEO gel.

Time (Days)	30 ± 2 °C/65 ± 5% RH			40 ± 2 °C/75 ± 5% RH		
	Appearance	pH	Drug Content (%)	Appearance	pH	Drug Content (%)
1	Homogeneous	5.85 ± 0.09	99.65 ± 0.08	Homogeneous	5.83 ± 0.07	99.67 ± 0.12
60	Homogeneous	5.57 ± 0.04	99.18 ± 0.43	Homogeneous	5.43 ± 0.15	98.91 ± 0.17
120 days	Homogeneous	5.48 ± 0.12	98.79 ± 0.66	Homogeneous	5.12 ± 0.07	98.56 ± 0.32

2.5. In Vitro Release Study

Figure 4 shows the release profile of AmB from the formulation. At the end of the experiment, an amount of 154.8 µg of AmB was released from the gel, which represents about 80% of the drug. The best fit of the experimental data was obtained with the Boltzmann sigmoidal model with a $r^2 = 0.9974$ and whose mathematical equation is:

$$Y = Bottom + (Top - Bottom)/1 + \exp\left(\frac{V50 - x}{Slope}\right) \quad (1)$$

where Y is the amount of released drug, Top and Bottom are the initial and final values of drug release, V50 is the time it takes to release half of the maximum amount susceptible to release and the Slope of the curve indicates the steepness.

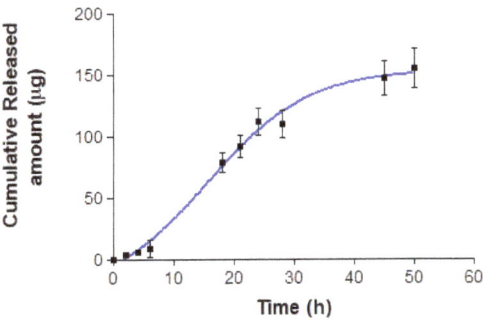

Figure 4. In vitro release profile of AmB from formulation. The cumulative amount released was plotted against time. Data represents mean ± SD ($n = 3$).

2.6. Ex Vivo Permeation Study

Ex vivo permeation studies of AmB + BGEO gel and AmB gel (*B. graveolens* essential oil-free AmB gel) were carried out in order to compare and evaluate the role of the *B. graveolens* essential oil in drug permeation. AmB was not detected in the aliquots extracted from the receptor compartment over a 24 h period of permeation assay in either of the two formulations. However, AmB was found inside the skin with a retention value of 997.78 µg/g skin/cm² for AmB + BGEO gel and 603.91 µg/g skin/cm² for AmB gel.

2.7. Efficacy Study: Antimicrobial Activity

The antimicrobial activity after 48 h is reported in Table 4 as Minimum Inhibitory Concentration (MIC) values against strains of *C. albicans*, *C. glabrata* and *C. parapsilosis*. The *B. graveolens* essential oil at concentrations of 6.25 to 12.50% (v/v) showed antimicrobial activity against the studied *Candida* strains. The AmB + BGEO gel exhibited the lowest MIC values (0.29, 0.39 and 0.58 µg/mL) compared with AmB gel (0.58, 0.58 and 1 µg/mL) against *C. albicans*, *C. glabrata* and *C. parapsilosis*, respectively.

Table 4. MIC against different cultures of *Candida* spp., Free AmB, AmB gel, AmB + BGEO gel and *B. graveolens* essential oil (BGEO) after incubation at 30 °C for 48 h (n = 3).

Tested Species	Origin	MIC (µg/mL)			% (v/v)
		Free AmB	AmB Gel	AmB + BGEO Gel	BGEO
C. albicans	ATCC 10231	0.15	0.58	0.29	12.50
C. grabrata	ATCC 66032	0.60	0.58	0.39	6.25
C. parapsilosis	ATCC 22019	0.30	1	0.58	12.50

2.8. Tolerance Studies

2.8.1. Cytotoxicity Studies by MTT Assay

The effect of different concentrations of AmB + BGEO gel on human keratinocytes was evaluated using MTT cytotoxicity assay. After 24 h of incubation, it was observed that the assayed dilutions of the formulation (1/50 to 1/2000) did not affect cell viability, which was close to 100% in relation to the control (Figure 5). Therefore, these results suggest that AmB + BGEO gel do not trigger toxicity in the cells.

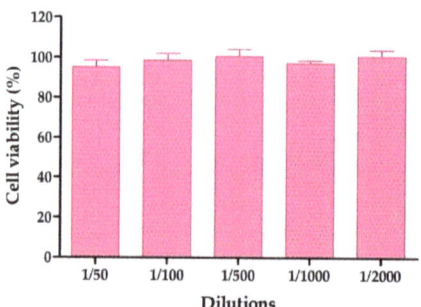

Figure 5. Percentage of cell viability of HaCaT cell line exposed to AmB + BGEO for 24 h at different concentrations.

2.8.2. In Vivo Tolerance Studies

No significant changes in the TEWL or SCH values with respect to the basal state were observed after 25 min of topical application of AmB + BGEO gel in the ventral area of the forearm of the volunteers (Figure 6). These results suggest that the formulation does not cause damage or irritation in the skin barrier.

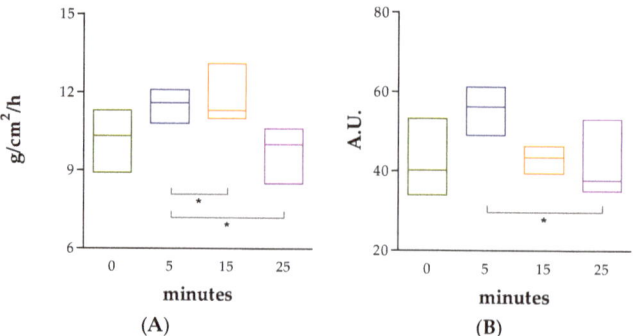

Figure 6. Tolerance studies in human individuals. (**A**) TEWL: Transepidermal water loss; (**B**) SCH: Stratum corneum hydration. Results are expressed as median, minimum and maximum (n = 12). Statistically significant differences: * $p < 0.05$.

3. Discussion

AmB is administered by intravenous infusion in the treatment of fungal infections [28]. This treatment causes several adverse effects including nausea, vomiting, rigors, fever, hypertension or hypotension, hypoxia and nephrotoxicity [16]. The incorporation of AmB into topical formulations could be used as a strategy to achieve a local effect in the skin without adverse systemic effects in the treatment of dermal candidiasis. However, its low aqueous solubility, great molecular weight (926 Da) and limited permeability of the SC to external substances, including drugs, could obstruct its penetration through the skin. In this study, the incorporation of *B. graveolens* essential oil into an AmB topical gel was carried out in order to promote drug permeation through the SC and its retention in human skin. The final formulation of AmB + BGEO gel (0.1%) was prepared using pharmaceutical excipients compatible with the drug (Table 2). This formulation was homogeneous with a pleasant citrus scent and had a slightly acidic pH value which assures non-irritating effects [29]. Determination of the flow properties of formulations, particularly those intended for skin application, provides important information about stability, sensory characteristics, spreadability and filling/dosing behavior [30]. A topical formulation should exhibit optimal viscosity and spreadability since a product too fluid or too viscous could be unpleasant or uncomfortable for patients [31,32]. Moreover, the viscosity and rheological behavior can modulate biopharmaceutical parameters such as release rates of drugs from their vehicles [33]. AmB + BGEO gel showed a mean viscosity of 5036 ± 45.71 mPa·s at 50 s^{-1} and a maximum extensibility of 27.81 cm^2, which suggest that this formulation is easy to apply (Figures 2 and 3). Rheological analysis and mathematical modeling confirmed the pseudoplastic behavior of AmB + BGEO gel and the presence of a hysteresis loop in the rheograms, suggesting thixotropic behavior [34]. These characteristics offer advantages for topical formulations since the viscosity decreases with friction, allowing for easy spreadability while returning to the initial state once the friction stops, which favors the residence in the treated area [35].

The stability studies at 30 and 40 °C for 120 days showed that AmB + BGEO gel maintained its homogeneous appearance and no significant changes in its pH values were detected after storage, showing values within the suitable range for skin application. Chemical stability was also observed with slight yet inconsequential changes in the quantified drug content, thus demonstrating high compatibility between the drug and the excipients (Table 3).

Interactions between the vehicle and drug define the release profile, which in turn affects the permeation rate of the drug [29]. In this research, the in vitro release study showed a released amount of 154.8 µg of AmB from the gel (Figure 4), which indicates that the vehicle is capable of releasing the drug without limiting skin permeation. According to the obtained r^2 value, the release kinetic of AmB from gel followed a Boltzmann sigmoidal model that is characterized by an initial phase of slow-or-negligible release (0–6 h) followed by a second phase of immediate-or-controlled release [36].

Ex vivo permeation studies are used to estimate the in vivo behavior of the formulation, since the composition and the physical properties of the carrier influence the amount of drug reaching the target area [30]. The success of topical treatment is contingent upon the ability of the drug to cross the SC as well as its distribution through the epidermis and dermis [37,38]. The results of this study showed that the drug does not reach the receptor compartment in either of the two formulations (AmB + BGEO gel and AmB gel) but is instead retained in the tissue, thereby promoting a local effect in the skin without adverse effects. However, a higher amount of drug retained inside the skin was observed in the AmB + BGEO gel (997.78 µg/g skin/cm^2) compared to AmB gel (603.91 µg/g skin/cm^2), suggesting that the incorporation of *B. graveolens* essential oil facilitated the penetration of the drug through the SC and its diffusion to the epidermis and dermis. This essential oil contains limonene, a lipophilic terpene reported to have a skin permeation-enhancing effect of both hydrophilic and lipophilic drugs [39]. The proposed mechanism of this effect is due to changes in the intercellular packing and disruption in lipid structures that involve the modification of SC from solvents, thus improving drug partitioning into the skin [40,41].

The efficacy study showed that AmB + BGEO gel exhibited a lower MIC value against strains of *C. albicans*, *C. glabrata* and *C. parapsilosis* and is consequently more effective than the formulation sans essential oil (AmB gel). Significant antimicrobial activity of *B. graveolens* essential oil against strains of *C. albicans* has been previously reported. This effect has been attributed to its terpene-rich composition, namely limonene, although the exact mechanism is not completely understood as of yet. Nevertheless, some studies support the idea that these compounds could cause membrane disruption which consequently induces the death of the fungus [42]. A number of studies have shown that natural secondary metabolites with low molecular weight ($\leq$500 g/mol) may act as adjuvants for antimicrobial drugs and thus potentiate its efficacy. Based on this approach, studies of combination therapy of antimicrobial drugs with terpenes have revealed promising effects against both susceptible and resistant pathogens [43]. In particular, essential oils such as *Citrus aurantium*, *Thymus kotschanus*, *myrtus communis* and *Mentha piperita* have shown a synergistic effect with clinical drugs including AmB, fluconazole, ketoconazole and meropenem [43–46]. In the current study, the combination of AmB with *B. graveolens* essential oil in a topical gel showed enhanced antifungal activity against *C. albicans*, *C. glabrata* and *C. parapsilosis*. These results indicate that the addition of *B. graveolens* essential oil in the formulation likely enhances the antimicrobial effect either due to its active compounds or a possible synergistic effect between its compounds and the drug.

The tolerability of AmB + BGEO gel was analyzed by in vitro and in vivo models. In vitro models are considered helpful to screen the toxicity of new formulations prior to the pre-clinical and clinical assessment. A variety of cell lines are frequently used for toxicity screening in a living system due to the cells being generally easy to cultivate, fast to grow and are sensitive to toxic irritation [47]. In this study, the tested dilutions of AmB + BGEO gel did not induce relevant cytotoxic effects on cells after 24 h of incubation, which confirms high biocompatibility between the developed formulation and human keratinocytes. This result was confirmed by evaluation of biomechanical skin properties including TEWL and SCH, which allow analysis of the integrity of the skin barrier after exposure to physical or chemical agents [30,48]. The results revealed an increase in TEWL and SCH values 5 min after topical application of AmB + BGEO gel; however, a tendency to return to the basal state was observed in both parameters after 25 min of assay, suggesting that AmB + BGEO gel does not cause irritation or damage to the skin surface of volunteers.

4. Materials and Methods

4.1. Materials

Amphotericin B (potency of 864 µg/mg) was purchased from Acofarma® (Barcelona, Spain). *B. graveolens* essential oil was provided by the Unit Operations Laboratory of the Universidad Técnica Particular de Loja [25]. Dimethyl Sulfoxide (DMSO) was obtained from Alfa Aesar (Thermo Fisher, Karlsruhe, DE-BW, Germany). Glycerin, propylene glycol 400 and castor oil were supplied by Sigma-Aldrich (Madrid, Spain). Capric Triglyceride (Labrafac™ lipophile WL 1349), polyglyceryl-3 dioleate (Plurol® oleique CC497), diethylene glycol monoethyl ether (Transcutol® P), and propylene glycol monolaurate-type II (Lauroglycol™ 90) were obtained from Gatefossé (Saint-Priest, France). Carboxymethylcellulose (CMC), carbopol® 940, sodium benzoate, parabens, and citric acid were obtained from Fagron Ibérica (Barcelona, Spain). HaCaT cell line was purchased from Cell Line Services (Eppelheim, DE-BW, Germany) and the reagents used for cell cultures were obtained from Gibco (Carcavelos, Lisbon, Portugal). The reagents for the MTT assay were obtained from Invitrogen Alfagene® (Carcavelos, Lisbon, Portugal). A Millipore Milli-Q® water purification system (Millipore Corporation; Burlington, MA, USA) was used. Finally, the chemicals and reagents were of analytical grade.

4.2. High-Performance Liquid Chromatography (HPLC)

AmB was quantified by a previously validated HPLC method [49]. The assay was carried out using a Waters HPLC with 2487 (UV/Vis) Detector & 717 Plus Autosampler (Waters, Milford, MA, USA). The mobile phase was a mixture of acetonitrile and glacial acetic acid 3.75% (65:35, v/v) filtered with a 0.45 μm PVDF membrane filter (Millipore Corp., Madrid, Spain). The assay was performed using a Kromasil C18 column (250 mm, 4.6 mm and 5 μm). The mobile phase was pumped at a flow rate of 0.5 mL/min and the injection volume was 10 μL. Finally, the elute was analyzed at 407 nm (wavelength of maximum absorbance of AmB).

4.3. Solubility Studies

The solubility of AmB in various solvents including DMSO, glycerin, propylene glycol 400, castor oil, Labrafac™ lipophile WL 1349, Plurol® oleique CC497 and Lauroglycol™ 90 was evaluated using an excess of AmB and mixing by magnetic stirring for 30 min at 1500 rpm. The samples were equilibrated for 24 h and subsequently centrifuged at 9000 rpm for 10 min. The supernatant was extracted and diluted with methanol in order to quantify the dissolved AmB using a UV-Visible DR 6000 spectrophotometer (Hach®, Düsseldorf, DE-NW, Germany).

4.4. Formulation: Design and Analysis of 2^3 Factorial Experiment

In this study, a 2^3 factorial experiment was designed to examine the influence of three factors: the type of polymer (A), humectant (B) and preservative (C) at two levels, which are indicated by the signs "+" and "−" in Table 5 [50].

Table 5. Factors studied in the factorial experimental design and their levels.

Factors	Levels	
	(+)	(−)
A: Polymer	Carboxymethylcellulose	Carbopol
B: Cosolvent	Glycerin	Propylene glycol 400
C: Preservative	Sodium benzoate	Parabens

Eight different formulations were obtained with the 2^3 factorial experiment using the ingredients at concentrations in accordance with the Handbook of Pharmaceutical Excipients and published data about efficacy and safety [51,52]. Furthermore, each formulation was composed of AmB (0.1%), BGEO (2%), DMSO (5%) and purified water. The pH was adjusted using citric acid (0.25%) in the CMC formulations and triethanolamine (1%) in the carbopol 940 formulations (Table 6).

Table 6. Formulations developed from the 2^3 factorial experiment.

Component	%	F1	F2	F3	F4	F5	F6	F7	F8
CMC	3	*		*		*		*	
Carbopol 940	1		*		*		*		*
Glycerin	20	*	*			*	*		
Propylene glycol 400	20			*	*			*	*
Sodium benzoate	0.02		*		*	*			*
Parabens	0.02	*		*			*	*	
Citric acid	0.20	*		*		*		*	
Triethanolamine	1		*		*		*		*
AmB	0.1	*	*	*	*	*	*	*	*
DMSO	5	*	*	*	*	*	*	*	*
BGEO	2	*	*	*	*	*	*	*	*
Water	sq	*	*	*	*	*	*	*	*

BGEO = *Bursera graveolens* essential oil, CMC = Carboxymethylcelullose, AmB = Amphotericin B, DMSO = Dimethyl Sulfoxide, sq = Sufficient quantity, * presence of the component (featured in the left-most column).

In order to prepare the gels, polymers were hydrated for 30 min in water (mix 1). AmB was dissolved in DMSO under magnetic stirring for 10 min immediately followed by adding cosolvent and *B. graveolens* essential oil (mix 2). Citric acid and preservatives were dissolved in water (mix 3). Finally, mix 1 and 3 were mixed at 850 rpm using a IKA ULTRA-TURRAX T50 (Staufen, Germany) for 10 min, after which mix 2 was incorporated under the same stirring conditions. The final formulation was selected based on physical and chemical stability after 60 days of storage at 30 °C.

4.5. Characterization of AmB + BGEO Gel

The pH of AmB gel was determined using a pH meter GLP 22 (Crison Instruments, Barcelona, Spain).

Viscosity and rheological behavior of AmB gel were evaluated with a Haake Rheostress 1 rotational rheometer (Thermo Fisher Scientific, Kalsruhe, Germany) equipped with a cone–plate sensor system including a fixed bottom plate and a Haake C60/2Ti movable top cone (60 mm diameter, 2° angle, 0.105 mm gap). AmB gel was tested in duplicate 24 h after preparation. Viscosity values and flow curves were recorded during the ramp-up period from 0 to 50 s^{-1} (3 min), constant shear rate period of 50 s^{-1} (1 min), and a ramp-down period from 50 to 0 s^{-1} (3 min). Obtained data from the flow curve were fitted to different mathematical models including Newtonian, Bingham, Ostwald-de-Waele, Cross, Casson and Herschel–Bulkley. The model that best statistically describes the experimental data was selected according to the correlation coefficient value (r). Viscosity mean value (mPa·s) was determined at 50 s^{-1} from the constant shear rate period of viscosity curve. The determination of the disturbance of the microstructure during the test or "apparent thixotropy" (Pa/s) was evaluated by determining the area of the hysteresis loop.

The extensibility of AmB gel was analyzed in triplicate following the previously described method [53]. A sample of 1 g of formulation was placed on the center of the base plate of an extensometer. Afterwards, a glass plate (7.93 g) was placed on the sample without sliding and a series of weights (27.89, 57.82, 107.69, 157.55, 207.46, 237.50 and 307.69 g) were added at 1 min intervals. The extended area of the sample was recorded and then fitted to mathematical models using GraphPad Prism® version 6.0 (GraphPad Software Inc., San Diego, CA, USA).

The drug content in the gel was determined by dissolving 100 mg of AmB gel in 5 mL of DMSO:methanol (1:1, v/v). After vortexing for 2 min, the solution was filtered and analyzed by HPLC method described in Section 4.2.

4.6. Stability Studies

After manufacturing, AmB + BGEO gel samples were stored at pre-established conditions of temperature and relative humidity (RH) in accordance with the Q1A(R2) ICH (International Conference on Harmonisation) Guidelines: 30 ± 2 °C/65 ± 5% RH and 40 ± 2 °C/75 ± 5% RH for 4 months [54]. Physical and chemical characterization of the formulation were carried out before and after storage in the aforementioned conditions using the method described in Section 4.5.

4.7. In Vitro Release Study

The release study of AmB from gel was performed using Franz diffusion cells of 13 mL and an effective diffusion area of 2.54 cm^2 (FDC 400; Crown Grass, Somerville, NJ, USA). The receptor medium (RM) was a mixture of NN-dimethyl formamide, methanol and water (55:5:40, v/v). The conditions of the experiment were maintained at 32 °C and under continuous stirring in order to achieve sink conditions. A 0.45 μm nylon membrane was mounted between the donor and receptor compartments. A sample of 200 mg of AmB + BGEO gel was placed in the donor compartment and aliquots of 300 μL were collected from receptor compartment and replaced with the same volume of fresh RM at predetermined time intervals (2, 4, 6, 18, 21 and 24 h). The released amount of AmB (μg) from the formulation was determined by HPLC (Section 4.2) and plotted versus time (h) using GraphPad Prism® 6.0 (GraphPad Software Inc., San Diego, CA, USA, 2014). The experiment was carried out in triplicate and data are represented as mean ± SD. Data from the release curve were fitted to several kinetic models including first order, Higuchi, Hyperbolic, Weibull and Korsmeyer–Peppa. Finally, the model with the highest coefficient of determination (r^2) was selected.

4.8. Ex Vivo Permeation Study

The permeation studies were carried out using AmB + BGEO gel and AmB gel (*B. graveolens* essential oil-free AmB gel developed with the same qualitative and quantitative formula only without the incorporation of the essential oil) in order to compare and evaluate the role of the *B. graveolens* essential oil in drug permeation. These ex vivo permeation studies were carried out in Franz diffusion cells of 6 mL (0.64 cm^2 diffusion area) using human skin obtained during an abdominal lipectomy of a healthy 38-year-old woman (Hospital of Barcelona, SCIAS, Barcelona, Spain). To that end, a written informed consent was provided by the volunteer in accordance with the Ethical Committee of the Hospital of Barcelona (number 001, dated 20 January 2016). To guarantee the integrity of the skin samples, Transepidermal water loss (TEWL) was measured using a Tewameter TM 300 (Courage & Khazaka Electronics GmbH; Cologne, Germany) and only those with results below 10 g/m^{2}h were used. Skin samples (0.4 mm thick) were mounted between the donor and receptor compartments. Transcutol® P was used as receptor medium (RM) which was kept at 32 °C and under stirring to guarantee sink conditions. A sample of 200 mg of AmB + BGEO gel or AmB gel was placed in the donor compartment in contact with the outer surface of skin. Aliquots of 300 µL were collected from the receptor compartment and replaced with the same volume of fresh RM at predetermined time intervals (2, 6, 18, 24, 28, 45 and 50 h). These aliquots were analyzed by HPLC (Section 4.2). Following permeation studies, these skin samples were removed from the Franz diffusion cells, washed with distilled water and cut along the edges in order to retain only the permeation area. Afterwards, skin samples were weighed and immersed in 1 mL of DMSO during 20 min under cold sonication using an ultrasonic bath in order to extract AmB retained in the skin (Qret, µg drug/g tissue/cm^2). Finally, the resulting solution was filtered and analyzed by HPLC.

4.9. Efficacy Study: Antimicrobial Activity

The efficacy of the formulation was evaluated by determination of Minimum Inhibitory Concentration (MIC), which is defined as the lowest concentration of an antimicrobial agent necessary to inhibit the growth of a microorganism. The MIC was calculated by the broth microdilution method against three different strains of *Candida* spp. including *C. albicans* ATCC 10231, *C. glabrata* ATCC 66032 and *C. parapsilosis* ATCC 22019 (American Type Culture Collection, Manassas, VA, USA). This assay was carried out according to the guidelines outlined by the European Committee on Antimicrobial Susceptibility Testing (EUCAST) and the CLSI Reference Method M27-A3 [55,56].

A synthetic medium containing RPMI-1640, glutamine, pH indicator without bicarbonate and glucose 2% w/v: RPMI-1640 2% G (Invitrogen, Madrid, Spain) was used as culture medium. The yeast strains were first cultured on a Sabouraud Dextrose Agar Medium (Invitrogen, Madrid, Spain) at 30 °C for 48 h. The inoculums were prepared by suspending yeast colonies in sterile $\frac{1}{4}$ Ringer's solution to achieve a density equivalent to 0.5 McFarland standards and counting in a Neubauer Chamber (1 to 5 × 10^6 Colony Forming Unit, CFU/mL). Subsequently, a 1:10 dilution (1 to 5 × 10^5 CFU/mL) was prepared to be used as the final inoculum.

A solution of AmB previously dissolved in DMSO (Free AmB) as well as samples of AmB + BGEO and AmB gel (*B. graveolens* essential oil-free AmB gel) were evaluated to perform a comparative analysis. The inoculum was used as a positive control and the culture medium as a negative control.

The experiment was performed using 96-well microdilution plates making serial double dilutions of the samples under analysis from 37.5 µg/mL to 0.0002 µg/mL for the formulations and 100% to 0.04% for the *B. graveolens* essential oil. Finally, 100 µL of the inoculum was added. Plates were read at t 0, 24 and 48 h after incubation at 30 °C with a microplate reader model 680 (Bio-Rad, Madrid, Spain) at 620 nm.

4.10. Tolerance Studies

4.10.1. Cytotoxicity Studies by MTT Method

In vitro MTT cytotoxicy assay were performed using the human keratinocytes cell line HaCaT. Cells were adjusted at 2×10^5 cell/mL, seeded in 96-well plate for 24 h in Dubelcco's Modified Eagle's Medium (DMEM) with high glucose content buffered with 25 mM HEPES, and supplemented with 1% non-essential amino acids, 100 U/mL penicillin, 100 g/mL streptomycin and 10% heat inactivated Fetal Bovine Serum (FBS). Next, the cells were incubated with different dilutions of the AmB + BGEO gel ranging from 1/50 to 1/2000 for 24 h. Later, the HaCaT cells were washed with 1% sterile PBS and incubated with MTT (Sigma-Aldrich Chemical Co, St. Louis, MO, USA) solution (2.5 mg/mL) for 2 h at 37 °C. The medium was then carefully removed and 0.1 mL of solubilization reagent (99% DMSO) was added to lyse the cells and dissolve the purple MTT crystals. Cell viability was measured at 570 nm in a microplate photometer Varioskan TM LUX (Thermo Scientific, Waltham, MA, USA). A negative control was processed in parallel for comparison. The results were expressed as percentage of cell survival relative to the control (untreated HaCaT cells; 100% viability) using the following equation:

$$\% \text{ Cell viability} = \frac{\text{Abs sample}}{\text{Abs control}} \times 100 \qquad (2)$$

4.10.2. In Vivo Tolerance

Measurements of transepidermal water loss (TEWL) and stratum corneum hydration (SCH) of the ventral area of the forearm of 12 volunteers (6 men and 6 women; ages between 20 and 35 years) with healthy skin were performed with prior written informed consent. This study was approved by the Ethics Committee of the University of Barcelona (IRB00003099) in accordance with the principles from the Declaration of Helsinki.

The time intervals of each measurement were 5, 15 and 25 min after absorption of AmB + BGEO gel in the application area. Readings were recorded using a Tewameter® TM300 and Corneometer® 825 (Courage & Khazaka Electronics GmbH, Cologne, Germany) for TEWL and SCH, respectively. For TEWL measurements, the probe was pressed and held on the skin for 2 min and the results are expressed as $g/cm^2/h$. For the SCH values, the probe was pressed on the skin to measure the dielectric constant of the skin where measurements were given in arbitrary units (AU). The results of TEWL and SCH were recorded as the median, minimum and maximum ($n = 12$).

5. Conclusions

In conclusion, the present study provides evidence that the topical gel of AmB enriched with *B. graveolens* essential oil offers appropriate characteristics for skin application including biocompatible values of pH, pseudoplastic behavior, optimal spreadability and acceptable tolerability, all of which make it an appealing and suitable formulation for human use. Furthermore, the incorporation of *B. graveolens* essential oil improved the biopharmaceutical profile of the drug, facilitating its penetration through the SC and its retention into the skin and consequently promoting a local effect in the target area linked to enhanced antifungal activity against *C.albicans*, *C. glabrata* and *C. parapsilosis*. Therefore, this formulation could constitute a promising alternative in the treatment of cutaneous candidiasis which encourages further research to explore its use in clinical practice.

Author Contributions: L.C.E. carried out all the experiments, analyzed the data/results, and wrote the paper; P.C.G. realized the in vivo tolerance studies and wrote the paper; L.S. carried out the biopharmaceutical and rheological studies and wrote the paper; N.B. developed the antimicrobial activity studies; N.D.-G. realized the cytotoxicity assay; B.C.-T. carried out the 2^3 factorial experiment; and A.C.C. conceived and designed all the experiments. All authors have read and agreed to the published version of the manuscript.

Funding: This research received no external funding.

Institutional Review Board Statement: The study was conducted according to the guidelines of the Declaration of Helsinki, and approved by the Institutional Review Board (or Ethics Committee) of University of Barcelona (IRB00003099, dated 30 January 2019).

Informed Consent Statement: Informed consent was obtained from all subjects involved in the study.

Data Availability Statement: Data is contained within the article.

Acknowledgments: L.C.E. acknowledges the support of the Universidad Técnica Particular de Loja and the Secretaría de Educación Superior, Ciencia, Tecnología e Innovación (SENESCYT—Ecuador). The authors would like to express their gratitude to Eduardo Valarezo for his provision of the *B. graveolens* essential oil. Finally, the authors also acknowledge Jonathan Proctor for his review of the use of the English language.

Conflicts of Interest: The authors declare no conflict of interest.

References

1. Watts, C.J.; Wagner, D.K.; Sohnle, P.G. Fungal Infections, Cutaneous. In *Encyclopedia of Microbiology*, 3rd ed.; Elsevier: New York, NY, USA, 2009; pp. 382–388.
2. Havlickova, B.; Czaika, V.A.; Friedrich, M. Epidemiological Trends in Skin Mycoses Worldwide. *Mycoses* **2008**, *51*, 2–15. [CrossRef]
3. Permana, A.D.; Paredes, A.J.; Volpe-Zanutto, F.; Anjani, Q.K.; Utomo, E.; Donnelly, R.F. Dissolving microneedle-mediated dermal delivery of itraconazole nanocrystals for improved treatment of cutaneous candidiasis. *Eur. J. Pharm. Biopharm.* **2020**, *154*, 50–61. [CrossRef] [PubMed]
4. Palese, E.; Nudo, M.; Zino, G.; Devirgiliis, V.; Carbotti, M.; Cinelli, E.; Rodio, D.M.; Bressan, A.; Prezioso, C.; Ambrosi, C.; et al. Cutaneous candidiasis caused by Candida albicans in a young non-immunosuppressed patient: An unusual presentation. *Int. J. Immunopathol. Pharm.* **2018**, *32*, 2058738418781368. [CrossRef] [PubMed]
5. Pappas, P.G.; Rex, J.H.; Sobel, J.D.; Filler, S.G.; Dismukes, W.E.; Walsh, T.J.; Edwards, J.E. Guidelines for Treatment of Candidiasis. *Clin. Infect. Dis.* **2004**, *38*, 161–189. [CrossRef] [PubMed]
6. Taudorf, E.H.; Jemec, G.B.E.; Hay, R.J.; Saunte, D.M.L. Cutaneous candidiasis—An evidence-based review of topical and systemic treatments to inform clinical practice. *J. Eur. Acad. Derm. Venereol.* **2019**, *33*, 1863–1873. [CrossRef] [PubMed]
7. Zhang, A.Y.; Camp, W.L.; Elewski, B.E. Advances in topical and systemic antifungals. *Derm. Clin.* **2007**, *25*, 165–183. [CrossRef] [PubMed]
8. Morio, F.; Jensen, R.H.; Le Pape, P.; Arendrup, M.C. Molecular basis of antifungal drug resistance in yeasts. *Int. J. Antimicrob. Agents* **2017**, *50*, 599–606. [CrossRef]
9. Cannon, R.D.; Lamping, E.; Holmes, A.R.; Niimi, K.; Tanabe, K.; Niimi, M.; Monk, B.C. Candida albicans drug resistance another way to cope with stress. *Microbiology* **2007**, *153*, 3211–3217. [CrossRef]
10. Bhattacharya, S.; Sae-Tia, S.; Fries, B.C. Candidiasis and Mechanisms of Antifungal Resistance. *Antibiotics* **2020**, *9*, 312. [CrossRef]
11. Carolus, H.; Pierson, S.; Lagrou, K.; Van Dijck, P. Amphotericin B and Other Polyenes-Discovery, Clinical Use, Mode of Action and Drug Resistance. *J. Fungi* **2020**, *6*, 321. [CrossRef]
12. Yamamoto, T.; Umegawa, Y.; Tsuchikawa, H.; Hanashima, S.; Matsumori, N.; Funahashi, K.; Seo, S.; Shinoda, W.; Murata, M. The Amphotericin B-Ergosterol Complex Spans a Lipid Bilayer as a Single-Length Assembly. *Biochemistry* **2019**, *58*, 5188–5196. [CrossRef] [PubMed]
13. Noor, A.; Preuss, C.V. *Antifungal Membrane Function Inhibitors (Amphotericin B)*; StatPearls Publishing: Treasure Island, FL, USA, 2020.
14. Chang, Y.-L.; Yu, S.-J.; Heitman, J.; Wellington, M.; Chen, Y.-L. New Facets of Antifungal Therapy. *Virulence* **2016**, *8*, 222–236. [CrossRef]
15. Ito, J.I.; Hooshmand-Rad, R. Treatment of Candida Infections with Amphotericin B Lipid Complex. *Clin. Infect. Dis.* **2005**, *40*, 384–391. [CrossRef]
16. Laniado-Laborin, R.; Cabrales-Vargas, M.N. Amphotericin B: Side effects and toxicity. *Rev. Iberoam. Micol.* **2009**, *26*, 223–227. [CrossRef] [PubMed]
17. Fernandez-Garcia, R.; de Pablo, E.; Ballesteros, M.P.; Serrano, D.R. Unmet clinical needs in the treatment of systemic fungal infections: The role of amphotericin B and drug targeting. *Int. J. Pharm.* **2017**, *525*, 139–148. [CrossRef]
18. Lopez-Castillo, C.; Rodriguez-Fernandez, C.; Cordoba, M.; Torrado, J.J. Permeability Characteristics of a New Antifungal Topical Amphotericin B Formulation with gamma-Cyclodextrins. *Molecules* **2018**, *23*, 3349. [CrossRef] [PubMed]

19. Sosa, L.; Calpena, A.C.; Silva-Abreu, M.; Espinoza, L.C.; Rincon, M.; Bozal, N.; Domenech, O.; Rodriguez-Lagunas, M.J.; Clares, B. Thermoreversible Gel-Loaded Amphotericin B for the Treatment of Dermal and Vaginal Candidiasis. *Pharmaceutics* **2019**, *11*, 312. [CrossRef]
20. Carvajal-Vidal, P.; Mallandrich, M.; Garcia, M.L.; Calpena, A.C. Effect of Different Skin Penetration Promoters in Halobetasol Propionate Permeation and Retention in Human Skin. *Int. J. Mol. Sci.* **2017**, *18*, 2475. [CrossRef]
21. Karande, P.; Jain, A.; Ergun, K.; Kispersky, V.; Mitragotri, S. Design Principles of Chemical Penetration Enhancers for Transdermal Drug Delivery. *Proc. Natl. Acad. Sci. USA* **2005**, *102*, 4688–4693. [CrossRef]
22. Chen, J.; Jiang, Q.D.; Wu, Y.M.; Liu, P.; Yao, J.H.; Lu, Q.; Zhang, H.; Duan, J.A. Potential of Essential Oils as Penetration Enhancers for Transdermal Administration of Ibuprofen to Treat Dysmenorrhoea. *Molecules* **2015**, *20*, 18219–18236. [CrossRef] [PubMed]
23. Herman, A.; Herman, A.P. Essential oils and their constituents as skin penetration enhancer for transdermal drug delivery: A review. *J. Pharm. Pharmacol.* **2015**, *67*, 473–485. [CrossRef]
24. Monzotea, L.; Hillb, G.; Cuellarc, A.; Scullc, R.; Setzerb, W. Chemical Composition and Anti-proliferative Properties of Bursera graveolens Essential Oil. *Nat. Prod. Commun.* **2012**, *7*, 1531–1534. [CrossRef]
25. Rey-Valeirón, C.; Guzmán, L.; Saa, L.R.; López-Vargas, J.; Valarezo, E. Acaricidal activity of essential oils of Bursera graveolens (Kunth) Triana & Planch and Schinus molle L. on unengorged larvae of cattle tick Rhipicephalus (Boophilus) microplus (Acari:Ixodidae). *J. Essent. Oil Res.* **2017**, *29*, 344–350. [CrossRef]
26. Carrión-Paladines, V.; Fries, A.; Caballero, R.E.; Pérez Daniëls, P.; García-Ruiz, R. Biodegradation of Residues from the Palo Santo (Bursera graveolens) Essential Oil Extraction and Their Potential for Enzyme Production Using Native Xylaria Fungi from Southern Ecuador. *Fermentation* **2019**, *5*, 76. [CrossRef]
27. Young, D.G.; Chao, S.; Casablanca, H.; Bertrand, M.-C.; Minga, D. Essential Oil of Bursera graveolens (Kunth) Triana et Planch from Ecuador. *J. Essent. Oil Res.* **2007**, *19*, 525–526. [CrossRef]
28. Tutaj, K.; Szlazak, R.; Szalapata, K.; Starzyk, J.; Luchowski, R.; Grudzinski, W.; Osinska-Jaroszuk, M.; Jarosz-Wilkolazka, A.; Szuster-Ciesielska, A.; Gruszecki, W.I. Amphotericin B-silver hybrid nanoparticles: Synthesis, properties and antifungal activity. *Nanomedicine* **2016**, *12*, 1095–1103. [CrossRef]
29. Welin-Berger, K.; Neelissen, J.; Bergenstahl, B. In vitro permeation profile of a local anaesthetic compound from topical formulations with different rheological behaviour—Verified by in vivo efficacy data. *Eur. J. Pharm. Sci.* **2001**, *14*, 229–236. [CrossRef]
30. Espinoza, L.C.; Silva-Abreu, M.; Calpena, A.C.; Rodriguez-Lagunas, M.J.; Fabrega, M.J.; Garduno-Ramirez, M.L.; Clares, B. Nanoemulsion strategy of pioglitazone for the treatment of skin inflammatory diseases. *Nanomedicine* **2019**, *19*, 115–125. [CrossRef]
31. Sengupta, P.; Chatterjee, B. Potential and future scope of nanoemulgel formulation for topical delivery of lipophilic drugs. *Int. J. Pharm.* **2017**, *526*, 353–365. [CrossRef] [PubMed]
32. Espinoza, L.C.; Vera-Garcia, R.; Silva-Abreu, M.; Domenech, O.; Badia, J.; Rodriguez-Lagunas, M.J.; Clares, B.; Calpena, A.C. Topical Pioglitazone Nanoformulation for the Treatment of Atopic Dermatitis: Design, Characterization and Efficacy in Hairless Mouse Model. *Pharmaceutics* **2020**, *12*, 255. [CrossRef] [PubMed]
33. Nastiti, C.; Ponto, T.; Abd, E.; Grice, J.E.; Benson, H.A.E.; Roberts, M.S. Topical Nano and Microemulsions for Skin Delivery. *Pharmaceutics* **2017**, *9*, 37. [CrossRef]
34. Suner-Carbo, J.; Calpena-Campmany, A.; Halbaut-Bellowa, L.; Clares-Naveros, B.; Rodriguez-Lagunas, M.J.; Barbolini, E.; Zamarbide-Losada, J.; Boix-Montanes, A. Biopharmaceutical Development of a Bifonazole Multiple Emulsion for Enhanced Epidermal Delivery. *Pharmaceutics* **2019**, *11*, 66. [CrossRef]
35. Berenguer, D.; Alcover, M.M.; Sessa, M.; Halbaut, L.; Guillen, C.; Boix-Montanes, A.; Fisa, R.; Calpena-Campmany, A.C.; Riera, C.; Sosa, L. Topical Amphotericin B Semisolid Dosage Form for Cutaneous Leishmaniasis: Physicochemical Characterization, Ex Vivo Skin Permeation and Biological Activity. *Pharmaceutics* **2020**, *12*, 149. [CrossRef]
36. Asghar, L.F.; Chandran, S. Design and evaluation of matrix base with sigmoidal release profile for colon-specific delivery using a combination of Eudragit and non-ionic cellulose ether polymers. *Drug Deliv. Transl. Res.* **2011**, *1*, 132–146. [CrossRef] [PubMed]
37. Hagen, M.; Baker, M. Skin penetration and tissue permeation after topical administration of diclofenac. *Curr. Med. Res. Opin.* **2017**, *33*, 1623–1634. [CrossRef]
38. Marwah, H.; Garg, T.; Goyal, A.K.; Rath, G. Permeation enhancer strategies in transdermal drug delivery. *Drug Deliv.* **2016**, *23*, 564–578. [CrossRef] [PubMed]
39. Lu, W.C.; Chiang, B.H.; Huang, D.W.; Li, P.H. Skin permeation of D-limonene-based nanoemulsions as a transdermal carrier prepared by ultrasonic emulsification. *Ultrason. Sonochem.* **2014**, *21*, 826–832. [CrossRef] [PubMed]
40. Yang, Z.; Teng, Y.; Wang, H.; Hou, H. Enhancement of skin permeation of bufalin by limonene via reservoir type transdermal patch: Formulation design and biopharmaceutical evaluation. *Int. J. Pharm.* **2013**, *447*, 231–240. [CrossRef]
41. Lim, P.F.; Liu, X.Y.; Kang, L.; Ho, P.C.; Chan, Y.W.; Chan, S.Y. Limonene GP1/PG organogel as a vehicle in transdermal delivery of haloperidol. *Int. J. Pharm.* **2006**, *311*, 157–164. [CrossRef]
42. Mendez, A.H.S.; Cornejo, C.G.F.; Coral, M.F.C.; Arnedo, M.C.A. Chemical Composition, Antimicrobial and Antioxidant Activities of the Essential Oil of Bursera graveolens (Burseraceae) From Perú. *Indian J. Pharm. Educ. Res.* **2017**, *51*, 429–436. [CrossRef]
43. Mahizan, N.A.; Yang, S.K.; Moo, C.L.; Song, A.A.; Chong, C.M.; Chong, C.W.; Abusheilaibi, A.; Lim, S.E.; Lai, K.S. Terpene Derivatives as a Potential Agent against Antimicrobial Resistance (AMR) Pathogens. *Molecules* **2019**, *24*, 2631. [CrossRef]
44. Nidhi, P.; Rolta, R.; Kumar, V.; Dev, K.; Sourirajan, A. Synergistic potential of Citrus aurantium L. essential oil with antibiotics against Candida albicans. *J. Ethnopharmacol.* **2020**, *262*, 113135. [CrossRef]

45. Muslim, S.N.; Hussin, Z.S. Chemical compounds and synergistic antifungal properties of Thymus kotschanus essential oil plus ketoconazole against Candida spp. *Gene Rep.* **2020**, *21*, 100916. [CrossRef]
46. Mahboubi, M.; Ghazian Bidgoli, F. In vitro synergistic efficacy of combination of amphotericin B with Myrtus communis essential oil against clinical isolates of Candida albicans. *Phytomedicine* **2010**, *17*, 771–774. [CrossRef]
47. Scherliess, R. The MTT assay as tool to evaluate and compare excipient toxicity in vitro on respiratory epithelial cells. *Int. J. Pharm.* **2011**, *411*, 98–105. [CrossRef]
48. Sarango-Granda, P.; Silva-Abreu, M.; Calpena, A.C.; Halbaut, L.; Fabrega, M.J.; Rodriguez-Lagunas, M.J.; Diaz-Garrido, N.; Badia, J.; Espinoza, L.C. Apremilast Microemulsion as Topical Therapy for Local Inflammation: Design, Characterization and Efficacy Evaluation. *Pharmaceuticals* **2020**, *13*, 484. [CrossRef]
49. Sosa, L.; Clares, B.; Alvarado, H.L.; Bozal, N.; Domenech, O.; Calpena, A.C. Amphotericin B releasing topical nanoemulsion for the treatment of candidiasis and aspergillosis. *Nanomedicine* **2017**, *13*, 2303–2312. [CrossRef]
50. Costa, G.M.D.A.; Alves, G.d.A.D.; Maia Campos, P.M.B.G. Application of design of experiments in the development of cosmetic formulation based on natural ingredients. *Int. J. Phytocosmetics Nat. Ingred.* **2019**, *6*, 4. [CrossRef]
51. Rowe, R.; Sheskey, P.; Owen, S. *Handbook of Pharmaceutical Excipients*, 5th ed.; Pharmaceutical Press: London, UK, 2006.
52. Tisserand, R.; Young, R. *Essential Oil Safety: A Guide for Health Care Professionals*, 2nd ed.; Churchill Livingstone Elsevier: London, UK, 2014.
53. Campana-Seoane, M.; Peleteiro, A.; Laguna, R.; Otero-Espinar, F.J. Bioadhesive emulsions for control release of progesterone resistant to vaginal fluids clearance. *Int. J. Pharm.* **2014**, *477*, 495–505. [CrossRef] [PubMed]
54. ICH. Stability Testing of New Drug Substances and Products Q1A(R2). In *International Conference on Harmonisation of Technical Requirements for Registration of Pharmaceuticals for Human Use*; ICH: Geneva, Switzerland, 2003.
55. Subcommittee on Antifungal Susceptibility Testing (AFST) of the ESCMID European Committee for Antimicrobial Susceptibility Testing (EUCAST). EUCAST Definitive Document EDef 7.1: Method for the determination of broth dilution MICs of antifungal agents for fermentative yeasts. *Clin. Microbiol. Infect.* **2008**, *14*, 398–405. [CrossRef] [PubMed]
56. Clinical and Laboratory Standards Institute, CLSI. *Reference Method for Broth Dilution Antifungal Susceptibility Testing of Yeast*, 3rd ed.; Document M27-A3; Clinical and Laboratory Standards Institute: Villanova, PA, USA, 2008; Volume 28, ISBN 1-56238-666-2.

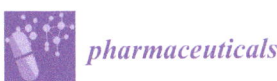

Article

Enhanced Anticancer Activity of *Hymenocardia acida* Stem Bark Extract Loaded into PLGA Nanoparticles

Oluwasegun Adedokun [1], Epole N. Ntungwe [2,3], Cláudia Viegas [4,5,6], Bunyamin Adesina Ayinde [7], Luciano Barboni [8], Filippo Maggi [9], Lucilia Saraiva [10], Patrícia Rijo [2,11,*] and Pedro Fonte [4,5,12,13,*]

1. Department of Pharmacognosy, Igbinedion University, Benin 23401, Nigeria; adedokun.oluwasegun@iuokada.edu.ng
2. Research Center for Biosciences & Health Technologies (CBIOS), Universidade Lusófona de Humanidades e Tecnologias, 1749-024 Lisboa, Portugal; epole.ntungwe@ulusofona.pt
3. Department of Biomedical Sciences, Faculty of Pharmacy, University of Alcalá de Henares, 28805 Alcalá de Henares, Spain
4. Department of Chemistry and Pharmacy, Faculty of Sciences and Technology, University of Algarve, Gambelas Campus, 8005-139 Faro, Portugal; viegas.claudiasofia@gmail.com
5. Center for Marine Sciences (CCMAR), University of Algarve, 8005-139 Faro, Portugal
6. Faculty of Medicine and Biomedical Sciences (FMCB), University of Algarve, 8005-139 Faro, Portugal
7. Department of Pharmacognosy, University of Benin, Benin 23401, Nigeria; baayinde@uniben.edu
8. School of Science and Technology, Chemistry Division, University of Camerino, 62032 Camerino, Italy; luciano.barboni@unicam.it
9. Chemistry Interdisciplinary Project (ChIP), School of Pharmacy, University of Camerino, 62032 Camerino, Italy; filippo.maggi@unicam.it
10. LAQV/REQUIMTE, Laboratório de Microbiologia, Departamento de Ciências Biológicas, Faculdade de Farmácia, Universidade do Porto, 4050-313 Porto, Portugal; lucilia.saraiva@ff.up.pt
11. Instituto de Investigação do Medicamento (iMed.ULisboa), Faculdade de Farmácia, Universidade de Lisboa, 1649-003 Lisboa, Portugal
12. iBB-Institute for Bioengineering and Biosciences, Department of Bioengineering, Instituto, Superior Técnico, Universidade de Lisboa, 1049-001 Lisboa, Portugal
13. Associate Laboratory i4HB–Institute for Health and Bioeconomy at Instituto Superior Técnico, Universidade de Lisboa, Av. Rovisco Pais, 1049-001 Lisboa, Portugal
* Correspondence: patricia.rijo@ulusofona.pt (P.R.); prfonte@ualg.pt (P.F.)

Abstract: *Hymenocardia acida* (H. acida) is an African well-known shrub recognized for numerous medicinal properties, including its cancer management potential. The advent of nanotechnology in delivering bioactive medicinal plant extract with poor solubility has improved the drug delivery system, for a better therapeutic value of several drugs from natural origins. This study aimed to evaluate the anticancer properties of *H. acida* using human lung (H460), breast (MCF-7), and colon (HCT 116) cancer cell lines as well as the production, characterization, and cytotoxicity study of *H. acida* loaded into PLGA nanoparticles. Benchtop models of *Saccharomyces cerevisiae* and *Raniceps ranninus* were used for preliminary toxicity evaluation. Notable cytotoxic activity in benchtop models and human cancer cell lines was observed for *H. acida* crude extract. The PLGA nanoparticles loading *H. acida* had a size of about 200 nm and an association efficiency of above 60%, making them suitable to be delivered by different routes. The outcomes from this research showed that *H. acida* has anticancer activity as claimed from an ethnomedical point of view; however, a loss in activity was noted upon encapsulation, due to the sustained release of the drug.

Keywords: anticancer activity; cytotoxicity; *Hymenocardia acida*; nanoencapsulation; nanoparticle; plant extract; PLGA

1. Introduction

Cancer is generally referred to as a lethal disease characterized by the uncontrolled growth and replication of cancer cells. It can occur in most organs of the multicellular organism and is reported as one of the major public health challenges. Additionally, it is the principal cause of morbidity worldwide among all age groups [1–4]. Cancer is the second leading cause of death in developing countries and the leading cause of death in developed countries [5]. Population growth, aging as well as the adoption of lifestyles associated with smoking, drinking, lack of physical exercise, and consumption of chemically contaminated foods have caused an increase in cancer incidence in developing nations [2,6,7]. Statistical reports show that by the year 2000, 10 million new cases of cancer had emerged with an increase of 25% every decade. Mortality rates associated with cancer might increase from 6 million to 16 million between the years 2000 and 2050, with 17 million and 7 million novel cases from developing and developed countries, respectively [8–10].

The management of cancer has been challenging despite the numerous methods of modern treatments available. These include radiotherapy, surgery, immunotherapy, and chemotherapy which can be used alone or in combination. Localized cancers are usually treated by surgery and radiation while cancer cells that have metastasized to other parts of the body are treated using chemotherapy, such as alkylating agents, antibiotics, hormones, and antimetabolites [8,10,11].

Despite the cytotoxic attributes of chemotherapeutic agents, they have significant limitations. For example, they display numerous side effects by affecting proliferating normal cells localized in the hair, bone marrow, and gastrointestinal tract. Other limitations include low absorption rate, development of secondary malignancy, high cost of drug/treatment, insolubility, instability, and tumor drug resistance.

All these limitations impose the search for natural drugs with improved efficacy, selectivity, reduced toxicity, and low secondary effects inherent in cancer management [12].

Plants are natural sources of drugs and have been used as medicines for at least 60,000 years. They can produce secondary metabolites with a wide range of pharmacological properties, including anticancer activity. They can be used as crude and/or their derived natural products or compounds and have been useful in cancer treatment, research, and development [13–15]. *Hymemocardia acida* Tul (Hymenocardiaceae) is a dioecious and deciduous shrub, mostly found in the Savannah region of the Southwestern part of Nigeria, normally 6–10 m in height. It is characterized by contorted and stunted growth, and it is widely known and used in African trado-medicine. It is called "heart-fruit" in English, "enanche" in Idoma, "ikalaga" in Igbo, "ii-kwarto" in Tiv, "emela" in Etulo, "Uchuo" in Igede, "jan yaro" in Hausa, "yawa satoje" in Fulani, and "Orunpa" in Yoruba [16–18]. Ethnomedicinal information suggests that the plant is used traditionally to treat hemorrhoids, chest pain, eye infection, migraine, skin diseases, and several infections, and as a poultice to treat abscesses and tumors [16,17,19]. Phytochemical studies indicate that these therapeutic applications result from their varied composition of secondary metabolites such as alkaloids, terpenoids, glycosides, flavonoids, saponins, and tannins [17].

Although experimental findings have shown that many natural products have a strong therapeutic value, their poor solubility and bioavailability (at the target organ) have been a challenge over time. Another problem associated with the use of conventional plant extract-based formulations is the presence of toxicity to other organs and tissues. To overcome this, some scientists have used the "green chemistry" approach to nanoparticle production that includes clean, non-toxic, and environmentally friendly methods. NP synthesized via green synthetic routes are highly water soluble, biocompatible, and less toxic [20]. Other strategies using hybrid systems combining nanoparticles and ionic liquids may be also used to improve the delivery of poorly soluble drugs [21,22].

Nanotechnology by the nanoencapsulation of natural products in a polymer to improve drug delivery to cancer targets has gained considerable interest over the past decades [17,23,24]. Thus, polymer-based drug delivery systems allow the control of drug release, enhance effective drug solubility, minimize drug degradation, contribute to reduced drug toxicity, and facilitate control of drug uptake, which significantly contributes to the therapeutic efficiency of a drug. Poly (lactic-co-glycolic acid) (PLGA) based nanoencapsulation has been shown to possess numerous advantages over other conventional delivery devices based on high biocompatibility, biodegradability, drug protection from degradation, sustained and controlled drug release, linkage of other molecules with PLGA for better interaction with biological materials, and the possibility to target specific organs or cells. Furthermore, PLGA will be degraded into nontoxic substances and the breakdown products are lactic acid and glycolic acid, which are hydrophilic, diffusible, and rapidly metabolized in the human body [25–27]. PLGA has also shown good results in improving the bioavailability of drugs delivered by the oral route, a non-invasive route that may be promising in cancer treatment [28], hence, the choice of PLGA base encapsulation in this research.

This research, therefore, aims to evaluate the cytotoxic activity of crude *H. acida* methanol stem extract using both benchtop assays as well as human cancer cell lines (breast, colon, and lung cancer cell lines). Additionally, nanoencapsulation of the extract was carried out using the sulforhodamine B (SRB) assay and reviewing comparative studies on the nanoencapsulated extract and crude extract on breast, colon, and lung cancer cell lines. This method allows the determination of the cell density, based on the measurement of cellular protein content and the cytotoxicity screening of compounds with adherent effect to 96-well format [29].

2. Results and Discussion

Surgery and or radiotherapy have been great tools for the management of diverse forms of cancer if diagnosed early. Studies have shown that half of all cancer patients use some form of integrative therapy when cancer cells are not responding to medical procedures to reduce pain as well as improve the overall wellbeing of the patients.

The use of medicinal plants for the treatment of diverse diseases, including cancer, cannot be overemphasized as they have served as the source for compounds of therapeutic importance [30]. Medicinal plants are a source for lead compounds and highly bioactive drugs useful in the management of diseases associated with man and animals [30,31]. Recent studies have shown that 55% of chemotherapeutics are directly or indirectly from natural products [32]. Side effects associated with present cancer therapeutics and increasing cancer cases have prompted the search for novel anticancer agents of plant extract or isolated compounds of natural origin, which needs to be studied using both in vitro and in vivo cytotoxicity models [30,33].

2.1. In Vitro Cytotoxicity Assay of H. acida Using R. ranninus

In this study, tadpoles (*R. ranninus*) were used in the in vitro cytotoxicity assay of *H. acida* crude extract due to their accessibility, mostly in the rainy season, allowing the simulation of a complete multicellular organism. The *H. acida* extract was exposed to *R. ranninus* for 24 h at a concentration range of 20–400 µg/mL. The cytotoxic potential against this model was verified by a reduction in the movement of the tadpoles and confirmed with consequent cessation of movement. The results reveal a significant difference in cytotoxicity activity ($p \leq 0.05$) in all concentrations of *H. acida* examined relative to 5% DMSO (negative control), which has no cytotoxic effect on *R. ranninus*. Moreover, at a concentration of 20 µg/mL, the *H. acida* extract showed 89.52 ± 1.52% bioactivity while concentrations at 40–400 µg/mL indicated 100.00 ± 0.00% cytotoxic potential against *R. ranninus* (Figure 1).

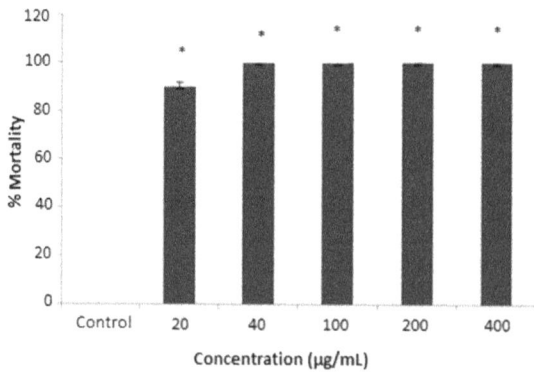

Figure 1. Effect of crude *Hymenocardia acida* (*H. acida*) extract on % *Raniceps ranninus* (*R. ranninus*) mortality at concentrations ranging from 20–400 µg/mL–an index of cytotoxic effect. A 5% DMSO solution was used as negative control. Each bar represents the mean ± SEM of 10 (ten) independent experiments ($n = 10$). Samples with superscript * indicate a significant difference at $p < 0.05$ relative to the negative control.

2.2. In Vitro Cytotoxicity Activity of Crude H. Acida Using S. cerevisiae

The yeast *S. cerevisiae* is one of the widely used eukaryotic models. Its rapid growth and ease of manipulation to evaluate multiple biological effects induced by the drugs under consideration make it a suitable model for cytotoxicity study [34]. In vitro preliminary cytotoxicity study on the crude stem bark extract of *H. acida* was performed against *S. cerevisiae* using nystatin as positive control and 2% DMSO in YPD as blank. The growth rate of *S. cerevisiae* in the blank was considered to be 100%, that is, a zero percentage of inhibition, so its absorbance was maximum at 300 min (0.328). The cells were exposed to *H. acida* extract and nystatin at different concentrations (7.81 to 500 µg/mL) and the absorbance of the specific cell growth rates was measured from 0 to 300 min.

According to the results (Table 1), *H. acida* extract showed a concentration-dependent effect. The extract significantly inhibited *S. cerevisiae* growth in all the concentrations tested over time when compared with Nystatin and negative control (DMSO). Overall, the percentage growth inhibition ranges from 71.70 to 100%. At a concentration of 500 µg/mL, 100% of inhibition was observed similar to Nystatin.

Table 1. General toxicity effect of crude extract of *H. acida* on the percentage of growth inhibition of *S. cerevisiae*.

Concentration (µg/mL)	% Growth Inhibition		
	DMSO [a]	Nystatin [b]	*H. acida* Crude
7.81	12.67 ± 1.21	97.25 ± 1.02 *	90.30 ± 0.99 *
15.6	16.80 ± 1.08	98.21 ± 0.98 *	71.70 ± 1.12
31.2	17.60 ± 0.01	98.78 ± 2.17 *	95.70 ± 1.10 *
62.5	30.73 ± 1.12	99.35 ± 2.92 *	95.40 ± 2.08 *
125	31.20 ± 1.03	99.59 ± 1.87 *	96.56 ± 1.98 *
250	33.84 ± 1.03	99.71 ± 1.34 *	96.98 ± 2.11 *
500	33.91 ± 1.10	100.00 ± 0.00 *	100.00 ± 0.00 *

The values above are presented by mean ± SEM of three replicates ($n = 3$). Values with superscript * indicate a significant difference at $p < 0.05$ when compared to the corresponding percentage inhibition of solvent (DMSO [a]) for each concentration using one-way analysis of variance (ANOVA) and complemented with the Krustal–Wallis test (non-parametric), [b] = positive control, and [a] = negative control.

Considering that the higher the percentage growth of inhibition, the higher the general toxicity of the extract, we can conclude that *H. acida* extract is toxic against S. *cerevisiae* and *R. ranninus*. The correlation between the results of these two organisms validates their use for preliminary toxicity studies. These results can be supported by the composition of *H. acida* in cyclopeptide alkaloids, namely in hymenocardine, found by Tuenter et al. (2016). In their studies, this compound present in the root bark of *H. acida* showed cytotoxicity activity against MRC-5 cells (human lung fibroblasts) with an IC_{50} value of 51.1 ± 17.2 µM [35]. Moreover, an in vivo study carried out by Sowemimo et al. (2007) showed that *H. acida* steam bark extract is toxic to brine shrimps and caused chromosomal damage in rat lymphocytes, and consequently that it is mutagenic and has cytotoxic activity [31].

2.3. Phytochemical Study of H. acida

To understand the chemical composition of the bioactive *H. acida* crude extract, and to identify the main compound responsible for the tested bioactivity, this extract was subjected to several chromatographic techniques. 3β- lup-20(29)-en-3ol (Lupeol) was isolated from this extract (as a colorless crystal, mp 212–214 °C) and its structure was confirmed through a comparison of its spectroscopic data (Supplementary Materials) to those described in the literature (Figure 2) [36–38].

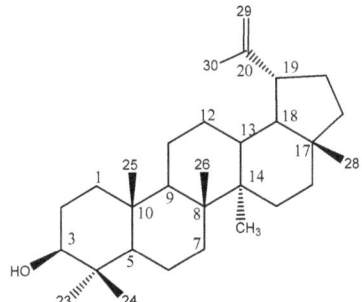

Figure 2. Lupeol isolated from *H. acida*.

2.4. H. acida-Loaded PLGA Nanoparticles Production and Characterization

PLGA nanoparticles are used to improve the pharmacokinetics, stability, and delivery of the extract [33]. Therefore, to enhance the drug delivery and therapeutic potentials of *H. acida* crude extract, *H. acida* nanoparticles (HA-Np) and blank nanoparticles (unloaded Np, negative control) were produced and characterized [39].

The mean hydrodynamic particle size of both HA-Np and unloaded Np were 210 ± 3 nm and 193 ± 2 nm, respectively, which showed good method robustness and ability to obtain a nanoparticle size suitable for different delivery routes [40–42]. The nanoparticles were further observed by scanning electron microscopy (SEM) to confirm the nanoparticles size and evaluate its morphology (Figure 3). The nanoparticles presented a spherical shape and smooth surface characteristic of PLGA nanoparticles [43]. No relevant differences were observed between unloaded and HA-Np, demonstrating the robustness of the production method.

The PdI of the nanoparticles was also determined. Small values of PdI (near to zero) were desirable because this indicates a uniform size distribution and a monodisperse nanoparticle formulation [44]. In the case of HA-Np, a PdI of 0.231 ± 0.050 was obtained to 0.100 ± 0.010 observed in unloaded Np, which implies more heterogeneity between the HA-Np particles and a polydisperse formulation as shown in Table 2. Similar results for nanoparticle size distribution and PdI were obtained by our group in the encapsulation of other drugs [42,45]. Although, this is an expected known result for loaded Np because the particles have to contain the volume of the extract of *H. acida* [40].

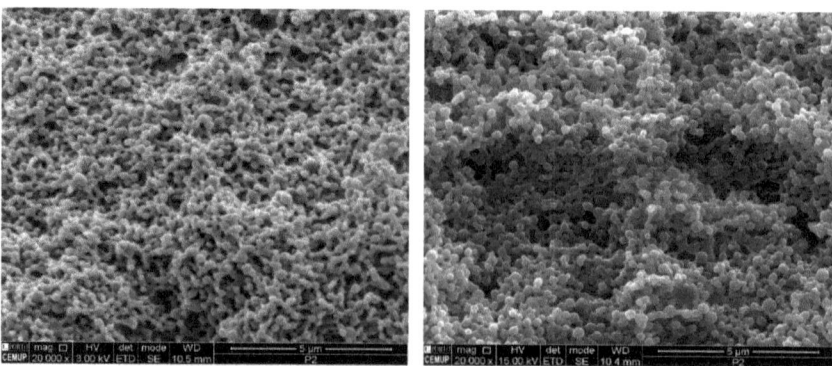

Figure 3. SEM microphotographs of unloaded PLGA Np (**left**) and *H. acida*-loaded PLGA nanoparticles (**right**).

Table 2. Physical–chemical properties and characterization of blank nanoparticles (unloaded Np) and *H. acida* nanoparticles (HA-Np) ($n = 3$, mean ± SEM). Results are significantly different ($p < 0.05$).

Parameter	Unloaded Np	HA-Np
Particle size (nm)	210 ± 3	193 ± 2
Polydispersity índex (PdI)	0.100 ± 0.010	0.231 ± 0.050
%AE	Not Applicable	61.71 ± 2.17%
Homogeneity	Homogenous	Homogenous
Colour	Whitish	Milky
Diffusion constant (D) (cm^2/sec)	2.34 × 10^8 ± 0.07	2.55 × 10^8 ± 0.09
Refractive Index	1.33 ± 0.01	1.33 ± 0.11
Viscosity (cP)	0.890 ± 0.110	0.888 ± 0.170

The diffusion constant describes the quantity of a substance that is diffusing from one region to another through a unit cross-section per unit time when the volume–concentration gradient is constant. A higher diffusion constant of 2.34 × 10^8 ± 0.07 was observed in *H. acida* nanoparticles (HA-Np) relative to unloaded Np 2.55 × 10^8 ± 0.09, which implies a faster rate of diffusion due to the small particle size of HA-Np. Although the diffusion constant is a physical constant that depends on molecular size, temperature (high surface area to volume ratio), pressure, and other properties of the diffusing substance, a reduced diffusion constant of HA-Np will enhance rapid contact of nanoparticle to the targeted receptor for improved drug delivery. Additionally, both unloaded Np as well as HA-Np nanoparticles obtained were homogenous in aspect and form a homogenous colloidal formulation. Moreover, 61.71 ± 2.17% association efficiency was observed, which is a very good achievement. A similar refractive index of 1.33 ± 0.01 was observed in both blank-Np as well as HA-Np, which implies that light waves will pass through both particles in a vacuum by 1.3328 times slower, which also showed a good nanoparticle formulation as shown in Table 2.

To confirm that the extract is incorporated in the polymeric matrix of the PLGA nanoparticles and to assess drug–polymer interactions upon encapsulation, FTIR analysis of *H. acida* extract, unloaded Np, and HA-Np was carried out (Figure 4). The FTIR analysis is a powerful non-invasive technique to assess the structure of NP and its content [46]. Their data also confirms that the extract is incorporated in the polymeric matrix of the PLGA nanoparticles because the transmittance band in the range 3100–3600 cm^{-1} present in the *H. acida* extract is reflected slightly in the HA-Np spectrum. Another characteristic band of the extract is found at 1600 cm^{-1} in the HA-Np spectrum. On the other hand, in the HA-Np spectrum, the bands related to the nanoparticles at the 1000–1600 cm^{-1} zone are attenuated.

All these bands confirm that *H. acida* extract is incorporated in the polymeric matrix of the PLGA nanoparticles. It is also possible to check the spectra of both unloaded Np as well as HA-Np, the intense band relative to the carbonyl groups present in the two monomers of PLGA (C = O stretching vibrations) around 1750 cm^{-1}, the band relative to ester bond (C-O-C stretching vibrations) around 1186 cm^{-1} and the band relative to C–H stretches around 2285–3010 cm^{-1} which does not appear in the *H. acida* extract spectrum [25,40].

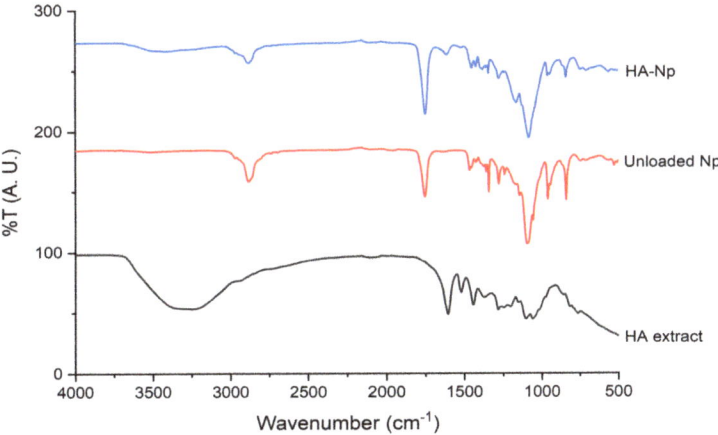

Figure 4. ATR-FTIR spectra of crude extract of *H. acida* (HA extract), blank nanoparticles (unloaded Np), and *H. acida* nanoparticles (HA-Np).

2.5. Cytotoxic Effect of H. acida and PLGA Nanoparticles on Human Cancer Cell Lines

PLGA is an FDA-approved polymer known for its biomedical applications in drug delivery due to its versatility, biodegradability, and biocompatibility. It is used extensively to prepare nanoparticles to deliver a wide range of therapeutic agents, including active pharmacological molecules, peptides, and nucleic acids [47].

The PLGA nanoparticles were produced to protect the *H. acida* extracts and to allow controlled release of the extracts into the target cells. Therefore, it is important that the stability and also cytotoxic effect of the *H. acida* extracts are maintained and that the release of the contents of the PLGA nanoparticles occurs promptly. The in vitro cytotoxicity of the *H. acida* extract and HA-Np nanoparticles was assessed using Sulfordiamine (SRB) assay. The results for the cytotoxic effect of *H. acida* crude extract and HA-Np on colon colorectal carcinoma (H460), human breast adenocarcinoma (MCF-7), and lung cancer carcinoma (HCT116) using this assay are shown in Table 3.

Table 3. Cytotoxic effect (IC$_{50}$ (µg/mL)) of *H. acida* nanoparticles in H460, MCF-7, and HCT116 cell lines of *H. acida* and *H. acida* nanoparticles using sulforhodamine B assay after 48 h of treatment. Data are presented by mean ± SEM (n = 4).

	Cancer Cell Lines (IC$_{50}$ (µg/mL))		
	H460	MCF-7	HCT116
H. acida crude	20.80 ± 6.10	38.70 ± 0.80	42.90 ± 0.20
HA-Np	>50	>50	>50
Doxorubicin	0.29 ± 2.32	0.08 ± 4.10	0.05 ± 3.24

H. acida crude extract had an IC$_{50}$ (µg/mL) of 20.80 ± 6.10 in the human lung (H460) cancer cell line, 38.70 ± 0.80 in MCF-7, and 42.90 ± 0.20, in colon (HCT116) cancer cell lines. The results obtained for cancer cell lines subjected to *H. acida* extract reveal a good cytotoxic effect of this extract, specifically in the H460 human lung cancer cell line. These results are in comparison with those obtained by Calhelha et al. [48]. The cytotoxic effect (in GI_{50} values, μg/mL) of Portuguese propolis samples (collected in Aljezur) against the lung (NCI-H460), breast (MCF7), and colon (HCT15) cancer cell lines (37 ± 1, 47 ± 2, and 50 ± 11) once again affirm the potential that *H. acida* extract is cytotoxic. Those results from *H. acida* were also comparable with the study proceeded by Sharma et al. [49], which reveals similar results from the anticancer activity of essential oil from *Cymbopogon flexuosus* in lung cancer cell lines (IC_{50} values varied from 49.7 to 79.0 μg/mL for each line) and in colon cancer cell lines (IC_{50} values varied from 4.2–60.2 μg/mL for each line). Thus, although the mechanisms by which *H. acida* has cytotoxic effects are unknown, it appears that its extracts have an impact on cell viability, and thus in cancer treatment. This impact of the extract on cell viability could be partly explained due to the presence of the isolated lupeol. Lupeol is shown to have cytotoxicity in different cancer cell lines. The anti-leukemic activity of this compound was tested against the K562 cells and it was shown to decrease cell viability [50]. Similar results were observed in other studies against different cancer cell lines where lupeol was cytotoxic against MCF-7, Caco-2, SW620, KATO-III, HCT-116 cell lines [51–54]. Lupeol can thus contribute to the cytotoxicity of *H. acida* extracts.

However, an $IC_{50} > 50$ for HA-Nps was observed in all human cancer cell lines, which means a poor activity of *H. acida* loaded in PLGA nanoparticles. One hypothesis for this loss of inactivity might be a result of the delayed release of the drugs (*H. acida*) from the PLGA nanoparticles. To overcome this loss of activity, a lower PLGA concentration could be used since this will result in a thinner cover of the Nps, and the production of highly porous nanoparticles making it easier to release the content [26]. Another hypothesis for this loss of cytotoxic effect of *H. acida* loaded in PLGA nanoparticles could be due to some loss of stability of the extracts during the encapsulation process, and consequently loss of efficacy.

Contrary to our results for the activity of HA-Np, recently, Adlravan et al., in their study on the potential cytotoxic activity of *Nasturtium officinale* extract non-nanoencapsulated (free NOE) and PLGA/PEG nanoencapsulated (NOE-loaded) in human lung carcinoma A549 cells, found that NOE-loaded showed better cytotoxic effects than free NOE. This work reinforces the idea that the nanoencapsulation of the extracts improves the anticancer effects of the therapies, as well as allows a sustained and controlled release of NOE constituents from nanoparticles and increases intracellular concentrations. On the other hand, free NOE easily diffuses through the lipid bilayers, being more rapidly eliminated, leading to lower cytotoxicity on target cells [55].

Based on the above results, additional studies should be performed on the in vitro release study for HA-Np to understand if the extract is difficult to release from the HA-Np. Other concentrations of PLGA or combinations of polymers should also be studied since encapsulation of extracts into nanoparticles is known to be a promising strategy to enhance therapeutic efficiency, and consequently overcome these challenges.

3. Materials and Methods

3.1. Materials and Cell Lines

(3-(4,5-dimethyl-2-thiazolyl)-2,5-diphenyl-2H-tetrazolium bromide) (MTT), rhodamine 123 (Rho123), 5-fluorouracil, Pluronic F-68, and dimethylsulfoxide (DMSO) were from Sigma–Aldrich Chemie GmbH (Paris, France). PLGA Resomer® RG 503 H (was obtained from Evonik Industries, Essen, Germany. Phosphate buffer saline (PBS) was from Merck (Darmstadt, Germany). Fetal bovine serum (FBS) was from Gibco, Alfagene, Carcavelos, Portugal. RPMI-1640 medium (Roswell Park Memorial Institut), DMEM (Dulbecco's Modified Eagle Medium), penicillin–streptomycin solution, antibiotic–antimycotic solution, L-glutamine, and trypsin/EDTA were from PAA (Vienna, Austria). *Saccharomyces cerevisiae* (ATCC 2601) cell culture, yeast extract peptone (YPD), HCT-116 (lung), MCF-7 (breast), and H460 (colon) human cancer cell lines were from the National Cancer Institute (Frederick, MD, USA). All other chemicals used in this study were of analytical grade and were purchased locally.

Cell Culture Maintenance

The cells were grown and maintained in an appropriate medium, pH 7.4, supplemented with 10% fetal calf serum, glutamine (2 mM), penicillin (100 units/mL), and streptomycin (100 µg/mL). The cell cultures were grown in a carbon dioxide incubator (Heraeus, GmbH, Germany) at 37 °C with 90% humidity and 5% CO_2 [56,57].

All cancer cells were cultured in RPMI-1640 medium with ultraglutamine (Lonza, VWR, Carnaxide, Portugal), and supplemented with 10% FBS. Cells were maintained at 37 °C in a humidified atmosphere of 5% CO_2.

3.2. Botanical Authentication and Extraction

H. acida stem barks were collected from the Iwo community in Osun State, Nigeria. Botanical identification and authentication were carried out at the herbarium section of the University of Benin by Prof. MacDonald Idu (Professor of Phytomedicine and Taxonomy). The voucher specimen (UBH-R633) was deposited at the herbarium unit. The plant was grounded to a coarse powder using a laboratory milling machine. The extraction was carried out in methanol using 1.2 kg of the plant powder and the plant extract was obtained using a Soxhlet apparatus. The crude extract obtained was concentrated using Heidolph Rotavapor (LABORATA 4000) with a speed set at 120 rpm and a reduced temperature of 40 °C. The concentrated extract was removed from the round bottom flask with methanol and poured into weighed beakers [58].

3.3. In Vitro Cytotoxicity Assay Using R. ranninus (Tadpoles)

A preliminary cytotoxicity study was carried out on crude stem extract of *H. acida* using *R. ranninus*. The organisms were collected from pounds at Olomo beach, Uhonmora village, Edo State. Ten *R. ranninus* of similar sizes were placed into different beakers containing 30 mL of the freshwater from the habitat of tadpoles. The volume was completed up to 49 mL with distilled water and the extract was added to a total volume of 50 mL. The extract was tested at 20, 40, 100, 200, and 400 µg/mL dissolved in 5% DMSO. The experimental procedure was performed in triplicate and a control assay was performed using 50 mL containing 1 mL of 5% DMSO in distilled water [23,56,59]. The mortality rates of the tadpoles were observed for a maximum of 24 h.

3.4. Isolation and Structural Characterization of Lupeol

About 51.90 g of aqueous fraction of *H. acida* was subjected to vacuum liquid chromatography (VLC) using dichloromethane, ethylactetae, and methanol in increasing order of polarity. This yielded four (A to D) VLC fractions, based on similarities in their analytical TLC profile, A (1; 1.13 g), B (2–3; 1.89 g), C (4–6; 4.88 g), and D (7–8; 41.15 g). B was further fractionated by normal phase open column chromatography using Silica gel G (kieselgel 70–230 mesh size) and dichloromethane, ethylactetae, and methanol as eluent with increasing polarity. Detection was carried out using non-destructive (visible light and UV light (254 and 365 nm)) followed by spraying with concentrated sulphuric acid and heating at 110 °C. This resulted in seven fractions (BF12–8). Fraction BF3 obtained from column chromatography was subjected to a series of purification using preparative-TLC and this resulted in a colorless crystal, lupeol (12.4 mg).

The 1D and 2D NMR analysis of the compound were carried out using a Bruker Fourier spectrometer (600 MHz). The compound was dissolved in deuterated chloroform. ^1H and ^{13}C chemical shifts are expressed in part per million (ppm) while coupling constant (*J*) as Hertz (Hz) (Supplementary Materials).

3.5. In Vitro Cytotoxicity Assay Using Saccharomyces Cerevisiae

Further preliminary cytotoxicity study was carried out on the crude stem extract of *H. acida* using *Saccharomyces cerevisiae* (*S. cerevisiae*). Approximately 1.0×10^7 cells per mL of *S. cerevisiae* cell cultures were obtained by inoculating *S. cerevisiae* grown on YPD medium (yeast extract 1%, peptone 0.5%, and glucose 2%) containing 1.5% agar into 20 mL of YPD and placed into an incubator 30 °C without agitation for 16–20 h. About 0.5×10^6 cells were transferred into 4 mL disposable cuvettes containing YPD medium and aliquots of stock solution of plant extract to obtain concentrations of 7.81 µg/mL, 15.6 µg/mL, 31.2 µg/mL, 62.5 µg/mL, 125 µg/mL, 250 µg/mL, and 500 µg/mL to a total volume of 2.2 mL. Nystatin, a known antifungal was used as the positive control while YPD medium and 5% DMSO were used as the negative controls. The cuvettes were incubated in a Heidolph Incubator 1000 with a shaker at 30 °C and 230 rpm agitation to ensure homogeneous suspensions for 5 h. Initial absorbance was measured at the start time (0 min) and every 60 min. The assay was performed in triplicates for each concentration. The reproducibility of the results was analyzed by repeating the assay on three different days. The absorbance at 525 nm of each sample (cell cultures) over the time (0–300 min) was measured. Growth curves were obtained from the number of cells per mL of YPD medium over time; the percentage growth inhibition rate of *S. cerevisiae* in the presence of *H. acida* stem extract and nystatin was determined. Statistical analysis was performed using one-way analysis of variance (ANOVA) and the Krustal–Wallis test (non-parametric) for comparison between groups. The values are presented as mean ± SEM; significant difference at $p < 0.05$ was considered. [57].

3.6. Production of H. acida Loaded PLGA Nanoparticles

H. acida loaded PLGA nanoparticles (HA-Np) were produced by solvent-evaporation o/w single emulsion technique [60]. Crude extract containing 20 mg of *H. acida* was added to 5 mL acetone: methanol (8:2), along with 50 mg PLGA resulting in *H. acida* organic solution. Then, this organic phase solution was added in a dropwise manner into a 10 mL aqueous solution containing the stabilizer Pluronic F-68 1% (w/v). This mixture was sonicated for 30 s at 70% of amplitude in a Q125 Sonicator (QSonica Sonicators, Newtown, CT, USA). The formed emulsion was then subjected to evaporation under reduced pressure for organic solvent removal. The formulations were washed three times and resuspended in ultrapure water. Then, the samples were freeze-dried for further use. Blank nanoparticles (unloaded Np) were also produced following the same procedure.

3.7. H. acida Loaded PLGA Nanoparticles Characterization

The freeze-dried samples were reconstituted with ultrapure water at the desired concentration and were lightly shaken in a vortex for 2 min for complete homogenization. The mean hydrodynamic particle size, polydispersity index (PdI), diffusion constant (D) and refractive index, and viscosity (cP) were evaluated by dynamic light scattering (DLS) using a Malvern Zetasizer Nano ZS ZS (Malvern Instruments, UK). Each sample of unloaded Np and HA-Np formulation was analyzed in triplicate at 25 °C.

The drug loading into PLGA nanoparticles was quantified by evaluating the association efficiency percentage (%AE) by an indirect method, where the amount of *H. acida* encapsulated into PLGA nanoparticles was calculated by the difference between the total amount of *H. acida* extract used in the nanoparticle formulation and considering the free *H. acida* amount in the supernatant after centrifugation of HA-Np formulation in HERMLE Z323K ultracentrifuge at $15,000 \times g$ during 20 min at 4 °C. The quantification of free *H. acida* in the supernatant was performed by Folin–Ciocalteu's method by using a UV-Visible spectrophotometer.

The %AE of HA-Np was determined by the following Equation (1):

$$\%AE = \frac{Total\ amount\ of\ H.acida - Free\ H.acida\ in\ supernatant}{Total\ amount\ of\ H.acida} \times 100 \qquad (1)$$

The morphology of the PLGA nanoparticles was evaluated by SEM using a FEI Quanta 400 FEG SEM (FEI, Hillsboro, OR, USA). In a prior observation, the nanoparticles were placed on metal stubs, and vacuum-coated with a layer of Gold/Palladium for 60 s with a current of 15 mA.

3.8. Fourier Transform Infrared Spectroscopy Spectroscopy

The *H. acida* extract, HA-Np, and unloaded Np were evaluated by ATR-FTIR. All spectra were collected from 64 scans, in the 4000–500 cm^{-1} range at 4 cm^{-1} resolutions, on an ABB MB3000 FTIR (Zurich, Switzerland). All spectra were area-normalized for comparison using the Origin 8 software (OriginLab Corporation, Northampton, MA, USA).

3.9. In Vitro Cytotoxicity Assay against Human Cancer Cell Lines

The crude extract and nanoencapsulated *H. acida* extract were subjected to in vitro cytotoxicity assay using human cancer cell lines involving semiautomatic procedure using sulforhodamine-B (SRB) assay, as described earlier [29,30,61,62]. They were tested in different cancer cell lines: colon colorectal carcinoma (HCT116), human breast adenocarcinoma (MCF-7), and lung cancer carcinoma (H460). The procedure involves growing human cancer cell lines in tissue culture flasks at a temperature of 37 °C, 5% CO_2 as well as 90% relative humidity in a complete growth medium. Flasks with a subconfluent stage of growth were selected and cells were harvested by treatment with trypsin-EDTA.

Cells were plated in 96-well plates at a density of 10,000 cells/100 µL cells/well and incubated for 24 h. *H. acida* and encapsulated samples were added to the 96-well plates. The extracts were tested at 10, 30, and 100 µg/mL, and prepared in DMSO (the final DMSO concentrations were between 0.001% (lowest) and 0.5% (highest)). The effect of the samples was analyzed following 48 h incubation, using the sulforhodamine B (SRB) assay. Briefly, following fixation with 10% trichloroacetic acid from Scharlau (Sigma–Aldrich, Sintra, Portugal), plates were stained with 0.4% SRB from Sigma–Aldrich (Sintra, Portugal) and washed with 1% acetic acid. The bound dye was then solubilized with 10 mM Tris Base and the absorbance was measured at 540 nm in a microplate reader (Biotek Instruments Inc., Synergy, MX, USA). The concentration of *H acida* and nanoencapsulated *H. acida* extract that causes a 50% reduction in the net protein increase in cells (IC_{50}) was determined. Data are mean ± SEM of 4–5 independent experiments [62].

3.10. Statistical Analysis

All data collected from the entire study were analyzed using *Microsoft Excel* and GraphPad Prism 7 (developed by Dr. Harvey Motulsky, San Diego, USA). Relevant tables, charts, and descriptive statistics were used to present the pertinent points of the study. Data were expressed as the mean ± SEM. The data were subjected to statistical analysis using one-way analysis of variance (ANOVA) and complemented with the Krustal–Wallis test (non-parametric).

4. Conclusions

H. acida possesses significant toxicity in *S. cerevisiae* and *R. ranninus* models. It had the highest cytotoxicity (IC_{50} of 20.80 ± 6.10 µg/mL) against the lung cancer cell lines. The solubility of this extract was successfully improved through nanoencapsulation. However, a loss in cytotoxicity was observed with IC_{50} = >50 for all the human cancer cell lines tested. This may be due to the sustained delay in the release of the extract from the nanoencapsulation. The present results show that *H. acida* can be a promising source for possible anticancer compounds. Further research is ongoing to identify more bioactive principles using bio-guided isolation procedures, identify the mechanism of action and structure–activity relationship in the bioactive principle(s), and improve the methods for encapsulation and controlled delivery.

Supplementary Materials: Lupeol NMR Data. The following are available online at https://www.mdpi.com/xxx/s1, Figure S1: ^{1}H-NMR spectrum of lupeol, Figure S2: ^{13}C spectra of Lupeol, Figure S3: HSQC spectrum of Lupeol, Figure S4: COSY spectrum of Lupeol, Figure S5: HMBC spectrum of Lupeol, Figure S6: Compound isolated from *H. acida* suggested to be 3β- lup-20(29)-en-3ol (Lupeol), Figure S7: Numbering and melting point of Lupeol isolated from *H. acida*.

Author Contributions: Conceptualization, P.R. and P.F.; methodology, O.A., E.N.N., C.V., B.A.A. and L.S.; validation, P.R. and P.F.; investigation, O.A., E.N.N., C.V., B.A.A., L.B., F.M. and L.S.; writing—original draft preparation, O.A. and E.N.N.; writing—review and editing, P.R. and P.F.; visualization, P.R. and P.F.; supervision, P.R. and P.F.; funding acquisition, P.R. and P.F. All authors have read and agreed to the published version of the manuscript.

Funding: This work was funded by national funds from Fundação para a Ciência e a Tecnologia (FCT) in the scope of the projects UIDB/04326/2020, UIDP/04326/2020 from CBIOS – Research Center for Biosciences and Health Technologies, and LA/P/0101/2020 of the Research Unit Center for Marine Sciences–CCMAR, and UIDB/04565/2020 and UIDP/04565/2020 of the Research Unit Institute for Bioengineering and Biosciences–iBB, UIDB/50006/2020 (LAQV/REQUIMTE) and the project LA/P/0140/2020 of the Associate Laboratory Institute for Health and Bioeconomy-i4HB. Cláudia Viegas also would like to thank FCT, Portugal for the Ph.D. grant (2020.08839.BD). Oluwasegun Adedokun thanks the fellowship from PADDIC – ALIES supervised by Patricia Rijo.

Institutional Review Board Statement: Not Applicable.

Informed Consent Statement: Not Applicable.

Data Availability Statement: Data is contained within the article and Supplementary Materials.

Conflicts of Interest: The authors declare no conflict of interest.

References

1. WHO. W.H.O. Cancer Control Programme. Available online: http://www.who.int/cancer/en/ (accessed on 20 March 2022).
2. Sung, H.; Ferlay, J.; Siegel, R.L.; Laversanne, M.; Soerjomataram, I.; Jemal, A.; Bray, F. Global Cancer Statistics 2020: GLOBOCAN Estimates of Incidence and Mortality Worldwide for 36 Cancers in 185 Countries. *CA Cancer J. Clin.* **2021**, *71*, 209–249. [CrossRef] [PubMed]
3. Hassanpour, S.H.; Dehghani, M. Review of cancer from perspective of molecular. *J. Cancer Res. Pract.* **2017**, *4*, 127–129. [CrossRef]
4. Ayati, A.; Moghimi, S.; Salarinejad, S.; Safavi, M.; Pouramiri, B.; Foroumadi, A. A review on progression of epidermal growth factor receptor (EGFR) inhibitors as an efficient approach in cancer targeted therapy. *Bioorg. Chem.* **2020**, *99*, 103811. [CrossRef] [PubMed]
5. WHO. Health Topics/Cancer. Available online: https://www.who.int/health-topics/cancer#tab=tab_1 (accessed on 30 March 2021).
6. Bray, F.; Ferlay, J.; Soerjomataram, I.; Siegel, R.L.; Torre, L.A.; Jemal, A. Global cancer statistics 2018: GLOBOCAN estimates of incidence and mortality worldwide for 36 cancers in 185 countries. *CA Cancer J. Clin.* **2018**, *68*, 394–424. [CrossRef]
7. Fidler, M.M.; Bray, F.; Soerjomataram, I. The global cancer burden and human development: A review. *Scand. J. Public Health* **2018**, *46*, 27–36. [CrossRef]
8. McGuire, S. World Cancer Report 2014. Geneva, Switzerland: World Health Organization, International Agency for Research on Cancer, WHO Press, 2015. *Adv. Nutr.* **2016**, *7*, 418–419. [CrossRef]
9. Murray, C.J.L.; Lopez, A.D. The global burden of disease: A comprehensive assessment of mortality and disability from diseases, injuries, and risk factors in 1990 and projected to 2020. In *Global Burden of Disease and Injury Series*; World Health Organization: Geneva, Switzerland, 1996; Volume xxxii, p. 990.
10. Schwartsmann, G.; Ratain, M.J.; Cragg, G.M.; Wong, J.E.; Saijo, N.; Parkinson, D.R.; Fujiwara, Y.; Pazdur, R.; Newman, D.J.; Dagher, R.; et al. Anticancer drug discovery and development throughout the world. *J. Clin. Oncol. Off. J. Am. Soc. Clin. Oncol.* **2002**, *20*, 47S–59S.
11. Burger, A.M.; Fiebig, H.-H. Preclinical Screening for New Anticancer Agents. In *Handbook of Anticancer Pharmacokinetics and Pharmacodynamics*; Figg, W.D., McLeod, H.L., Eds.; Humana Press: Totowa, NJ, USA, 2004; pp. 29–44. ISBN 978-1-59259-734-5.
12. Carr, C.; Ng, J.; Wigmore, T. The side effects of chemotherapeutic agents. *Curr. Anaesth. Crit. Care* **2008**, *19*, 70–79. [CrossRef]
13. Newman, D.J.; Cragg, G.M.; Snader, K.M. The influence of natural products upon drug discovery. *Nat. Prod. Rep.* **2000**, *17*, 215–234. [CrossRef]
14. Watt, J.M.; Breyer Brandwijk, M.G. *Medicinal and Poisonous Plants of South and Eastern Africa*, 2nd ed.; E. S. Livingstone Ltd.: Edinburgh, UK, 1962.
15. Caparica, R.; Júlio, A.; Araújo, M.E.M.; Baby, A.R.; Fonte, P.; Costa, J.G.; Santos de Almeida, T. Anticancer activity of rutin and its combination with ionic liquids on renal cells. *Biomolecules* **2020**, *10*, 233. [CrossRef]
16. Ibrahim, H.; Sani, F.S.; Danladi, B.H.; Ahmadu, A.A. Phytochemical and antisickling studies of the leaves of *Hymenocardia acida* Tul (Euphorbiaceae). *Pak. J. Biol. Sci.* **2007**, *10*, 788–791. [CrossRef] [PubMed]
17. Tor-Anyin, T.A.; Shimbe, R.Y.; Anyam, J.V. Phytochemical and Medicinal activities of *Hymenocardia acida* Tul (Euphorbiaceae): A Review. *J. Nat. Prod. Plant Resour.* **2013**, *3*, 11–16.

18. Olotu, P.N.; Olotu, I.A.; Kambasha, M.B.; Ahmed, A.; Ajima, U.; Ohemu, T.L.; Okwori, V.A.; Dafam, D.G.; David, J.; Ameh, E.G.; et al. Culture and Traditional Medicine Practice among the Idoma People of Otukpo Local Government Area of Benue State, Nigeria. *Int. Res. J. Pharm.* **2017**, *8*, 33–39. [CrossRef]
19. Starks, C.M.; Williams, R.B.; Norman, V.L.; Rice, S.M.; O'Neil-Johnson, M.; Lawrence, J.A.; Eldridge, G.R. Antibacterial chromene and chromane stilbenoids from *Hymenocardia acida*. *Phytochemistry* **2014**, *98*, 216–222. [CrossRef] [PubMed]
20. Hussain, A.; Oves, M.; Alajmi, M.F.; Hussain, I.; Amir, S.; Ahmed, J.; Rehman, T.; El-Seedi, H.R.; Ali, I. Biogenesis of ZnO nanoparticles using: Pandanus odorifer leaf extract: Anticancer and antimicrobial activities. *RSC Adv.* **2019**, *9*, 15357–15369. [CrossRef]
21. Júlio, A.; Costa Lima, S.A.; Reis, S.; Santos de Almeida, T.; Fonte, P. Development of ionic liquid-polymer nanoparticle hybrid systems for delivery of poorly soluble drugs. *J. Drug Deliv. Sci. Technol.* **2020**, *56*, 100915. [CrossRef]
22. Júlio, A.; Caparica, R.; Costa Lima, S.A.; Fernandes, A.S.; Rosado, C.; Prazeres, D.M.F.; Reis, S.; Santos de Almeida, T.; Fonte, P. Ionic Liquid-Polymer Nanoparticle Hybrid Systems as New Tools to Deliver Poorly Soluble Drugs. *Nanomaterials* **2019**, *9*, 1148. [CrossRef]
23. Narayan, S. Curcumin, A Multi-Functional Chemopreventive Agent, Blocks Growth of Colon Cancer Cells by Targeting β-Catenin-Mediated Transactivation and Cell–Cell Adhesion Pathways. *J. Mol. Histol.* **2004**, *35*, 301–307. [CrossRef]
24. Armendáriz-Barragán, B.; Zafar, N.; Badri, W.; Galindo-Rodríguez, S.A.; Kabbaj, D.; Fessi, H.; Elaissari, A. Plant extracts: From encapsulation to application. *Expert Opin. Drug Deliv.* **2016**, *13*, 1165–1175. [CrossRef]
25. Singh, G.; Kaur, T.; Kaur, R.; Kaur, A. Recent biomedical applications and patents on biodegradable polymer PLGA. *Int. J. Pharmacol. Pharm. Sci.* **2014**, *1*, 30–42.
26. Sousa, F.; Castro, P.; Fonte, P.; Kennedy, P.J.; Neves-Petersen, M.T.; Sarmento, B. Nanoparticles for the delivery of therapeutic antibodies: Dogma or promising strategy? *Expert Opin. Drug Deliv.* **2017**, *14*, 1163–1176. [CrossRef] [PubMed]
27. Danhier, F.; Ansorena, E.; Silva, J.M.; Coco, R.; Le Breton, A.; Préat, V. PLGA-based nanoparticles: An overview of biomedical applications. *J. Control. Release* **2012**, *161*, 505–522. [CrossRef] [PubMed]
28. Macedo, A.; Castro, P.M.; Roque, L.; Thomé, N.G.; Reis, C.; Pintado, M.M.; Fonte, P. Novel and revisited approaches in nanoparticle systems for buccal drug delivery. *J. Control. Release* **2020**, *320*, 125–141. [CrossRef] [PubMed]
29. Vichai, V.; Kirtikara, K. Sulforhodamine B colorimetric assay for cytotoxicity screening. *Nat. Protoc.* **2006**, *1*, 1112–1116. [CrossRef] [PubMed]
30. Martin-Cordero, C.; Leon-Gonzalez, A.J.; Calderon-Montano, J.M.; Burgos-Moron, E.; Lopez-Lazaro, M. Pro-oxidant natural products as anticancer agents. *Curr. Drug Targets* **2012**, *13*, 1006–1028. [CrossRef]
31. Sowemimo, A.A.; Fakoya, F.A.; Awopetu, I.; Omobuwajo, O.R.; Adesanya, S.A. Toxicity and mutagenic activity of some selected Nigerian plants. *J. Ethnopharmacol.* **2007**, *113*, 427–432. [CrossRef] [PubMed]
32. Cragg, G.M.; Pezzuto, J.M. Natural Products as a Vital Source for the Discovery of Cancer Chemotherapeutic and Chemopreventive Agents. *Med. Princ. Pract.* **2016**, *25*, 41–59. [CrossRef]
33. Mohanraj, V.J.; Chen, Y. Nanoparticles—A review. *Trop. J. Pharm. Res.* **2007**, *5*, 561–573. [CrossRef]
34. Rimpiläinen, T.; Nunes, A.; Calado, R.; Fernandes, A.S.; Andrade, J.; Ntungwe, E.; Spengler, G.; Szemerédi, N.; Rodrigues, J.; Gomes, J.P.; et al. Increased antibacterial properties of indoline-derived phenolic Mannich bases. *Eur. J. Med. Chem.* **2021**, *220*, 113459. [CrossRef]
35. Tuenter, E.; Exarchou, V.; Baldé, A.; Cos, P.; Maes, L.; Apers, S.; Pieters, L. Cyclopeptide Alkaloids from Hymenocardia acida. *J. Nat. Prod.* **2016**, *79*, 1746–1751. [CrossRef]
36. Silva, A.T.M.; Magalhães, C.G.; Duarte, L.P.; Mussel, W.N.; Ruiz, A.L.; Shiozawa, L.; Carvalho, J.E.; Trindade, I.C.; Vieira Filho, S.A. Lupeol and its esters: NMR, powder XRD data and in vitro evaluation of cancer cell growth. *Braz. J. Pharm. Sci.* **2017**, *53*, e00251. [CrossRef]
37. Igoli, O.J.; Gray, A.I. Friedelanone and other triterpenoids from hymenocardia acida. *Int. J. Phys. Sci.* **2008**, *3*, 156–158, ISSN 1992-1950.
38. Jain, V.; Bari, S. Bari Isolation of Lupeol, Stigmasterol and Campesterol from Petroleum Ether Extract of Woody Stem of Wrightia tinctoria. *Asian J. Plant Sci.* **2010**, *9*, 163–167. [CrossRef]
39. Fonte, P.; Soares, S.; Sousa, F.; Costa, A.; Seabra, V.; Reis, S.; Sarmento, B. Stability Study Perspective of the Effect of Freeze-Drying Using Cryoprotectants on the Structure of Insulin Loaded into PLGA Nanoparticles. *Biomacromolecules* **2014**, *15*, 3753–3765. [CrossRef] [PubMed]
40. Sousa, F.; Cruz, A.; Fonte, P.; Pinto, I.M.; Neves-Petersen, M.T.; Sarmento, B. A new paradigm for antiangiogenic therapy through controlled release of bevacizumab from PLGA nanoparticles. *Sci. Rep.* **2017**, *7*, 3736. [CrossRef]
41. Fonte, P.; Soares, S.; Costa, A.; Andrade, J.C.; Seabra, V.; Reis, S.; Sarmento, B. Effect of cryoprotectants on the porosity and stability of insulin-loaded PLGA nanoparticles after freeze-drying. *Biomatter* **2012**, *2*, 329–339. [CrossRef]
42. Fonte, P.; Araújo, F.; Seabra, V.; Reis, S.; van de Weert, M.; Sarmento, B. Co-encapsulation of lyoprotectants improves the stability of protein-loaded PLGA nanoparticles upon lyophilization. *Int. J. Pharm.* **2015**, *496*, 850–862. [CrossRef]
43. Fonte, P.; Andrade, F.; Azevedo, C.; Pinto, J.; Seabra, V.; van de Weert, M.; Reis, S.; Sarmento, B. Effect of the Freezing Step in the Stability and Bioactivity of Protein-Loaded PLGA Nanoparticles Upon Lyophilization. *Pharm. Res.* **2016**, *33*, 2777–2793. [CrossRef]

44. Sousa, F.; Cruz, A.; Pinto, I.M.; Sarmento, B. Nanoparticles provide long-term stability of bevacizumab preserving its antiangiogenic activity. *Acta Biomater.* **2018**, *78*, 285–295. [CrossRef]
45. Fonte, P.; Lino, P.R.; Seabra, V.; Almeida, A.J.; Reis, S.; Sarmento, B. Annealing as a tool for the optimization of lyophilization and ensuring of the stability of protein-loaded PLGA nanoparticles. *Int. J. Pharm.* **2016**, *503*, 163–173. [CrossRef]
46. Sarmento, B.; Ferreira, D.C.; Jorgensen, L.; van de Weert, M. Probing insulin's secondary structure after entrapment into alginate/chitosan nanoparticles. *Eur. J. Pharm. Biopharm.* **2007**, *65*, 10–17. [CrossRef] [PubMed]
47. Ibrahim, W.N.; Rosli, L.M.B.M.; Doolaanea, A.A. Formulation, cellular uptake and cytotoxicity of thymoquinone-loaded plga nanoparticles in malignant melanoma cancer cells. *Int. J. Nanomed.* **2020**, *15*, 8059–8074. [CrossRef] [PubMed]
48. Calhelha, R.C.; Falcão, S.; Queiroz, M.J.R.P.; Vilas-Boas, M.; Ferreira, I.C.F.R. Cytotoxicity of portuguese propolis: The proximity of the in vitro doses for tumor and normal cell lines. *Biomed. Res. Int.* **2014**, *2014*, 897361. [CrossRef] [PubMed]
49. Sharma, P.R.; Mondhe, D.M.; Muthiah, S.; Pal, H.C.; Shahi, A.K.; Saxena, A.K.; Qazi, G.N. Anticancer activity of an essential oil from Cymbopogon flexuosus. *Chem.-Biol. Interact.* **2009**, *179*, 160–168. [CrossRef]
50. Machado, V.R.; Jacques, A.V.; Marceli, N.S.; Biavatti, M.W.; Santos-Silva, M.C. Anti-leukemic activity of semisynthetic derivatives of lupeol. *Nat. Prod. Res.* **2020**, *35*, 4494–4501. [CrossRef]
51. Quang, D.N.; Pham, C.T.; Le, L.T.K.; Ta, Q.N.; Dang, N.K.; Hoang, N.T.; Pham, D.H. Cytotoxic constituents from Helicteres hirsuta collected in Vietnam. *Nat. Prod. Res.* **2020**, *34*, 585–589. [CrossRef]
52. Ogunlaja, O.O.; Moodley, R.; Singh, M.; Baijnath, H.; Jonnalagadda, S.B. Cytotoxic activity of the bioactive principles from Ficus burtt-davyi. *J. Environ. Sci. Health Part B* **2018**, *53*, 261–275. [CrossRef]
53. Somwong, P.; Suttisri, R. Cytotoxic activity of the chemical constituents of Clerodendrum indicum and Clerodendrum villosum roots. *J. Integr. Med.* **2018**, *16*, 57–61. [CrossRef]
54. Ragasa, C.Y.; Cornelio, K.B. Triterpenes from Euphorbia hirta and their cytotoxicity. *Chin. J. Nat. Med.* **2013**, *11*, 528–533. [CrossRef]
55. Adlravan, E.; Nejati, K.; Karimi, M.A.; Mousazadeh, H.; Abbasi, A.; Dadashpour, M. Potential activity of free and PLGA/PEG nanoencapsulated nasturtium officinale extract in inducing cytotoxicity and apoptosis in human lung carcinoma A549 cells. *J. Drug Deliv. Sci. Technol.* **2021**, *61*, 102256. [CrossRef]
56. Samanta, S.; Pain, A.; Dutta, R.; Saxena, A.K.; Shanmugavel, M.; Pandita, R.M.; Qazi, G.N.; Sanyal, U. Antitumor activity of Nitronaphthal-NU, a novel mixed-function agent. *J. Exp. Ther. Oncol.* **2005**, *5*, 15–22. [PubMed]
57. Roberto, A.; Caetano, P.P. A high-throughput screening method for general cytotoxicity part I: Chemical toxicity. *Rev. Lusófona Ciênc. Tecnol. Saúde* **2005**, *2*, 95–100.
58. Mandal, S.C.; Mandal, V.; Das, A.K. *Essentials of Botanical Extraction*; Academic Press: Cambridge, MA, USA, 2015; pp. 1–207.
59. Ayinde, B.A.; Agbakwuru, U. Cytotoxic and growth inhibitory effects of the methanol extract Struchium sparganophora Ktze (Asteraceae) leaves. *Pharmacogn. Mag.* **2010**, *6*, 293–297. [CrossRef] [PubMed]
60. Paul, S.; Bhattacharyya, S.S.; Boujedaini, N.; Khuda-Bukhsh, A.R. Anticancer potentials of root extract of Polygala senega and its PLGA nanoparticles-encapsulated form. *Evid.-Based Complement. Altern. Med.* **2010**, *2011*, 517204. [CrossRef]
61. Skehan, P.; Storeng, R.; Scudiero, D.; Monks, A.; McMahon, J.; Vistica, D.; Warren, J.T.; Bokesch, H.; Kenney, S.; Boyd, M.R. New Colorimetric Cytotoxicity Assay for Anticancer-Drug Screening. *J. Natl. Cancer Inst.* **1990**, *82*, 1107–1112. [CrossRef]
62. Mothana, R.A.; Lindequist, U.; Gruenert, R.; Bednarski, P.J. Studies of the in vitro anticancer, antimicrobial and antioxidant potentials of selected Yemeni medicinal plants from the island Soqotra. *BMC Complement. Altern. Med.* **2009**, *9*, 7. [CrossRef]

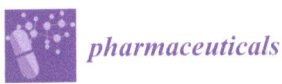 *pharmaceuticals*

Review

Linarin, a Glycosylated Flavonoid, with Potential Therapeutic Attributes: A Comprehensive Review

Javad Mottaghipisheh [1,*], Hadi Taghrir [2], Anahita Boveiri Dehsheikh [3], Kamiar Zomorodian [4], Cambyz Irajie [5], Mohammad Mahmoodi Sourestani [3] and Aida Iraji [6,7,*]

1. Center for Molecular Biosciences (CMBI), Institute of Pharmacy/Pharmacognosy, University of Innsbruck, Innrain 80-82, 6020 Innsbruck, Austria
2. Department of Medicinal Chemistry, Faculty of Pharmacy, Shiraz University of Medical Sciences, Shiraz 71468-64685, Iran; hadi_taghrir@yahoo.com
3. Department of Horticultural Science, Faculty of Agriculture, Shahid Chamran University of Ahvaz, Ahvaz 61357-43311, Iran; anahitaboveiri84@gmail.com (A.B.D.); m.mahmoodi@scu.ac.ir (M.M.S.)
4. Department of Medical Mycology and Parasitology, School of Medicine, Shiraz University of Medical Sciences, Shiraz 14336-71348, Iran; kzomorodian@gmail.com
5. Department of Medical Biotechnology, School of Advanced Medical Sciences and Technologies, Shiraz University of Medical Sciences, Shiraz 71348-14336, Iran; irajie@sums.ac.ir
6. Central Research laboratory, Shiraz University of Medical Sciences, Shiraz 71348-14336, Iran
7. Stem Cells Technology Research Center, Shiraz University of Medical Sciences, Shiraz 71348-14336, Iran
* Correspondence: javad.mottaghipisheh@uibk.ac.at (J.M.); iraji@sums.ac.ir (A.I.)

Abstract: Many flavonoids, as eminent phenolic compounds, have been commercialized and consumed as dietary supplements due to their incredible human health benefits. In the present study, a bioactive flavone glycoside linarin (LN) was designated to comprehensively overview its phytochemical and biological properties. LN has been characterized abundantly in the *Cirsium*, *Micromeria*, and *Buddleja* species belonging to Asteraceae, Lamiaceae, and Scrophulariaceae families, respectively. Biological assessments exhibited promising activities of LN, particularly, the remedial effects on central nervous system (CNS) disorders, whereas the remarkable sleep enhancing and sedative effects as well as AChE (acetylcholinesterase) inhibitory activity were highlighted. Of note, LN has indicated promising anti osteoblast proliferation and differentiation, thus a bone formation effect. Further biological and pharmacological assessments of LN and its optimized semi-synthetic derivatives, specifically its therapeutic characteristics on osteoarthritis and osteoporosis, might lead to uncovering potential drug candidates.

Keywords: flavonoids; linarin; chemotaxonomy; phytochemistry; bioactivities

1. Introduction

The application of plants for medicinal purposes is as old as humanity itself. Since many of them are considered as functional foods and extensively consumed in folk medicine, their biological and phytochemical assessments are pivotal attitudes [1,2]. By developing human knowledge, the study of plant constituents has led to the discovery of secondary metabolites (phytochemicals) as the major compounds responsible for the bioactivities. These biosynthesized compounds (both volatile and non-volatile) mostly possess defensive roles in plants to assist surviving them against abiotic and biotic stressors [3,4].

Investigation of phytoconstituents has been the target of many researchers in order to determine their health benefits. So far, many phytochemicals have been developed and consumed as successful drugs for the treatment of a diverse range of ailments and disorders, specifically cancer types [5–7]. Among the varied phytochemical classifications, flavonoids have been introduced as one of the largest natural phenolic compounds with broad valuable biological properties [8,9]. Based on the chemical structures, these compounds are divided into six main subclasses: flavones, flavanones, flavonols, flavan-3-ols, isoflavones, and anthocyanins [10,11]. Even though the phytochemical and biological characteristics of these compounds are being studied [11,12], they are still interesting target molecules to be explored.

Linarin (syn. acacetin 7-O-rhamnosyl(1'''→6'')glucoside, or acacetin 7-O-rutinoside), as a glycosylated flavone (Figure 1), has been identified from various plant species mainly belonging to the Asteraceae and Lamiaceae families. Regarding the potent bioactivities of this flavonoid reported by several experiments, and the importance of flavonoid consumption as drugs and/or supplements, the present study aims at comprehensively collecting all the phytochemical (i.e., chemotaxonomy and phytochemistry) and biological reports of this flavonoid.

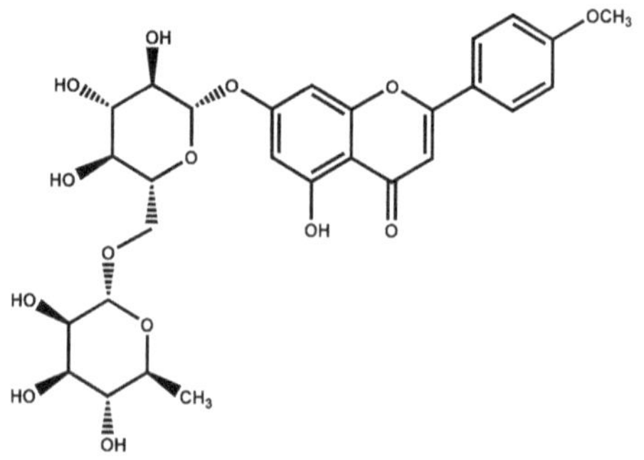

Figure 1. The chemical structure of linarin.

The scientific databases including Web of Science, SciFinder, and PubMed were used to find the correlated data by utilizing the keyword of "linarin" within the English-language papers (access date: 25 May 2021).

2. Phytochemistry and Chemotaxonomy of Linarin

So far, among the 13 plant families containing linarin (LN), Asteraceae and Lamiaceae have been identified as the richest ones. The most LN contents have been reported in various *Cirsium* spp.; however, this compound has also been isolated from the genus *Micromeria* and *Buddleja* belonging to Lamiaceae and Scrophulariaceae, respectively. This glycosylated flavone has mainly been isolated and characterized from alcoholic (methanolic and ethanolic) and hydro-alcoholic extracts. In the following sections, the available data on the phytochemistry of this compound are discussed in detail (Tables S1 and S2).

2.1. Isolation of Linarin from Plant Species

2.1.1. Asteraceae

LN has been isolated from diverse parts of *Cirsium* spp. By utilizing column chromatography on silica gel (CC) as the final separation step, this compound has been isolated from the methanolic extract of *C. arvense* aerial parts [13]. From the roots of *C. arvense* subsp. *vestitum* via application of vacuum column chromatography [14], and flowers of *C. canum* (L.) using reverse-phase high-performance liquid chromatography (RP-HPLC), LN has been isolated [15].

C. japonicum can be considered as one of the richest plant species of LN. Sephadex® LH-20 (SLH) has been applied to the isolation or purification of many flavonoid derivatives [12]. This technique has been employed to isolate LN from the aerial parts of *C. japonicum* [16].

Zhang et al. (2018) isolated LN from *C. japonicum* [17]; in addition, liquid chromatography-mass spectrometry (LC-MS/MS) was implemented to characterize it from the hydro-ethanolic (70%) extract [18]. Preparative-HPLC has been exploited to isolate LN from the ethanolic fraction of *C. japonicum* var. *maackii* [19]. Moreover, the methanolic extract of *C. japonicum* var. *ussuriense* (Regel) Kitam. ex Ohwi obtained from the aerial parts has been subjected to isolate LN by applying the solvent system of $CHCl_3$–MeOH–H_2O (25:8:5) in CC on silica gel [20].

LN has been isolated from three other *Cirsium* species: from the leaf and flower methanolic extract of *C. rivulare* using preparative-HPLC [21]; from the flower methanolic fraction of *C. setidens* applying CC on Silica gel [22]; and from the aerial arts using liquid chromatography (LC) [23] and hydro-ethanolic extracts of *C. setosum* (Willd.) MB. (utilizing HPLC) [24]; however, LN has also been identified from the ethanolic extract of this species by applying ultra-performance liquid chromatography-mass spectrometry (UPLC–MS) [25].

Chrysanthemum species are considered as one of the major sources of LN. It has been isolated from the methanolic extracts of *Chrysanthemum boreale* (Makino) Makino flowers by utilizing CC on silica [26,27], and the hydro-ethanolic (95%) fractions obtained from the *Chrysanthemum morifolium* Ramat flowers [28].

C. indicum, famed as "Ye Ju Hua" in China, has a long history in the treatment of inflammation, hypertension, and respiratory diseases in traditional Chinese and Korean medicine; furthermore, it is traditionally used in tea preparations, tinctures, creams, and lotions [29].

This plant species (*C. indicum*) has been implemented to isolate LN conducted by several studies. It has also been isolated from its flower, using mostly CC on silica gel [30–33], from the dichloromethane extracts of aerial part and methanolic soluble-fraction of the whole part via application of CC on silica gel [34,35].

The purification of LN was also carried out by the solid-liquid extraction method from the hydroethanolic (75%) extract of the same plant species through utilization of various solvents including petroleum ether, ethyl acetate, ethanol, and water [36]. The whole herb and its aerial parts of *C. zawadskii* var. *latilobum* (Maxim.) Kitam. has been reported to possess LN, whereas CC on silica gel was used [37,38].

In the study of Li et al. (2016), high-speed counter-current chromatography (HSCCC) was applied in order to isolate this flavonoid from the hydro-ethanolic extract (80%) of *Flos Chrysanthemi indici* [39], however, it has also been identified from this species as reported by three other groups [40–42].

The whole part methanolic extract of *Artemisia capillaris* Thunb. has been chromatographed by CC on silica gel using CH_2Cl_2–MeOH (20:1) as solvent systems leading to isolate LN [43]; moreover, this compound was identified in a rare species *Picnomon acarna* (L.) Cass., where its aerial parts were separated in CC [44].

2.1.2. Lamiaceae

Lamiaceae (syn. Labiatae), a large plant family consisting of perennial or annual herbaceous plants and shrubs, is majorly known for their aromatic characteristics [45]. Various genus belonging to this family are considered as natural flavonoid sources including LN. Among them, different species of *Mentha*, *Micromeria*, and *Satureja* can be mentioned.

LN has previously been isolated from the hydro-methanolic (80%) extracts of the flower [46] and aerial parts [47] of *Mentha arvensis* L.; however, it has been reported in *M. haplocalyx* Briq. in the ethyl acetate extracts of the aerial parts of three other *Mentha* species comprising *M. spicata*, *M. piperita*, and *M. villosonervata*, where CC on silica gel was applied as the final chromatography step [48].

Dai et al. (2008) isolated LN from a hydro-ethanolic (75%) soluble-fraction of *Dracocephalum peregrinum* L. aerial parts by hiring extensive chromatographic techniques [49]. This flavone has previously been isolated and characterized from other following species: ethanolic extract of *Leonurus japonicus* Houtt. aerial parts (via CC on silica gel CH_2Cl_2–MeOH (100:1–0:100) [50] as well as the leaves of methanolic extracts of *Calamintha officinalis* Moench [51] and *Calamintha glandulosa* (Req.) Benth. [52], where in the later study, semiprep-HPLC was utilized as the final separation step by using H_2O–ACN (50 to 100%). LN has further been reported in the *Ziziphora clinopodioides* Lam. herb methanolic extract [53].

2.1.3. Scrophulariaceae

The plants belonging to Scrophulariaceae can be considered as the third natural source of LN. Among them *Buddleja* spp. are the richest ones. Previously, from the leaf methanolic extract of *Buddleja davidii* Franch., LN was isolated by the utilization of centrifugal partition chromatography (CPC) and the solvent system of $CHCl_3$–MeOH–H_2O (45:33:22) [54]. El-Domiaty et al. (2009) also purified LN from the whole part hydro-ethanolic (95%) extract of *Buddleja asiatica* Lour., while CC on silica gel was used to separate it [55].

Buddleja cordata Kunth was subjected to isolate its phytoconstituents and LN was isolated and characterized from the leaves [56] and whole parts [57]. In three other investigations, LN was isolated from mostly alcoholic extracts of the flowers of *Buddleja officinalis* Maxim [58–60]. CC on silica gel using $CHCl_3$–MeOH with ratios of 19:1, 9:1, 8:2 were applied to isolate LN from the aerial parts of *Buddleja scordioides* Kunth [61]. This compound was isolated from two *Linaria* species *L. japonica*, *L. vulgaris*, and *L. kurdica* subsp. *eriocaly*, while the whole parts were chromatographed [62–64].

2.1.4. Miscellaneous Plants

LN has been isolated from the whole part methanolic extract of *Exacum macranthum* Arn. ex Griseb. (Gentianaceae) via the recrystallization method [65]. This phytochemical has also been isolated and identified from *Lobelia chinensis* Lour. (Campanulaceae) [66], *Ginkgo biloba* L. (Ginkgoaceae) [67], *Bombax malabaricum* DC. (Malvaceae) [68], *Avena sativa* L.(Poaceae) [69], *Thalictrum aquilegiifolium* L. [70], and *Coptis chinensis* Franch [71] (Ranunculaceae), *Zanthoxylum affine* Kunth (Rutaceae) [72] and *Lippia rubella* (Moldenke) T.R.S.Silva & Salimena (Verbenaceae) [73].

2.2. Quantification and Qualification Analysis of Linarin in Plants

By utilization of extensive analytical methods, LN has been qualified and quantified in plant species. So far, the plants belonging to Asteraceae, Lamiaceae, Scrophulariaceae, and Valerianaceae have been reported to be rich in LN content. Table S2 comprehensively lists all the information regarding the fingerprinting analysis of this compound throughout the plant species, however, the following sections describe them in brief.

2.2.1. Asteraceae

Plants in the Asteraceae family, particularly *Cirsium* spp. and *Chrysanthemum* spp., have been characterized as the richest herbal sources of LN. It has been identified throughout six species of the *Cirsium* genus; HPLC coupled to an ultraviolet (UV) detector was used to qualify this compound in the methanolic extract of *C. arvense* [13], along with the report by Demirta et al. (2017), which quantified LN from its root via HPLC-MS (MicroTOF-Q) [14].

The LN content of various soluble-fraction extracted from the flower part of *Cirsium canum* (L.) All. has formerly been analyzed by HPLC-DAD (HPLC-diode array detector). Consequently, the hydro-methanolic (50%) and dichloromethane extracts possessed the highest and lowest contents with 121.75 and 1.94 µg/g, respectively [15].

Cirsiumjaponicum (Thunb.) Fisch. ex DC., Japanese field thistle, is renowned in Chinese pharmacopeia for the treatment of inflammation and bleeding [16] as well as application in Korean folk medicine as a uretic as well as antihemorrhagic and antihepatitic medication [74]. Nonetheless, Ganzera et al. (2005) analyzed pectolinarin as the main phytoconstituent of the *C. japonicum* methanolic aerial part extract, and LN was also quantified with a significant content of 0.26–1.15 mg/100 g through different plant samples by employing HPLC-MS [16].

From the alcoholic extracts of two different *C. japonicum* varieties (*C. japonicum* var. *maackii* Maxim and *C. japonicum* var. *ussuriense* (Regel) Kitam. ex Ohwi), LN was detected by employing HPLC-UV [19,20]. Moreover, the mixture of LN and pectolinarin was compared with the methanolic extracts obtained from the leaf (170 mg/g) and flower (20 mg/g) parts of *Cirsium rivulare* (Jacq.) All., whereas HPLC-UV was utilized as the analytical tool [21].

The methanolic extract of *Cirsiumsetidens*(Dunn) Nakai was phytochemically analyzed through HPLC-UV and a significant LN concentration of 120.3 mg/g was measured [22].

Cirsiumsetosum (Willd.) Besser ex M.Bieb. has further been elaborated to possess phytochemical contents in four studies. The LN content range of 0.3–2 mg/100 g has been recorded through analysis with HPLC-MS [16]. The methanolic soluble partitions of *Hemistepta lyrate* (Bunge) Bunge flower extracted from different plant samples were analytically assessed, and LN was subsequently quantified (0.06–4.26 mg/g) [26].

In a comparative phytochemical analysis of the ethanolic extract obtained from the *Chrysanthemum morifolium* Ramat. flower, LN was qualified and quantified in three cultivars by using HPLC-DAD-ESI/MS with the contents ranging from 0.117 to 0.583 mg/g [28]. HPLC-DAD analysis of the *Chrysanthemum zawadskii* var. *latilobum* (Maxim.) Kitam. extract showed LN as the marker compound with a 22.8 mg/g extract [75].

Chrysanthemum indicum L., as an edible medicinal plant, is famed for its consumption as a food supplement and herbal tea. It has a diverse range of therapeutic applications, specifically in Chinese and Korean folk medicine, for the treatment of immune-related disorders, to heal several infectious diseases, and hypertension symptoms [31]. In several studies reporting its phytoconstituents, LN has also been characterized as the major compounds. He et al. (2016) qualified this compound in the flower methanolic extract via utilization of HPLC-DAD [31].

In a comparative investigation, the phytochemical content of different parts of *C. ndicum* dichloromethane extract was analyzed. As the result, the leaf extract contained the highest LN content (1.47 g/100 g) compared to its stem and flower parts (0.65 g/100 g) [35]. In a similar study, HPLC-MS application led to the fingerprinting analysis of various *C. indicum* parts collected from China; consequently, the root and flower parts indicated the highest and lowest LN amounts (0.344 and 0.052 µg/mg FW), respectively [34]. Furthermore, the hydro-ethanolic extract (75%) of several *C. indicum* samples was phytochemically assessed by HPLC-DAD, and a diverse range of LN concentrations (2.08–55.68%) was recorded [36]. Apart from a qualification study, in which the LN content was determined in the flower methanolic extract of *C. indicum* [32], hydro-ethanolic partition (95%) of the flower and bud parts contained 48.3 mg/g, whilst acetonitrile and water (in formic acid 0.1%) in HPLC-DAD was used as the solvent system [30].

The flower hydro-ethanolic extract (80%) was analyzed via HPLC-UV and LN was accordingly quantified (32.8 mg/g) [39]. The impacts of several extraction conditions on LN contents of the *C. indicum* flower ethanolic extract [40] have been explored; the highest LN yield (88.11%) was measured in the plant samples extracted with 80% ethanol, 2 h of extraction, extraction frequency of three, and solvent to material ratio of 12 mL/g [40].

HPLC-DAD-MS was formerly employed to analyze LN in the hydro-methanolic (60%) extract of *C. indicum* [41]; in addition, a method for fingerprinting analysis of its methanolic extract via HPLC-DAD was introduced by Jung et al. (2012), where it contained 14.6–15.3 µg/g [42].

2.2.2. Lamiaceae

Lamiaceae, as the second richest LN natural source, has been analytically investigated by diverse groups. The occurrence of this flavone glycoside has been confirmed in various *Mentha* species. The flower methanolic fraction of *M. arvensis* was formerly analyzed and 6% of LN content was reported [46]. In a quantification measurement, the hydromethanolic (80%) extract of aerial parts of *M. arvensis* was subjected to HPLC-DAD and UPLC-ESI/Q-TOF/MS, and the LN presence was validated [47].

This compound was further detected in the *Menthahaplocalyx* (Briq.) Trautm. extract (via HPLC-MS/MS) [76]; furthermore, Erenler et al. (2018) comparatively analyzed the ethyl acetate aerial part extracts of three other *Mentha* species including *M. haplocalyx*, *Menthaspicata* L., and *Mentra x piperita* L. The highest and lowest LN contents were observed in *M. spicata* and *M. piperita* samples with 42.21 and 0.04 mg/g, respectively [48].

Marin et al. (2001), by using HPLC-UV, detected LN in the leaf hydro-methanolic (80%) extracts of the following plant species: *Acinos arvensis* ssp. *villosus*, *Acinos. Hungaricus* (Simonk.) Šilic, *Calamintha glandulosa* (Req.) Benth., *Micromeria albanica* (K.Malý) Šilić, *Micromeria cristata* (Hampe) Griseb., *Micromeria dalmatica* Benth., *Micromeria juliana* (L.) Benth. ex Rchb., *Micromeria thymifolia* (Scop.) Fritsch, *Satureja cuneifolia* Ten., *Satureja kitaibelii* Wierzb. ex Heuff., and *Satureja montana* ssp. *montana*. Moreover, the leaf hydro-methanolic fraction of *Calamintha officinalis* Moench was phytochemically analyzed through HPLC-UV and water–acetonitrile, and methanol as solvents, and LN with a concentration of 0.27 mg/g was identified [51].

The chemical composition of *Ziziphora clinopodioides* Lam. has further been studied analytically; UPLC-Q-TOF-MS was utilized to detect LN from its hydro-ethanolic (70%) extract [77] as well as the quantification analysis of the herb methanolic fraction, where by applying RP-RRLC (RP-rapid resolution liquid chromatography), the LN contents were detected (3.15–20.55 mg/g) [53].

2.2.3. Scrophulariaceae

Buddleja spp. has been analytically elaborated in the case of its phytoconstituents; consequently, LN was detected as one of the main compounds. Fan et al. (2008) identified LN in the leaf methanolic fractions of *Buddleja davidii* Franch. and *Buddleja nitida* Benth., where LC-MS/MS was used. LN concentration of the ethanolic extracts (70%) was assessed in the leaf and in vitro culture samples of *Buddleja cordata* Kunth including white and green callus and root samples by using HPLC-DAD, and the highest content was detected in the leaf ethanolic extract (41.81 ± 5.21 mg/g) [56]. The hydro-ethanolic (70%) fraction of *Buddleja officinalis* Maxim. flower was analyzed via utilization of UHPLC-LTQ-Orbitrap, and LN was consequently qualified [59]. The lyophilized infusion prepared from *Linaria vulgaris* Mill. has previously been experimented through HPLC-UV and LN was quantified with a significant content of 3.84 g/kg drug [63].

2.2.4. Valerianaceae

Valeriana spp. has been characterized for its LN content. In [78], by applying HPLC-DAD, they analytically investigated six *Valeriana* species (*Valeriana edulis* Nutt., *Valeriana officinalis* L., *Valeriana jatamansi* Jones, *Valeriana procera* Kunth, and *Valeriana sitchensis* Bong.), with the highest and lowest LN content detected in the methanolic extracts of *V. jatamansi* and *V. edulis* with 0.24 and <0.002%, respectively.

2.2.5. Miscellaneous Plants

The methanolic extracts of the *Lobelia chinensis* Lour. herb belonging to the Campanulaceae family were characterized for its phytochemicals by two analytical tools (LC-MS and HPLC-DAD-MS), and LN was qualified [66]. The hydro-ethanolic (70%) fractions extracted from the inflorescence part of *Coptis chinensis* Franch. (Ranunculaceae family) were assessed via HPLC-MS and LN was identified as the main compounds [71]. Moreover, Rios et al. (2018) identified LN in the hexane, acetone, and methanolic extracts of *Zanthoxylum affine* Kunth (Rutaceae) aerial parts, whilst HPLC−Q-TOF-MS was employed with water and methanol as the solvent systems [72].

3. Biological Properties of LN

Generally, LN is still a relatively un-investigated drug resource. As a result, in this section, the therapeutic potential of LN and LN containing plants is summarized in Figure 2 and are classified according to which could be useful for potential clinical applications (Table S3).

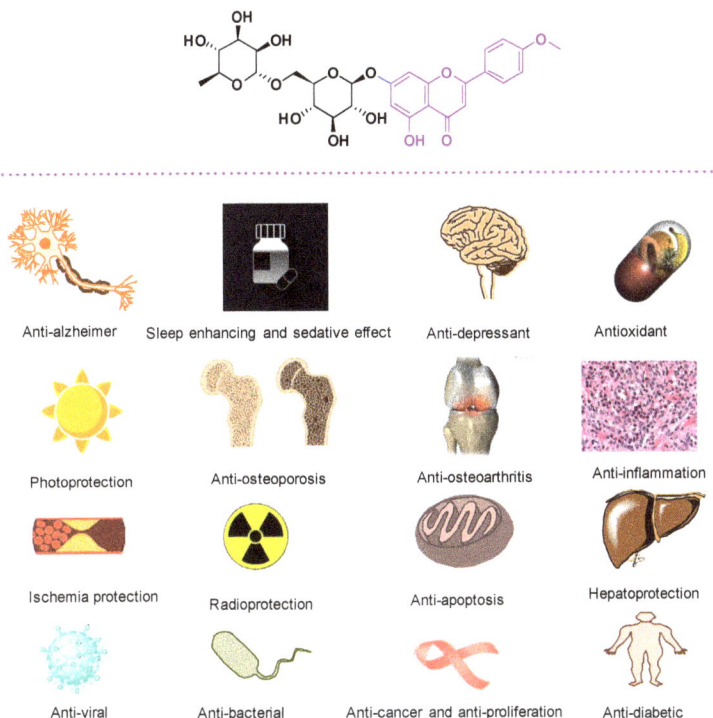

Figure 2. Summary of the biological activities of LN.

3.1. Anti-Alzheimer Properties

One of the most successful strategies to target Alzheimer's disease is the development of agents that effectively interact with key enzymes involved in cholinergic dysfunction, especially acetylcholinesterase (AChE). This enzyme terminates the action of acetylcholine neurotransmitters and reduces the information transfer across the synapse [79]. Inhibitory potential of LN against AChE extracted from *B. davidii* was evaluated. Bioautographic assessment on LN and related flavonoids showed that the 4′-OMe group as well as the 7-substituted on the B-ring increased the inhibitory potency [54].

Feng et al. (2017) evaluated the AChE inhibitory potential of LN both in vitro and in vivo. In vitro assays using Ellman's colorimetric method exhibited an IC_{50} of 3.801 ± 1.149 μM [9]. A molecular docking study showed that the 4′-methoxy group and the 7-O-sugar moiety of LN might be essential for AChE inhibition. Furthermore, ex-vivo study on mice showed that intraperitoneal administration of LN at doses of 35, 70, and 140 mg/kg decreased the AChE activity on the cortex and hippocampus of mice, where the inhibition effects of LN at the high dose were similar to huperzine A as the positive control (0.5 mg/kg) [80].

Pan et al. (2019) reported that 16.7 μg/mL and 50 μg/mL of LN (92% pure) had prominent AChE inhibition in zebrafish [81]. In addition, this compound could significantly improve the recovery of dyskinesia in Alzheimer's disease (animal model). The hydroxyl groups of LN showed strong hydrogen bond interactions with residues Tyr130, Asn85, Trp84, and Asp72 at the anionic subsite of AChE; however, the methoxy flavone segment of LN exhibited π–π interactions with residues Phe331, Trp279, and Phe290 of the peripheral anionic site [81]. The summary of the structure–activity relationship (SAR) of LN against AChE is presented in Figure 3.

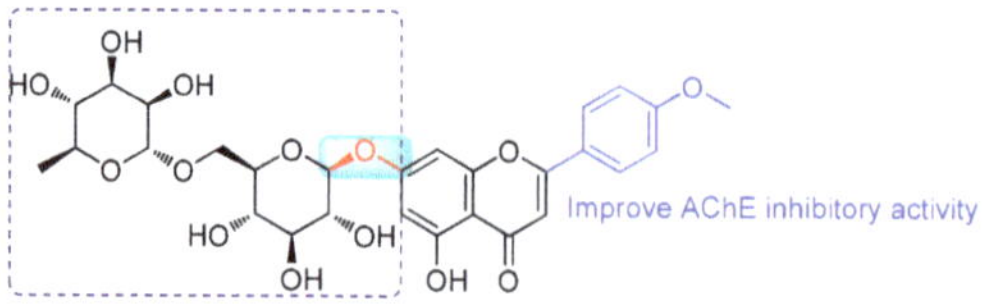

Figure 3. Structure–activity relationship of LN against AChE.

3.2. Antioxidant Properties

It is well-documented that oxidative stress and neurodegeneration are destructive in central nervous system (CNS) disorders such as Parkinson's disease and Alzheimer's disease, and protection of cells from oxidative stress toxicity might be beneficial in the abovementioned diseases. In this regard, Santos et al. exhibited the neuroprotective action of the *V. officinalis* extract in neuroblastoma SH-SY5Y of Parkinson's disease. To determine the mechanism of action, in silico molecular docking and molecular dynamics evaluations on apigenin, LN, hesperidin, and valeric acid as the main compounds of *Valeriana* against hub gene transcripts were performed. Specifically, LN fitted strongly to sulfonylurea receptor-1 (SUR1). The ligand mainly interacted with SER 857, accepting one hydrogen bond and donating two. Most likely, LN can relieve the effects of oxidative stress during ATP depletion due to its ability to binding to SUR1 [82].

The high-performance liquid chromatography-electrospray ionization–mass spectrometry (HPLC–ESI–MS) analysis of *C. japonicum* exhibited chlorogenic acid, LN, and pectolinarin as the main compounds. Furthermore, the protective effect of *C. japonicum* on adrenal pheochromocytoma (PC12) cells in vitro and *Caenorhabditis elegans* (in vivo) were also assessed. The cell viability showed a steady increase until 50 μg/mL and then decreased. Pre-treatment of extracts in PC12 cells significantly prevented intracellular ROS accumulation in comparison to the H_2O_2 treated control ($p < 0.05$). Under normal growth conditions, treatment with 50 and 100 μg/mL *C. japonicum* extract for 96 h greatly reduced intracellular ROS levels by 37% and 39%, respectively, compared to the control [83].

In the other study, the neuroprotective effect of LN against H_2O_2-induced oxidative stress in rat hippocampal neurons was assessed. The results showed that H_2O_2 at 400 μM markedly increased the number of apoptotic neurons, while treatment of the neurons with LN significantly reduced the cell death induced by H_2O_2 [84].

3.3. Sleep Enhancing and Sedative Effect

A set of flavonoid glycosides was evaluated for the sedative, sleeping, and locomotor activity. The following potencies were consequently reported 2S-hesperidin > LN > rutin > diosmin\cong 2S-neohesperidin > gossypin ~ 2S-naringin. The SAR proposed the important role of the 1→6 bond between rhamnose and glucose while changing the bond to 1→2, a remarkable decrease in the activity [85].

Nugroho et al. (2013) reported that LN isolated from the *C. boreale* methanolic extract possessed sedative and sleep-enhancing properties [86]. In detail, 10 and 20 mg/kg LN reduced the latency time for the loss of righting reflex caused by pentobarbital injection and delayed the total duration of sleeping time to around 100 min in mice [86].

3.4. Anti-Osteoporosis Activity

The potential application of LN (isolated from *B. officinalis*) in the response against oxidative stress on osteoblastic MC3T3-E1 cells exposed to H_2O_2 was evaluated. LN (0.2 μg/mL) significantly increased cell survival, alkaline phosphatase (ALP) activity, collagen content, calcium deposition, and osteocalcin secretion, whereas it decreased the production of the receptor activator of nuclear factor-kB ligand (RANKL), protein carbonyl (PCO), and malondialdehyde (MDA) of osteoblastic MC3T3-E1 cells in the presence of hydrogen peroxide. It was shown that LN exerts antiresorptive actions through the reduction of RANKL and oxidative damage [58]. With more focus toward the antioxidant potential of LN, in another study, the antiosteoporosis activity of *Flos Chrysanthemi indici* on bone loss in ovariectomized mice was evaluated. All isolated compounds including acacetin, apigenin, luteolin, and LN enhanced the differentiation and proliferation of osteoblasts in MC3T3-E1 cells. They also improved the mRNA levels of runt-related transcription factor 2 (RUNX2), osteocalcin (OCN), osteopontin (OPN), and type I collagen. The AKT signaling pathway was also activated in MC3T3-E1 cells by the four compounds [39].

Li et al. (2016) comprehensively evaluated the molecular mechanism pathway of LN on osteoblast differentiation. First, extracted LN from *Flos Chrysanthemi indici* was assessed on MC3T3-E1 cells (a mouse osteoblastic cell line), and next, the osteoprotective effect of LN in mice was evaluated. LN upregulated osteogenesis-related gene expression including that of ALP, OCN, RUNX2, bone sialoprotein (BSP), and type I collagen. Additionally, it was shown that LN enhanced osteoblast proliferation and differentiation in MC3T3-E1 cells dose-dependently through enhanced ALP activity and mineralization of the extracellular matrix by activating the BMP-2/RUNX2 pathway through protein kinase A signaling in vitro, promoting osteoid gene expression and protecting against OVX-induced bone loss in vivo [87].

In addition, a reducing impact of LN on the RANKL-induced macrophage differentiation into multinucleated osteoclasts and osteoclastic bone resorption through reducing lacunar acidification and bone matrix degradation has been demonstrated. Moreover, LN reduced the transmigration and focal contact of osteoclasts to bone matrix-mimicking RGD peptide, which was accomplished by inhibiting the induction of integrins, integrin-associated proteins of paxillin, and gelsolin, cdc42, and CD44 involved in the formation of actin rings [88].

3.5. Osteoarthritis Treatment

Osteoarthritis is an age-related joint disease characterized by the degeneration of articular cartilage and chronic pain. Recent studies have confirmed the potential role of anti-inflammatory agents to target osteoarthritis. The LN treatment suppressed lipopolysaccharide (LPS), causing the overproduction of nitric oxide (NO), prostaglandin E2 (PGE2), IL-6, and TNF-α in chondrocyte. In addition, the LPS-stimulated expression of cyclooxygenase-2 (COX-2) and inducible nitric oxide nitrate (iNOS) was decreased by LN pre-treatment. The mechanism of action showed the suppression of Toll-like receptor 4 (TLR4)/myeloid differentiation protein-2 (MD-2) dipolymer complex formation and subsequently intervened in nuclear factor kappa-B (NF-κB) activation [89].

The osteoarthritis mechanism of action of *C. zawadskii* var. *latilobum* extract revealed that the matrix metalloproteinases-1 (MMP-1), MMP-3, MMP-9 and MMP-13 expressions were inhibited by the dose-dependent extract, while expressions of the ECM synthetic genes, COL2A1 and ACAN, and the transcription factor SOX9 were increased to normal condition by the extract treatment dose-dependently. It would be interesting to note that SOX9 is a repressor of ECM-degrading aggrecanases, disintegrin, and metalloproteinase with thrombospondin motifs-4 (ADAMTS-4) and ADAMTS-5, and this extract considerably reduced the levels of these enzymes; it is worth mentioning that these potencies can remarkably be correlated to the LN content of the extract possessing 22.8 mg/g [75].

3.6. Ischemia Protection

In the other study, the effect of LN to inhibit ischemia-reperfusion injury was also evaluated. The primary study confirmed the low toxicity of LN ($\leq$30 μM) against normal H9C2 cells. Further assessments showed that LN could protect myocardial tissue from the injury of ischemia-reperfusion related to activation of the Nrf-2 and PI3 K/Akt signaling pathway. Meanwhile, the antioxidative enzymes, regulated by Nrf-2, were enhanced against the oxidative stress caused by hypoxia-reoxygenation. Importantly, with the inhibition of oxidative stress, some proliferation and apoptosis-related proteins such as NF-κB and cytochrome C were adjusted to support the viability of cells [90].

Furthermore, the anti-inflammatory effect of LN during ischemia-reperfusion-acute kidney injuries was assessed. LN inhibited the acute kidney injury in an in vivo ischemia-reperfusion injury model and decreased the expression of interleukin-12 (IL-12) p40 in in vivo and in vitro models. Evaluation on the mechanism of action of LN identified E26 oncogene homolog 2 (ETS2) protein transcription factor for its regulatory action on IL-12 p40 according to microarray analysis and protein–protein interaction. In addition, in silico study showed that the contact area ETS2 is highly conserved and located on a PPI domain of ETS2, which designates that LN may alter the interaction with synergistic proteins in the regulation of IL-12 p40 expression [91].

3.7. Anti-Inflammation Activity

Anti-inflammatory assessment of forty-two identified compounds from *Chrysanthemi indici* showed that LN, 3,5-dicaffeoylquinic acid, and luteolin with good biocompatibility could be considered as the important contributors to the anti-inflammatory effect of this plant, which decreased levels of NO, TNF-α, IL-6, and PGE2 in RAW264.7 macrophage cells treated with LPS [92].

In another study, the pelvic inflammatory disease with dampness-heat stasis syndrome was investigated and showed that LN at 8–32 μM can significantly inhibit the NO release in a concentration-dependent manner. Results also confirmed that the inhibitory effects on NO production were not due to the cytotoxicity but strong inhibition of NO production. However, the rapid response of LN on the release of TNF-α upon LPS stimulation for 2 h was not significant [93].

3.8. Photoprotective Properties

Acevedo et al. (2005) studied the photoprotective properties of the methanolic extract of *Buddleja scordioides* as well as verbascoside, LN, and linarin peracetate against UV-B induced cell death using *E. coli* as a cell model. Linarin peracetate (2 mg/mL) protected bacteria efficiently with cell death after 125–250 min, while LN reached cell death until 40–80 min. Interestingly, the sun protection factor (SPF) in guinea pigs was 9 ± 0.3 in the LN (2 mg/cm^2) receiving group, while linarin acetate showed a SPF of 5 ± 0.2. The methanolic extract had the smallest SPF (3 ± 0.09), probably due to the low concentration of the photoprotective compound [61].

Examination of the photoprotective properties of *Buddleja cordata* against UVB-induced skin damage in SKH-1 hairless mice showed that 200 μL of 2 mg/mL extract successfully reduced the redness of UVB irradiation to around 120 within 24 h of UV exposure compared to the untreated group with a redness of 300 [94].

3.9. Radioprotection

In another study, LN isolated from *Chrysanthemum morifolium* flowers significantly decreased the IR-induced cell migration and invasion at a concentration of 5 μM in A549 (human lung cancer cells). LN affected cell viability with an IC$_{50}$ value of 282 μM. The mechanism was confirmed via inhibiting NF-κB and IκB-α phosphorylation as well as MMP-9 downregulation [95].

3.10. Anti-Apoptosis Potential

The liver injury and hepatic fibrosis caused by the co-treatment with D-galactosamine (GalN)/lipopolysaccharide (LPS) have been extensively approved. Apoptosis is an important cellular pathological process in GalN/LPS-induced liver injury.

In a study conducted by JooKim et al., the cytoprotective mechanisms of LN against GalN/LPS-induced hepatic failure in mice were evaluated. After 6 h of GalN/LPS injection, the serum levels of alanine aminotransferase, aspartate aminotransferase, TNF-α, IL-6, and interferon-γ as well as TLR4 and interleukin-1 receptor-associated kinase (IRAK) expression were significantly elevated.

LN (50 mg/kg) treatment reversed the lethality induced by GalN/LPS via decreasing the levels of TLR4, IRAK, and suppressing the serum release and hepatic mRNA expression of TNF-α, IL-6, and IFN-γ. In the TUNEL assay, in which the apoptotic cells were monitored, LN also suppressed the increase in the number of apoptotic cells and reduced the cytosolic release of cytochrome c and caspase-3 cleavage.

LN administration increased the level of anti-apoptotic Bcl-xL and ratio of p-STAT3/STAT3 protein. Furthermore, LN attenuated the expression of FAS-associated death domain and caspase-8, and reduced the pro-apoptotic Bim phosphorylation induced by GalN/LPS.

These results confirmed the potential properties of LN to suppress TNF-α-mediated apoptotic pathways and pro-apoptotic Bim phosphorylation as well as enhance STAT3 activity and increase anti-apoptotic Bcl-xL levels [33].

3.11. Hepatoprotective Function

HPLC-MS analysis of the *Coptis chinensis* inflorescence extract detected 18 flavonoids and alkaloids derivatives including magnoflorine, thebaine, anonarine 5-OH berberine, jateorhizine, columbamine, coptisine, epiberberine, palmatine, berberine, worenine, and LN. Cell viability assessment of *Coptis chinensis* inflorescence extract and LN in HepG2 cells exhibited IC_{50} values of 291.15 and 83.88 μg/mL, respectively. Next, the hepatoprotective function of *C. chinensis* and LN showed the reduction in reactive oxygen species (ROS) generation induced by CCl_4 in HepG2 cells. LN could also phosphorylate mitogen-activated protein kinases (MAPKs) and upregulate Kelth-like ECH-associated protein (Keap1). The pathways of MAPKs and Keap1 lead to the separation of Keap1 and nuclear factor (erythroid-derived 2)-like 2 (Nrf2). Note that the free Nrf2 transferred to the nucleus and enhanced the expression of phase II detoxification enzymes [71].

3.12. Non-Alcoholic Steatohepatitis Effect

Nonalcoholic steatohepatitis (NASH), known as liver inflammation and damage caused by a buildup of fat in the liver, is recognized as a common cause of elevated liver enzymes [96]. Investigations of high-fat high-cholesterol diet in rats showed that LN could suppress the expression of mRNA levels of hepatic inflammation cytokines including monocyte chemotactic protein and TNF-α as well as chemokine ligand 1 (CXCL1). A high dose of LN-extract (60 mg/kg) significantly lowered the serum alanine aminotransferase (ALT) and aspartate aminotransferase (AST) and inhibited the activation of the c-Jun N-terminal kinase (JNK) induced by a high-fat high-cholesterol diet [97].

3.13. Anti-Diabetic Effects

The anti-diabetic effects of the *Chrysanthemum zawadskii* extract at different doses (125, 250, and 500 mg/kg body weight) were investigated every day for five or six weeks. The extraction was standardized and showed 1.32 ± 0.22 mg LN/g extract. Subsequently, the extract significantly decreased fasting blood glucose levels in streptozotocin and streptozotocin and high fat diet-induced diabetic models, even at low doses. In addition, glucose tolerance and insulin tolerance were improved by increasing insulin levels and decreasing hemoglobin A1c (HbA1c) levels in serum [98].

Yang-Ji et al. (2016) also demonstrated that the *Chrysanthemum zawadskii* extract could effectively inhibit the lipase and α-glucosidase enzymes to target the diabetic. This potency might well be correlated with the LN content [99].

Similarly, molecular docking, molecular dynamic, conceptual DFT, and pharmacophore mapping studies against α-amylase and α-glucosidase illustrated that LN could be a beneficial preventative and possibly therapeutic agent against diabetes [100].

3.14. Analgesic and Anti-Pyretic Properties

Martlnez-Vázquez et al. (1996) evaluated the potential analgesic and antipyretic activities of aqueous extract of leaves of *Buddleia cordata* as well as its main compound LN in animal models [101]. The oral administration of an aqueous extract of *B. cordata* and

LN showed a dose-dependent antipyretic activity. Aqueous extract and LN (100 mg/kg) remarkably increased the reaction time of mice by 70% and 55% on heat-induced pain, respectively. Similarly, the antipyretic effect of LN was better than that of the aqueous extract in the yeast-induced hyperthermia test. Three hours after the treatment, LN displayed maximal inhibitory effect with the average temperature being reduced by 1.8 °C (50 mg/kg) and 2.0 °C (100 mg/kg), whilst the extract reduced hyperthermia by 1.4 and 1.9 °C at 100 and 200 mg/kg, respectively [101].

3.15. Spasmolytic Properties

So far, many studies have approved the remarkable antispasmodic effects of the flavonoids presented in diverse plant species [102–104]. LN also showed an acceptable effect investigated by one study. Phytochemical investigation of the hydro-ethanolic extract of *L. japonicus* resulted in the extraction of three flavonoid glycosides named spinosin, LN, and apigenin-7-O-β-D-glucopyranoside as well as four cyclopeptides and nine alkaloids. These compounds were used in the uterine contraction assay. The findings demonstrated that the flavonoid glycosides (spinosin, LN, and apigenin-7-O-β-D-glucopyranoside) at 50 μM inhibited the contraction of the uterine smooth muscle strips significantly; viscerally, cyclopeptides and alkaloids increased contraction of uterine smooth muscle [50].

3.16. Treatment of Chronic Venous Hypertension

In a previous experiment, 100 mg/kg/day MPFF (diosmetin, hesperidin, LN, and isorhoifolin) in a chronic venous hypertension animal model showed significant prevention of capillary rarefaction and inflammatory cascade by decreasing the number of sticking leukocytes. MPFF reduced the enlargement of venular diameter as well as maintained venous tone [105].

3.17. Anti-Bacterial Activity

Corn mint (*Mentha arvensis*) provides a good source of LN and rosmarinic acid. The methanolic extract inhibited the growth of *Chlamydia pneumoniae* CWL-029 in vitro in a dose-dependent manner. The antichlamydial effect of LN showed complete growth inhibition of strain bacterium *Chlamydia pneumoniae*, and inhibited the growth of strain K7 by >60% at 100 μM. Administration of *M. arvensis* extract (20 mg/kg, 3 days) was able to significantly diminish the inflammatory parameters related to *C. pneumoniae* infection in mice ($p = 0.019$) [47].

3.18. Anti-Viral Activity

Virus is a threat to public health due to its high mutation rate and resistance to existing drugs. Recently, the antiviral activity of LN was investigated to develop new antiviral agents. Evaluation of the flavonoid prescription drug baicalin-linarin-icariinnotoginsenoside R1 was assessed on duck virus hepatitis (DVH) caused by duck hepatitis A virus type 1 (DHAV-1). The mentioned drug showed an anti-DHAV-1 ability with T and B lymphocyte-promoting effects. It also inhibited DHAV-1 reproduction by suppressing its adsorption and release. The mechanism of this antiviral effect showed that the drug at 5 μg/mL increased T and B lymphocyte proliferation. Moreover, according to the in vivo study, the drug stimulated total anti-DHAV-1 antibody secretion in ducklings at the dosage of 4 mg per duckling, but had no significant stimulation impact on the IL-2 and IFN-c secretion [106].

In another study, Chen et al. (2017) assessed the baicalin-LN-icariin-notoginsenoside R1 on DHAV-1 as well as its hepatoprotective and antioxidative potencies. Results showed that the DHAV-1 inhibitory rate of this multi-therapy was 69.3% at 20 μg/mL. The survival rate of ducklings treated by 3 mg drug per duckling (once a day for five days) was about 35.5%, which was significantly higher than that of the virus control (0.0%). Additionally, the degree of oxidative stress, the serum MDA, SOD, CAT, and GSH-Px levels at 8 and 54 h were measured and demonstrated a significant reduction compared to the blank and virus groups, which showed the reduction of oxidative stress in the infected duck [107].

Human immunodeficiency virus (HIV) is an infection that attacks the body's immune system, specifically the white blood cells called CD4. The development of anti-HIV-1 drugs has gained much attention nowadays [108]. It has been shown that human γδ T cells (lymphocytes) consist of Vδ1-TCR-expressing Vδ1+ T cells and Vδ2-TCR-expressing Vδ2+ T cells, which play pivotal roles in bridging innate and adaptive immunity. It was proposed that stimulation Vδ1+ T cells may constitute a new class of anti-HIV drugs, targeting the mucosal compartment to suppress the R5-type of HIV-1. Yonekawa et al. (2019) reported that LN at 100 µg/mL and some flavonoid glycosides, which have both rutinose at the A ring and methoxy substitution at the B ring, can activate host Vδ1+ T cells in HIV patients and can contribute to limiting the R5-type of HIV-1 replication. LN stimulated PBMC-derived Vδ1+ T cells to secrete chemokines MIP-1α, MIP-1β, and RANTES and cytokines such as IL-5 and IL-13, which may improve the immune system [109]. Figure 4 exhibits the structure–activity relationship of LN against HIV.

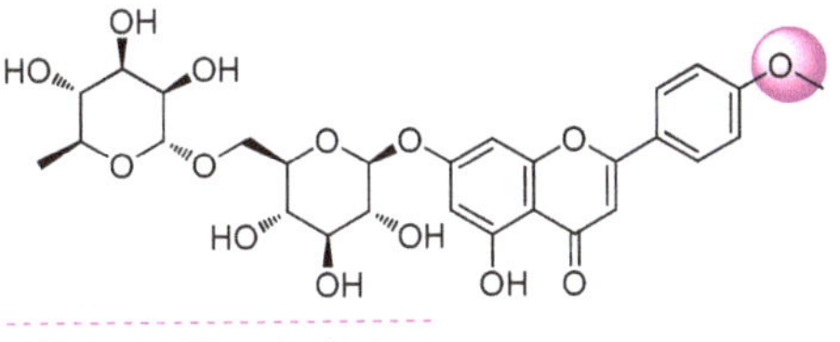

Figure 4. Structure–activity relationship of LN against HIV.

In another study, virtual screening on Chinese medicinal compounds was applied to discover novel natural drugs against the influenza A virus using Naïve Bayesian classifiers, and mt-QSAR models. In the selected set, LN exhibited a significant reduction in TNF-α expression to around 40 pg/mL compared to the control group with ~80 pg/mL, whereas it may regulate the expression of cytokines and chemokines, which represent direct and indirect suppression of influenza A [110].

3.19. Anti-Cancer and Anti-Proliferative Activity

Cancer is one of the major causes of death worldwide, affecting more than 14.1 million people worldwide [111]. Over the past few years, attention has been paid to find potent natural products as anticancer therapeutic agents [79,112,113].

Flavonoids are known to be one of the most popular groups of bioactive phytochemicals with anticancer activity; however, limited study has been conducted to evaluate the activity of LN as anticancer agents [79].

The methanolic extract of *Chrysanthemum indicum* and purified LN exerted antiproliferative activity against human non-small cell lung cancer cells via suppression of Akt activation and induction of cyclin-dependent kinase inhibitor p27Kip1, as evidenced by cell cycle analysis and treatment with LY294002. These findings may indicate the anticancer potential of LN as the core functional constituent of *C. indicum* [114].

Glioma is the most common form of malignant brain cancer with a high mortality rate in humans. NF-κB activity is a common phenomenon in various cancers, resulting in abnormal cell proliferation, malignant transformation, or resistance to cell death. Previously, the anti-cancer role of LN in glioma was tested in vitro and in vivo. LN suppressed glioma cell proliferation and migration by inducing apoptosis, which was through reducing the cell cycle-related signals including survivin, p-Rb, and cyclin D1, while promoting p21, Bax, caspase-3, and poly (ADP-ribose) polymerase (PARP) activation. LN also showed an increase in P53 as an essential tumor suppressor. Moreover, it reduced cellular proliferation of glioma through p53 upregulation and NF-κB/p65-downregulation, thereby inhibiting glioma cell growth [115].

The cytotoxicity of *Jatropha pelargoniifolia* loaded chitosan nanoparticles against A549 human lung adenocarcinoma cells (IC$_{50}$ = 13.17 µM) was higher than that of the free extract

(IC_{50} = 25.16 µM) and comparable to that of methotrexate (IC_{50} = 11.84 µM) as an anticancer drug [116].

Oral squamous cell carcinoma is characterized by overexpression of Akt1 (RAC-alpha serine/threonine-protein kinase) and Akt2 (RAC-beta serine/threonine-protein kinase). It was reported that Akt1 and Akt2 inhibitors can lead to oral squamous cell carcinoma treatment with no affinity toward monoamine oxidase B (MAOB). In silico studies introduced LN as inhibitors of Akt1 and Akt2 with strong binding affinities of 11.5 kcal/mol and 11.1 kcal/mol, respectively, with no affinity toward MAOB, which can be an ideal candidate for oral squamous cell carcinoma treatment [117].

3.20. Negative Biological Results of LN

3.20.1. Estrogenic Activity

The estrogenic activity of six chemical constituents (apigenin, hispidulin, cirsimaritin, cirsimarin, pectolinarin, and LN) isolated from *Cirsium japonicum* on MCF-7 cells was assessed. Among them, hispidulin and cirsimaritin showed strong estrogen receptor transactivation, while the rest of the compounds had weaker or relatively no effects. The SAR confirmed that estrogen receptor transactivation increases as the number of –OH groups in the flavonoid structure increased [19].

3.20.2. Anti-Fungal Effect

Combined chromatographic techniques were implemented in the phytochemical analysis of *Lippia rubella*, leading to the isolation of several compounds such as lippiarubelloside A and lippiarubelloside B, verbascoside as well as LN. Inhibitory evaluation of LN against some fungal strains such as *Candida albicans* (ATCC 10231) and *Candida parasilopsis* (ATCC 22019) asserted no significant activity (MIC >125 µg/mL), and moderate effects against *Cryptococcus neoformans* and *Cryptococcus neoformans* (MIC: 125 µg/mL) [73].

3.20.3. Anti-Depressant Properties

Depression is a mental health disorder characterized by loss of interest, pleasure, with feelings of sadness, low self-worth, and tiredness, which disturbed sleep or appetite, leading to suicide in severe cases. The exact mechanism of depression is still unknown, and most of the antidepressants act as inhibitors of intracellular monoamine (exp, norepinephrine) reuptake. Additionally, it has been shown the gamma-aminobutyric acid (GABA) levels as well as cortical GABAA receptors decreased in patients with depression.

In this regard, the norepinephrine reuptake of *Cirsium japonicum* and its major constituents (linarin, pectolinarin, chlorogenic acid, luteolin) were evaluated. *Cirsium japonicum* showed an antidepressant effect by significantly reducing the immobile behavior of mice in the forced swimming test, without enhancing locomotor activity in the open-field test. In addition, the *C. japonicum* extract had no effect on monoamine uptake while significantly promoting Cl^- ion influx in human neuroblastoma cells and modulating the GABAA receptor. Further evaluation showed that among the major constituents of the *C. japonicum* extract, only luteolin produced antidepressant activity as a positive modulator of the GABA-mediated Cl^- ion channel complex and LN was almost inactive [118]. Results showed that the antidepressant effect of *Cirsium japonicum* could be due to the luteolin constituent.

4. Perspectives

Anti-SARS-CoV-2 (COVID-19) Effect

Severe acute respiratory syndrome-coronavirus 2 (SARS-CoV-2) is a RNA airborne virus infection known as the pathogen responsible for coronavirus disease 2019 (COVID-19) [119]. Millions of COVID-19 patients have been reported thus far; however, there is no concrete evidence on the effectiveness and safety of the specific treatment against SARS-CoV-2 [120,121]. One area that has been affected immensely is the investigation of natural remedies as medications and/or supportive therapies to treat patients with

COVID-19 infection. Mostly, antiviral drugs directly target the infecting pathogen to halt its development [122]. In the case of SARS-CoV-2, the influence of active substances of medicinal plants were surveyed in inhibiting four important druggable targets including S and N proteins, 3CLpro, and RdRp. RdRp controls the replication of SARS-CoV-2 while 3CLpro is the main protease of the virus. Moreover, N and S proteins are responsible for SARS-CoV-2 assembly and attachment, respectively. Molecular docking outcomes of the study revealed that LN, amentoflavone, (-)-catechin gallate, and hypericin had an affinity for these basic proteins, which possess an effective role in SARS-CoV-2 infection [123].

5. Conclusions

Investigation of plant secondary metabolites with valuable impacts on human health is an attractive and broad research area. Flavonoids, a large family of phenolic compounds due to their pivotal therapeutic effects, have been the subject of many studies. Nowadays, their diverse derivatives are widely consumed as dietary supplements. Although the most renowned flavonoids (i.e., apigenin, luteolin, hispidulin, kaempferol, myricetin, quercetin, naringenin, etc.) are aglycosylated [124], the glycosylated forms are also of interest. It is believed that the glycosylation of flavonoids can lead to the development of their biological features by reducing the probable toxicity and increasing their bioavailability [125].

The present context overviewed a very promising but not well-investigated glycosylated flavone named LN. From the phytochemical viewpoint, the plant genus *Cirsium*, *Micromeria*, *Buddleja*, and *Chrysanthemum* are the major natural sources of LN. This compound demonstrated promising bioactivities through the studies carried out in vitro and in vivo. The encouraging properties of LN have been shown through osteoblast proliferation and differentiation with high anti-arthritis and antiosteoporosis potencies; however, its effect on the treatment of CNS disorders have also been pointed out.

Further phytochemical investigations of different natural sources leading to the isolation and identification of LN as well as exploring the optimized extraction methods can support the implementation of its bioactivity assessments. Complementary biological and pharmacological evaluations (particularly toxicity and clinical trials) of LN and its derivatives are proposed in future in order to develop potential natural-based drugs/supplements with the least side effects.

Supplementary Materials: The followings are available online at https://www.mdpi.com/article/10.3390/ph14111104/s1, Table S1: Isolation and identification of linarin from plant species; Table S2: Identification and characterization of linarin from plant species; Table S3: Biological properties of linarin. References [126–138] are cited in the supplementary materials.

Author Contributions: Conceptualization, methodology, writing, and supervision by J.M.; Data collection by H.T., A.B.D. and M.M.S.; Investigation and writing by K.Z., C.I. and A.I. were performed. All authors have read and agreed to the published version of the manuscript.

Funding: This research received no external funding.

Institutional Review Board Statement: Not applicable.

Informed Consent Statement: Not applicable.

Data Availability Statement: Not applicable.

Acknowledgments: The authors wish to thank the support of the Vice-Chancellor for Research of Shiraz University of Medical Sciences (Grant No. 24425). This agency was not involved in the design of the study and collection, analysis, and interpretation of data as well as in writing the manuscript.

Conflicts of Interest: The authors declare no conflict of interest.

References

1. Mottaghipisheh, J.; Kiss, T.; Tóth, B.; Csupor, D. The *Prangos* genus: A comprehensive review on traditional use, phytochemistry, and pharmacological activities. *Phytochem. Rev.* **2020**, *19*, 1449–1470. [CrossRef]

2. Mottaghipisheh, J.; Maghsoudlou, M.T.; Valizadeh, J.; Arjomandi, R. Antioxidant activity and chemical composition of the essential oil of *Ducrosia anethifolia* (DC.) Boiss. from Neyriz. *J. Med. Plants By-Prod.* **2014**, *2*, 215–218.
3. Dehsheikh, A.B.; Sourestani, M.M.; Dehsheikh, P.B.; Mottaghipisheh, J.; Vitalini, S.; Iriti, M. Monoterpenes: Essential oil components with valuable features. *Mini-Rev. Med. Chem.* **2020**, *20*, 958–974. [CrossRef] [PubMed]
4. Bhattacharya, A. High-temperature stress and metabolism of secondary metabolites in plants. In *Effect of High Temperature on Crop Productivity and Metabolism of Macro Molecules*; Elsevier: London, UK, 2019; pp. 391–484.
5. Kwok, K.K.; Vincent, E.C.; Gibson, J.N. Antineoplastic drugs. In *Pharmacology and Therapeutics for Dentistry*; Elsevier: Amsterdam, The Netherlands, 2017; pp. 530–562.
6. Pullaiah, T.; Raveendran, V. Camptothecin: Chemistry, biosynthesis, analogs, and chemical synthesis. In *Camptothecin and Camptothecin Producing Plants*; Elsevier: Amsterdam, The Netherlands, 2020; pp. 47–101.
7. Dockery, L.; Daniel, M.-C. Dendronized Systems for the Delivery of Chemotherapeutics. *Adv. Cancer Res.* **2018**, *139*, 85–120. [PubMed]
8. Panche, A.N.; Diwan, A.D.; Chandra, S.R. Flavonoids: An overview. *J. Nutr. Sci.* **2016**, *5*, e47. [CrossRef]
9. Feng, W.; Hao, Z.; Li, M. Isolation and structure identification of flavonoids. In *Flavonoids—From Biosynthesis to Human Health*; InTech: Rijeka, Croatia, 2017; pp. 17–23.
10. Yamagata, K. Metabolic syndrome: Preventive effects of dietary flavonoids. *Stud. Nat. Prod. Chem.* **2019**, *60*, 1–28.
11. Mottaghipisheh, J.; Stuppner, H. A comprehensive review on chemotaxonomic and phytochemical aspects of homoisoflavonoids, as rare flavonoid derivatives. *Int. J. Mol. Sci.* **2021**, *22*, 2735. [CrossRef]
12. Mottaghipisheh, J.; Iriti, M. Sephadex® LH-20, isolation, and purification of flavonoids from plant species: A comprehensive review. *Molecules* **2020**, *25*, 4146. [CrossRef]
13. Arai, M.A.; Tanaka, M.; Tanouchi, K.; Ishikawa, N.; Ahmed, F.; Sadhu, S.K.; Ishibashi, M. Hes1-binding compounds isolated by Target Protein Oriented Natural Products Isolation (TPO-NAPI). *J. Nat. Prod.* **2017**, *80*, 538–543. [CrossRef]
14. Demirtas, I.; Tufekci, A.R.; Yaglioglu, A.S.; Elmastas, M. Studies on the antioxidant and antiproliferative potentials of *Cirsium arvense* subsp. *vestitum*. *J. Food Biochem.* **2017**, *41*, e12299. [CrossRef]
15. Kozyra, M.; Biernasiuk, A.; Malm, A.; Chowaniec, M. Chemical compositions and antibacterial activity of extracts obtained from the inflorescences of *Cirsium canum* (L.) all. *Nat. Prod. Res.* **2015**, *29*, 2059–2063. [CrossRef] [PubMed]
16. Ganzera, M.; Pöcher, A.; Stuppner, H. Differentiation of *Cirsium japonicum* and *C. setosum* by TLC and HPLC-MS. *Phytochem. Anal.* **2005**, *16*, 205–209. [CrossRef] [PubMed]
17. Ma, Q.; Jiang, J.-G.; Zhang, X.-M.; Zhu, W. Identification of luteolin 7-O-β-D-glucuronide from *Cirsium japonicum* and its anti-inflammatory mechanism. *J. Funct. Foods* **2018**, *46*, 521–528. [CrossRef]
18. Zhang, Z.; Jia, P.; Zhang, X.; Zhang, Q.; Yang, H.; Shi, H.; Zhang, L. LC–MS/MS determination and pharmacokinetic study of seven flavonoids in rat plasma after oral administration of *Cirsium japonicum* DC. extract. *J. Ethnopharmacol.* **2014**, *158*, 66–75. [CrossRef] [PubMed]
19. Lee, D.; Jung, Y.; Baek, J.Y.; Shin, M.S.; Lee, S.; Hahm, D.H.; Lee, S.C.; Shim, J.S.; Kim, S.N.; Kang, K.S. Cirsimaritin contributes to the estrogenic activity of *Cirsium japonicum* var. *maackii* through the activation of estrogen receptor α. *Bull. Korean Chem. Soc.* **2017**, *38*, 1486–1490. [CrossRef]
20. Han, H.-S.; Shin, J.-S.; Lee, S.-B.; Park, J.C.; Lee, K.-T. Cirsimarin, a flavone glucoside from the aerial part of *Cirsium japonicum* var. *ussuriense* (Regel) Kitam. ex Ohwi, suppresses the JAK/STAT and IRF-3 signaling pathway in LPS-stimulated RAW 264.7 macrophages. *Chem. Biol. Interact.* **2018**, *293*, 38–47. [CrossRef]
21. Walesiuk, A.; Nazaruk, J.; Braszko, J.J. Pro-cognitive effects of *Cirsium rivulare* extracts in rats. *J. Ethnopharmacol.* **2010**, *129*, 261–266. [CrossRef] [PubMed]
22. Jeong, G.H.; Park, E.K.; Kim, T.H. New anti-glycative flavonoids from *Cirsium setidens* with potent radical scavenging activities. *Phytochem. Lett.* **2018**, *26*, 115–119. [CrossRef]
23. Lu, Y.; Song, W.; Liang, X.; Wei, D.; Zhang, X. Chemical fingerprint and quantitative analysis of *Cirsium setosum* by LC. *Chromatographia* **2009**, *70*, 125–131. [CrossRef]
24. Sun, Q.; Chang, L.; Ren, Y.; Cao, L.; Sun, Y.; Du, Y.; Shi, X.; Wang, Q.; Zhang, L. Simultaneous analysis of 11 main active components in *Cirsium setosum* based on HPLC-ESI-MS/MS and combined with statistical methods. *J. Sep. Sci.* **2012**, *35*, 2897–2907. [CrossRef]
25. Wang, B.; Lv, D.; Huang, P.; Yan, F.; Liu, C.; Liu, H. Optimization, evaluation and identification of flavonoids in *Cirsium setosum* (Willd.) MB by using response surface methodology. *J. Food Meas. Charact.* **2019**, *13*, 1175–1184. [CrossRef]
26. Nugroho, A.; Lim, S.C.; Byeon, J.S.; Choi, J.S.; Park, H.J. Simultaneous quantification and validation of caffeoylquinic acids and flavonoids in *Hemistepta lyrata* and peroxynitrite-scavenging activity. *J. Pharm. Biomed. Anal.* **2013**, *76*, 139–144. [CrossRef] [PubMed]
27. Shin, K.H.; Kang, S.S.; Seo, E.A.; Shin, S.W. Isolation of aldose reductase inhibitors from the flowers of *Chrysanthemum boreale*. *Arch. Pharm. Res.* **1995**, *18*, 65–68. [CrossRef]
28. Han, A.R.; Kim, H.Y.; So, Y.; Nam, B.; Lee, I.S.; Nam, J.W.; Jo, Y.D.; Kim, S.H.; Kim, J.B.; Kang, S.Y.; et al. Quantification of antioxidant phenolic compounds in a new *Chrysanthemum* cultivar by high-performance liquid chromatography with diode array detection and electrospray ionization mass spectrometry. *Int. J. Anal. Chem.* **2017**, *2017*, 1–8. [CrossRef]

29. Dasgupta, A. Antiinflammatory herbal supplements. In *Translational Inflammation*; Elsevier: Amsterdam, The Netherlands, 2019; pp. 69–91.
30. Wu, X.L.; Li, C.W.; Chen, H.M.; Su, Z.Q.; Zhao, X.N.; Chen, J.N.; Lai, X.P.; Zhang, X.J.; Su, Z.R. Anti-inflammatory effect of supercritical-carbon dioxide fluid extract from flowers and buds of *Chrysanthemum indicum* Linnén. *Evid.-Based Complement. Altern. Med.* **2013**, *2013*, 413237. [CrossRef] [PubMed]
31. He, J.; Wu, X.; Kuang, Y.; Wang, T.; Bi, K.; Li, Q. Quality assessment of *Chrysanthemum indicum* Flower by simultaneous quantification of six major ingredients using a single reference standard combined with HPLC fingerprint analysis. *Asian J. Pharm. Sci.* **2016**, *11*, 265–272. [CrossRef]
32. Seo, D.W.; Cho, Y.R.; Kim, W.; Eom, S.H. Phytochemical linarin enriched in the flower of *Chrysanthemum indicum* inhibits proliferation of A549 human alveolar basal epithelial cells through suppression of the Akt-dependent signaling pathway. *J. Med. Food* **2013**, *16*, 1086–1094. [CrossRef]
33. Kim, S.J.; Cho, H.I.; Kim, S.J.; Park, J.H.; Kim, J.S.; Kim, Y.H.; Lee, S.K.; Kwak, J.H.; Lee, S.M. Protective effect of linarin against D-galactosamine and lipopolysaccharide-induced fulminant hepatic failure. *Eur. J. Pharmacol.* **2014**, *738*, 66–73. [CrossRef] [PubMed]
34. Jiang, Y.; Ji, X.; Duan, L.; Ye, P.; Yang, J.; Zhan, R.; Chen, W.; Ma, D. Gene mining and identification of a flavone synthase II involved in flavones biosynthesis by transcriptomic analysis and targeted flavonoid profiling in *Chrysanthemum indicum* L. *Ind. Crops Prod.* **2019**, *134*, 244–256. [CrossRef]
35. Hwang, S.; Paek, J.; Lim, S. Simultaneous ultra performance liquid chromatography determination and antioxidant activity of linarin, luteolin, chlorogenic acid and apigenin in different parts of compositae species. *Molecules* **2016**, *21*, 1609. [CrossRef] [PubMed]
36. Qiaoshan, Y.; Suhong, C.; Minxia, S.; Wenjia, M.; Bo, L.; Guiyuan, L. Preparative purification of linarin extracts from *Dendranthema indicum* flowers and evaluation of its antihypertensive effect. *Evid.-Based Complement. Altern. Med.* **2014**, *2014*, 394276. [CrossRef]
37. Shin, H.J.; Lee, S.Y.; Kim, J.S.; Lee, S.; Choi, R.J.; Chung, H.S.; Kim, Y.S.; Kang, S.S. Sesquiterpenes and other constituents from *Dendranthema zawadskii* var. latilobum. *Chem. Pharm. Bull.* **2012**, *60*, 306–314. [CrossRef]
38. Singh, R.P.; Agrawal, P.; Yim, D.; Agarwal, C.; Agarwal, R. Acacetin inhibits cell growth and cell cycle progression, and induces apoptosis in human prostate cancer cells: Structure-activity relationship with linarin and linarin acetate. *Carcinogenesis* **2005**, *26*, 845–854. [CrossRef]
39. Li, J.; Lin, X.; Zhang, Y.; Liu, W.; Mi, X.; Zhang, J.; Su, J. Preparative purification of bioactive compounds from *Flos Chrysanthemi indici* and evaluation of its antiosteoporosis effect. *Evid.-Based Complement. Altern. Med.* **2016**, *2016*, 2587201. [CrossRef] [PubMed]
40. Pan, H.; Zhang, Q.; Cui, K.; Chen, G.; Liu, X.; Wang, L. Optimization of extraction of linarin from *Flos Chrysanthemi indici* by response surface methodology and artificial neural network. *J. Sep. Sci.* **2017**, *40*, 2062–2070. [CrossRef] [PubMed]
41. Wang, S.; Hao, L.-J.; Zhu, J.-J.; Wang, Z.-M.; Zhang, X.; Song, X. Comparative evaluation of *Chrysanthemum Flos* from different origins by HPLC-DAD-MS n and relative response factors. *Food Anal. Methods* **2015**, *8*, 40–51. [CrossRef]
42. Zhang, Q.; Li, J.; Wang, C.; Sun, W.; Zhang, Z.; Cheng, W. A gradient HPLC method for the quality control of chlorogenic acid, linarin and luteolin in *Flos Chrysanthemi indici* suppository. *J. Pharm. Biomed. Anal.* **2007**, *43*, 753–757. [CrossRef]
43. Jung, H.A.; Park, J.J.; Islam, M.N.; Jin, S.E.; Min, B.S.; Lee, J.H.; Sohn, H.S.; Choi, J.S. Inhibitory activity of coumarins from *Artemisia capillaris* against advanced glycation endproduct formation. *Arch. Pharm. Res.* **2012**, *35*, 1021–1035. [CrossRef]
44. Laskaris, G.G.; Gournelis, D.C.; Kokkalou, E. Phenolics of *Picnomon acarna*. *J. Nat. Prod.* **1995**, *58*, 1248–1250. [CrossRef]
45. Kokkini, S.; Karousou, R.; Hanlidou, E. HERBS I Herbs of the Labiatae. In *Encyclopedia of Food Sciences and Nutrition*; Elsevier: Amsterdam, The Netherlands, 2003; pp. 3082–3090.
46. Oinonen, P.P.; Jokela, J.K.; Hatakka, A.I.; Vuorela, P.M. Linarin, a selective acetylcholinesterase inhibitor from *Mentha arvensis*. *Fitoterapia* **2006**, *77*, 429–434. [CrossRef]
47. Salin, O.; Törmäkangas, L.; Leinonen, M.; Saario, E.; Hagström, M.; Ketola, R.A.; Saikku, P.; Vuorela, H.; Vuorela, P.M. Corn mint (*Mentha arvensis*) extract diminishes acute *Chlamydia pneumoniae* infection in vitro and in vivo. *J. Agric. Food Chem.* **2011**, *59*, 12836–12842. [CrossRef]
48. Erenler, R.; Telci, İ.; Elmastas, M.; Aksit, H.; Gul, F.; Tufekci, A.R.; Demirtas, İ.; Kayir, Ö. Quantification of flavonoids isolated from *Mentha spicata* in selected clones of Turkish mint landraces. *Turk. J. Chem.* **2018**, *42*, 1695–1705. [CrossRef]
49. Dai, L.-M.; Zhao, C.-C.; Jin, H.-Z.; Tang, J.; Shen, Y.-H.; Li, H.-L.; Peng, C.-Y.; Zhang, W.-D. A new ferulic acid ester and other constituents from *Dracocephalum peregrinum*. *Arch. Pharm. Res.* **2008**, *31*, 1325–1329. [CrossRef] [PubMed]
50. Liu, J.; Peng, C.; Zhou, Q.-M.; Guo, L.; Liu, Z.-H.; Xiong, L. Alkaloids and flavonoid glycosides from the aerial parts of *Leonurus japonicus* and their opposite effects on uterine smooth muscle. *Phytochemistry* **2018**, *145*, 128–136. [CrossRef] [PubMed]
51. Monforte, M.T.; Lanuzza, F.; Pergolizzi, S.; Mondello, F.; Tzakou, O.; Galati, E.M. Protective effect of *Calamintha officinalis* Moench leaves against alcohol-induced gastric mucosa injury in rats. Macroscopic, histologic and phytochemical analysis. *Phyther. Res.* **2012**, *26*, 839–844. [CrossRef] [PubMed]
52. Marin, P.D.; Grayer, R.J.; Veitch, N.C.; Kite, G.C.; Harborne, J.B. Acacetin glycosides as taxonomic markers in *Calamintha* and *Micromeria*. *Phytochemistry* **2001**, *58*, 943–947. [CrossRef]
53. Tian, S.; Yu, Q.; Xin, L.; Zhou, Z.S.; Upur, H. Chemical fingerprinting by RP-RRLC-DAD and principal component analysis of *Ziziphora clinopodioides* from different locations. *Nat. Prod. Commun.* **2012**, *7*, 1181–1184. [CrossRef]

54. Fan, P.; Hay, A.E.; Marston, A.; Hostettmann, K. Acetylcholinesterase-inhibitory activity of Linarin from *Buddleja davidii*, structure-activity relationships of related flavonoids, and chemical investigation of *Buddleja nitida*. *Pharm. Biol.* **2008**, *46*, 596–601. [CrossRef]
55. El-Domiaty, M.M.; Wink, M.; Aal, M.M.A.; Abou-Hashem, M.M.; Abd-Alla, R.H. Antihepatotoxic activity and chemical constituents of *Buddleja asiatica* Lour. *Z. Naturforsch. C* **2009**, *64*, 11–19. [CrossRef] [PubMed]
56. Estrada-Zúñiga, M.E.; Cruz-Sosa, F.; Rodríguez-Monroy, M.; Verde-Calvo, J.R.; Vernon-Carter, E.J. Phenylpropanoid production in callus and cell suspension cultures of *Buddleja cordata* Kunth. *Plant. Cell Tissue Organ. Cult.* **2009**, *97*, 39–47. [CrossRef]
57. Rodríguez-Zaragoza, S.; Ordaz, C.; Avila, G.; Muñoz, J.L.; Arciniegas, A.; De Vivar, A.R. In vitro evaluation of the amebicidal activity of *Buddleia cordata* (Loganiaceae, H.B.K.) on several strains of Acanthamoeba. *J. Ethnopharmacol.* **1999**, *66*, 327–334. [CrossRef]
58. Kim, Y.H.; Lee, Y.S.; Choi, E.M. Linarin isolated from *Buddleja officinalis* prevents hydrogen peroxide-induced dysfunction in osteoblastic MC3T3-E1 cells. *Cell. Immunol.* **2011**, *268*, 112–116. [CrossRef]
59. Sun, M.; Luo, Z.; Liu, Y.; Yang, R.; Lu, L.; Yu, G.; Ma, X.; Liu, A.; Guo, Y.; Zhao, H. Identification of the major components of *Buddleja officinalis* extract and their metabolites in rat urine by UHPLC-LTQ-orbitrap. *J. Food Sci.* **2016**, *81*, H2587–H2596. [CrossRef]
60. Tai, B.H.; Jung, B.Y.; Cuong, N.M.; Linh, P.T.; Tung, N.H.; Nhiem, N.X.; Huong, T.T.; Anh, N.T.; Kim, J.A.; Kim, S.K.; et al. Total peroxynitrite scavenging capacity of phenylethanoid and flavonoid glycosides from the flowers of *Buddleja officinalis*. *Biol. Pharm. Bull.* **2009**, *32*, 1952–1956. [CrossRef]
61. Avila Acevedo, J.G.; Castañeda, C.M.C.; Benitez, F.J.C.; Durán, D.A.; Barroso, V.R.; Martínez, C.G.; Muñoz, L.J.L.; Martínez, C.A.; Romo de Vivar, A. Photoprotective activity of *Buddleja scordioides*. *Fitoterapia* **2005**, *76*, 301–309. [CrossRef]
62. Otsuka, H. Isolation of isolinariins A and B, new flavonoid glycosides from *Linaria japonica*. *J. Nat. Prod.* **1992**, *55*, 1252–1255. [CrossRef]
63. Vrchovská, V.; Spilková, J.; Valentão, P.; Sousa, C.; Andrade, P.B.; Seabra, R.M. Assessing the antioxidative properties and chemical composition of *Linaria vulgaris* infusion. *Nat. Prod. Res.* **2008**, *22*, 735–746. [CrossRef]
64. Aydoğrdu, İ.; Zihnioğrlu, F.; Karayildirim, T.; Gülcemal, D.; Alankuş-Çalışkan, Ö.; Bedir, E. α-glucosidase inhibitory constituents of *Linaria kurdica* subsp. eriocalyx. *Nat. Prod. Commun.* **2010**, *5*, 841–844. [CrossRef]
65. Leslie Gunatilaka, A.; Sotheeswaran, S.; Balasubramaniam, S.; Indumathie Chandrasekara, A.; Badra Sriyani, H. Linarin, a flavone glycoside from *Exacum macranthum*. *Planta Med.* **1980**, *39*, 66–72. [CrossRef]
66. Zhou, Y.; Wang, Y.; Wang, R.; Guo, F.; Yan, C. Two-dimensional liquid chromatography coupled with mass spectrometry for the analysis of *Lobelia chinensis* Lour. using an ESI/APCI multimode ion source. *J. Sep. Sci.* **2008**, *31*, 2388–2394. [CrossRef]
67. Wang, T.; Xiao, J.; Hou, H.; Li, P.; Yuan, Z.; Xu, H.; Liu, R.; Li, Q.; Bi, K. Development of an ultra-fast liquid chromatography–tandem mass spectrometry method for simultaneous determination of seven flavonoids in rat plasma: Application to a comparative pharmacokinetic investigation of *Ginkgo biloba* extract and single pure ginkgo. *J. Chromatogr. B* **2017**, *1060*, 173–181. [CrossRef]
68. El-Hagrassi, A.M.; Ali, M.M.; Osman, A.F.; Shaaban, M. Phytochemical investigation and biological studies of *Bombax malabaricum* flowers. *Nat. Prod. Res.* **2011**, *25*, 141–151. [CrossRef] [PubMed]
69. Zhang, W.-K.; Xu, J.-K.; Zhang, L.; Du, G.-H. Flavonoids from the bran of *Avena sativa*. *Chin. J. Nat. Med.* **2012**, *10*, 110–114. [CrossRef]
70. Ina, H.; Iida, H. Linarin monoacetate from *Thalictrum aquilegifolium*. *Phytochemistry* **1981**, *20*, 1176–1177. [CrossRef]
71. Ma, B.-X.; Meng, X.-S.; Tong, J.; Ge, L.-L.; Zhou, G.; Wang, Y.-W. Protective effects of *Coptis chinensis* inflorescence extract and linarin against carbon tetrachloride-induced damage in HepG2 cells through the MAPK/Keap1-Nrf2 pathway. *Food Funct.* **2018**, *9*, 2353–2361. [CrossRef]
72. Rios, M.Y.; Córdova-Albores, L.C.; Ramírez-Cisneros, M.Á.; King-DÍaz, B.; Lotina-Hennsen, B.; Rivera, I.L.; Miranda-Sánchez, D. Phytotoxic potential of *Zanthoxylum affine* and its major compound linarin as a possible natural herbicide. *ACS Omega* **2018**, *3*, 14779–14787. [CrossRef] [PubMed]
73. Martins, G.R.; da Fonseca, T.S.; Martínez-Fructuoso, L.; Simas, R.C.; Silva, F.T.; Salimena, F.R.G.; Alviano, D.S.; Alviano, C.S.; Leitão, G.G.; Pereda-Miranda, R.; et al. Antifungal phenylpropanoid glycosides from *Lippia rubella*. *J. Nat. Prod.* **2019**, *82*, 566–572. [CrossRef]
74. Liu, S.; Luo, X.; Li, D.; Zhang, J.; Qiu, D.; Liu, W.; She, L.; Yang, Z. Tumor inhibition and improved immunity in mice treated with flavone from *Cirsium japonicum* DC. *Int. Immunopharmacol.* **2006**, *6*, 1387–1393. [CrossRef]
75. Byun, J.-H.; Choi, C.-W.; Jang, M.-J.; Lim, S.H.; Han, H.J.; Choung, S.-Y. Anti-osteoarthritic mechanisms of *Chrysanthemum zawadskii* var. *latilobum* in MIA-induced osteoarthritic rats and interleukin-1β-induced SW1353 human chondrocytes. *Medicina (B. Aires).* **2020**, *56*, 685. [CrossRef]
76. Chen, X.; Zhang, S.; Xuan, Z.; Ge, D.; Chen, X.; Zhang, J.; Wang, Q.; Wu, Y.; Liu, B. The phenolic fraction of *Mentha haplocalyx* and its constituent linarin ameliorate inflammatory response through inactivation of NF-kB and MAPKs in lipopolysaccharide-induced RAW264.7 cells. *Molecules* **2017**, *22*, 811. [CrossRef]
77. Zhang, X.-M.; An, D.-Q.; Guo, L.-L.; Yang, N.-H.; Zhang, H. Identification and screening of active components from *Ziziphora clinopodioides* Lam. in regulating autophagy. *Nat. Prod. Res.* **2019**, *33*, 2549–2553. [CrossRef]

78. Navarrete, A.; Avula, B.; Choi, Y.-W.; Khan, I.A. Chemical fingerprinting of valeriana species: Simultaneous determination of valerenic acids, flavonoids, and phenylpropanoids using liquid chromatography with ultraviolet detection. *J. AOAC Int.* **2006**, *89*, 8–15. [CrossRef]
79. Srivastava, S.; Ahmad, R.; Khare, S.K. Alzheimer's disease and its treatment by different approaches: A review. *Eur. J. Med. Chem.* **2021**, *216*, 113320. [CrossRef]
80. Feng, X.; Wang, X.; Liu, Y.; Di, X. Linarin inhibits the acetylcholinesterase activity in-vitro and ex-vivo. *Iran. J. Pharm. Res.* **2015**, *14*, 949–954. [CrossRef] [PubMed]
81. Pan, H.; Zhang, J.; Wang, Y.; Cui, K.; Cao, Y.; Wang, L.; Wu, Y. Linarin improves the dyskinesia recovery in Alzheimer's disease zebrafish by inhibiting the acetylcholinesterase activity. *Life Sci.* **2019**, *222*, 112–116. [CrossRef] [PubMed]
82. Santos, G.; Giraldez-Alvarez, L.D.; Ávila-Rodriguez, M.; Capani, F.; Galembeck, E.; Neto, A.G.; Barreto, G.E.; Andrade, B. SUR1 receptor interaction with hesperidin and linarin predicts possible mechanisms of action of *Valeriana officinalis* in Parkinson. *Front. Aging Neurosci.* **2016**, *8*, 1–12. [CrossRef]
83. Jang, M.; Kim, K.-H.; Kim, G.-H. Antioxidant capacity of thistle (*Cirsium japonicum*) in various drying methods and their protection effect on neuronal PC12 cells and *Caenorhabditis elegans*. *Antioxidants* **2020**, *9*, 200. [CrossRef] [PubMed]
84. Zeng, J.; Hu, W.; Li, H.; Liu, J.; Zhang, P.; Gu, Y.; Yu, Y.; Wang, W.; Wei, Y. Purification of linarin and hesperidin from *Mentha haplocalyx* by aqueous two-phase flotation coupled with preparative HPLC and evaluation of the neuroprotective effect of linarin. *J. Sep. Sci.* **2021**, *44*, 2496–2503. [CrossRef]
85. Fernández, S.P.; Wasowski, C.; Loscalzo, L.M.; Granger, R.E.; Johnston, G.A.R.; Paladini, A.C.; Marder, M. Central nervous system depressant action of flavonoid glycosides. *Eur. J. Pharmacol.* **2006**, *539*, 168–176. [CrossRef]
86. Nugroho, A.; Lim, S.C.; Choi, J.; Park, H.J. Identification and quantification of the sedative and anticonvulsant flavone glycoside from *Chrysanthemum boreale*. *Arch. Pharm. Res.* **2013**, *36*, 51–60. [CrossRef]
87. Li, J.; Hao, L.; Wu, J.; Zhang, J.; Su, J. Linarin promotes osteogenic differentiation by activating the BMP-2/RUNX2 pathway via protein kinase A signaling. *Int. J. Mol. Med.* **2016**, *37*, 901–910. [CrossRef] [PubMed]
88. Kim, S.-I.; Kim, Y.H.; Kang, B.G.; Kang, M.K.; Lee, E.J.; Kim, D.Y.; Oh, H.; Oh, S.Y.; Na, W.; Lim, S.S.; et al. Linarin and its aglycone acacetin abrogate actin ring formation and focal contact to bone matrix of bone-resorbing osteoclasts through inhibition of αvβ3 integrin and core-linked CD44. *Phytomedicine* **2020**, *79*, 153351. [CrossRef] [PubMed]
89. Qi, W.; Chen, Y.; Sun, S.; Xu, X.; Zhan, J.; Yan, Z.; Shang, P.; Pan, X.; Liu, H. Inhibiting TLR4 signaling by linarin for preventing inflammatory response in osteoarthritis. *Aging (Albany NY)* **2021**, *13*, 5369–5382. [CrossRef]
90. Yu, Q.; Li, X.; Cao, X. Linarin could protect myocardial tissue from the injury of Ischemia-reperfusion through activating Nrf-2. *Biomed. Pharmacother.* **2017**, *90*, 1–7. [CrossRef] [PubMed]
91. Chengyu, Y.; Long, Z.; Bin, Z.; Hong, L.; Xuefei, S.; Congjuan, L.; Caixia, C.; Yan, X. Linarin protects the kidney against ischemia/reperfusion injury via the inhibition of bioactive ETS2/IL-12. *Biol. Pharm. Bull.* **2021**, *44*, 25–31. [CrossRef]
92. Tian, D.; Yang, Y.; Yu, M.; Han, Z.Z.; Wei, M.; Zhang, H.W.; Jia, H.M.; Zou, Z.M. Anti-inflammatory chemical constituents of *Flos Chrysanthemi indici* determined by UPLC-MS/MS integrated with network pharmacology. *Food Funct.* **2020**, *11*, 6340–6351. [CrossRef] [PubMed]
93. Hu, L.; Chen, Y.; Chen, T.; Huang, D.; Li, S.; Cui, S. A systematic study of mechanism of *Sargentodoxa cuneata* and *Patrinia scabiosifolia* against pelvic inflammatory disease with dampness-heat stasis syndrome via network pharmacology approach. *Front. Pharmacol.* **2020**, *11*, 1856. [CrossRef]
94. Acevedo, J.G.A.; Espinosa González, A.M.; y Campos, D.M.D.M.; Benitez Flores, J.d.C.; Delgado, T.H.; Maya, S.F.; Contreras, J.C.; López, J.L.M.; García Bores, A.M. Photoprotection of *Buddleja cordata* extract against UVB-induced skin damage in SKH-1 hairless mice. *BMC Complement. Altern. Med.* **2014**, *14*, 1–9. [CrossRef]
95. Jung, C.-H.; Han, A.-R.; Chung, H.-J.; Ha, I.-H.; Um, H.-D. Linarin inhibits radiation-induced cancer invasion by downregulating MMP-9 expression via the suppression of NF-κB activation in human non-small-cell lung cancer A549. *Nat. Prod. Res.* **2019**, *33*, 3582–3586. [CrossRef]
96. Peng, C.; Stewart, A.G.; Woodman, O.L.; Ritchie, R.H.; Qin, C.X. Non-alcoholic steatohepatitis: A review of its mechanism, models and medical treatments. *Front. Pharmacol.* **2020**, *11*, 1864. [CrossRef]
97. Zhuang, Z.J.; Shan, C.W.; Li, B.; Pang, M.X.; Wang, H.; Luo, Y.; Liu, Y.L.; Song, Y.; Wang, N.N.; Chen, S.H.; et al. Linarin enriched extract attenuates liver injury and inflammation induced by high-fat high-cholesterol diet in rats. *Evid.-Based Complement. Altern. Med.* **2017**, *2017*, 4701570. [CrossRef]
98. Kim, Y.J.; Kim, H.K.; Lee, H.S. Hypoglycemic effect of standardized *Chrysanthemum zawadskii* ethanol extract in high-fat diet/streptozotocin-induced diabetic mice and rats. *Food Sci. Biotechnol.* **2018**, *27*, 1771–1779. [CrossRef] [PubMed]
99. Kim, Y.-J.; Kim, S.-E.; Lee, H.S.; Hong, S.-Y.; Kim, S.-E.; Kim, Y.J.; Lee, J.H.; Park, S.J.; Kim, J.H.; Park, Y.-J.; et al. Comparison of linarin content and biological activity in ethanol extraction of *Chrysanthemum zawadskii*. *J. Korean Soc. Food Sci. Nutr.* **2016**, *45*, 1414–1421. [CrossRef]
100. Chenafa, H.; Mesli, F.; Daoud, I.; Achiri, R.; Ghalem, S.; Neghra, A. In silico design of enzyme α-amylase and α-glucosidase inhibitors using molecular docking, molecular dynamic, conceptual DFT investigation and pharmacophore modelling. *J. Biomol. Struct. Dyn.* **2021**, 1–22. [CrossRef] [PubMed]
101. Martínez-Vázquez, M.; Ramírez Apan, T.O.; Aguilar, M.H.; Bye, R. Analgesic and antipyretic activities of an aqueous extract and of the flavone linarin of *Buddleia cordata*. *Planta Med.* **1996**, *62*, 137–140. [CrossRef]

102. Sándor, Z.; Mottaghipisheh, J.; Veres, K.; Hohmann, J.; Bencsik, T.; Horváth, A.; Kelemen, D.; Papp, R.; Barthó, L.; Csupor, D. Evidence supports tradition: The in vitro effects of roman chamomile on smooth muscles. *Front. Pharmacol.* **2018**, *9*, 323. [CrossRef]
103. Ghayur, M.N.; Khan, H.; Gilani, A.H. Antispasmodic, bronchodilator and vasodilator activities of (+)-catechin, a naturally occurring flavonoid. *Arch. Pharm. Res.* **2007**, *30*, 970–975. [CrossRef]
104. Mendel, M.; Chłopecka, M.; Dziekan, N.; Karlik, W. Antispasmodic effect of selected *Citrus* flavonoids on rat isolated jejunum specimens. *Eur. J. Pharmacol.* **2016**, *791*, 640–646. [CrossRef] [PubMed]
105. das Graças, C.; de Souza, M.; Cyrino, F.Z.; de Carvalho, J.J.; Blanc-Guillemaud, V.; Bouskela, E. Protective effects of Micronized Purified Flavonoid Fraction (MPFF) on a novel experimental model of chronic venous hypertension. *Eur. J. Vasc. Endovasc. Surg.* **2018**, *55*, 694–702. [CrossRef] [PubMed]
106. Chen, Y.; Zeng, L.; Yang, J.; Wang, Y.; Yao, F.; Wu, Y.; Wang, D.; Hu, Y.; Liu, J. Anti-DHAV-1 reproduction and immuno-regulatory effects of a flavonoid prescription on duck virus hepatitis. *Pharm. Biol.* **2017**, *55*, 1545–1552. [CrossRef] [PubMed]
107. Chen, Y.; Zeng, L.; Lu, Y.; Yang, Y.; Xu, M.; Wang, Y.; Liu, J. Treatment effect of a flavonoid prescription on duck virus hepatitis by its hepatoprotective and antioxidative ability. *Pharm. Biol.* **2017**, *55*, 198–205. [CrossRef]
108. Zarenezhad, E.; Farjam, M.; Iraji, A. Synthesis and biological activity of pyrimidines-containing hybrids: Focusing on pharmacological application. *J. Mol. Struct.* **2021**, *1230*, 129833. [CrossRef]
109. Yonekawa, M.; Shimizu, M.; Kaneko, A.; Matsumura, J.; Takahashi, H. Suppression of R5-type of HIV-1 in CD4 + NKT cells by Vδ1 + T cells activated by flavonoid glycosides, hesperidin and linarin. *Sci. Rep.* **2019**, *9*, 1–12. [CrossRef] [PubMed]
110. Xu, L.; Jiang, W.; Jia, H.; Zheng, L.; Xing, J.; Liu, A.; Du, G. Discovery of multitarget-directed ligands against influenza a virus from compound yizhihao through a predictive system for compound-protein interactions. *Front. Cell. Infect. Microbiol.* **2020**, *10*, 16. [CrossRef]
111. Fedotcheva, T.A.; Fedotcheva, N.I.; Shimanovsky, N.L. Progestins as anticancer drugs and chemosensitizers, new targets and applications. *Pharmaceutics* **2021**, *13*, 1616. [CrossRef]
112. Talib, W.H.; Alsayed, A.R.; Barakat, M.; Abu-Taha, M.I.; Mahmod, A.I. Targeting drug chemo-resistance in cancer using natural products. *Biomedicines* **2021**, *9*, 1353. [CrossRef]
113. Ailioaie, L.M.; Ailioaie, C.; Litscher, G. Latest innovations and nanotechnologies with curcumin as a nature-inspired photosensitizer applied in the photodynamic therapy of cancer. *Pharmaceutics* **2021**, *13*, 1562. [CrossRef] [PubMed]
114. Thaipong, K.; Boonprakob, U.; Crosby, K.; Cisneros-Zevallos, L.; Hawkins Byrne, D. Comparison of ABTS, DPPH, FRAP, and ORAC assays for estimating antioxidant activity from guava fruit extracts. *J. Food Compos. Anal.* **2006**, *19*, 669–675. [CrossRef]
115. Zhen, Z.G.; Ren, S.H.; Ji, H.M.; Ma, J.H.; Ding, X.M.; Feng, F.Q.; Chen, S.L.; Zou, P.; Ren, J.R.; Jia, L. Linarin suppresses glioma through inhibition of NF-κB/p65 and up-regulating p53 expression in vitro and in vivo. *Biomed. Pharmacother.* **2017**, *95*, 363–374. [CrossRef]
116. Alqahtani, M.S.; Al-Yousef, H.M.; Alqahtani, A.S.; Tabish Rehman, M.; AlAjmi, M.F.; Almarfidi, O.; Amina, M.; Alshememry, A.; Syed, R. Preparation, characterization, and in vitro-in silico biological activities of *Jatropha pelargoniifolia* extract loaded chitosan nanoparticles. *Int. J. Pharm.* **2021**, *606*, 120867. [CrossRef]
117. Sharif Siam, M.K.; Sarker, A.; Sayeem, M.M.S. In silico drug design and molecular docking studies targeting Akt1 (RAC-alpha serine/threonine-protein kinase) and Akt2 (RAC-beta serine/threonine-protein kinase) proteins and investigation of CYP (cytochrome P450) inhibitors against MAOB (monoamine oxidase B) for OSCC (oral squamous cell carcinoma) treatment. *J. Biomol. Struct. Dyn.* **2021**, *39*, 6467–6479. [CrossRef]
118. De La Peña, J.B.I.; Kim, C.A.; Lee, H.L.; Yoon, S.Y.; Kim, H.J.; Hong, E.Y.; Kim, G.H.; Ryu, J.H.; Lee, Y.S.; Kim, K.M.; et al. Luteolin mediates the antidepressant-like effects of *Cirsium japonicum* in mice, possibly through modulation of the GABAA receptor. *Arch. Pharm. Res.* **2014**, *37*, 263–269. [CrossRef]
119. Bouazzaoui, A.; Abdellatif, A.A.H.; Al-Allaf, F.A.; Bogari, N.M.; Al-Dehlawi, S.; Qari, S.H. Strategies for vaccination: Conventional vaccine approaches versus new-generation strategies in combination with adjuvants. *Pharmaceutics* **2021**, *13*, 140. [CrossRef] [PubMed]
120. Sheikh, A.B.; Pal, S.; Javed, N.; Shekhar, R. COVID-19 vaccination in developing nations: Challenges and opportunities for innovation. *Infect. Dis. Rep.* **2021**, *13*, 429–436. [CrossRef] [PubMed]
121. Jirjees, F.; Saad, A.K.; Al Hano, Z.; Hatahet, T.; Al Obaidi, H.; Dallal Bashi, Y.H. COVID-19 treatment guidelines: Do they really reflect best medical practices to manage the pandemic? *Infect. Dis. Rep.* **2021**, *13*, 259–284. [CrossRef]
122. Shah, S.A.A.; ul Hassan, S.S.; Bungau, S.; Si, Y.; Xu, H.; Rahman, M.H.; Behl, T.; Gitea, D.; Pavel, F.-M.; Corb Aron, R.A.; et al. Chemically diverse and biologically active secondary metabolites from marine *Phylum chlorophyta*. *Mar. Drugs* **2020**, *18*, 493. [CrossRef] [PubMed]
123. Mahmoudi, S.; Balmeh, N.; Mohammadi, N.; Sadeghian-Rizi, T. The novel drug discovery to combat COVID-19 by repressing important virus proteins involved in pathogenesis using medicinal herbal compounds. *Avicenna J. Med. Biotechnol.* **2021**, *13*, 108. [CrossRef]
124. Egert, S.; Rimbach, G. Which sources of flavonoids: Complex diets or dietary supplements? *Adv. Nutr.* **2011**, *2*, 8–14. [CrossRef] [PubMed]
125. Slámová, K.; Kapešová, J.; Valentová, K. "Sweet flavonoids": Glycosidase-catalyzed modifications. *Int. J. Mol. Sci.* **2018**, *19*, 2126. [CrossRef]

126. Fernández, S.; Wasowski, C.; Paladini, A.C.; Marder, M. Sedative and sleep-enhancing properties of linarin, a flavonoid-isolated from *Valeriana officinalis*. *Pharmacol. Biochem. Behav.* **2004**, *77*, 399–404. [CrossRef] [PubMed]
127. Chari, V.M.; Jordan, M.; Wagner, H.; Thies, P.W. A 13C-NMR study of the structure of an acyllinarin from *Valeriana wallichii*. *Phytochemistry* **1977**, *16*, 1110–1112. [CrossRef]
128. Martínez-Vázquez, M.; Ramírez Apan, T.O.; Lastra, A.L.; Bye, R. A comparative study of the analgesic and anti-inflammatory activities of pectolinarin isolated from *Cirsium subcoriaceum* and linarin isolated from *Buddleia cordata*. *Planta Med.* **1998**, *64*, 134–137. [CrossRef] [PubMed]
129. Han, S.; Sung, K.; Yim, D.; Lee, S.; Lee, C.; Ha, N.; Kim, K. The effect of linarin on LPS-induced cytokine production and nitric oxide inhibition in murine macrophages cell line RAW264.7. *Arch. Pharm. Res.* **2002**, *25*, 170–177. [CrossRef] [PubMed]
130. Shim, S.; Kang, H.; Sun, H.; Lee, Y.; Park, J.; Chun, S. Isolation and identification of flavonoids from *Gujeolcho* (*Chrysanthemum zawadskii* var. *latilobum*) as inhibitor of histamine release. *Food Sci. Biotechnol.* **2012**, *21*, 613–617. [CrossRef]
131. Xu, Z.; Sun, X.; Lan, Y.; Han, C.; Zhang, Y.; Chen, G. Linarin sensitizes tumor necrosis factor-related apoptosis (TRAIL)-induced ligand-triggered apoptosis in human glioma cells and in xenograft nude mice. *Biomed. Pharmacother.* **2017**, *95*, 1607–1618. [CrossRef] [PubMed]
132. Lv, G.-Y.; Zhang, Y.-P.; Gao, J.-L.; Yu, J.-J.; Lei, J.; Zhang, Z.-R.; Li, B.; Zhan, R.-J.; Chen, S.-H. Combined antihypertensive effect of luteolin and buddleoside enriched extracts in spontaneously hypertensive rats. *J. Ethnopharmacol.* **2013**, *150*, 507–513. [CrossRef] [PubMed]
133. Kim, B.; Lee, J.H.; Seo, M.J.; Eom, S.H.; Kim, W. Linarin down-regulates phagocytosis, pro-inflammatory cytokine production, and activation marker expression in RAW264.7 macrophages. *Food Sci. Biotechnol.* **2016**, *25*, 1437–1442. [CrossRef] [PubMed]
134. Kim, A.R.; Kim, H.S.; Kim, D.K.; Lee, J.H.; Yoo, Y.H.; Kim, J.Y.; Park, S.K.; Nam, S.T.; Kim, H.W.; Park, Y.H.; et al. The extract of *Chrysanthemum zawadskii* var. *latilobum* ameliorates collagen-induced arthritis in mice. *Evid.-Based Complement. Altern. Med.* **2016**, *2016*, 3915013. [CrossRef]
135. Han, X.; Wu, Y.I.-C.; Meng, M.; Sun, Q.-S.; Gao, S.-M.; Sun, H. Linarin prevents LPS-induced acute lung injury by suppressing oxidative stress and inflammation via inhibition of TXNIP/NLRP3 and NF-κB pathways. *Int. J. Mol. Med.* **2018**, *42*, 1460–1472. [CrossRef]
136. Xie, G.; Yang, J.; Wei, X.; Xu, Q.; Qin, M. Separation of acteoside and linarin from *Buddlejae Flos* by high-speed countercurrent chromatography and their anti-inflammatory activities. *J. Sep. Sci.* **2020**, *48*, 1–8. [CrossRef]
137. Benitez, F.J.C.; Acevedo, J.G.A.; Castan, C.M.C.; Dura, D.A.; Barroso, V.R.; Martı, C.G.; Vivar, A.R. De Photoprotective activity of *Buddleja scordioides*. *Fitoterapia* **2005**, *76*, 301–309. [CrossRef]
138. Chow, N.; Fretz, M.; Hamburger, M.; Butterweck, V. Telemetry as a tool to measure sedative effects of a valerian root extract and its single constituents in mice. *Planta Med.* **2011**, *77*, 795–803. [CrossRef] [PubMed]

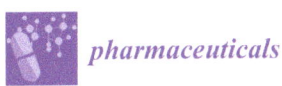

Review

Flavonoids from the Genus *Euphorbia*: Isolation, Structure, Pharmacological Activities and Structure–Activity Relationships

Douglas Kemboi Magozwi [1,2,*], Mmabatho Dinala [1], Nthabiseng Mokwana [1], Xavier Siwe-Noundou [2,*], Rui W. M. Krause [2], Molahlehi Sonopo [3], Lyndy J. McGaw [4], Wilma A. Augustyn [1] and Vuyelwa Jacqueline Tembu [1,*]

[1] Department of Chemistry, Tshwane University of Technology, Pretoria 0001, South Africa; dinalamabatho@gmail.com (M.D.); nthabi.mokwana@gmail.com (N.M.); AugustynW@tut.ac.za (W.A.A.)
[2] Department of Chemistry, Rhodes University, Grahamstown 6140, South Africa; r.krause@ru.ac.za
[3] Radiochemistry, South African Nuclear Energy Corporation, Pelindaba, Brits R104, South Africa; sonopom@yahoo.com
[4] Phytomedicine Programme, Department of Paraclinical Sciences, University of Pretoria, Private Bag X04 Onderstepoort 0110, Pretoria 0001, South Africa; lyndy.mcgaw@up.ac.za
* Correspondence: kemboidouglas01@gmail.com (D.K.M.); X.siwenoundou@ru.ac.za (X.S.-N.); TembuVJ@tut.ac.za (V.J.T.); Tel.: +27-12-382-6288 (V.J.T.)

Abstract: Plants of the genus *Euphorbia* are widely distributed across temperate, tropical and subtropical regions of South America, Asia and Africa with established Ayurvedic, Chinese and Malay ethnomedical records. The present review reports the isolation, occurrence, phytochemistry, biological properties, therapeutic potential and structure–activity relationship of *Euphorbia* flavonoids for the period covering 2000–2020, while identifying potential areas for future studies aimed at development of new therapeutic agents from these plants. The findings suggest that the extracts and isolated flavonoids possess anticancer, antiproliferative, antimalarial, antibacterial, anti-venom, anti-inflammatory, anti-hepatitis and antioxidant properties and have different mechanisms of action against cancer cells. Of the investigated species, over 80 different types of flavonoids have been isolated to date. Most of the isolated flavonoids were flavonols and comprised simple O-substitution patterns, C-methylation and prenylation. Others had a glycoside, glycosidic linkages and a carbohydrate attached at either C-3 or C-7, and were designated as D-glucose, L-rhamnose or glucorhamnose. The structure–activity relationship studies showed that methylation of the hydroxyl groups on C-3 or C-7 reduces the activities while glycosylation loses the activity and that the parent skeletal structure is essential in retaining the activity. These constituents can therefore offer potential alternative scaffolds towards development of new *Euphorbia*-based therapeutic agents.

Keywords: *Euphorbia*; flavonoids; pharmacological activities; structure–activity relationship

1. Introduction

Euphorbia species are used in traditional medicine for the treatment of various diseases. Plants of the *Euphorbia* genus are common herbs that are applied in the treatment of respiratory diseases, healing of wounds, relieving skin irritations, indigestion, inflammation, microbial infestations and also as a food source [1–4]. Prehistorical records show that *Euphorbia* species were used in the treatment of scorpion and snake bites, liver diseases, respiratory disorders, asthma and rheumatism in the Chinese and Ayurveda medicine systems [3,4].

The medicinal applications of these species have been attributed to the presence of diverse secondary metabolites such as flavonoids and terpenes [5–7]. The abundance of these chemical constituents in *Euphorbia* species qualifies them as a rich source of therapeutic natural products possessing various pharmacological activities. These constituents can provide potential lead molecules for drug discovery. The genus *Euphorbia* is also among the largest of genera in the *spurge* family, and consists of several other subsections and subgenera, having more than 2000 species [8,9] with promising research potential.

Flavonoids are among the dominant constituents of *Euphorbia* species after macrocyclic diterpenes and triterpenoids [4,10]. Flavonoids mainly occur as isoflavonoids (3-phenylbenzopyrans), neoflavonoids (4-phenylbenzopyrans), chalcones [7,11], flavonols, flavanone, flavanonol, flavanol and anthocyanidins [11]. These constituents are structurally and biogenetically related as they share a common precursor, the chalcone [11,12]. They have also been reported to possess various pharmacological activities [12–14] and have promising therapeutic potential.

Apart from their biological functions in protecting plant species against herbivores and other pathogens as well as acting as stress-protecting agents, they also perform important pharmacological activities in humans. Reports indicate that plant flavonoids exhibit anti-ulcer, antidepressant, antimicrobial, antiviral, antibacterial, anti-diabetic, anti-inflammatory, anti-agiogenic [15], antiproliferative [16–22] and anticancer [6] activities in vitro. Even though they have not been classified as nutrients, the intake of flavonoids is considered to be significant for human health [23]. They are also used as natural dyes as well as for cosmetics and skin-care products [16,24]. Related studies have shown that flavonoids from the *Euphorbia* species also have a wide range of pharmacological activities such as cytotoxic, anti-inflammatory properties and tumor-promoting abilities [25,26].

Furthermore, various reports have stated the significance of flavonoids in metabolism of the thyroid hormone, which is commonly reported to be vitamin P and is considered useful in counteracting hemorrhage [27]. They are also functional foods for promotion of good health and prevention of diseases [27]. As a result, significant efforts have been made in isolation, identification and characterization of flavonoids from the latex, aerial parts, roots, stems, seeds, stem bark and whole plant extracts of some *Euphorbia* species since early times [28,29]. Indeed, several reviews have been published about the role and significance of plant flavonoids as a source of bioactive compounds. For instance, in 2019, Avtar and Bhawna [20] reviewed the chemistry and pharmacology of flavonoids, while Dieter [30] reported the significance of flavonoids in plant resistance to microbial attack.

Similarly, Muhammad et al. [7] reviewed the significance of flavonoids as prospective neuroprotectants in ageing associated with neurological disorders, while Ali et al. [31] reported the therapeutic role of flavonoids in bowel diseases. In addition, the role of plant flavonoids in cancer and apoptosis mechanisms was also reported [32], as well as the commercial application of flavonoids as anti-infective agents [14]. Efforts have also been made to review the occurrence of flavonoids in medicinal plants. For example, Bathelemy et al. [33] reported the occurrence, classification and biological activities of flavonoids from African medicinal plants, while Panche et al. [34] and Shashank and Abhay [35] reported the occurrence of flavonoids in selected species of different plant families. In addition, Nigel and Renee [36] reviewed over 796 naturally occurring flavonols, dihydroflavonols, chalcones, dihydrochalcones, aurones and anthocyanins.

However, even though other reports have reviewed the phytochemical constituents of *Euphorbia* species, most of the published reviews have exclusively focused on ethnomedicinal uses [2–6], isolated diterpenes [10], essential oils and triterpenoids [4]. For example, Goel et al. [37] reviewed the structural diversity of phorbol esters while Shi et al. [38] reported the pharmacological activities and chemical constituents of *Euphorbia* species. In addition, Andrea and co-authors reviewed the structural diversity of *Euphorbia* diterpenes covering the period 2008–2012, and their pharmacological activities [10], while Kemboi et al. [4] reported the ethnomedicinal uses and the structural diversity of *Euphorbia* triterpenoids. Rojas et al. [39] reviewed the phytochemical and functional properties of *E. antisyphilitica* Zucc, while Yang et al. [40] described the traditional uses, phytochemistry and pharmacological aspects of *E. ebracteolata* Hayata. In general, reports on *Euphorbia* species have exclusively focused on isolated diterpenes and triterpenes with limited reference to flavonoids, and other phenolic constituents such as flavonoids over the past two decades, and there is no report of isolated *Euphorbia* flavonoids within this period. Hence, in order to gain a more comprehensive understanding of *Euphorbia* flavonoids, the current review reports the occurrence, isolation, structure, pharmacological activities and the therapeutic potential of flavonoids of the genus *Euphorbia* covering the period 2000–2020. Harnessing this information can provide an updated database of compounds of the *Euphorbia* species that may provide potential hits for drug discovery or developing a useful pharmacopeia, as well as assisting in explaining the observed synergistic effect of the crude extracts.

2. Literature Sources and Search Strategy

Information about the *Euphorbia* flavonoids, their chemistry, biosynthesis, structure, biological activities, structure–activity relationships and potential therapeutic value was obtained through an online literature search using terms such as '*Euphorbia* flavonoids', '*Euphorbia* constituents', 'biological activities of *Euphorbia* flavonoids', 'therapeutic potential' and 'structure–activity relationship of *Euphorbia* flavonoids' using online databases such as Scopus, Scifinder, Wiley online, Springer Link, Science Direct, PubMed, and Google Scholar. The online search was customized between the years 2000 and 2020 which resulted into over 400 reports about *Euphorbia*, mainly in the English language that were easily accessible. Of these over 100 reports relevant to the study that described studies on isolation and elucidation of known and novel *Euphorbia* flavonoids, their biological activities, therapeutic potential and the structure–activity relationships were selected. The retrieved information was critically analyzed and searched for descriptions of previously described *Euphorbia* flavonoids, their occurrence (extraction solvent and plant part used), structures, their biological activities, therapeutic potential, and structure–activity relationships. Additional information was obtained by reviewing and analyzing the cited references in the selected articles. Hence, the present review provide an account of the previous and the latest information on *Euphorbia* flavonoids isolated between January 2000 and December 2020, their pharmacological activities, therapeutic potential and structure–activity relationships.

3. Flavonoids

Flavonoids are natural compounds with various phenolic structures biosynthesized by plants [11]. Since the first isolation of a plant flavonoid, rutin, in 1930, there have been over 6000 different types of flavonoids identified from plant species to date [11,41]. The basic skeletal structure of flavonoids has 15 carbon atoms that are arranged to form a C_6-C_3-C_6 ring system. They are divided into different classes based on their molecular structures and the degree of oxidation and unsaturation of the linking chain at C-3. They are biosynthesized in plants via the shikimic acid pathway [11,12,16] as summarized in Figure 1.

The initial stage is the condensation of a *p*-coumaroyl-CoA molecule with 3 molecules of malonyl-CoA to give chalcone in the presence of the chalcone isomerase enzyme. Chalcone is further isomerized by chalcone flavanone isomerase enzyme (CHI) to form flavanone. Thereafter, the pathway diverges to several other branches to produce different classes of flavonoids such as flavonols, flavones, flavonones or their dihydroderivatives [11,12] as illustrated in Figure 1.

The position of the benzenoid substituent is the basis of their classification into 2-phenylbenzopyrans, isoflavonoids (3-phenylbenzopyrans), neoflavonoids (4- phenylbenzopyrans) and chalcones. However, flavonols differ from flavonones by the hydroxyl substituent at C-3' and C-2-C-3 double bonds (Havsteen, 1983). In most cases, flavonoids have the hydroxyl group at C-3, C-5, C-7, C-2', C-3', C- C-4', C-5'. For flavonoid glycosides, the glycosidic linkage is unusually located at C-3 or C-7 and the carbohydrate attached can either be D-glucose, L-rhamnose, glucorhamnose, galactose or arabinose [42]. As a consequence, flavonoids are divided into seven major groups [35,43] as in Figure 2. However, further information on classification and biosynthesis of plant flavonoids is not dealt with in this review as the references can be consulted for detailed information.

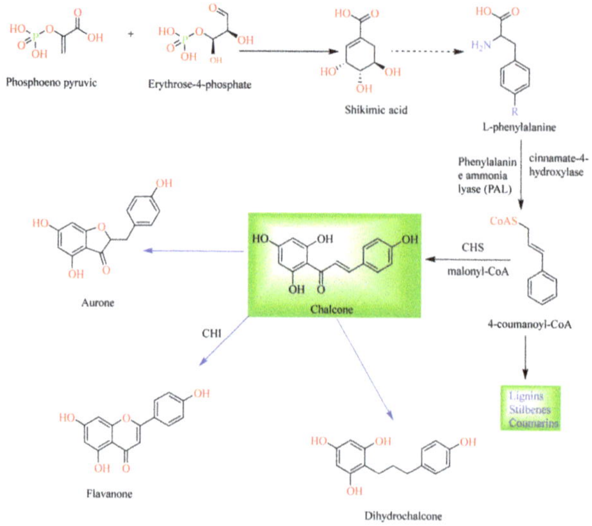

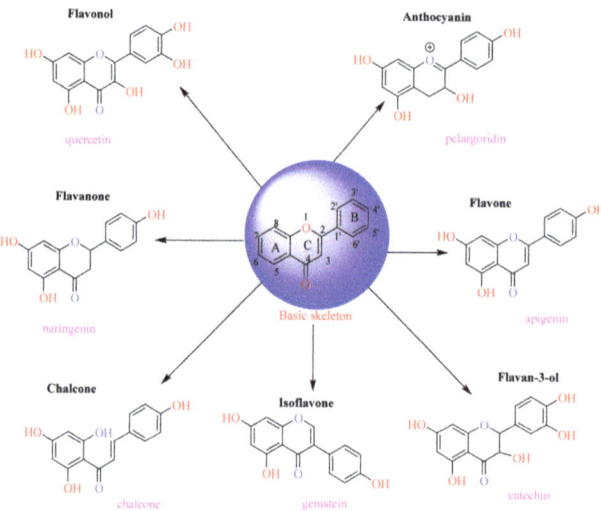

Figure 1. General biosynthetic pathway of flavonoids.

Figure 2. Representative structures of major classes of flavonoids.

4. Isolation of *Euphorbia* Flavonoids

Generally, flavonoids of the *Euphorbia* species are isolated using similar procedures as employed for other chemical constituents. Since all *Euphorbia* parts accumulate these constituents, the stems, aerial parts, roots, fruits, seeds, flowers and in some cases the whole plant are usually investigated. The aerial part is commonly studied since it is known to contain different phenolic compounds, especially flavonoids [44–46]. However, isolation of these constituents is a complex procedure, because they occur in small quantities as complex mixtures of sugars with similar or related structural parent skeletal framework. Thus, their isolation and identification require the use of a multistep method. The common procedure involves three main stages, including plant preparation, extraction and fractionation of the crude extracts into discrete portions of similar Rf values, and isolation/purification. The sample preparation mostly involves maceration of shade-dried and powdered plant material with methanol or ethanol at room temperature for several days. The resulted filtrates are concentrated under reduced pressure to afford crude extracts. The organic extracts are then subjected to column chromatography with differing step-gradient solvent systems as eluents. Thereafter, the concentrated fractions are monitored by thin-layer chromatography (TLC) using various solvent systems. In cases where the species are rich with flavonoids, the TLC chromatograms of the fractions that have been eluted display intense yellow or brown spots when stained with p-anisaldehyde-sulphuric acid mixture [7].

In some cases, due to trace levels and the complexity of these constituents, they are identified using updated techniques with better resolution and sensitivity such as ultraperformance liquid chromatography coupled with quadrupole tandem time of flight mass spectrometry (UPLC-Q-TOF-MS) or the more traditional techniques such as high-performance liquid chromatography mass spectrometry (HPLC-MS) or vacuum liquid chromatography (VLC) and rotation planar chromatography (RPC) over silica gel using step gradient elution [44].

5. Flavonoids Isolated from *Euphorbia* Species

The current report documents the isolation, identification, structure, biological activities, structure–activity relationships and the therapeutic potential of various types of flavonoids from more than 30 *Euphorbia* species in the past two decades as summarized in Table 1. Of the species that have been investigated, over 80 different types of flavonoids (**1–85**) have been isolated from the aerial parts, roots, seeds and whole plant of these species. Over 50 of these compounds were isolated from the aerial and roots extracts, representing about 90% of all flavonoids reported. It could therefore be suggested that the concentration of these chemical constituents is in the aerial and roots parts. Many of these compounds were derived from the ethanol or methanol extracts of these plant parts. Among the investigated species, *E. lunulata* (number of isolated flavonoids (n) = 33) [26,47], *E. humifusa* (n = 11) [48], *E. hirta* (n = 10) [49] and *E. tirucalli* (n = 8) [50] were frequently investigated species, with *E. lunulata* [26,47] recording the highest number of isolated flavonoids (n = 33). In contrast, *E. mygdaloides* [51], *E. paralias* [52], *E. stenoclada* [53], *E. altotibetic* [51,54], *E. allepica* [51,55] and *E. magalanta* [51] were the least-investigated species, having the least number of isolated flavonoids (n = 1). Others include *E. helioscopia* (n = 7) [56], *E. lathyris* (n = 3) [57], *E. humifusa* [58], *E. ebracteolata* (n = 4) [59] and *E. lunulata* [60]. Future studies should therefore be directed on these species, as they remain a promising source of bioactive constituents.

Most of the isolated flavonoids were flavonols and comprise simple *O*-substitution patterns, C-methylation, prenylation, and adducts of quercetin (**55**) and kaempferol (**30**). Others have a glycoside, glycosidic linkages and a carbohydrate attached at either C-3 or C-7, and have been designated as D-glucose such as kaempferol 3-*O*-glucoside (**31**), L-rhamnose such as kaempferol-3-L-rhamnoside (**37**), or glucorhamnose such as kaempferol-3-*O*-α-rhamnoside-*O*-β-D-glucopyranoside (**39**). Of these, prenylated and glycosylated flavonols remain the most abundant classes of reported flavonoids in the review period, representing about 80% of all reported flavonoids in *Euphorbia* species to date. However, flavanones and chalcones have also been reported within the review period. For instance, 2′,4,4′-trihydroxychalcone (**9**) [56], has been reported from *E. helioscopia*. In addition, Laila [48] reported the isolation of 3,5,3′-trihydroxy-6,7-D-methoxy-4′ (7″-hydroxygeranyl-1″-ether) flavone (**10**) and 5,7,8,3′,4′-pentahydroxy-3-methoxyflavone (**19**) from the methanol extracts of *E. paralais* and *E. retusa*, respectively. Reported literature also shows that the flavone category makes up the second-largest group of flavonoids of the *Euphorbia* species, and includes apigenin (**21**), *O*-methylated flavones such as acacetin (**20**) from *E. bivonae* as well as flavonoid glycosides such as rutin (**81**) from *E. guyoniana*, kaempferol-3-*O*-α-dirhamnoside-*O*-β-D-glucopyranoside (**39**) from *E. bivonae* and kaempferol-3-rutinoside (**15**) from *E. larica*, among others. Most of the studied species contain one or many different classes of these flavonoids. Table 1 gives a summary of the isolated flavonoids, their structures, occurrence and their pharmacological effect.

Table 1. Reported flavonoids from *Euphorbia* species.

No	Compound Structure and Name	Classification	Species Name	Plant Part, Solvent	Biological Effect	Reference
1.	R_1 = β-D-glucopyranoside quercetin 3-O-β-D-rutinoside	Glucosidic flavonol	E. microsciadia	Aerial, EtOH	Antiproliferative	[45]
2.	R_1 = α-L-rhamnopyranosyl(1-6)-β-D-glucopyranoside myricetin 3-O-β-D-galactopyranoside	Glucosidic flavonol	E. microsciadia	Aerial, EtOH	Antiproliferative	[45]
3.	R_1 = β-D-galactopyranoside quercetin 3-O-β-D-galactopyranoside	Glucosidic flavonol	E. microsciadia, E. heterophylla	Aerial, EtOH	Antiproliferative	[45,46]
4.	ampelopsin	Flavonol	E. tirucalli	Whole plant, EtOH	Antibacterial, antifungal	[50]
5.	myricetin	Flavonol	E. tirucalli	Whole plant, EtOH	Antibacterial, antifungal	[49]

Table 1. Cont.

No	Compound Structure and Name	Classification	Species Name	Plant Part, Solvent	Biological Effect	Reference
6.	R=β-D-glucopyr-anosyl-(2″→1‴)-O-α-L-rhamnopyranoside R₁=p-coumaroyl hirtacoumaroflavonoside (7-O-(p-coumaroyl)-5,7,4-trihydroxy-6-(3,3-dimethylallyl)-flavonol-3-O-β-D-glucopyr-anosyl-(2″→1‴)-O-α-L-rhamnopyranoside)	Carbohydrate flavonol	E. hirta	Roots, MeOH	Inhibitory activity (α-glucosidase)	[49]
7.	dimethoxyquercitrin	Glucosidic flavonol	E. hirta	Roots, MeOH	Inhibitory activity (α-glucosidase)	[49]
8.	2-(3,4-dihydroxy-5-methoxy-phenyl)-3,5-dihydroxy-6,7-dimethoxychromen-4-one	Flavonol	E. neriifolia	EtOH, leaves	Ant-oxidant	[61]
9.	2′,4,4′-trihydroxychalcone	Chalcone	E. helioscopia	Whole plant, EtOH	Not evaluated	[56]
10.	3,5,3′-trihydroxy-6,7-dimethoxy-4′(7″-hydroxygeranyl-1″-ether) flavone	Flavone	E. paralais	Whole plant, MeoH	Not evaluated	[48]

Table 1. Cont.

No	Compound Structure and Name	Classification	Species Name	Plant Part, Solvent	Biological Effect	Reference
11.	3,5,7-trihydroxi-2-(3′,4′,5′ trihidroxefenil)-2,3 dihidrobenzopiran-4-ona	Flavonol	E. tirucalli, E. helioscopia	Roots, EtOH	Antimicrobial	[50,56,62]
12.	3,5,7-trihydroxy-8-methoxyflavone	Flavone	E. lunulata	Aerial, EtOH		[26,47]
13.	3,5,7-trihydroxy-2-2(3′, 4′, 5′-trihydroxyphenyl) benzopyran-4-one	Flavonol	E. tirucalli	Roots, EtOH	Antimicrobial	[50,63]
14.	3-O-methylquercetin	Flavonol	E. lunulata	Aerial, EtOH	Antiproliferative	[25,26]
15.	kaempferol 3-O-rutinoside	Glucosidic flavonol	E. larica, E. virgata, E. mgalanta, E. helioscopia, E. bivonae, E. ebracteolata	Whole plant, EtOH	Not evaluated	[56,64–66]
16.	5,7,2′,5′-tetrahydroxyflavone	Flavone	E. lunulata	Aerial, EtOH	Antiproliferative	[25,26]

Table 1. Cont.

No	Compound Structure and Name	Classification	Species Name	Plant Part, Solvent	Biological Effect	Reference
17.	hirtaflavonoside-B (5,7,3',4'-trihyroxy-6-(3,3-dimethyl allyl)-8-9-iso-butenyl)-flavonol-3-O-β-D-glucosidase)	Glucosidic flavonol	E. hirta	Roots, MeOH	Inhibitory activity (α-glucosidase)	[49]
18.	6-methoxyapigenin	Flavone	E. larica, E. lunulata	Aerial, EtOH	Antiproliferative	[29,67]
19.	5,7,8,3',4'-pentahydroxy-3-methoxyflavone	Flavone	E. retusa	Whole plant, MeOH	Not evaluated	[48]
20.	acacetin	Flavone	E. bivonae	Roots, MeOH	Not evaluated	[66]
21.	apigenin	Flavone	E. lunulata, E. condylocarpa	Aerial, EtOH	Antiproliferative, antioxidant, anti-tumour, anti-inflammatory, antibacterial, antiproliferative	[25,26,68]
22.	apigenin-7-O-(6''-O-galloyl)-β-D-glucopyranoside R=-(6''-O-galloyl)-β-D-glucopyranoside)	Glucosidic flavone	E. humifusa	Whole plant, EtOH	Anti-HBV	[58]

Table 1. Cont.

No	Compound Structure and Name	Classification	Species Name	Plant Part, Solvent	Biological Effect	Reference
23.	R=O-β-D-Glc apigenin-7-O-β-D-glucoside	Glucosidic flavone	E. lunulata, E. humifusa	Aerial, EtOH	Anti-HBV	[26,54,58]
24.	aromadendrin	Flavonol	E. cuneate	Aerial, EtOH	Antiulcerogenic	[69]
25.	glabrone	Flavone	E. helioscopia	Whole plant, EtOH	Not evaluated	[56]
26.	hyperoside	Flavone	E. lunulata	Aerial, EtOH	Antiproliferative	[26,70]
27.	hyperin	Glucosidic flavonol	E. lunulata	Whole plant, C_3H_6O	Antiproliferative	[60]
28.	isoquercetin	Glucosidic flavonol	E. lunulata, E. tirucalli, E. ebracteolata	Aerial, EtOH	Antiproliferative	[25,26,50,71]

Table 1. Cont.

No	Compound Structure and Name	Classification	Species Name	Plant Part, Solvent	Biological Effect	Reference
29.	jaceosidin	Flavone	E. lunulata	Aerial, EtOH	Antiproliferative	[26,67]
30.	kaempferol	Flavonol	E. guyoniana, E. allepica, E. charnaesyce, E. rnagalanta, E. virgate, E. lunulata, E. hirta, E. wallichii	Aerial; C_3H_6O:MeOH, whole plant; Me_2CO_2, Leaf; EtOH	Not evaluated	[26,29,55, 72–74]
31.	kaempferol 3-O-glucoside	Glucosidic flavonol	E. guyoniana, E. rnagalanta, E. charnaesyce, E. virgata	Aerial, C_3H_6O:MeOH, Leaf; EtOH	Not evaluated	[29,72]
32.	kaempferol 3-O-β-D-glucopyranoside	Glucosidic flavonol	E. altotibetic, E. retusa	Whole plant		[54]
33.	R=O-β-D-glucopyranosyl-(1→4)-α-L-rhamnopyranosyl-(1→6)-β-D-galactopyranoside kaempferol 3-O-β-D-glucopyranosyl-(1→4)-α-L-rhamnopyranosyl-(1→6)-β-D-galactopyranoside	Carbohydrate flavonol	E. ebracteolata	Aerial, EtOH	Not evaluated	[59]
34.	isorhamnetin	Flavanone	E. hirta, E. guyoniana, E. charnaesyce, E. rnagalanta, E. amygdaloides	Aerial, C_3H_6O:MeOH, Leaf; EtOH	Not evaluated	[29,72,75]

Table 1. Cont.

No	Compound Structure and Name	Classification	Species Name	Plant Part, Solvent	Biological Effect	Reference
35.	kaempferol-3-O-β-D-glucuronide	Glucosidic flavonol	E. lathyris	Aerial, EtOH	Cytotoxic	[57]
36.	R=glucuronide kaempferol-3-glucuronide	Glucosidic flavonol	E. lathyris	Aerial, MeoH	Not evaluated	[51,57]
37.	R=O-L-Rh kaempferol-3-L-rhamnoside	Carbohydrate flavonol	E. lunulata	Aerial, EtOH	Antiproliferative	[26,70]
38.	R=O-(6″-O-Galloyl)-β-D-Glc kaempferol-3-O-(6″-galloyl)-β-D-glucoside	Carbohydrate flavonol	E. lunulata, E. fischeriana, E. esula	Aerial, EtOH	Antiproliferative	[26,76]
39.	R=O-α-dirha-O-β-D-glucopyranoside kaempferol-3-O-α-rhamnoside-O-β-D-glucopyranoside	Carbohydrate flavonol	E. bivonae	Roots, MeOH	Not evaluated	[66]
40.	R=O-β-D-Glc kaempferol-3-O-β-D-glucoside	Glucosidic flavonol	E. lunulata, E. fischeriana, E. esula	Aerial, EtOH	Antiproliferative	[26,76]

Table 1. Cont.

No	Compound Structure and Name	Classification	Species Name	Plant Part, Solvent	Biological Effect	Reference
41.	R=O-glucose-rhamnose 4′-O-methoxy-luteolin-7-O-rhamnoglucoside	Carbohydrate flavonol	E. cuneate	Aerial, EtOH	Antiulcerogenic	[69]
42.	R=O-β-glucopyranosyl kaempferol-3-β-D glucopyranosyl	Glucosidic flavonol	E. retusa	Whole plant, MeOH	Not evaluated	[48]
43.	R=O-β-D-Gal kaempferol-7-O-β-D-glucoside	Glucosidic flavonol	E. lunulata, E. fischeriana, E. esula	Aerial, EtOH	Antiproliferative	[26,76]
44.	licochalcone A	Chalcone	E. helioscopia	Whole plant, EtOH	Not evaluated	[56]
45.	licochalcone B	Chalcone	E. helioscopia	Whole plant, EtOH	Not evaluated	[56]
46.	luteolin	Flavone	E. lunulata, E. hirta, E. humifusa, E. bivonae	Aerial, whole plant, roots, EtOH,	Antiproliferative, Anti-HBV	[25,26,58,66,73]

Table 1. Cont.

No	Compound Structure and Name	Classification	Species Name	Plant Part, Solvent	Biological Effect	Reference
47.	R=O-(6''-O-coumaroyl)-β-D-glucopyranoside luteolin-7-O-(6''-O-coumaroyl)-β-D-glucopyranoside	Glucosidic flavonol	E. humifusa	Whole plant, EtOH	Anti-HBV	[58]
48.	R=O-(6''-trans-feruloyl)-β-D-glucopyranoside luteolin-7-O-(6''-O-trans-feruloyl)-β-D-glucopyranoside	Glucosidic flavonol	E. humifusa	Whole plant, EtOH	Anti-HBV	[58]
49.	R=glu luteolin-7-O-β-D-glucopyranoside	Glucosidic flavonol	E. humifusa	Whole plant, EtOH	Anti-HBV	[58]
50.	myricetin	Flavonol	E. lunulata, E. wallichii	Aerial, EtOH	Antiproliferative	[25,26,74]
51.	R=O-(2'', 3''-O-digalloyl)-β-D-Gal myricetin-3-O-(2'',3''-digalloyl)-β-D-galactopyranoside	Carbohydrate flavone	E. lunulata	Aerial, EtOH	Antiproliferative	[25,26]
52.	R=O-(2'''-galloyl)-β-D-Gal myricetin-3-O-(2''-galloyl)-β-D-galactopyranoside	Carbohydrate flavone	E. lunulata	Aerial, EtOH	Antiproliferative	[25,26]

Table 1. Cont.

No	Compound Structure and Name	Classification	Species Name	Plant Part, Solvent	Biological Effect	Reference
53.	myricitrin	Glucosidic flavone	E. lunulata	Aerial, EtOH	Antiproliferative	[25,26]
54.	naringenin-7-O-β-D-glucoside	Glucosidic flavone	E. lunulata	Aerial, EtOH		[26,54]
55.	quercetin	Flavonol	E. guyoniana, E. stenoclada, E. hirta, E. neriifolia, E. charnaesyce, E. rnagalanta, E. virgate, E. lunulata, E. humifusa, E. helioscopia, E. tirucalli	Aerial, leaves, C_3H_6O:MeOH, Leaf; EtOH	Antiproliferative, anti-HBV, antidiarrheal, anticancer, antimalarial, antibacterial, antifungal	[26,29,50, 53,58,62, 67,72,77]
56.	R=O-(2",3"-digalloyl)-β-D-Glc quercetin 3-O-(2',3'-digalloyl)-β-D-galactopyranoside	Carbohydrate flavonol	E. lunulata	Whole plant, C_3H_6O	Antiproliferative	[60]
57.	R=O-(2"-O-Galloyl)-β-D-Gal quercetin 3-O-(2'-galloyl)-β-D-galactopyranoside	Carbohydrate flavonol	E. lunulata	Whole plant, C_3H_6O	Antiproliferative	[60]
58.	R=O-(2",3"-digalloyl)-β-D-galactopyranoside quercetin 3-O-(2",3"-digalloyl)-β-D-galactopyranoside	Carbohydrate flavonol	E. lunulata	Roots, MeOH	Antiproliferation activity	[78]

Table 1. Cont.

No	Compound Structure and Name	Classification	Species Name	Plant Part, Solvent	Biological Effect	Reference
59.	quercetin 3-O-(2″-galloyl)-β-D-galactopyranoside	Carbhydrate flavonol	E. lunulata	Roots, MeOH	Antiproliferation activity	[78]
60.	quercetin 3-O-6″-(3-hydroxyl-3-methylglutaryl)-β-D-glucopyranoside	Glucosidic flavonol	E. ebracteolata	Aerial, EtOH	Not evaluated	[59]
61.	quercetin 3-O-6′-(3hydroxyl-3-methylglutaryl)-β-D-glucopyranoside	Glucosidic flavonol	E. ebracteolata	Aerial, MeOH	Not evaluated	[78,79]
62.	quercetin 3-O-glucoside	Glucosidic flavonol	E. guyoniana, E. charnaesyce, E. virgate, E. paralias, E. condylocarpa	Aerial, whole plant, C_3H_6O:MeOH, Leaf; EtOH	Anticancer against colon, breast, hepato cellular and lung cancer cell lines, inhibitory activities	[29,52,68,72]

Table 1. Cont.

No	Compound Structure and Name	Classification	Species Name	Plant Part, Solvent	Biological Effect	Reference
63.	R=O-α-L-rhamnopyranoside quercetin 3-O-α-L-rhamnopyranoside	Carbohydrate flavonol	E. heterophylla	Aerial, EtOH	Not evaluated	[46]
64.	quercetin 3-O-β-D-6″-malonate	Carbohydrate flavonol	E. heterophylla	Aerial, EtOH	Not evaluated	[46]
65.	R= glu quercetin 3-O-β-D-glucopyranoside	Glucosidic flavonol	E. paralias, E. humifusa, E. microsciadia, E. heterophylla, E. ebracteolata	Whole plant, Aerial, EtOH	Ant-HBV	[45,52,58,71]
66.	R=O-β-D-Glc quercetin-3-O-β-glucuronic	Glucosidic flavonol	E. lunulata, E. esula	Aerial, EtOH	Antiproliferative	[26,80]
67.	R=O-L-Rha quercetin-3-L-rhamnoside	Carbohydrate flavonol	E. lunulata	Aerial, EtOH	Antiproliferative	[26,70]
68.	R=(2″-galloyl)-β-D-galactopyranoside quercetin-3-O-(2″-galloyl)-β-D-galactopyranoside	Glucosidic flavonol	E. lunulata	Aerial, EtOH	Antiproliferative	[26,70]

Table 1. Cont.

No	Compound Structure and Name	Classification	Species Name	Plant Part, Solvent	Biological Effect	Reference
69.	R= O-(2″,3″-digalloyl)-β-D-Gal quercetin-3-O-(2″,3″-digalloyl)-β-D-galactopyranoside	Glucosidic flavonol	E. lunulata	Aerial, EtOH	Antiproliferative	[26,70]
70.	R=O-(6″-O-Galloyl)-β-D-Gal quercetin-3-O-(6″-galloyl)-β-D-galactopyranoside	Carbohydrate flavonol	E. lunulata	Aerial, EtOH		[26,54]
71.	R= rha(1→2)gal quercetin-3-O-α-L-rhamnosyl (1→6)-β-D-galactoside	Carbohydrate flavonol	E. humifusa	Whole plant, EtOH	Anti-HBV	[58]
72.	R=O-α-L-Rh quercetin-3-O-α-rhamnoside	Carbohydrate flavonol	E. hirta	Whole plant, MeOH	Anti-snake venom activity	[81]
73.	R= β-D-glucopyr-(1-4)-O-β-Lrha quercetin-3-O-β-D-glucopyranosyl-(1-4)-O-α-L-rhamnopyranoside	Carboydrate flavonol	E. drancunculoides	Aerial, EtOH	Cytotoxic	[82]

Table 1. Cont.

No	Compound Structure and Name	Classification	Species Name	Plant Part, Solvent	Biological Effect	Reference
74.	quercetin-3-O-β-D-galactoside (R= gal)	Glucosidic flavonol	E. humifusa,	Whole plant, EtOH,	Anti-HBV, cytotoxic	[58]
75.	quercetin-3-O-β-L-rhamnoside (R= β-L-rha)	Carbohydrate flavonol	E. lunulata, E. fischeriana, E. esula	Aerial, EtOH	Antiproliferative	[26,76]
76.	quercetin-7-O-β-D-glucoside (R=O-β-D-Glc)	Glucosidic flavonol	E. lunulata, E. fischeriana, E. esula	Aerial, EtOH	Antiproliferative	[26,76]
77.	quercetin 3-O-6″-(3-hydroxy-3-methylglutaryl)-β-D-glucopyranoside	Glucosidic flavonol	E. ebracteolata	leaves		[83]
78.	quercitrin	Glucosidic flavonol	E. stenoclada, E. tirucalli	Aerial, MeOH, EtOH	Antiproliferative, antibacterial, antifungal	[50,53]

Table 1. Cont.

No	Compound Structure and Name	Classification	Species Name	Plant Part, Solvent	Biological Effect	Reference
79.	pinocembrin	Flavone	E. hirta	Aerial, EtOH	Not evaluated	[75]
80.	rhamnetin-3-α-arabinofuranoside	Carbohydrate flavonol	E. lathyris, E-amygdaloides	Aerial, EtOH	Not evaluated	[51,75]
81.	rutin	Glucosidic flavonol	E. guyoniana, E. charnaesyce, E. rnagalanta, E. virgate, E. tirucalli, E. ebracteolata	Aerial, C_3H_6O:MeOH, Leaf; EtOH	Antibacterial, antifungal	[29,50,71,72]
82.	eriodictyol	Flavone	E. matabelensis	Stems, MeOH	Antiproliferative	[84]
83.	naringenin	Flavone	E. matabelensis	Stems, MeOH	Antiproliferative	[84]
84.	5,7,3′,4′-trihyroxy-6-(3,3–dimethyl allyl)-8-9-iso-butenyl)-flavonol-3-C-β-D-glucosidase	Glucosidic flavonol	E. hirta	Aerial, MeOH	Inhibitory activity (α-glucosidase)	[85]

Table 1. Cont.

No	Compound Structure and Name	Classification	Species Name	Plant Part, Solvent	Biological Effect	Reference
85.	R=apio(1→2)glu apigenin-7-O-β-D-apiofuranosyl(1→2)-β-D-glucopyranoside	Glucosidic flavonol	E. humifusa	Whole plant, EtOH	Anti-HBV	[58]
86.	R=β-D-glucoside isoaromadendrin-7-O-β-D-glucopyranoside (isosinemsin)	Glucosidic flavonol	E. cuneata	Whole plant, EtOH	Hypertensive	[86]

Some flavonoids such as rhamnetin-3-α-arabinofuranoside (80) from *E. amygdaloides*, kaempferol-3-glucuronide (36) from *E. lathyris* [52,57] and quercetin-3-O-β-D-glucopyranosyl-(1-4)-O-α-L-rhamnopyranoside (73) from *E. drancunculoides* were identified for the first time in these species. Phytochemical investigation of *E. humifusa* ethanol extracts resulted in isolation of 13 flavone glucosides. Among them were the uncommonly isolated apigenin-7-O-(6″-O-galloyl)-β-D-glucopyranoside (22), luteolin-7-O-β-D-glucopyranoside (49), luteolin-7-O-(6″-O-trans-feruloyl)-β-D-glucopyranoside (48) as well as luteolin-7-O-(6″-O-coumaroyl)-β-D-glucopyranoside (47). It was interesting to note that luteolin-7-O-(6″-O-trans-feruloyl)-β-D-glucopyranoside (48) and luteolin-7-O-(6″-O-coumaroyl)-β-D-glucopyranoside (47) had similar features as apigenin-7-O-(6″-O-galloyl)-β-D-glucopyranoside (22). The distinctive feature was that the parent structure of apigenin-7-O-(6″-O-galloyl)-β-D-glucopyranoside (22) was apigenin (21) with a galloyl substitution on glucoside, while luteolin-7-O-(6″-O-trans-feruloyl)-β-D-glucopyranoside (48) and luteolin-7-O-(6″-O-coumaroyl)-β-D-glucopyranoside (47) was luteolin (46) with a feruloyl and coumaroyl substituent on the parent ring system, respectively [58].

In addition, flavonoids named kaempferol-3-O-β-D-glucopyranosyl-(1→4)-α-L-rhamnopyranosyl-(1→6)-β-D-galactopyranoside (33) and quercetin 3-O-6″-(3-hydroxyl-3-methylglutaryl)-β-D-glucopyranoside (60) from *E. ebracteolata* were reported for the first time by Xin et al. [59]. This showed the structural diversity of *Euphorbia* flavonoids. A limited number of chalcones have also been isolated from *Euphorbia* species. For instance, licochalcone A (44), 2′,4,4′-trihydroxychalcone (9), licochalcone B (45), and glabrone (25) were isolated from *E. helioscopia* [56]. Most of these flavonoids were identified from the aerial extracts, which also reported significant pharmacological activities. Chemical investigation of the ethanolic root extracts of *E. tirucalli* using chromatographic procedures led to the isolation of a previously unreported flavonoid called myricetin (5) [50]. In addition, previously unreported quercetin 3-O-(2′,3′-digalloyl)-β-D-galactopyranoside (56) was isolated from the acetone whole plant extract of *E. lunulata* [60]. This compound showed weak antiproliferative activities and was found to mimic insulin that is bound with the galloyl group at the galactosyl moiety. Hence, it could become one of the seed molecules that can be used for the development of a nonpeptidyl insulin alternative medicine [60].

6. Biological Studies, Structure–Activity Relationship and Therapeutic Potential

6.1. Cytotoxic Studies

In vitro evaluation of the ethanolic extract of *E. stenoclada* for its antiproliferative activity against human airway smooth muscle cells (HASMC) was conducted by Chaabi et al. [53]. The results showed that the ethanolic extract abolished completely the interleukin-1β (IL-1β)-induced proliferation of HASMC with IC_{50} of 0.73 ± 0.08 µg/mL. However, there was reduced activity of the fractionated crude extracts, suggesting that the crude extract was active due to the synergetic effect of multiple compounds. In addition, no cytotoxic effects were exhibited up to 20 µg/mL. Quercetin (**55**), the major constituent isolated from this extract, showed moderate activity with IC_{50} of 0.49 ± 0.12 µg/mL.

The structure–activity relationship studies using methylated and glycosylated flavonols showed that methylation reduces the antiproliferative activities, while glycosylation lost the activity [53]. For all the quercetin heterosides used, none of them exhibited any activity on the 1β (IL-1β)-induced proliferation of HASMC, an indication that the presence of the hydroxyl group at C-3 is key in retaining the activity, as its substitution resulted in low activity or complete loss of it. In addition, methylation of any of the hydroxyl groups of flavonol also had a negative effect on the activity. This was the case even at higher concentrations, suggesting that the free hydroxyl groups of quercetin (**55**) are all important in retaining its activity and that its substitution by methylation and glycosylation results in a lowering or loss of its activity [53]. It was also found to have a relaxant effect on guinea pig trachea pre-contracted with histamine [78,87] as well as in vitro inhibition of histamine release from the rat peritoneal mast cells by 95–97% [88]. This shows the therapeutic potential of quercetin (**55**) as a promising antiasthmatic agent.

Analysis of the anticancer activities of the flavonoid rich extract of *E. lunulata* showed that it could inhibit the growth of Lewis lung cancer cells in mice and the rabbit serum. It was also shown to significantly inhibit the proliferation of lung cancer cells (A549) in a concentration–time dependent manner. For instance, at a concentration of 20% for 72 h, the proliferation rate of lung cancer cells was 39.08% [89]. The authors suggested that the plant extract could induce cell apoptosis by cell arrest in G1 phase. In addition, Gao et al. [90] found that the hexane extract of *E. lunulata* could inhibit the proliferation of human hepatoma (Hep-G2) cells also in a time–concentration dependent manner in vitro, with an inhibition rate of 0.063 at 2.5 µg/mL and 0.69 at 80 µg/mL after 48 h. This was further related to the mitochondrial pathways and/or cellular pathways of apoptosis.

The flavonoids eriodictyol (**82**) and naringenin (**83**) isolated from *E. metabelensis* tested negative on human normal cells (HeLa), breast cancer (MCF-7) and epithelial human breast cancer (MDA-MB-231) cell lines, and G-protein-gated inwardly rectifying potassium (GIRK) channel-blocking activities in vitro. The IC_{50} values for naringenin (**83**) were reported as 12.43 µM for HeLa, 5.78 µM for MCF-7, and 19.13 µM for MDA-MB-231 cells. Its blocking activity on GIRK channels was reported to be weak with inhibition of $12.18\% \pm 1.39$ for eriodictyol (**82**) and $13.50\% \pm 2.69$ for naringenin (**83**), at 10.00 µM. Despite the negative effect, these compounds possess promising anti-inflammatory, anti-allergenic, antimicrobial, and antioxidant properties [77,84,91–93].

Phytochemical analysis of 15 *Euphorbia* species revealed the presence of flavonoids from the methanol aerial extracts [51]. The plant extracts were evaluated for their in vitro anticancer properties against human liver cancer (HepG-2) and breast cancer (MCF-7) cell lines. The methanol extract of *E. lactea* exhibited good anticancer activities against HepG-2 and MCF-7 cell lines with IC_{50} of 5.20 and 5.10 µg/mL, respectively. Previous anticancer assays of ethanolic extracts from the same species displayed significant activities against a hepatic cancer cell line (HEp-2) with IC_{50} of 89.00 µg/mL [94]. In addition, similar studies have shown that the extract of *E. lactea* displayed anticancer and anti-migratory activities toward cellosaurus (HN22) cells [95]. It was also observed that the extracts of *E. officinarum* and *E. royleana* showed significant activities against human colon cancer adenocarcinoma cell lines (Caco-2) [51]. This was the first assay on the cytotoxicity of *E. officinarum* against these cancer cell lines. Methanol extracts of *E. trigona* reported moderate cytotoxicity against MCF-7 and Caco-2 cells, while previous studies on the latex of *E. trigona* against colon cancer cell lines (HT-29) were found to be inactive [96]. Notably, among the tested *Euphorbia* extracts, only *E. horrida*, *E. tirucalli* and *E. ingens* were inactive against all three tested cell lines. In contrast, previous studies reported good cytotoxic effects of *E. tirucalli* butanol extract against MCF-7 cells as well as against human leukocytes, with IC_{50} of between 100 and 150 µg/mL [97]. The observed anticancer activities were attributed to the presence of identified phenolic and flavonoid constituents in the plant extracts.

Chemical investigation of *E. paralias* whole-plant extracts afforded quercetin-3-*O*-β-D-glucoside (**62**). This compound exhibited moderate toxicity against human liver cancer (HepG-2) and human lung cancer (A549) cells with IC_{50} values of 41 and 36 µM, respectively [52]. It also displayed the ability to inhibit the glutamine synthase enzyme with IC_{50} of 40 µM. Due to the fact that this enzyme is a potential target in the development of new antimycobacterial agents and that it plays an important role as a virulent factor of *Mycobacterium tuberculosis*, quercetin-3-*O*-β-D-glucoside (**62**) could be suggested for development as a potential antituberculotic agent [52]. In addition, Salehi et al. [77] reported the antidiarrheal activities of quercitrin (**78**) isolated from *E. hirta* decoction in mice at doses of 50 mg/kg.

Cheng et al. [62] found that *E. helioscopia* had a high concentration of quercetin (**55**) flavonoid. Evaluation of the extracts showed that it effectively inhibited the growth of HepG2 (human hepatocellular carcinoma lines) at 50 µg/mL in vivo ($p < 0.01$).

Flavonoids show anti-inflammatory and antiproliferative properties through several mechanisms of action such as inhibition of protein kinase and transcription factors, inhibition of phosphodiesterase impact on arachidonic acid metabolisms and effects in immune system, among others. Since protein kinases are essential in signal transduction during cell activation in inflammation, some flavonoids are known to target multiple central kinases involved in the processes of multiple signaling pathways [98]. Flavonoids have also been reported to inhibit kinases such as protein kinase C, phosphatidylinositol kinase, phosphoinositol kinase, tyrosine kinase or cyclin-dependent kinase-4 [99,100]. They are suggested to modulate protein kinases by inhibiting the transcription factors, such as nuclear factor kappa-light chain enhancer of activated B cells (NF-κB) [101], which regulates different chemokines, cytokines and cell adhesion molecules that are involved in inflammation. For example, quercetin (**55**) has been used as an effective colorectal cancer agent and has been shown to exhibit different mechanisms of action, among them antioxidant activity, cell-cycle arrest, modulation of estrogen receptors, increase in apoptosis, inhibition of metastasis, regulation of signaling pathways and angiogenesis [102]. Luteolin (**46**) has shown anticancer activities in hepatocellular carcinoma (HCC) through a pro-apoptotic process and cell-cycle arrest at the G2/M stage [103].

In respect to the inhibition of phosphodiesterase enzyme impact on arachidonic acid metabolisms, flavonoids are known to inhibit the phosphodiesterases signals such as cAMP phosphodiesterase which is a key messenger molecule that regulates cell functions during inflammation stages. Flavonoids have the potential to block phosphodiesterases cAMP degradation and prolong cAMP signaling of the enzyme, thereby exhibiting anti-inflammatory properties [104]. Kaempferol (**30**) was found to stimulate body antioxidants against free radicals that may cause cancer [105], while myricetin (**5**) showed significant anti-inflammatory and anticancer activities by targeting different metabolic pathways in mitochondria that may result in cancer-cell death [106]. Furthermore, the synthetic polylactic-co-glycolic acid (PLGA) nanoparticles from the flavonoid hesperidin decreased the cell viability against C6 glioma cells [106,107]. In addition, the most common benzofuranone, an anticancer flavonoid, was found to have different mechanisms of action against cancer cells as it has multiple targets such as acting on cyclin dependent kinase, adenosine receptor, histone deacetylase, microtubules, telomerase and sirtuins [108].

During inflammation, arachidonic acid is produced from the phospholipids of the plasma membranes by the phospholipase A2 (PLA2) enzyme. The acid is then oxidized by different oxygenases enzymes to produce thromboxanes, leukotrienes prostaglandins and other inflammatory mediators [109]. Flavonoids can inhibit such enzymes that are involved in this process (metabolism of arachidonic acid) and hence reduce the discharge of inflammatory mediators resulting from this pathway. Flavonoids are further suggested to inhibit the biosynthesis of thromboxanes, prostaglandins and leukotrienes by inhibition of the phospholipase A2 (PLA2) [110,111] and cyclooxygenase (COX) [112] enzymes.

Flavonoids can also inhibit maturation of dendritic cells (DCs) by suppressing maturation markers such as CD80, CD86, which are relevant for CD4+T lymphocytes cell activation [113,114]. Flavonoids influence the inflammatory response of dendritic cells by modulation of the iron metabolism [115]. Other studies have shown that some flavonoids decrease the discharge of histamine or prostaglandin from mast cells or can lead to inhibition of pro-inflammatory cytokines or chemokine production in neutrophils, mast cells and other immune cells [116–118]. It has also been demonstrated that flavonoids can bind to cytokine receptors such as the IL-17RA subunit of the IL-17 receptor, leading to the attenuation in its signaling. They can also inhibit the downstream signaling from receptors such as the high affinity receptor and other receptors at the site of inflammation [119].

6.2. Antioxidant Activities

Phytochemical investigation of *E. neriifolia* resulted in identification of the 2-(3,4-dihydroxy-5-methoxy-phenyl)-3,5-dihydroxy-6,7-dimethoxychromen-4-one (**8**) flavonoid from the leaf ethanol extract. This compound scavenged free radicals and reactive oxygen species (ROS), and inhibited lipid peroxidation with antioxidant activity of 76.15% compared to ascorbic acid at 75.6%. This suggests that compound (**8**) may have anticancer potential if such activity can be replicated in vivo. The high concentration of such flavonoids in *E. neriifolia* has been predicted to be responsible for the observed antioxidative mechanisms, which may be useful therapeutically, as oxidation has been implicated in causing several degenerative diseases [61].

A previous study by the same group reported that the pre-hepato-carcinogenesis, which is commonly induced by N-nitrosodiethylamine (DENA), was inhibited by the 70% hydro-ethanolic (v/v) extract of *E. neriifolia* and by the isolated flavonoid (**8**) [120]. These bioactive constituents, especially flavonoids and saponins, are known to neutralize the free radicals and other metabolic intermediate products that are highly reactive due to the presence of an unpaired electron. Hence, they are attributed to the observed protective histological effects. These findings could therefore be essential in validation of the ethnomedicinal uses and therapeutic potential of this plant.

Phytochemical investigation of *E. lathyris* showed that the root extract has the highest concentration of rutin flavonoids. However, the antioxidant evaluation of the testa, root and seed extracts showed that 2,2-diphenyl-1-picrylhydrazyl (DPPH) free-radical scavenging activity was highest for the testa extracts (61.29 ± 0.29 mmol Trolox/100 g dry weight of free compounds), while the highest ferric-reducing antioxidant power was shown by the seed extracts (1927.43 ± 52.13 mg $FeSO_4$/100 g dry weight of free compounds). It was also established that the DPPH free-radical scavenging activities are dependent on the total phenolic content for different parts of *E. lathyris* extracts, which means that the higher the concentration of flavonoids and other phenolic compounds, the higher is the activity [121].

The postulated mechanism of action of these flavonoids as antioxidants is protection against lipid peroxidation that results in cell death. Quercetin (**55**), a free radical scavenger, was found to exert a protective effect. Furthermore, it was found to prevent free-radical-induced tissue damage in different ways. The most common is suggested to be the direct scavenging of free radicals. By doing so, the flavonoid, specifically quercetin (**55**), could inhibit the oxidized low-density lipoprotein (LDL) oxidation in vitro [122]. This action is known to protect against atherosclerosis. In addition, quercetin (**55**) can offer other potential therapeutic application in the prevention and treatment of allergies, fever and asthma. It was also found to work better when it is used in combination with bromelain [122]. Indeed, flavonoids such as quercetin (**55**) are common in foods such as apples, onions, tea, nuts, berries, cauliflower and cabbage among others. They can therefore provide many health-promoting benefits such as improving cardiovascular health, treatment of eye diseases, arthritis and, allergic disorders, as well as reducing the risk of cancers. Chemical analysis of the ethyl acetate aerial extracts of *E. geniculata* resulted in isolation of rutin (**81**), quercetin-3-*O*-rhamnoside (**75**), quercetin-3-*O*-β-D- glucopyranoside (**65**), and quercetin (**55**). The nephroprotective potential of the plant extract was further evaluated in male rats with thioacetamide-induced kidney injury. The results showed marked nephrotoxicity and were suggested to be through the alteration of kidney biomarkers and improving the redox status of the tissue, hence bringing the serum biochemical parameters to normal levels [123].

Within the larger *Euphorbiaceae* species, other genera have been reported to contain antioxidant flavonoids. For instance, chemical analysis of *Croton* species; *C. andinus*, *C. argentines*, *C. catamarcensis*, *C. cordobensis*, *C. curiosus*, *C. lachnostachyus*, *C. lanatus*, *C. saltensis* and *C. serratifolius* revealed the presence of *O*-glycosides flavonols, including kaempferol, quercetin and isorhamnetin as well as flavones such as apigenin. There was a significant degree ($p > 0.05$) of correlation between relative abundances of phenolic content and quercetin derivatives in these species, with the reducing antioxidant potential [124].

6.3. Anti-Hepatitis Activities

All the isolated flavonoids from *E. humifusa* were evaluated for their anti-HBV activity in vitro [58]. The compounds were assayed for their anti-HBV potential by observing the inhibitory secretion of hepatitis B surface antigen (HBsAg) and hepatitis B e-antigen (HBVe, HBeAg) in HBV-infected HepG-2 cells, at a non-cytotoxic concentration. The flavonoids apigenin-7-*O*-β-D-glucopyranoside (**23**) and apigenin-7-*O*-(6″-*O*-galloyl)-β-D-glucopyranoside (**22**) significantly blocked the secretion of HBsAg and HBeAg in a dose-dependent manner. Apigenin-7-*O*-β-D-glucopyranoside (**23**) inhibited HBsAg secretion and HBeAg secretion by 77.2% and 55.5%, respectively, at a non-cytotoxic concentration of 40 µgmL^{-1}, This was slightly higher than that of apigenin-7-*O*-(6″-*O*-galloyl)-β-D-glucopyranoside (**23**) with inhibition of 82.2% and 65.6% for HBsAg and HBeAg secretion, respectively, at non-cytotoxic concentrations of 80 µgmL^{-1}. Apigenin-7-*O*-(6″-*O*-galloyl)-β-D-glucopyranoside (**22**) has a similar structure to apigenin-7-*O*-β-D-glucopyranoside (**23**) except for the substitution of a galloyl group on C-6 of glucoside. Therefore, it was postulated that the galloyl group could be important in retaining the anti-HBV activity [58].

In contrast, luteolin-7-*O*-β-D-glucopyranoside (**49**) and luteolin-7-*O*-(6″-*O*-trans-feruloyl)-β-D-glucopyranoside (**48**) showed weaker anti-HBV activity, as they had 50% and 33.9% secretion inhibition of HBsAg and HBeAg, respectively, at a non-cytotoxic concentration of 30 µgmL^{-1}. In addition, luteolin-7-*O*-(6″-*O*-coumaroyl)-β-D-glucopyranoside (**48**) displayed weak activity with secretion inhibition of HBsAg and HBeAg at 18.6% and 58.9% at a concentration of 80 µgmL^{-1}. Luteolin (**46**), and quercetin (**55**), on the other hand, were inactive in relation to their high cytotoxicity. In addition apigenin-7-*O*-β-D-apiofuranosyl (1→2)-β-D-glucopyranoside (**85**), quercetin-3-*O*-α-L-rhamnosyl(1→6)-β-D-galactoside (**84**), quercetin-3-*O*-β-D-glucopyranoside (**65**) and quercetin-3-*O*-β-D-galactoside (**74**) (quercetin glucoside) showed no effect. The structure–activity relationship studies revealed that the parent structure (Figure 3) was essential to the anti-HBV activity of these compounds. It was also established that the number of glucosides in the parent structure could significantly influence their cytotoxicity. Furthermore, substitution of an acyl moiety for the glucoside is also important in retaining the anti-HBV activities of these compounds [58].

Analysis of the aerial part extracts of *E. microsciadia* resulted in isolation of four (**1–3, 65**) flavonoids for the first time from this species [45]. These compounds were further evaluated for their immunomodulatory activities in vitro. The results showed lower lymphocyte suppression activity for all the flavonoids compared to prednisolone, the standard drug. It was also established that the suppressive activities of flavonoids having a hydroxyl group at both C-3′-and C-4′ in their B-ring such as quercetin 3-*O*-β-D-galactopyranoside (**3**) were more active than those with C-3′, C-4′ and C-5′ hydroxyl substitution as in myricetin 3-*O*-β-D-galactopyranoside (**2**). In addition, quercetin 3-*O*-β-D-rutinoside and myricetin 3-

O-β-D-galactopyranoside (**2**) were inactive even at a higher concentration of 50 µg/mL [45]. It can therefore be rationalized that the hydroxyl groups at C-3, C-3', C-4', C-5' and the parent structure are essential in retaining the activities and that glycosylation and methylation of these hydroxyl groups lowers the activity. Hence, they can be considered as key pharmacopheric elements of flavonoids as illustrated in Figure 3.

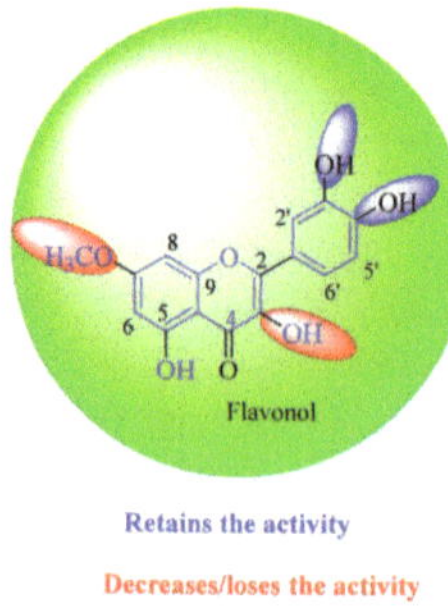

Group	Antibacterial	Anticancer	Anti-inflammatory	Antioxidant
Number of OH	Increase	Increase	Increase	Increase
O-Me	Decrease	Increase	Increase	Increase
C_2=C_3	Retains	Retains	Retains	Retains
3-OH	Increase	Increase	Increase	Increase
Glycosylation	Increase	Decrease	Decrease	Decrease
3'-OH	Increase	Increase	Increase	Increase
4'-OH	Increase	Increase	-	Increase
5'-OH	Decrease	-	Decrease	Decrease

Figure 3. Summary of key pharmacopheric elements of flavonoids.

This was in agreement with previous reports that showed reduction of in vitro biological activities of the glycosylated form of these flavonoids [125]. Glycosylation of quercetin flavonoids reduces the in vitro biological activities compared to their corresponding aglycone forms. The lymphocyte antiproliferative activities of these compounds suggests that the type and the size of the sugar moiety influences the suppression activity on the T-cells. In other similar studies, using five different cell lines (colorectal adenocarcinoma (HT-29), lung carcinoma (A549), breast cancer (MCF-7), hepatocellular carcinoma (HepG-2) and colorectal carcinoma (HCT-116)), quercetin 3-O-β-D-galactopyranoside (**2**) showed the highest growth inhibitory rate of 20% in HT-29 and HepG-2, while rutin (**81**) recorded an inhibitory rate of 15% [126]. Flavonoids have also been suggested to have the capability to inhibit the production of superoxide enzymes such as xanthine oxidase and protein kinase C (PKC). PKC plays a significant role in the activation of T-cells. Hence, the inhibition of PKC by these compounds could be suggested to be their mechanism of action for the observed lymphocyte antiproliferative activities [126].

6.4. Anti-Venom Activities

Quercetin-3-O-rhamnoside (**72**) from the methanol extract of *E. hirta* demonstrated inhibition of the protease, phospholipase (PLA$_2$), hyaluronidase and hemolytic activity of lyophilized snake venom. There was also an increase in survival time of mice that were injected with a mixture of snake venom with quercetin-3-O-rhamnoside (**72**). An increase in concentration of quercetin led to a reduction in edema to 107%, suggesting the inflammation inhibition that is caused by the venom. This could validate the medicinal application of this species traditionally in treating snake and scorpion poisoning [2,4]. Exploring such multifunctional plant molecules with anti-venom activities could further help in development of alternative and complementary medicine for snake- and scorpion-bite treatments, particularly in rural areas where the distribution of snake antivenom is not available. Furthermore, in silico molecular-docking analysis showed that quercetin-3-O-rhamnoside (**72**) interacts more efficiently through hydrogen bonds. The presence of a sugar substituent in quercetin-3-O-rhamnoside (**72**) was found to enhance the enzyme-ligand interactions. This was supported by findings of molecular dynamic simulations in vitro that showed the presence of various amino acid residues at the substrate binding sites of quercetin-3-O-rhamnoside (**72**) over quercetin (**55**). This study can therefore provide a scientific basis for the use of *E. hirta* extracts in traditional medicines [81]. In a related study, two *Jatropha* (*Euphorbiaceae*) species showed marked anti-edematogenic activities. While there was no observed difference when the extracts of the two species (*J. mollissima* and *J. gossypiifolia*) were administered by oral route ($p > 0.05$), through the intraperitoneal route *J. gossypiifolia* exhibited promising anti-edematogenic activity ($p < 0.001$) higher than *J. mollissima*. In antimicrobial studies, only *J. gossypiifolia* displayed antibacterial activity against *Staphylococcus aureus*, *Staphylococcus epidermidis* and *Bacillus cereus* with MIC value of 6.0 μg/μL compared to Vancomycin with MIC value of 0.5 μg/μL [127].

6.5. Antimalarial Activities

The methanol extract of *E. hirta* aerial parts exhibited 90% growth inhibition against *Plasmodium falciparum* at 5 μg/mL and displayed low toxicity against multidrug-resistant KB 3-1 cells [16]. This demonstrates the potential of this plant as an antimalarial agent, which supports the traditional uses in treatment of microbial infections [2]. Moreover, from this extract through a bio-guided methodology, flavonols were identified as quercitrin (**78**), and myricitrin (**53**). These flavonoids were able to inhibit the proliferation of the protozoan parasite responsible for malaria disease, *Plasmodium falciparum* strains FCR-3 (cycloguanil-resistant from Gambia) and CDC1 (chloroquine sensitive), with similar IC_{50} values 2.50 to 11.60 μM, respectively [16]. Antiplasmodial studies of ethanol extracts of the *E. hirta* whole plant showed that the flavonoid rich ethanol extracts did not suppress the chloroquine-sensitive strains of *Plasmodium* in vivo. The extract reduced the parasetemia levels at 44.36% compared to Camosunate (68.35%) [128]. Moreover, in vivo studies on the effects of flavonoids on mean arterial blood pressure and heart rate in albino rats showed that isoaromadendrin-7-O-β-D-glucopyranoside (isosinemsin) isolated from *E. cuneata* exhibited a decrease in blood pressure and heart rate at 16.6 mmHg and 16.6%, respectively [87].

6.6. Antibacterial and Antifungal Activities

Evaluation of extracts and isolated compounds from *E. tirucalli* displayed significant antibacterial and antifungal activities of the extracts against *Staphylococcus aureus* ATCC 6538, *S. brasiliensis* UFPE 121, *E. coli* ATCC 8739 and *C. albicans* UFPE 0231, with minimum inhibition (MIC) values ranging between 256 to 1024 μg/mL. Ampelopsin (**4**) was the most active compound with MIC value of 16 μg/mL against *E. coli* ATCC 8739, compared to tetracycline, with MIC value of 32 μg/mL. This demonstrates the antibacterial potential of *Euphorbia* flavonoids compared to conventional antibiotics. In antifungal studies, myricetin (**5**) showed the highest activity compared to amphotericin B against *C. albicans* UFPE 0231 with MIC value of 32 μg/mL compared to amphotericin B (16 μg/mL) [50]. Similarly, chemical profiling of the hexane extract of *E. royleana* revealed high phenolic and flavonoid contents and displayed significant antimicrobial activities [129]. The extract exhibited antifungal activity against *Aspergillus niger* and antibacterial activity against the Gram-positive bacteria *Bacillus subtilis* [129]. In addition, antibacterial evaluation of *E. guyoniana* extracts showed that the strains used were more sensitive to the flavonoids fractions of *E. guyoniana* with MICs varying from 1.47 to 61.78 mg/mL in the order of *Staphylococcus aureus* > *Streptococcus faecalis* > *Escherichia coli* [130].

In related studies, antibacterial activities of flavonoids from other genera in the Euphorbiaceae family have been reported. For instance, kaempferol 7-O-β-D-(6″-O-cumaroyl)-glucopyranoside, isolated from *Croton piauhiensis* (Euphorbiaceae) leaves, was evaluated for its antibacterial activities. The intrinsic antimicrobial activities and enhancement properties of this compound against *Pseudomonas aeruginosa Escherichia coli* and *Staphylococcus aureus* strains were further investigated. The results revealed that kaempferol 7-O-β-D-(6″-O-cumaroyl)-glucopyranoside had no antibacterial activity against strains tested at concentrations <1024 μg/mL. The combination of kaempferol 7-O-β-D-(6″-O-cumaroyl)-glucopyranoside at a concentration of 128 μg/mL with gentamicin exhibited synergistic effects against *S. aureus* and *E. coli* and also reduced the minimum inhibition (MIC) from 16 μg/mL to 4 μg/mL and 8 μg/mL, respectively [131]. In contrast, Ali et al. [132] showed that 5-7-dihydroxyflavone from *Oroxylum indicum* inhibited the growth of Gram-negative bacteria such as *E. coli* and *P. aeruginosa*. In the same study, the authors reported that the baicalein flavonoid exhibited weak activities against Gram-positive bacteria such as *Bacillus subtilis* and *S. aureus*. The weak activity was attributed to the presence of a new group at C-6. The activities with synergistic effects were attributed to the hydroxyl phenyl groups that have high affinity for proteins [133].

Even though the mechanisms of action of various *Euphorbia* flavonoids have not been fully explored, various mechanisms of action of plant flavonoids have previously been fronted. Flavones are suggested to form a complex with components of the cell wall and thus inhibit further adhesions or microbial growth. For instance, licoflavone C isolated from *Retama raetam* flowers was found to be active against *E. coli* via formation of complexes with extracellular and soluble proteins with MIC value of 7.81 µg/mL [134]. Other postulated mechanisms include inhibition of bacterial enzymes (such as tyrosyl-tRNA synthetase) [135], inhibition of bacterial efflux pump and rise in the susceptibility of existing antibiotics [136], change in cytoplasmic membrane function, nucleic acid synthesis inhibition, decrease in cell attachment, inhibition of energy metabolism, formation of biofilm, changing in membrane permeability, attenuation of the pathogenicity [137,138], damage of the cytoplasmic membrane [137,138], inhibition of nucleic acid synthesis (for instance, the inhibition of DNA gyrase from *E. coli* by quercetin (**55**), and apigenin (**21**) [139]) among others, as summarized in Figure 4. It was further established that the combination of apigenin and ceftazidime damages the cytoplasmic membrane of ceftazidime-resistant enterobacter cloacae, leading to subsequent leakage of intracellular components [140].

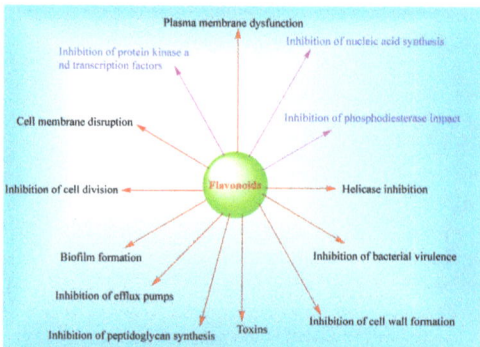

Figure 4. Summary of antibacterial and antifungal mechanisms of actions of flavonoids.

7. Conclusions and Future Perspectives

The extensive utilization of *Euphorbia* species in traditional and complementary medicines for treatment of various diseased conditions has led to increased interest in their phytochemistry and in vitro as well as in vivo studies using cells and animal models. The present review comprises a detailed phytopharmacological account of information available on *Euphorbia* flavonoids between 2000 and 2020. The findings suggest that the extracts and isolated flavonoids possess anticancer, antiproliferative, antimalarial, antibacterial, antivenom, anti-inflammatory, anti-hepatitis and antioxidant properties. Of these, antioxidant and anticancer activities are the most studied biological activities, partly due to the ethnomedicinal application of these species as anticancer agents. Indeed, it is widely accepted that the crude extracts have a synergetic effect compared to individual bioactive compounds. Nonetheless, only a handful of studies assessed the pharmacological potential of *Euphorbia* flavonoids as most studies employed the whole crude extracts. This limits the translational value as researchers are not equipped to determine whether the observed activities are related to the actions of a single bioactive compound or the synergy between multiple constituents present. It was also reported that these flavonoids possess different mechanisms of action against cancer cells. For instance, quercetin exhibited different mechanisms of action such as antioxidant activity, cell-cycle arrest and modulation of estrogen receptors among others. This is essential towards development of a potent anticancer agent. Of the investigated species, over 80 different types of flavonoids have been isolated from the aerial parts, roots, seeds and whole plant of these species. Most of the isolated flavonoids were flavonols and comprised simple O-substitution patterns, C-methylation and prenylation. Others had glycoside, glycosidic linkages and a carbohydrate attached at either C-3 or C-7, and were designated as D-glucose, L-rhamnose or glucorhamnose. A limited number of chalcones were also reported. The structure–activity relationship studies showed that methylation of hydroxyl groups at C-3 or C-7 reduces the activities, while glycosylation results in loss of activity. These constituents can therefore offer a potential alternative for development of therapeutic agents based on the *Euphorbia* species.

While the overall findings suggest a promising future with an abundance of therapeutic potential of the *Euphorbia* species, there are still many aspects of research on these species that need to be considered. These include using species from different ecological zones, adoption of high throughput screening strategies and metabolomics tools for discovery of new bioactive compounds in complex plant matrices, toxicological studies, detailed mechanistic studies and molecular analysis. Furthermore, the current evidence is largely limited to the unverified ethnomedicinal application of these species in folk medicine and their pharmacological studies in vitro. Essentially, more robust scientific studies are needed before confirmatory decisions can be made on the therapeutic potential of flavonoids from *Euphorbia* species.

Author Contributions: Conceptualization, D.K.M. and V.J.T. Literature search D.K.M., M.D., and N.M. Writing and draft preparation D.K.M. Review and editing W.A.A., M.S., L.J.M., R.W., M.K., X.S.-N. and V.J.T. Supervision, V.J.T. All authors have read and agreed to the published version of the manuscript.

Funding: This project was supported by NRF-TWAS, South Africa. National Research Foundation Research grant under grant numbers (99358) and Tshwane University of Technology, Pretoria, South Africa.

Institutional Review Board Statement: Not applicable.

Informed Consent Statement: Not applicable.

Data Availability Statement: Not applicable.

Conflicts of Interest: The authors declare no conflict of interest.

References

1. De Montellano, B.O. Empirical Aztec medicine. *Science* **1975**, *188*, 215–220. [CrossRef] [PubMed]
2. Madeleine, E.; Olwen, M.; Grace, C.; Haris, S.L.; Niclas, N.; Henrik, T.; Nina, R. Global medicinal uses of *Euphorbia* L. (*Euphorbiaceae*). *J. Ethnopharmacol.* **2015**, *76*, 90–101. [CrossRef]
3. Hooper, M. *Major Herbs of Ayurveda*; Elsevier Health Sciences: Amsterdam, The Netherlands, 2002; pp. 340–345.
4. Kemboi, D.; Xolani, P.; Moses, L.; Jacqueline, T. A review of the ethnomedicinal uses, biological activities and triterpenoids of *Euphorbia* species. *Molecules* **2020**, *25*, 4019. [CrossRef] [PubMed]
5. Islam, M.T.; Mata, O.; Aguiar, R.S.; Paz, M.C.J.; Alencar, M.B.; Melo-Cavalcante, A.C. Therapeutic potential of essential oils focusing on diterpenes. *Phytother. Res.* **2016**, *30*, 1420–1444. [CrossRef]
6. Mihail, A.; Viktorija, M.; Liljana, K.G.; Liljana, G.T. Review of the anticancer and cytotoxic activity of some species from the genus *Euphorbia*. *Agric. Conspec. Sci.* **2019**, *84*, 11–23. Available online: https://hrcak.srce.hr/file/318988 (accessed on 1 July 2020).
7. Muhammad, A.; Abdul, S.; Muhammad, J.; Farhat, U.; Muhammad, O.; Ikram, U.; Jawad, A.; Muhammad, S. Flavonoids as prospective neuroprotectants and their therapeutic propensity in aging associated neurological disorders. *Front. Aging Neurosci.* **2019**, 1–20. [CrossRef]
8. Scholz, A. Euphorbiaceae. In *Syllabus der Planzenfamilien*; Engler, A., Ed.; Gebrüder Borntrager: Berlin, Germany, 1964; pp. 255–261.
9. Webster, G.L. Classification of the *Euphorbiaceae*. *Ann. Mol. Bot. Gard.* **1994**, *81*, 3–32. [CrossRef]
10. Andrea, V.; Judit, H. *Euphorbia* diterpenes: Isolation, structure, biological activity, and synthesis (2008–2012). *Chem Rev.* **2014**, *114*, 8579–8612. [CrossRef]
11. Nabavi, S.M.; Samec, D.; Tomczyk, M.; Milella, L.; Russo, D.; Habtemariam, S.; Suntar, I.; Rastrelli, L.; Daglia, M.; Xiao, J. Flavonoid biosynthetic pathways in plants: Versatile targets for metabolic engineering. *Biotechnol. Adv.* **2018**. [CrossRef]

12. Scarano, A.; Chieppa, M.; Santino, A. Looking at flavonoid biodiversity in horticultural crops: A colored mine with nutritional benefits. *Plants* **2018**, *7*, 98. [CrossRef]
13. Sudhakaran, M.; Sardesai, S.; Dose, A.I. Flavonoids: New frontier for immuno-regulation and breast cancer control. *Antioxidants* **2019**, *8*, 103. [CrossRef]
14. Pretorius, J.C. Flavonoids: A review of its commercial application potential as anti-infective agents. *Anti-Infect. Agents Curr. Med. Chem.* **2003**, *2*, 335–353. [CrossRef]
15. Zhao, K.; Yuan, Y.; Lin, B.; Miao, Z.; Li, Z.; Guo, Q.; Lu, N. LW-215, a newly synthesized flavonoid, exhibits potent anti-angiogenic activity in vitro and in vivo. *J. Pharmacol. Sci.* **2018**, *642*, 533–541. [CrossRef]
16. Liu, J.; Wang, X.; Yong, H.; Kan, J.; Jin, C. Recent advances in flavonoid-grafted polysaccharides: Synthesis, structural characterization, bioactivities and potential applications. *Int. J. Biol. Macromol.* **2018**, *116*, 1011–1025. [CrossRef]
17. Camero, C.M.; Germanò, M.P.; Rapisarda, A.; D'Angelo, V.; Amira, S.; Benchikh, F.; Braca, A.; De Leo, M. Anti-angiogenic activity of iridoids from *Galium tunetanum*. *Rev. Bras. Farm.* **2018**, *28*, 374–377. [CrossRef]
18. Patel, K.; Kumar, V.; Rahman, M.; Verma, A.; Patel, D.K. New insights into the medicinal importance, physiological functions and bioanalytical aspects of an important bioactive compound of foods 'Hyperin': Health benefits of the past, the present, the future. *Beni-Suef Univ. J. Basic Appl. Sci.* **2018**, *7*, 31–42. [CrossRef]
19. Zamora-Ros, R.; Guinó, E.; Alonso, M.H.; Vidal, C.; Barenys, M.; Soriano, A.; Moreno, V. Dietary flavonoids, lignans and colorectal cancer prognosis. *Sci. Rep.* **2015**, *5*, 14148. [CrossRef]
20. Avtar, C.; Bhawna, G. Chemistry and Pharmacology of flavonoids—A review. *Indian J. Pharm. Edu. Res.* **2019**, *53*, 8–20. Available online: https://www.ijper.org/article/918 (accessed on 23 February 2021).
21. Reale, G.; Russo, G.I.; di Mauro, M.; Regis, F.; Campisi, D.; Giudice, A.L.; Marranzano, M.; Ragusa, R.; Castelli, T.; Cimino, S. Association between dietary flavonoids intake and prostate cancer risk: A case-control study in Sicily. Complement. *Ther. Med.* **2018**, *39*, 14–18. [CrossRef]
22. Rienks, J.; Barbaresko, J.; Nothlings, U. Association of isoflavone biomarkers with risk of chronic disease and mortality: A systematic review and meta-analysis of observational studies. *Nutr. Rev.* **2017**, *75*, 616–641. [CrossRef]
23. Darband, S.G.; Kaviani, M.; Yousefi, B.; Sadighparvar, S.; Pakdel, F.G.; Attari, J.A.; Mohebbi, I.; Naderi, S.; Majidinia, M. Quercetin: A functional dietary flavonoid with potential chemo-preventive properties in colorectal cancer. *J. Cell. Physiol.* **2018**, *233*, 6544–6560. [CrossRef] [PubMed]
24. Danihelová, M.; Viskupiˇcová, J.; Šturdík, E. Lipophilization of flavonoids for their food, therapeutic and cosmetic applications. *Acta Chim.* **2012**, *5*, 59–69. [CrossRef]
25. Yang, Z.-G.; Jia, L.-N.; Shen, Y.; Ohmura, A.; Kitanaka, S. Inhibitory effects of constituents from *Euphorbia lunulata* on differentiation of 3T3-L1 cells and nitric oxide production in RAW264.7 cells. *Molecules* **2011**, *16*, 8305–8318. [CrossRef] [PubMed]
26. Yuwei, W.; Xiao, Y.; Lingna, W.; Fang, Z.; Yongqing, Z. Research progress on chemical constituents and anticancer pharmacological activities of *Euphorbia lunulata* Bunge. *Bio. Med. Res. Int.* **2020**, 1–11. [CrossRef]
27. Caballero, B.; Trugo, L.; Finglas, P. *Encyclopedia of Food Sciences and Nutrition*, 2nd ed.; Academic Press: London, UK, 2003.
28. Sotnikova, O.M.; Chagovets, R.K.; Litvinenko, V.I. New flavanone compounds from *Euphorbia stepposa*. *Chem. Nat. Compd.* **1968**, *4*, 71–74. [CrossRef]
29. Ulubelen, A.; Öksüz, S.; Halfon, B.; Aynehchi, Y.; Mabry, T.J. Flavonoids from *Euphorbia larica*, *E. virgata*, *E. chamaesyce* and *E. magalanta*. *J. Nat. Prod.* **1983**, *46*, 598. [CrossRef]
30. Dieter, T. Significance of flavonoids in plant resistance: A review. *Environ. Chem. Lett.* **2006**, *4*, 147–157. [CrossRef]
31. Ali, S.; Behrad, D.; Farzaneh, H.; Azadeh, M.; Antoni, S.; Seyed, F.; Leo, R.; Seyed, M.; Anupam, B. Therapeutic potential of flavonoids in inflammatory bowel disease: A comprehensive review. *World J. Gastroenterol.* **2017**, *23*, 5097–5114. [CrossRef]
32. Mariam, A.; Samson, M.; Elizabeth, V.; Sharon, V.; Peter, K.; Alena, L.; Dietrich, B. Flavonoids in cancer and apoptosis. *Cancers* **2019**, *11*, 28. [CrossRef]
33. Bathelemy, N.; Ghislain, W.; Justin, K.; Pantaleon, A.; Tchoukoua, A.; Aimé, G.; Igor, K.; Bonaventure, T.; Berhanu, M.; Victor, K. Flavonoids and related compounds from the medicinal plants of Africa. *J. Med. Plant. Res.* **2019**. [CrossRef]
34. Panche, A.N.; Diwan, A.D.; Chandra, S.R. Flavonoids: An overview. *Sci. World J.* **2013**, *16*. [CrossRef]
35. Shashank, K.; Abhay, K. Chemistry and biological activities of flavonoids: An Overview. *Sci. World J.* **2013**, 1–16. [CrossRef]
36. Nigel, C.; Renee, J. Flavonoids and their glycosides, including anthocyanins. *Nat. Prod. Rep.* **2011**, *28*, 1626. [CrossRef]
37. Goel, G.; Makkar, S.; Francis, G.; Becker, K. Phorbol esters: Structure, biological activity, and toxicity in animals. *Int. J. Toxicol.* **2007**, *26*, 279. [CrossRef]
38. Shi, Q.W.; Su, X.H.; Kiyota, H. Chemical and pharmacological research of the plants in genus *Euphorbia*. *Chem. Rev.* **2008**, *108*, 4295. [CrossRef]
39. Rojas, R.; Tafolla-Arellano, J.C.; Martínez-Ávila, G.C.G. *Euphorbia antisyphilitica* Zucc: A Source of Phytochemicals with Potential Applications in Industry. *Plants* **2021**, *10*, 8. [CrossRef]
40. Yang, T.; Jun, H.; Yu, Y.; Wen-Wen, L.; Cong-Yuan, X.; Jie-Kun, X.; Wei-Ku, Z. *Euphorbia ebracteolata* Hayata (Euphorbiaceae): A systematic review of its traditional uses, botany, phytochemistry, pharmacology, toxicology, and quality control. *Phytochemistry* **2021**, *186*, 112736. [CrossRef]
41. Agati, G.; Azzarello, E.; Pollastri, S.; Tattini, M. Flavonoids as antioxidants in plants: Location and functional significance. *Plant Sci.* **2012**, *196*, 67–76. [CrossRef]

42. Middleton, E. The flavonoids. *Trends Pharmacol. Sci.* **1984**, *5*, 335–338.
43. Murphy, K.; Chronopoulos, A.; Singh, I. Dietary flavanols and procyanidin oligomers from cocoa (Theobroma cacao) inhibit platelet function. *Am. J. Clin. Nutr.* **2003**, *77*, 1466–1473. [CrossRef]
44. Ke, L.; Hang, F.; Peipei, Y.; Lingguang, Y.; Qiang, X.; Xiang, L.; Liwei, S.; Yujun, L. Structure-activity relationship of eight high content flavonoids analyzed with a preliminary assign-score method and their contribution to antioxidant ability of flavonoids-rich extract from *Scutellaria*. *Arab. J. Chem.* **2018**, *11*, 159–170. [CrossRef]
45. Syed, M.; Ghanadiana, A.; Suleiman, A.; Sumaira, H.; Omer, A.; Jean, J. Flavonol glycosides from *Euphorbia microsciadia* Bioss with their immunomodulatory activities. *Iran. J. Pharm. Res.* **2012**, *11*, 925–930. Available online: https://pubmed.ncbi.nlm.nih.gov/24250520/ (accessed on 14 January 2021).
46. De-freitsa, T.J.B.; Silva, A.J.; Kuster, R. Isolation and characterization of polyphenols from *Euphorbia heterophylla* L. (Euphorbiaceae) leaves. *Rev. Fitos* **2019**, *13*, 49–60. [CrossRef]
47. Zhang, W.J. *Study on Chemical Constituents and Antitumor Activity of Euphorbia Lunulata Bge*; Huaqiao University: Quanzhou, China, 2016.
48. Laila, A.-G. Study on Flavonoids and Triterpenoids content of some *Euphorbiaceae* plants. *J. Life Sci.* **2011**, *5*, 100–107. Available online: https://www.researchgate.net/publication/273351317 (accessed on 14 January 2021).
49. Sheliya, M.A.; Rayhana, B.; Ali, A.; Pillai, K.K.; Aeri, V.; Sharmam, R. Inhibition of α-glucosidase by new prenylated flavonoids from *Euphorbia hirta* l. herbs. *J. Ethnopharmacol.* **2015**, *176*, 1–8. [CrossRef]
50. Maria, D.; Luziene, A.C.; Emily, C.; Bruno, O.; M´arcia, V.; Lívia, N.C.; Renata, M. Bioactivity flavonoids from roots of *Euphorbia tirucalli* L. *Phytochem. Lett.* **2021**, *41*, 186–192. [CrossRef]
51. Seham, S.; Raba, M.; Ahmed, F.; Nadia, M.; Sameh, F.; Mohamed, N.; Usama, R.A.; Elham, A. Cytotoxic activity and metabolic profiling of fifteen *Euphorbia* Species. *Metabolites* **2021**, *11*, 15. [CrossRef]
52. Safwat, N.A.; Kashef, M.T.; Aziz, R.K.; Amer, K.F.; Ramadan, M.A. Quercetin 3-O-glucoside recovered from the wild Egyptian Sahara plant, *Euphorbia paralias* L., inhibits glutamine synthetase and has antimycobacterial activity. *Tuberculosis* **2017**, *108*, 106–113. [CrossRef]
53. Chaabi, M.; Freund-Michel, V.; Frossard, N.; Randriantsoa, A.; Andriantsitohaina, R.; Lobstein, A. Anti-proliferative effect of *Euphorbia stenoclada* in human airway smooth muscle cells in culture. *J. Ethnopharmacol.* **2007**, *109*, 134–139. Available online: https://www.sciencedirect.com/science/article/pii/S0378874106003539 (accessed on 14 January 2021). [CrossRef]
54. Li, R.; Wang, J.; Wu, H.X.; Li, L.; Wang, N.L. Isolation, identification and activity determination of antioxidant active components in *Euphorbia lunulata* Bunge. *J. Shenyang Pharm. Univ.* **2011**, *28*, 25–29.
55. Sevil, O.; Faliha, G.; Long-Ze, L.; Roberto, R.; Gil, J.M.; Pezzuto, M.; Geoffrey, A.C. Aleppicatines A and B from *Euphorbia allepica*. *Phytochemistry* **1996**, *42*, 473–478.
56. Wen, Z.; Yue-Wei, G. Chemical studies on the constituents of the chinese medicinal herb *Euphorbia helioscopia* L. *Chem. Pharm. Bull.* **2006**, *54*, 1037–1039. Available online: https://pubmed.ncbi.nlm.nih.gov/16819227/ (accessed on 14 January 2021).
57. Dumkow, K. Kaempferol-3-glucuronide and quercetin-3-glucuronide, principal flavonoids of *Euphorbia lathyris* L. and their separation on acetylated polyamide. *Z. Naturforsch* **1969**, *24*, 358. [CrossRef]
58. Ying, T.; Li-Min, S.; Xi-Qiao, L.; Bin Li, Q.; Jun-Xing, D. Anti-HBV active flavone glucosides from *Euphorbia humifusa* Willd. *Fitoterapia* **2010**, *81*, 799–802. [CrossRef]
59. Liu, X.; Ye, W.; Yu, B.; Zhao, S.; Wu, H.; Che, C. Two new flavonol glycosides from *Gymnema sylvestre* and *Euphorbia ebracteolata*. *Carbohydr. Res.* **2004**, *339*, 891–895. [CrossRef]
60. Tadahiro, N.; Li-Yan, W.; Kouji, K.; Susumu, K. Flavonoids that mimic human ligands from the whole plants of *Euphorbia lunulata*. *Chem. Pharm. Bull.* **2005**, *53*, 305–308. Available online: https://pubmed.ncbi.nlm.nih.gov/15744103/ (accessed on 24 January 2021).
61. Veena, S.; Pracheta, J. Extraction, isolation and identification of flavonoid from *Euphorbia neriifolia* leaves. *Arab. J. Chem.* **2017**, *10*, 509–514. [CrossRef]
62. Cheng, J.; Han, W.; Wang, Z.; Shao, Y.; Wang, Y.; Zhang, Y.; Li, Z.; Xu, X.; Zhang, Y. Hepatocellular carcinoma growth is inhibited by *Euphorbia helioscopia* L. extract in nude mice xenografts. *Bio. Med. Res. Int.* **2015**, 1–9. [CrossRef]
63. Abu-reidah, I.M.; Ali-shtayeh, M.S.; Jamous, R.M.; Arr´aez-rom´an, D.; Segura-carretero, A. HPLC–DAD–ESI-MS/MS screening of bioactive components from *Rhus coriaria* L. (Sumac) fruits. *Food Chem.* **2015**, *166*, 179–191. [CrossRef]
64. Markham, K.R.; Ternai, B. 13C NMR of flavonoids-ii flavonoids other than flavone and flavonol aglycones. *Tetrahedron* **1976**, *32*, 2607–2612. [CrossRef]
65. Ahn, B.T.; Lee, K.S. Phenolic compounds from *Euphorbia ebracteolata*. *Saengyak Hakhoechi* **1996**, *27*, 136–141.
66. Heba, I.; Abd, E.-M. Flavonoid and phenolic acid compounds in *Euphorbia bivonae* Steud roots. *Curr. Sci. Int.* **2015**, *4*, 668–676. Available online: http://www.curresweb.com/csi/csi/2015/668-676.pdf (accessed on 2 February 2021).
67. Liu, C.; Sun, H.; Wang, W.T. Study on chemical constituents of *Euphorbia lunulata* bge. *J. Chin. Med. Mater.* **2015**, *3*, 514–517.
68. Hassana, G.K.; Omera, M.A.; Babadoust, S.; Najata, D.D. Flavonoids from *Euphorbia condylocarpa* roots. *Int. J. Chem. Bio. Sci.* **2014**, *6*, 56–60. Available online: http://www.iscientific.org/wp-content/uploads/2018/02/8-IJCBS-14-06-05.pdf (accessed on 2 February 2021).
69. Amani, S.A.; Nabilah, A.; John, E.; Reham, M.; Mohamed, E. Antiulcerogenic activities of the extracts and isolated flavonoids of *Euphorbia cuneata* Vahl. *Phytother. Res.* **2013**, *27*, 126–130. [CrossRef]

70. Shang, T.M.; Wang, L.; Liang, X.T. Study on the chemical constituents of *Euphorbia Lunulata*. *J. Chem.* **1979**, *37*, 119–128.
71. Lee, S.C.; Ahn, B.T.; Park, W.Y.; Lee, S.H.; Ro, J.S.; Lee, K.S.; Ryu, E.K. Pharmacognostic study on *Euphorbia ebracteolata*. Flavonoid constituents. *Korean J. Pharmacogn.* **1992**, *23*, 126–131.
72. Tarek, B.; Hichema, A.; Khalfallaha, A.; Kabouchea, Z.; Kabouchea, I.; Jaime, B.; Christian, B. A New alkaloid and flavonoids from the aerial parts of *Euphorbia guyoniana*. *Nat. Prod. Commun.* **2010**, *5*, 1–3. Available online: https://pubmed.ncbi.nlm.nih.gov/20184016/ (accessed on 2 February 2021).
73. Wu, Y.; Qu, W.; Geng, D.; Liang, J.-Y.; Luo, Y.-L. Phenols and flavonoids from the aerial part of *Euphorbia hirta*. *Chin. J. Nat. Med.* **2012**, *10*, 40–42. [CrossRef]
74. Abida, T.; Ismat, N.; Hifsa, M. Isolation of flavonols from Euphorbia wallichii by preparative High Performance Liquid Chromatography. *Nat. Sci.* **2009**, *7*, 1–3. Available online: http://www.sciencepub.net/nature (accessed on 2 February 2021).
75. Mueller, R.; Pohl, R. Flavonol glycosides of *Euphorbia amygdaloides* and their quantitative determination at various stages of plant development. 5. Flavonoids of native *Euphorbiaceae*. *Planta Med.* **1970**, *18*, 114–129. [CrossRef]
76. Chai, G.S. Study on the chemical constituents of the seeds of *Euphorbia Fischeriana* Steud and *Euphorbia Esula Linn*. Qiqihar University, Qiqihar, China. Chemo-prevention. *Food Chem.* **2013**, *138*, 2099–2107. [CrossRef]
77. Salehi, B.; Iriti, M.; Vitalini, E.; Antolak, H.; Pawlikowska, E.; Kręgiel, D.; Sharifi-rad, J.; Oyeleye, S.I.; Ademiluyi, A.O.; Czopek, K.; et al. *Euphorbia*-derived natural products with potential for use in health maintenance. *Biomolecules* **2019**, *9*, 337. [CrossRef]
78. Ozbílgín, S.; Saltan, G. Uses of some *Euphorbia* species in traditional medicine in turkey and their biological activities. *Turk. J. Pharm. Sci.* **2012**, *9*, 241–256.
79. Liu, Z.G.; Li, Z.L.; Bai, J.; Meng, D.L.; Li, N.; Pei, Y.H.; Zhao, F.; Hua, H.M. Anti-inflammatory diterpenoids from the roots of *Euphorbia ebracteolata*. *J. Nat. Prod.* **2014**, *77*, 792–799. [CrossRef]
80. Halaweish, F.; Kronberg, S.; Rice, J. Rodent and ruminant ingestive response to flavonoids in *Euphorbia esula*. *J. Chem. Ecol.* **2003**, *5*, 1073–1082. [CrossRef]
81. Kadiyala, G.; Anbarasu, K.; Kadali, R.; Jayanthi, S.; Vishwanath, B.S.; Gurunathan, J. Quercetin-3-O-rhamnoside from *Euphorbia hirta* protects against snake venom induced toxicity. *Biochim. Biophys. Acta* **2016**, *1860*, 1528–1540. [CrossRef]
82. Noori, M.; Chehreghani, A.; Kaveh, M. Flavonoids of 17 species of *Euphorbia* (Euphorbiaceae). *Iran. Toxicol. Environ. Chem.* **2009**, *91*, 631–641. [CrossRef]
83. Byung, T.A.; Kapjin, O.; Jai, S.R.; Kyong, S.L. A New Flavonoid from *Euphorbia ebracteolata*. *Planta Med.* **1996**, *62*, 383–384.
84. Reham, H.; Norbert, K.; Peter, W.; Ágnes, K.; István, Z.; Péter, O.; László, T.; Judit, H.; Andrea, V. Isolation and pharmacological investigation of compounds from *Euphorbia matabelensis*. *Nat. Prod. Commun.* **2019**, 1–5. [CrossRef]
85. Martinez, V.M.; Ramirez, A.T.; Lazcano, M.; Bye, R. Anti-inflammatory Active Compounds from then-hexane extract of *Euphorbia hirta*. *J. Mex. Chem. Soc.* **1999**, *43*, 103–105.
86. Bahar, A.; Tawfeq, A.; Jaber, S.m.; Kehel, T. Isolation, antihypertensive activity and structure activity relationship of flavonoids from medicinal plants. *Indian J. Chem.* **2005**, *44*, 400–404. Available online: http://nopr.niscair.res.in/bitstream/123456789/8947/1/IJCB%2044B(2)%20400-404.pdf (accessed on 2 February 2021).
87. Ko, W.C.; Wang, H.L.; Lei, C.B.; Shih, C.H.; Chung, M.I.; Lin, C.N. Mechanisms of relaxant action of 3-O-methylquercetin in isolated guinea pig trachea. *Planta Medica* **2002**, *68*, 30–35. [CrossRef]
88. Haggag, E.G.; Abou-Moustafa, M.A.; Boucher, W.; Theoharides, T.C. The effect of herbal water-extract on histamine release from mast cells and on allergic asthma. *J. Herb. Pharmacother.* **2003**, *3*, 41–54. Available online: https://pubmed.ncbi.nlm.nih.gov/15277119/ (accessed on 2 February 2021). [CrossRef]
89. Jiang, S. *The Inhibition of Lung Cancer Active Ingredient Extracts of Euphorbia Lunulata and Its Mechanism*; Ocean University of China: Qingdao, China, 2011.
90. Gao, F.; Fu, Z.; Tian, H.; He, Z. The *Euphorbia lunulata* extract inhibits proliferation of human hepatoma Hep-G2 cells and induces apoptosis. *J. BUON* **2013**, *18*, 491–495. Available online: https://www.ncbi.nlm.nih.gov/pubmed/23818367 (accessed on 2 February 2021).
91. Hameed, A.; Hafizur, R.M.; Hussain, N. Eriodictyol stimulates insulin secretion through cAMP/PKA signaling pathway in mice islets. *Eur. J. Pharmacol.* **2018**, *820*, 245–255. [CrossRef]
92. Campos, P.M.; Prudente, A.S.; Horinouchi, C.D. Inhibitory effect of GB-2a (I3-naringenin-II8-eriodictyol) on melanogenesis. *J. Ethnopharmacol.* **2015**, *174*, 224–229. [CrossRef]
93. Lee, J.K. Anti-inflammatory effects of eriodictyol in lipopolysaccharide-stimulated raw 264.7 murine macrophages. *Arch. Pharm. Res.* **2011**, *34*, 671–679. [CrossRef]
94. Whelan, L.C.; Ryan, M.F. Ethanolic extracts of Euphorbia and other ethnobotanical species as inhibitors of human tumour cellgrowth. *Phytomedicine* **2003**, *10*, 53–58. [CrossRef]
95. Wongprayoon, P.; Charoensuksai, P. Cytotoxic and anti-migratory activities from hydroalcoholic extract of *Euphorbia lactea* Haw against HN22 cell line. *Thai J. Pharm. Sci.* **2018**, *13*, 69–77. [CrossRef]
96. Villanueva, J.; Quirós, L.M.; Castañón, S. Purification and partial characterization of a ribosome-inactivating protein from the latex of *Euphorbia trigona* Miller with cytotoxic activity toward human cancer cell lines. *Phytomedicine* **2015**, *22*, 689–695. [CrossRef] [PubMed]

97. Waczuk, E.P.; Kamdem, J.P.; Abolaji, A.O.; Meinerz, D.F.; Bueno, D.C.; do Nascimento Gonzaga, T.K.; do Canto Dorow, T.S.; Boligon, A.A.; Athayde, M.L.; da Rocha, J.B.T. *Euphorbia tirucalli* aqueous extract induces cytotoxicity, genotoxicity and changes in antioxidant gene expression in human leukocytes. *Toxicol. Res.* **2015**, *4*, 739–748. [CrossRef]
98. Hou, D.X.; Kumamoto, T. Flavonoids as protein kinase inhibitors for cancer chemoprevention: Direct binding and molecular modeling. *Antioxid. Redox Signal.* **2010**, *13*, 691–719. [CrossRef] [PubMed]
99. Lolli, G.; Cozza, G.; Mazzorana, M.; Tibaldi, E.; Cesaro, L.; Donella-Deana, A.; Pinna, L.A. Inhibition of protein kinase CK2 by flavonoids and tyrphostins. A structural insight. *Biochemistry* **2012**, *51*, 6097–6107. [CrossRef] [PubMed]
100. Yokoyama, T.; Kosaka, Y.; Mizuguchi, M. Structural insight into the interactions between death-associated protein kinase 1 and natural flavonoids. *J. Med. Chem.* **2015**, *58*, 7400–7408. [CrossRef]
101. Peng, H.L.; Huang, W.C.; Cheng, S.C.; Liou, C.J. Fisetin inhibits the generation of inflammatory mediators in interleukin-1β-induced human lung epithelial cells by suppressing the Nf-κb and Erk1/2 pathways. *Int. Immunopharmacol.* **2018**, *60*, 202–210. [CrossRef]
102. Atashpour, S.; Fouladdel, S.; Movahhed, T.K.; Barzegar, E.; Ghahremani, M.H.; Ostad, S.N.; Azizi, E. Quercetin induces cell cycle arrest and apoptosis in CD133+ cancer stem cells of human colorectal HT29 cancer cell line and enhances anticancer effects of doxorubicin. *Iran. J. Basic Med. Sci.* **2015**, *18*, 635. Available online: https://www.ncbi.nlm.nih.gov/pubmed/26351552 (accessed on 10 February 2021).
103. Yang, P.-W.; Lu, Z.-Y.; Pan, Q.; Chen, T.-T.; Feng, X.-J.; Wang, S.-M.; Pan, Y.-C.; Zhu, M.-H.; Zhang, S.-H. MicroRNA-6809-5p mediates luteolin-induced anticancer effects against hepatoma by targeting flotillin. *Phytomedicine* **2019**, *57*, 18–29. [CrossRef]
104. Guo, Y.Q.; Tang, G.H.; Lou, L.L.; Li, W.; Zhang, B.; Liu, B.; Yin, S. Prenylated flavonoids as potent phosphodiesterase-4 inhibitors from *Morus alba*: Isolation, modification, and structure-activity relationship study. *Eur. J. Med. Chem.* **2018**, *144*, 758–766. [CrossRef]
105. Choene, M.; Motadi, L. Validation of the antiproliferative effects of *Euphorbia tirucalli* extracts in breast cancer cell lines. *Mol. Biol.* **2016**, *50*, 98–110. [CrossRef]
106. Devi, K.P.; Rajavel, T.; Nabavi, S.F.; Setzer, W.N.; Ahmadi, A.; Mansouri, K.; Nabavi, S.M. Hesperidin: A promising anticancer agent from nature. *Ind. Crops Prod.* **2015**, *76*, 582–589. [CrossRef]
107. Ersoz, M.; Erdemir, A.; Duranoglu, D.; Uzunoglu, D.; Arasoglu, T.; Derman, S.; Mansuroglu, B. Comparative evaluation of hesperetin loaded nanoparticles for anticancer activity against C6 glioma cancer cells. *Artif. Cells Nanomed. Biotechnol.* **2019**, *47*, 319–329. [CrossRef]
108. Alsayari, A.; Muhsinah, A.B.; Hassan, M.Z.; Ahsan, M.J.; Alshehri, J.A.; Begum, N. Aurone: A biologically attractive scaffold as anticancer agent. *Eur. J. Med. Chem.* **2019**, *166*, 417–431. [CrossRef]
109. Yahfoufi, N.; Alsadi, N.; Jambi, M.; Matar, C. The immunomodulatory and anti-inflammatory role of polyphenols. *Nutrients* **2018**, *10*, 1618. [CrossRef]
110. Kumar, R.; Caruso, I.P.; Ullah, A.; Cornelio, M.L.; Fossey, M.A. Exploring the binding mechanism of flavonoid quercetin to phospholipase A2: Fluorescence spectroscopy and computational approach. *Eur. J. Exp. Biol.* **2017**, *7*, 33. [CrossRef]
111. Novo, M.; Hessel, H.; Fabri, C.; Ramos da Cruz Costa, C.; de Oliveira Toyama, D.; Domingues Passero, L.F.; Dalastra Laurenti, M.; Hikari Toyama, M. Evaluation of rhamnetin as an inhibitor of the pharmacological effect of secretory phospholipase A2. *Molecules* **2017**, *22*, 1441. [CrossRef]
112. González Mosquera, D.M.; Hernández Ortega, Y.; Fernández, P.L.; González, Y.; Doens, D.; Vander Heyden, Y.; Pieters, L. Flavonoids from Boldoa purpurascens inhibit proinflammatory cytokines (TNF-α and IL-6) and the expression of COX-2. *Phytother. Res.* **2018**, *32*, 1750–1754. [CrossRef]
113. Li, Y.; Yu, Q.; Zhao, W.; Zhang, J.; Liu, W.; Huang, M.; Zeng, X. Oligomeric proanthocyanidins attenuate airway inflammation in asthma by inhibiting dendritic cells maturation. *Mol. Immunol.* **2017**, *91*, 209–217. [CrossRef]
114. Lin, X.; Lin, C.H.; Zhao, T.; Zuo, D.; Ye, Z.; Liu, L.; Lin, M.T. Quercetin protects against heat stroke-induced myocardial injury in male rats: Antioxidative and anti-inflammatory mechanisms. *Chemico-Biol. Interact.* **2017**, *265*, 47–54. [CrossRef]
115. Galleggiante, V.; De Santis, S.; Cavalcanti, E.; Scarano, A.; De Benedictis, M.; Serino, G.; Chieppa, M. Dendritic cells modulate iron homeostasis and inflammatory abilities following quercetin exposure. *Curr. Pharm. Des.* **2017**, *23*, 2139–2146. [CrossRef]
116. Gong, J.H.; Shin, D.; Han, S.Y.; Kim, J.L.; Kang, Y.H. Kaempferol suppresses eosionphil infiltration and airway inflammation in airway epithelial cells and in mice with allergic asthma. *J. Nutr.* **2011**, *142*, 47–56. [CrossRef] [PubMed]
117. Weng, Z.; Patel, A.B.; Panagiotidou, S.; Theoharides, T.C. The novel flavone tetramethoxyluteolin is a potent inhibitor of human mast cells. *J. Allergy Clin. Immunol.* **2015**, *135*, 1044–1052. [CrossRef] [PubMed]
118. Weng, Z.; Zhang, B.; Asadi, S.; Sismanopoulos, N.; Butcher, A.; Fu, X.; Theoharides, T.C. Quercetin is more effective than cromolyn in blocking human mast cell cytokine release and inhibits contact dermatitis and photosensitivity in humans. *PLoS ONE* **2012**, *7*. [CrossRef] [PubMed]
119. Kim, D.H.; Jung, W.S.; Kim, M.E.; Lee, H.W.; Youn, H.Y.; Seon, J.K.; Lee, J.S. Genistein inhibits pro-inflammatory cytokines in human mast cell activation through the inhibition of the ERK pathway. *Int. J. Mol. Med.* **2014**, *34*, 1669–1674. [CrossRef]
120. Veena, S.; Pracheta, J. Protective assessment of *Euphorbia neriifolia* and its isolated flavonoid against N nitrosodiethylamine-induced Hepatic carcinogenesis in male mice: A histopathological analysis. *Toxicol. Int.* **2015**, 1–8. [CrossRef]
121. Lizhen, Z.; Chu, W.; Qiuxia, M.; Qin, T.; Yu, N.; Wei, N. Phytochemicals of *Euphorbia lathyris* L. and their antioxidant activities. *Molecules* **2017**, *22*, 1335. [CrossRef]

122. Kerry, N.L.; Abbey, M. Red wine and fractionated phenolic compounds prepared from red wine inhibits low density lipoprotein oxidation in vitro. *Atherosclerosis* **1997**, *135*, 93–102. Available online: https://pubmed.ncbi.nlm.nih.gov/9395277/ (accessed on 1 March 2021). [CrossRef]
123. Hanan, M.; Ali, S.; Afaf, E.A.; Sayed, A.E.; Wagdi, I.A.; Wafaa, H.B.; Hanaa, M. Nephroprotective and antioxidant activities of ethyl acetate fraction of *Euphorbia geniculata* Ortega family *Euphorbiaceae*. *Arab. J. Chem.* **2020**, *13*, 7843–7850. [CrossRef]
124. Claudia, M.; Furlan, K.; Pereira, S.; Martha, D.; Sedano-Partida, L.; Barbosa, D.; Deborah, Y.A.C.; Maria, L.; Giuseppina, N.; Paul, E.; et al. Flavonoids and antioxidant potential of nine Argentinian species of Croton (Euphorbiaceae). *Braz. J. Bot.* **2015**, *38*, 693–702. [CrossRef]
125. Mishra, B.; Priyadarsini, K.; Kumar, M.; Unnikrishnan, M.; Mohan, H. Effect of *O*-glycosilation on the antioxidant activity, free radical reactions of a plant flavonoid, chrysoeriol. *Bioorg. Med. Chem.* **2003**, *11*, 2677–2685. [CrossRef]
126. You, H.J.; Ahn, H.J.; Ji, G.E. Transformation of rutin to antiproliferative quercetin-3-glucoside by *Aspergillus niger*. *J. Agric. Food Chem.* **2010**, *58*, 10886–10892. [CrossRef]
127. Juliana, F.; Jacyra, A.S.; Júlia, M.F.; Angela, K.C.; Yamara, A.S.M.; Elizabeth, C.G.; Denise, V.T.; Arnóbio, A.S.; Silvana, M.Z.; Matheus, F. Comparison of two *Jatropha* species (*Euphorbiaceae*) used popularly to treat snakebites in Northeastern Brazil: Chemical profile, inhibitory activity against Bothrops erythromelas venom and antibacterial activity. *J. Ethnopharmacol.* **2018**, *213*, 12–20. [CrossRef]
128. Ajayi, E.I.O.; Adeleke, M.A.; Adewumi, T.Y.; Adeyemi, A.A. Antiplasmodial activities of ethanol extracts of *Euphorbia hirta* whole plant and *Vernonia amygdalina* leaves in *Plasmodium berghei*-infected mice. *J. Taibah Univ. Sci.* **2017**, *11*, 831–835. [CrossRef]
129. Ashraf, A.; sarfraz, R.A.; Rashid, M.A.; Shahid, M. Antioxidant, antimicrobial, antitumor, and cytotoxic activities of an important medicinal plant (*Euphorbia royleana*) from Pakistan. *J. Food Drug Anal.* **2015**, *23*, 109–115. [CrossRef]
130. Boumaza, S.; Bouchenak, O.; Yahiaoui, K.; Toubal, S.; El haddad, D.; Arab, K. Effect of the aqueous extract of *Euphorbia guyoniana* (*euphorbiaceae*) on pathogenic bacteria from land-based sources. *Appl. Ecol. Environ. Res.* **2018**, *16*, 3767–3781. [CrossRef]
131. Beatriz, G.; Hélcio, S.; Paulo, N.; Bandeira, T.; Helena, S.; Rodrigues, C.; Matos, F.; Nascimento, G.C.; de Carvalho, R.; Braz-Filhoe, M.R.; et al. Coutinhoa Evaluation of antibacterial and enhancement of antibiotic action by the flavonoid kaempferol 7-O-β-D-(6″-O-cumaroyl)-glucopyranoside isolated from *Croton piauhiensis müll*. *Microb. Pathog.* **2020**, *143*, 104144. [CrossRef]
132. Ali, M.; Mat Houghton, P.J.; Raman, A.; Hoult, J.R.S. Antimicrobial and anti-inflammatory activities of extracts and constituents of *Oroxylum indicum* (L.) Vent. *Phytomedicine* **1998**, *5*, 375–381. [CrossRef]
133. Alcaráz, L.E.; Blanco, S.E.; Puig, O.N.; Tomás, F.; Ferretti, F.H. Antibacterial activity of flavonoids against methicillin-resistant Staphylococcus aureus strains. *J. Theor. Biol.* **2000**, *205*, 231–240. [CrossRef]
134. Edziri, H.; Mastouri, M.; Mahjoub, M.A.; Mighri, Z.; Mahjoub, A.; Verschaeve, L. Antibacterial, antifungal and cytotoxic activities of two flavonoids from *Retama raetam* flowers. *Molecules* **2012**, *17*, 7284–7293. [CrossRef]
135. Jamil, S. Antimicrobial Flavonoids from Artocarpus anisophyllus Miq and Artocarpus lowii King. *J. Teknol.* **2014**, *71*, 95–99. [CrossRef]
136. Farooq, S.; Wahab, A.T.; Fozing, C.; Rahman, A.U.; Choudhary, M.I. Artonin I inhibits multidrug resistance in Staphylococcus aureus and potentiates the action of inactive antibiotics in vitro. *J. Appl. Microbiol.* **2014**, *117*, 996–1011. [CrossRef]
137. Cushnie, T.T.; Lamb, A.J. Detection of galangin-induced cytoplasmic membrane damage in Staphylococcus aureus by measuring potassium loss. *J. Ethnopharmacol.* **2005**, *101*, 243–248. [CrossRef]
138. Cushnie, T.T.; Lamb, A.J. Recent advances in understanding the antibacterial properties of flavonoids. *Int. J. Antimicrob. Agents* **2011**, *38*, 99–107. [CrossRef]
139. Ohemeng, K.A.; Schwender, C.F.; Fu, K.P.; Barrett, J.F. DNA gyrase inhibitory and antibacterial activity of some flavones. *Bioorg. Med. Chem. Lett.* **1993**, *3*, 225–230. [CrossRef]
140. Xie, Y.; Yang, W.; Tang, F.; Chen, X.; Ren, L. Antibacterial activities of flavonoids: Structure-activity relationship and mechanism. *Curr. Med. Chem.* **2015**, *22*, 132–149. [CrossRef]

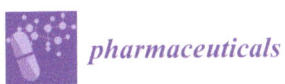

Review

Pharmacological Activity of *Garcinia indica* (Kokum): An Updated Review

Sung Ho Lim [1], Ho Seon Lee [1], Chang Hoon Lee [2] and Chang-Ik Choi [1,*]

1. Integrated Research Institute for Drug Development, College of Pharmacy, Dongguk University-Seoul, Goyang 10326, Korea; 93sho617@naver.com (S.H.L.); ghtjsrhtn@naver.com (H.S.L.)
2. BK21 FOUR Team and Integrated Research Institute for Drug Development, College of Pharmacy, Dongguk University-Seoul, Goyang 10326, Korea; uatheone@dongguk.edu
* Correspondence: cichoi@dongguk.edu; Tel.: +82-31-961-5230

Abstract: *Garcinia indica* (commonly known as kokum), belonging to the Clusiaceae family (mangosteen family), is a tropical evergreen tree distributed in certain regions of India. It has been used in culinary and industrial applications for a variety of purposes, including acidulant in curries, pickles, health drinks, wine, and butter. In particular, *G. indica* has been used in traditional medicine to treat inflammation, dermatitis, and diarrhea, and to promote digestion. According to several studies, various phytochemicals such as garcinol, hydroxycitric acid (HCA), cyanidin-3-sambubioside, and cyanidin-3-glucoside were isolated from *G. indica*, and their pharmacological activities were published. This review highlights recent updates on the various pharmacological activities of *G. indica*. These studies reported that *G. indica* has antioxidant, anti-obesity, anti-arthritic, anti-inflammatory, antibacterial, hepatoprotective, cardioprotective, antidepressant and anxiolytic effects both in vitro and in vivo. These findings, together with previously published reports of pharmacological activity of various components isolated from *G. indica*, suggest its potential as a promising therapeutic agent to prevent various diseases.

Keywords: *Garcinia indica*; kokum; wild mangosteen; pharmacological activity

1. Introduction

The use of medicinal herbs as medicine is the oldest form of medical treatment known to humanity and has been used in all cultures throughout history [1]. Since time immemorial, humans have recognized their dependence on nature for healthy living, and have relied on a variety of plant resources for medicine to cure numerous diseases [2]. This indigenous knowledge, passed down from generation to generation in different parts of the world, has contributed significantly to the development of traditional medical systems [3], as well as provided a scientific basis for their traditional uses by exploring various biologically active natural products [4]. For instance, between 1981 and 2014, about 26% of new chemical entities were natural products or derived from natural products [5]. They are widely used in the prevention and treatment of clinical diseases as they have the unique advantages of low toxicity and side effects compared with chemical drugs [6]. Among medicinal plants, Clusiaceae contains approximately 50 genera and 600 species [7], and has been extensively used in ethnomedicine to treat a number of disease conditions, including wounds, ulcers, dysentery, cancer, inflammation, and infection [8,9].

Garcinia belongs to the Clusiaceae family (Mangosteen family) and has multiple application in the culinary, pharmaceutical, and industrial fields [10]. The plants are distributed around the world including tropical Asia, Africa, and Western Polynesia [11]. In the last few decades, they have received considerable attention and extracts of different plant parts of the Garcinia species, e.g., *Garcinia brasiliensis*, *G. cambogia*, *G. gardneriana*, *G. pedunculata*, and *G. mangstana* have demonstrated potential effectiveness in the prevention and treatment of non-transmissible chronic diseases [12]. Furthermore, it was reported that they contain a wide range of biologically active metabolites and that the chemical compositions of their extracts are rich in bioactive molecules including hydroxycitric acid (HCA), bioflavonoids, procyanidines and polyisoprenylated benzophenone derivatives including garcinol, xanthochymol and guttiferone isoforms [9,13]. These compounds have been implicated in biological activities such as antioxidant [14], anticancer [15,16], and antiviral effects [17]. In particular, the major bioactive ingredients such as garcinol, HCA, and cyanidin-3-glucoside have been isolated (Figure 1), characterized and evaluated for their therapeutic properties. For example, garcinol showed anti-inflammatory effects by regulating various signaling pathways, molecular binding, and gene expression contributing to inflammation, such as inhibition of the cyclooxygenase-2, 5-lipoxygenase and inducible nitric oxide synthase synthesis [18–20]. Also, garcinol was reported to have antioxidant effects through high free-radical, superoxide anion (O^{2-}) scavenging activity [21,22], and to have neuroprotective properties by functioning as a histone acetyltransferase inhibitor (HAT) [23]. In addition, recent studies demonstrated its anticancer effects by inducing apoptosis and cell cycle arrest, inhibiting of angiogenesis, and regulating of gene expression in oncogenic cells [24].

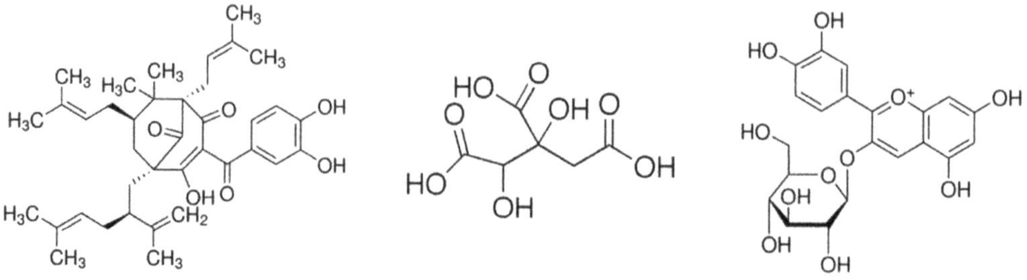

Figure 1. Chemical structure of bioactive ingredients isolated from *G. indica*.

Garcinia indica is a plant native to certain regions of India [25]. It is an underexploited slender evergreen tree and is known as wild mangosteen, kokum, and goa butter tree [26]. All parts of *G. indica*, i.e., fruits, rind, seeds, etc., have been used in various culinary, industrial and pharmaceutical applications, as well as fruit drinks and food [27]. Its pharmacological properties including antioxidant [28], anti-inflammatory activity [29], antimicrobial [30], anticancer [31], and anti-obesity [32] effects have been reported. The present review aims to discuss these recent studies and update the pharmacological properties of *G. indica*.

2. Methodology

We collected scientific literature on the origin, medicinal uses, and pharmacological activity of *G. indica* published in the English language up till 2021 from PubMed, Google Scholar, and Web of Science. The search terms were "*Garcinia indica*", "kokum", "pharmacological activity", "antioxidant", "anti-obesity", "anti-inflammatory", and "anti-diabetic".

As a result of the literature research, various pharmacological activities of *G. indica* were reported and reviewed [33–35], and a total of 7 papers were additionally reported recently. We comprehensively reviewed and updated the study design, results, and interpretation of each paper.

3. Pharmacological Properties of *G. indica*

A summary of the pharmacological properties of *G. indica* is described in Table 1.

Table 1. Summary of pharmacological studies for *Garcinia indica*.

Pharmacological Activity	Tested Substance	In Vitro/In Vivo	Model	Dose/Concentration	Ref.
Antioxidant	Aqueous extract	In vivo	Wister albino rats	400 and 800 mg/kg	[36]
	Fruit extract	In vitro	-	1.5 mM	[37]
	Garcinol-enriched fraction	In vivo	C57BL/6 male mice	25, 50, and 100 mg/kg	[38]
	Aqueous extract	In vitro	-	-	[39]
		In vivo	Wister albino rats	250 and 500 mg/kg	
	G. indica fruit rind powder	In vivo	Swiss albino mice, Wister rats	0.5, 1, and 2% w/w	[40]
Anti-obesity	Garcinol-enriched fraction	In vivo	C57BL/6 male mice	25, 50, and 100 mg/kg	[38]
	Fruit extract	In vitro	3T3-L1 preadipocytes	1 and 2 µg/mL	[41]
		In vivo	C57BL/6 male mice	0.01% w/w	
Anti-arthritic	Garcinol-enriched fraction	In vivo	Male Wistar rats	10 mg/kg	[42]
Anti-inflammatory	Garcinol-enriched fraction	In vivo	C57BL/6 male mice	25, 50, and 100 mg/kg	[38]
Antidepressant and anxiolytic effect	*G. indica* fruit rind powder	In vivo	Swiss albino mice, Wister rats	0.5, 1, and 2%	[40]
Antibacterial	Fruit extract	In vitro	-	1.5 mM	[37]
Hepatoprotective	Aqueous extract	In vivo	Wister albino rats	400 and 800 mg/kg	[36]
Cardioprotective	Garcinol-enriched fraction	In vivo	C57BL/6 male mice	25, 50, and 100 mg/kg	[38]
	Aqueous extract	In vivo	Wister albino rats	250 and 500 mg/kg	[39]

3.1. Antioxidant Effects

The overproduction of oxidants can cause oxidative damage to biomolecules such as lipids, DNA, and proteins, increasing the risk of cancer, and cardiovascular and other diseases [43,44]. Antioxidants may reduce oxidative stress through various mechanisms [45]. In the past few years, there have been many reports on the antioxidant activity of *G. indica* [46–53]. Panda V et al. [36] reported the antioxidant effect of aqueous extracts of *G. indica* in an animal model of oxidative stress induced with ethanol (EtOH). Malondialdehyde (MDA), a lipid peroxidation marker, was elevated in the EtOH-treated group compared with the normal group. Treatment with the aqueous extracts of *G. indica* reversed these results. The reduced glutathione (GSH) level in the EtOH-treated group was significantly reduced compared with the normal group ($p < 0.001$). Treatment of the EtOH-treated group with aqueous extracts of *G. indica* (400 and 800 mg/kg) significantly restored the decreased levels of GSH ($p < 0.05$ and $p < 0.01$, respectively). In addition, superoxide dismutase (SOD) and catalase (CAT) activities were also markedly lower in the EtOH-treated group compared with the normal group ($p < 0.01$). The reduction in SOD and CAT activity levels were improved in a dose-dependent manner when treated with the aqueous extracts of *G. indica*. In particular, the high-dose group treated with 800 mg/kg of aqueous extracts of *G. indica* recovered to near normal levels. Furthermore, treatment with aqueous extracts of *G. indica* significantly ameliorated glutathione peroxidase and glutathione reductase activity, which were decreased by EtOH treatment ($p < 0.01$).

Nanobiotechnology is a new field of research related to the convergence of biology and nanotechnology [54]. A recent study successfully demonstrated the use of plant extracts for the biogenic synthesis of silver nanoparticles (AgNPs) with antioxidant activity [55]. However, the synthesis of AgNPs was mainly achieved by physical and chemical methods of metal nanoparticle synthesis, which includes the use of hazardous chemicals that limit their potential use in biomedical applications [56]. To overcome these disadvantages, biosynthesis using various biological agents such as bacteria, fungi, plants, and their extracts is a green chemistry approach that is inexpensive, does not use hazardous chemicals, and has excellent biocompatibility and low toxicity [57]. Sangaonkar, G.M. et al. [37] optimized parameters for a simple, stable and benign biosynthesis method of AgNPs using *G. indica* fruit extract. Then, they performed 1,1-diphenyl-2-picrylhydrazyl (DPPH) free-radical scavenging, reducing power activity, and hydrogen peroxide and nitric oxide (NO) radical scavenging activity to evaluate the potential antioxidant activity of AgNPs biologically synthesized with *G. indica* fruit extract. They found that the tested range of AgNPs (20, 40, 60, 80, and 100 μg/mL) inhibited DPPH activity in a dose-dependent manner and exhibited a 57% inhibitory effect at the maximum concentration. Similar to the DPPH activity, the NO radical scavenging activity of AgNPs was confirmed to be dose-dependent, but lower compared with the DPPH activity. Furthermore, A 100 μg/mL AgNPs, which was less than half of the dose of butylated hydroxytoluene used as a positive control, resulted in 27% NO radical scavenging. Similar to DPPH and NO radical scavenging activity, the inhibitory response of biological AgNPs to reducing power was increased in a dose-dependent manner. Whereas, as a result of H_2O_2 radical scavenging activity, the inhibitory activity of AgNPs at the highest concentration was 65%, which was similar to the inhibitory activity of 72% using the same test concentration of standard ascorbic acid. In conclusion, *G. indica* fruit extract containing significant amounts of natural antioxidants such as HCA can be used in environmentally friendly AgNPs, preventing the use of toxic chemicals. Therefore, *G. indica* has important applications in biomedical fields as a good source of reducing and capping agents.

Barve, K. [38] performed lipid peroxide, GSH, CAT, and SOD assays using C57BL/6 male mice to measure the antioxidant activity of the garcinol-enriched fraction (GEF). This fraction was prepared from the hexane extract of *G. indica*. The extracts were loaded on a silica column, and hexane and ethyl acetate were eluted in ascending order of polarity to obtain various fractions by flash chromatography at a flow rate of 15 mL/min. The collected fractions (12 mL) were confirmed for the presence of garcinol by thin-layer chromatography, and this flash chromatography procedure was repeated 3 times to obtain sufficient GEF. Lipid peroxidation and changes in the oxido-redox state were measured for enzymatic and non-enzymatic markers. Lipid peroxide, an indicator of oxidative stress, was twice as high in disease-induced animals fed a modified Western diet compared with normal animals ($p < 0.001$). Simvastatin treatment was used as a positive control and animals treated with GEF (50 and 100 mg/kg) showed significantly reduced effects ($p < 0.05$ and $p < 0.01$, respectively), although they were higher than those in normal animals. GSH levels in disease-induced animals were significantly depleted compared with those in normal animals ($p < 0.001$). Treatment with GEF (25, 50, and 100 mg/kg) strikingly ameliorated depleted GSH levels in a dose-dependent manner, although this did not reach normal levels. CAT and SOD activity levels were significantly reduced in disease-induced animals ($p < 0.001$ and $p < 0.0001$, respectively). GEF treatment at 25 mg/kg reversed CAT activity levels, but this did not reach statistical significance. However, GEF treatment at 50 and 100 mg/kg significantly restored the CAT activity levels to levels similar to those of normal animals. Of note, only 100 mg/kg GEF treatment significantly increased the SOD activity level.

In another study conducted by Patel et al. [39], the IC_{50} value for the DPPH scavenging activity of an aqueous extract of *G. indica* was estimated to be 231.85 ± 21.56 μg/mL. They also used animal models to measure biomarkers related to oxidative stress, including SOD, CAT, and thiobarbituric acid reactive substance (TBARS). The group treated with 85 mg/kg of isoprenaline (ISO) showed significantly reduced SOD and CAT values (5.38 ± 0.31 unit/g of tissue and 0.54 ± 0.02 μmol of H_2O_2 consumed/min/g of tissue, respectively) compared to the normal group (13.55 ± 0.62 unit/g of tissue and 2.66 ± 0.24 μmol of H_2O_2 consumed/min/g of tissue, respectively). Treatment of the ISO-induced toxicity group with an aqueous extract of *G. indica* at 250 and 500 mg/kg slightly restored the SOD levels (6.12 ± 0.93 and 7.56 ± 0.22 unit/g of tissue, respectively) and slightly improved the CAT levels (1.1 ± 0.17 and 1.08 ± 0.19 μmol of H_2O_2 consumed/min/g of tissue, respectively). Furthermore, treatment with ISO increased the TBARS level (3.82 ± 0.21 nmol MDA/g of tissue) compared with the normal group (1.65 ± 0.12 nmol MDA/g of tissue). The tested concentrations of aqueous extracts of *G. indica* did not affect these values (2.55 ± 0.25 and 2.17 ± 0.13 nmol MDA/g of tissue, respectively) and treatment of the normal control group with 500 mg/kg *G. indica* aqueous extract did not change the levels of any of the three biomarkers related to oxidative stress. They used the lower dose range because the antioxidant enzyme levels were not restored in the 250 and 500 mg/kg *G. indica*-treated groups.

Dhamija I et al. [40] measured antioxidant activity to elucidate the mechanism of antidepressant effect in various animal models. *G. indica* at 1% w/w significantly decreased monoamine oxidase levels (MAO-A and MAO-B) in brain homogenates, similar to a group treated with fluoxetine. By measuring the MDA concentration in the brain homogenate, a direct correlation was observed between the dose of *G. indica* and a decrease in the MDA level, suggesting a decrease in free-radical production.

3.2. Anti-Obesity Effects

Recently, as the prevalence of overweight and obesity has reached epidemic levels, the incidence of various comorbidities such as type 2 diabetes, cardiovascular disease, and cancer has rapidly increased, causing enormous health and economic burdens [58,59]. Medicines and bariatric surgery are the main strategies to prevent and treat obesity, but there are side effects [60]. For this reason, various natural products and their components are being tested to improve obesity with minimal side effects [61]. An anti-obesity effect of garcinol isolated from *G. indica* was reported [62–64].

As mentioned above, Barve, K. [38] confirmed the reduction of the oxidative stress response of GEF. In addition, he conducted research into the anti-obesity effects of GEF. C57BL/6 male mice were randomly divided into 6 groups of 6 mice each: Group 1 (normal control); Group 2 (disease-induced control by a modified Western diet); Group 3 (positive control receiving 8 mg/kg of simvastatin); and Groups 4, 5, and 6 (treated with 25, 50, and 100 mg/kg of GEF). Compared with Group 1, the weights of animals in all groups were significantly increased at 12 weeks. Group 2 weights continued to increase significantly until 16 weeks ($p < 0.05$), but those in Groups 3, 4, 5, and 6 treated with simvastatin and GEF decreased significantly from 12 to 16 weeks ($p < 0.001$ and $p < 0.0001$, respectively). Group 2 showed significant negative changes in the lipid profile indicative of disease induction. Groups 3, 4, 5, and 6 showed a decrease in the increased total cholesterol and triglyceride levels induced by a Western diet in a concentration-dependent manner, In particular, the values of Group 6 were similar to those of Group 1 ($p < 0.01$ and $p < 0.0001$, respectively). Furthermore, treatment with different concentrations of GEF elevated high-density cholesterol levels in a concentration-dependent manner and significantly decreased low density cholesterol levels to those of positive control levels ($p < 0.0001$).

Tung YC et al. [41] investigated the potential anti-obesity effects of *G. indica* fruit extract (GIE) in a 3T3-L1 cell model and high-fat diet (HFD)-induced obese animal model. First, 3T3-L1 preadipocytes were used for the following experiments after differentiation induced by differentiation medium (DMI) containing 5 μg/mL insulin, 0.5 mM 3-isobutylmethylxanthine, 1 μM dexamethasone, and 2 μM rosiglitazone. After confirming the lipid content by Oil Red O staining, the groups treated with 1 and 2 μg/mL GIE showed significantly reduced triglyceride levels to 63.5% and 65.6% without cytotoxic effects, compared with the group treated with only DMI. However, treatment with GIE in the tested range did not affect the amount of glycerol in the medium. The weights of C57BL/6 male mice fed a normal diet (ND) or HFD for 12 weeks were 27.5 and 37.4 g, respectively. The body weights of the group supplemented with 0.01% GIE in HFD were significantly reduced to 34.4 g ($p < 0.05$), and no effects on liver, kidney, or spleen weight were observed. A significantly reduced weight of mesenteric, perigonadal and retroperitoneal fat was noted in the group supplemented with GIE. Treatment with GIE also reduced the ratio of body fat compared with the HFD group. In addition, the histopathological examination of liver and the perigonadal adipose tissue of mice demonstrated that GIE treatment reduces the adipocyte size and liver fat accumulation. They further investigated the expressions of proteins related to adipogenesis, lipolysis and β-oxidation to elucidate the mechanisms involved in these effects. There was no significant difference in PPARγ and C/EBPα, proteins related to adipogenesis, between the ND and HFD groups, whereas PPARγ and C/EBPα protein levels were significantly decreased after supplementation with GIE compared with the HFD group. Although there was no significant difference in the protein levels of CPT-1A between the ND and HFD groups, supplementation with GIE was significantly elevated in the protein levels of CPT-1A compared to the HFD group. Moreover, a significant increase in PPARα protein levels was observed in the GIE supplemented group compared with the HFD group. These results suggest that GIE exerts anti-obesity effects in 3T3-L1 adipocytes and animal models by inhibiting adipogenesis and increasing β-oxidation.

3.3. Anti-Arthritic Activity

Arthritis is highly prevalent worldwide and can be divided into types, the most common of which are rheumatoid arthritis, osteoarthritis, psoriatic arthritis and inflammatory arthritis [65]. The exact cause of arthritis is not yet clear, and although it is commonly used to treat various types of anti-inflammatory arthritis, it is associated with serious side effects such as gastric bleeding and an increased risk of other cardiovascular problems [66]. Consequently, it is very important to explore effective and safe anti-arthritis drug candidates isolated from natural products.

Warriar, P. et al. [42] evaluated the anti-arthritic effects of GEF in rheumatoid arthritis. An extract (9 gm) of *G. indica* was adsorbed onto silica and loaded. Thereafter, fractions were obtained through stepwise gradient elution with n-hexane-ethyl acetate, including a fraction (800 mg) showing the maximum concentration of garcinol. A rat model of adjuvant arthritis (AA) was developed with a single injection of 0.1 mL of Complete Freund's Adjuvant (CFA). Rats were divided into 4 groups of 6 each as follows: Group 1 (normal control); Group 2 (disease control of CFA alone); Group 3 (positive control receiving 10 mg/kg of diclofenac sodium); Group 4 (treated with 10 mg/kg of GEF). To examine the major lesions and determine the effects of the therapeutic agents, the volume of the left hind paw of rats was measured on days 0, 1, 5, 12, 16, and 21 using an electronic transfusion meter. To determine the severity of the secondary lesions, the volume of the right hind paw was also measured. In addition, to evaluate the severity of AA, the ears, nose, tail, forepaws, and hind paws of the rats were visually examined for inflammatory lesions, and arthritis severity was scored according to the redness, swelling, and presence of nodules [67]. The CFA-treated group developed primary arthritis in the left hind paw, and compared with the normal group, a significant level of swelling was observed and maintained for 21 days ($p < 0.0001$). Treatment with GEF significantly suppressed paw swelling from days 5 to 21, similar to the positive control group, when compared with the disease control group. On the other hand, the GEF-treated group also had a decrease in the swelling of the right hind paw, but this was not statistically significant. CFA-treated rats showed a significant increase in the arthritis index compared with the control group, reaching a maximum at 5 days, and then gradually decreasing. The groups treated with 10 mg/mL of GEF and diclofenac had a significantly reduced arthritis index compared with the disease control animal group ($p < 0.01$). Treatment of CFA significantly reduced the stair climbing activity of all animals from days 5 to 21 compared with the normal group demonstrating the induction of hyperalgesia ($p < 0.0001$). However, the group treated with GEF and diclofenac had improved scores from days 12 and 16, which were significantly increased until day 21. In addition, the motility score, which was reduced by CFA treatment, steadily and significantly recovered from days 16 to 21 in the GEF-treated group. This study indicated that GEF has anti-arthritic activity in an animal model of arthritis induced with CFA.

3.4. Anti-Inflammatory Effects

Inflammation is the immune system's first biological response to infection, injury, or irritation [68]. There is evidence that anti-inflammatory effects are mediated through the modulation of various inflammatory cytokines [69]. Interleukin 6 (IL-6) is produced rapidly and transiently in response to infection and tissue damage and contributes to host defense through the stimulation of acute phase responses, as well as hematopoietic and immune responses [70]. A study conducted by Barve, K. [38] showed that, after 16 weeks, IL-6 levels in the plasma and thoracic aorta were significantly increased in induced hyperlipidemic animals compared with normal animals ($p < 0.0001$ and $p < 0.001$, respectively). In animals treated with 25 mg/kg GEF, IL-6 levels in the thoracic aorta were decreased but not significant, and IL-6 levels were significantly decreased in animals treated with 50 or 100 mg/kg GEF ($p < 0.01$). In addition, plasma IL-6 levels were significantly reduced in a dose-dependent manner by treatment with all concentrations of GEF ($p < 0.0001$).

3.5. Antidepressant and Anxiolytic Effects

Depression and anxiety are the most common mental disorders and are the leading cause of psychosocial dysfunction [71]. Pharmacotherapy is the first line treatment of these disorders, but it can impose some problems, including sedation and amnesia, causing tolerance, psychomotor effects, and dependence [72]. These considerations emphasized the importance of finding new psychopharmacological drugs with an immediate onset of action and fewer side effects [73]. In this regard, natural products represent promising candidates for the pharmacological treatment of these pathologies [74].

Dhamija, I. et al. [40] investigated the antidepressant and anti-anxiety effects of *G. indica* using mouse and rat models in which the rind of *G. indica* was triturated with a mortar and pestle and mixed with feed. Elevated plus maze (EPM), light–dark model (LDM), and hole-board tests (HBT) were used to evaluate anxiolytic effects, and the forced swim test (FST), tail suspension test (TST), reserpine-induced hypothermia model, measurement of locomotor activity, and estimations of biochemical were used as methods to measure antidepressant activity. Positive controls received 1 mg/kg diazepam (standard anxiolytic), 15 mg/kg imipramine and 20 mg/kg fluoxetine (standard antidepressant agents), and 0.5, 1, and 2% w/w of *G. indica* rind mixed into their food. In the LDM, a significant increase in the length of time animals stayed in the lighted compartments indicated anxiolytic activity and the reverse of this represented anxiogenic activity. In the HBT models, head-dipping behavior reflected the animal's emotional state. Administration of *G. indica* resulted in a significant increase in the length of time mice stayed in the light box in the LDM ($p < 0.05$). In addition, treatment with 0.5, 1, and 2% w/w of *G. indica* increased the number of head dips. In the EPM, anxiolytic effects were found in the state of open arms by increasing the length of stay and the number of entries. On the other hand, spending less time with arms outstretched reflected anxiety effect. *G. indica* at concentrations of 0.5, 1, and 2% w/w dose-dependently improved the time spent and number of entries in the open arms of the EPM ($p < 0.05$). Immobility refers to a condition in animals known as helplessness that can be converted by antidepressants such as fluoxetine and imipramine. A decrease in immobility indicates the absence of depression. *G. indica* at the concentrations tested in the FST and TST models significantly decreased animal immobility ($p < 0.05$). The rectal temperature in mouse using a reserpine-induced hypothermia model reflected the depletion of noradrenaline and serotonin in the brain, and 1% w/w *G. indica* significantly reversed the reserpine-induced hypothermia. ($p < 0.05$). These results indicate that *G. indica* fruit rind as a functional food exhibits significant antidepressant and anti-anxiety effects, without impairing motor activity and not involving CNS stimulation.

3.6. Antibacterial Activity

Bacterial resistance to antibiotics has rapidly increased and is one of the major threats to public health in the 21st century [75]. Natural products have historically been successful as a source of new antibiotics, and most existing classes of antibiotics are derived from natural compounds [76]. The potential for antibacterial effects of *G. indica* has been reported [77–79].

Sangaonkar, G.M. et al. [37] noted the antioxidant effect and the antibacterial effects of the biogenic synthesis of AgNPs using *G. indica* fruit extract. It was reported that

AgNPs exhibit potential antibacterial activity against methicillin resistant *Staphylococcus aureus* (MRSA) by a mechanism different from that of antibiotics [80]. Based on this potential effect of AgNPs, they tested the antimicrobial activity 20 μg/μL AgNPs against 7 bacterial pathogens (*Escherichia coli, Bacillus subtilis, Staphylococcus aureus, Pseudomonas aeruginosa, Salmonella enterica typhi, Proteus vulgaris, Serratia marcescens*) and found that it inhibited the growth of *E. coli, B. subtilis, S. aureus*, and *P. aeruginosa*, with a clear region of inhibition in the range of 12–15 mm. However, *S. enterica typhi, P. vulgaris,* and *S. marcescens* were not inhibited by AgNP treatment. As a result of measuring the minimum inhibitory concentration using the micro-broth dilution method reported by Siddiq et al. [81], the inhibitory power of AgNPs was estimated to be 20 mg/mL for *E. coli, B. subtilis,* and *S. aureus*, and 40 mg/mL for *P. aeruginosa*. In addition, the minimum bactericidal concentration for *E. coli, B. subtilis,* and *S. aureus* was the same as the minimum inhibitory concentration, and 160 mg/mL for *P. aeruginosa*. These results suggest that AgNPs biosynthesized with *G. indica* fruit extract have important applications in biomedical fields as an antibacterial agent.

3.7. Hepatoprotective Activity

As mentioned above, Panda, V. et al. [36] determined the antioxidant effects of *G. indica* through various mechanisms. Significantly increased levels of serum enzymes such as aspartate aminotransferase (AST), alanine aminotransferase (ALT), and alkaline phosphatase were observed in an EtOH-treated animal group compared with the normal animal group ($p < 0.001$). These activities were due to the release of enzymes into the blood following extensive liver damage caused by the EtOH. Treatment with 400 or 800 mg/kg aqueous extracts of *G. indica* reduced AST activity ($p < 0.001$). However, ALT and AST activities were significantly improved only in the 800 mg/kg of the *G. indica*-treated group, similar to treatment with silymarin, which protects hepatocytes from toxins ($p < 0.05$). Moreover, increased serum triglyceride (sTG) levels and decreased total protein (TP) and albumin (Alb) levels were observed in EtOH-fed rats compared with the normal group. These effects suggested the decreased activity of lipase enzyme responsible for lipoprotein uptake by extrahepatic tissues. Treatment with aqueous extracts of *G. indica* restored these increased sTG levels and decreased TP levels in a dose-dependent manner. However, treatment with aqueous extracts of *G. indica* ameliorated Alb levels, although this did not reach statistical significance. Finally, light microscopy histopathological studies of liver sections fixed in 10% buffered formalin, embedded in paraffin, cut to 5 μm, and stained with hematoxylin and eosin (H/E), showed a moderate-to-marked degree of histoarchitectural changes in animals treated with EtOH. There were moderate-to-severe abscesses and bleeding, and the central vein revealed congestion of sinusoids. Moderate mononuclear inflammatory infiltration was observed in all zones, and many hepatocytes showed degenerative changes. However, the group treated with 400 mg/kg aqueous extracts of *G. indica* had mild-to-moderate mononuclear inflammatory infiltration in all areas with moderate fat changes and few regenerated cells. In the group treated with 800 mg/kg aqueous extracts of *G. indica*, slight or minimal fat changes were present around the dilated central vein, and many regenerative cells were observed. This histology was similar to that of the silymarin-treated group, a proven hepatoprotective, with a tendency to be more normal compared with the group treated with 400 mg/kg aqueous extracts of *G. indica*. These findings suggest that the hepatoprotective effect of aqueous extracts of *G. indica* in ethanol-induced hepatotoxicity may be due to increased endogenous antioxidant levels and the inhibition of lipid peroxidation in the liver.

It is important to note that there are concerns about the risk of hepatotoxicity related to garcinia food supplements from a recent report by the Scientific Committee of the Spanish Agency for Food Safety and Nutrition (AESAN) [82]. As a result of several previous studies [83–85], *G. gummi-gutta* (*G. cambogia*) and HCA, its main active ingredient, can cause herb-induced hepatotoxicity (HILI) including elevated liver enzyme levels, hepatitis, cholestasis, and jaundice. Furthermore, these acute liver damages are known to persist even after discontinuation of their intake. Although no research results have been reported on the direct association between *G. indica* and acute liver injury, more scientific and clinical investigations on the effect of *G. indica* on liver health since *G. indica* also contain HCA.

3.8. Cardioprotective Activity

Atherosclerosis is one of the leading causes of cardiovascular disease, with significant mortality and morbidity worldwide. Barve, K. [38] calculated various indicators to predict the risk of atherosclerosis and subsequent cardiovascular disease using lipid values as follows: atherogenic index of plasma (AIP) = (log (triglycerides/high-density cholesterol)), cardiac risk ratio (CRR) = (total cholesterol/high-density cholesterol), atherogenic coefficient (AC) = (total cholesterol−high-density cholesterol/high-density cholesterol). The values of AIP, CPR, and AC were significantly higher at the end of 12 weeks in the group of animals fed a modified Western diet compared with the group of normal animals ($p < 0.01$, $p < 0.001$ and $p < 0.0001$, respectively). However, treatment with all tested concentrations of GEF significantly reduced these values ($p < 0.0001$), almost normalizing the levels, and attenuating the risk of atherosclerosis. Histopathological studies using light microscopy were performed by staining tissue sections of the thoracic aorta of mice with H/E. Then, lesions were scored for global pathological changes (lesion scores) as follows: score 0 = no change, score 1 = minimal changes, score 2 = minor changes, score 3 = moderate changes, and score 4 = significant changes. In the disease-induced animals, histopathological analysis of the aorta showed thickening of the vessel wall, and the lesion score of 3.33. Treatment with 25 or 50 mg/kg GEF improved some of these changes, resulting in a lesion score of 2.33, but this was not statistically significant. On the other hand, treatment with simvastatin or 100 mg/kg GEF showed completely normal vasculature with lesion scores of 0.66 and 1 ($p < 0.0001$ and $p < 0.001$, respectively).

Patel et al. [39] evaluated the cardioprotective effects of aqueous extracts of *G. indica* by ISO-induced myocardial injury in Wistar albino rats. The aqueous extract of *G. indica* did not affect the levels of cardiac injury markers including serum troponin I, lactate dehydrogenase, creatinine kinase-MB, ALT, AST, and uric acid, which were significantly increased by ISO treatment. In addition, histopathological analysis demonstrated that the animals treated with aqueous *G. indica* extract had improved edema, infiltration, and necrosis levels, but no statistical significance was observed compared with the ISO control group. The results of these experiments suggest that aqueous extracts of *G. indica* do not have a cardioprotective effect against myocardial damage, and further studies with larger sample sizes and higher dose ranges may be needed to evaluate its cardioprotective effects.

4. Pharmacological Effects of Garcinol, a Major Active Constituent from *G. indica*

As mentioned above, various pharmacological activities of extracts and fractions of *G. indica* have been reported [33]. *G. indica* contains a major active compound called garcinol. This component is a yellow-colored, fat soluble pigment found in the rinds of *G. indica* at a level of 2–3%, which can be separated from the fruit rinds by EtOH and hexane extraction [35]. Garcinol shows powerful antioxidant activity, since it contains both phenolic hydroxyl groups and a β-diketone moiety, and in this respect, it resembles the structure of curcumin [48]. In addition, like the various pharmacological activities of *G. indica* mentioned above, there are many reported mechanisms by which garcinol also acts as an antioxidant, anti-inflammatory, or anticancer effects. It inhibited free-radical DPPH and was shown to have antioxidant activity on arachidonic acid metabolism and NO radical synthesis. These activities are involved in inflammation and carcinogenesis. Garcinol effectively inhibited inducible nitric oxide synthase (iNOS) synthesis by suppressing the activation of nuclear factor NFκB, and diminished the production of extracellular signal-regulated kinase 1/2, cyclooxygenase-2, and prostaglandins. In addition, it inhibited the activation of 5-lipoxygenase, which is responsible for the production of inflammatory molecules such as leukotrienes. These actions have inspired studies on inflammation-related cancers. In addition to reducing inflammation, the mechanisms underlying anticancer effects such as induction of apoptosis, inhibition of cell growth and proliferation, stimulation of cell cycle arrest and prevention of cancer cell metastasis have been identified. Consequently, numerous preclinical studies have reviewed the antitumor potential of garcinol in a variety of oncological variants, including colon, breast, prostate, head, and neck cancer, and hepatocellular carcinoma [86,87]. Furthermore, the antioxidant and anti-inflammatory properties of garcinol could be extended to a neuroprotective role, and garcinol acts as a potent natural HAT inhibitor, and has presented promising results in molecular interactions studies against MAO-B and catechol-O-methyltransferase, as well as in L-DOPA-induced dyskinesia. It has recently been reported the ability of garcinol to modulate memory and cognition by affecting nerve growth and survival and altering the neurochemical state of the brain [88].

5. Conclusions

G. indica has various pharmacological activities including antioxidant, anti-obesity, anti-arthritis, anti-inflammatory, antibacterial, hepatoprotective, cardioprotective, anti-depressant and anti-anxiety effects. These characteristics are consistent with the previously reported activity of abundant phytochemical components such as garcinol, HCA, cyanidin-3-sambubioside and cyanidin-3-glucoside isolated from *G. indica*. These studies suggest the potential of *G. indica* as a promising therapeutic agent for controlling and preventing various diseases. However, given that most of the trials have been conducted either in vitro or in vivo, further study at the clinical level is needed to establish the efficacy and safety of *G. indica* in humans.

Author Contributions: Conceptualization, C.H.L. and C.-I.C.; methodology, S.H.L. and C.-I.C.; writing—original draft preparation, S.H.L. and H.S.L.; writing—review and editing, C.H.L. and C.-I.C.; supervision, C.H.L. and C.-I.C.; project administration, C.-I.C. All authors have read and agreed to the published version of the manuscript.

Funding: This research was supported by the BK21 FOUR program through the National Research Foundation (NRF) of Korea, funded by the Ministry of Education (MOE, Korea).

Institutional Review Board Statement: Not applicable.

Informed Consent Statement: Not applicable.

Data Availability Statement: Data are contained within the article.

Conflicts of Interest: The authors declare no conflict of interest.

References

1. Barnes, J.; Anderson, L.A.; Phillipson, J.D. *Herbal Medicines*, 3rd ed.; Pharmaceutical Press: London, UK, 2007; pp. 1–23.
2. Kunle, O.F.; Egharevba, H.O.; Ahmadu, P.O. Standardization of Herbal Medicines—A Review. *Int. J. Biodivers. Conserv.* **2012**, *4*, 101–112. [CrossRef]
3. Jachak, S.M.; Saklani, A. Challenges and Opportunities in Drug Discovery from Plants. *Curr. Sci.* **2007**, *92*, 1251–1257.
4. Imam, M.Z.; Akter, S. *Musa Paradisiaca* L. and *Musa Sapientum* L.: A Phytochemical and Pharmacological Review. *J. Appl. Pharm. Sci.* **2011**, *1*, 14–20.
5. Newman, D.J.; Cragg, G.M. Natural Products as Sources of New Drugs from 1981 to 2014. *J. Nat. Prod.* **2016**, *79*, 629–661. [CrossRef] [PubMed]
6. An, P.; Zhang, L.-J.; Peng, W.; Chen, Y.-Y.; Liu, Q.-P.; Luan, X.; Zhang, H. Natural Products Are an Important Source for Proteasome Regulating Agents. *Phytomedicine* **2021**, *93*, 153799. [CrossRef] [PubMed]
7. Di Stasi, L.C.; Hiruma-Lima, C.A. *Plantas Medicinais Na Amazônia e Na Mata Atlântica*, 2nd ed.; Editora Unesp: São Paulo, Brazil, 2002; pp. 87–112.
8. de Melo, M.S.; Quintans, J.d.S.S.; Araújo, A.A. de S.; Duarte, M.C.; Bonjardim, L.R.; Nogueira, P.C. de L.; Moraes, V.R. de S.; Araújo-Júnior, J.X. de; Ribeiro, Ê.A.N.; Quintans-Júnior, L.J. A Systematic Review for Anti-Inflammatory Property of Clusiaceae Family: A Preclinical Approach. *Evid.-Based Complement. Altern. Med.* **2014**, *2014*, e960258. [CrossRef]
9. Acuña, U.M.; Dastmalchi, K.; Basile, M.J.; Kennelly, E.J. Quantitative High-Performance Liquid Chromatography Photo-Diode Array (HPLC-PDA) Analysis of Benzophenones and Biflavonoids in Eight Garcinia Species. *J. Food Compos. Anal.* **2012**, *25*, 215–220. [CrossRef]

10. Hemshekhar, M.; Sunitha, K.; Santhosh, M.S.; Devaraja, S.; Kemparaju, K.; Vishwanath, B.S.; Niranjana, S.R.; Girish, K.S. An Overview on Genus Garcinia: Phytochemical and Therapeutical Aspects. *Phytochem. Rev.* **2011**, *10*, 325–351. [CrossRef]
11. Chen, T.-H.; Tsai, M.-J.; Fu, Y.-S.; Weng, C.-F. The Exploration of Natural Compounds for Anti-Diabetes from Distinctive Species Garcinia Linii with Comprehensive Review of the Garcinia Family. *Biomolecules* **2019**, *9*, 641. [CrossRef] [PubMed]
12. Do Espirito Santo, B.L.S.; Santana, L.F.; Kato Junior, W.H.; de Araújo, F.d.O.; Bogo, D.; Freitas, K. de C.; Guimarães, R. de C.A.; Hiane, P.A.; Pott, A.; Filiú, W.F. de O.; et al. Medicinal Potential of Garcinia Species and Their Compounds. *Molecules* **2020**, *25*, 4513. [CrossRef] [PubMed]
13. Rao, A.V.R.; Sarma, M.R.; Venkataraman, K.; Yemul, S.S. A Benzophenone and Xanthone with Unusual Hydroxylation Patterns from the Heartwood of Garcinia Pedunculata. *Phytochemistry* **1974**, *13*, 1241–1244. [CrossRef]
14. Yamaguchi, F.; Saito, M.; Ariga, T.; Yoshimura, Y.; Nakazawa, H. Free Radical Scavenging Activity and Antiulcer Activity of Garcinol from *Garcinia Indica* Fruit Rind. *J. Agric. Food Chem.* **2000**, *48*, 2320–2325. [CrossRef] [PubMed]
15. Ito, C.; Itoigawa, M.; Miyamoto, Y.; Onoda, S.; Rao, K.S.; Mukainaka, T.; Tokuda, H.; Nishino, H.; Furukawa, H. Polyprenylated Benzophenones from Garcinia Assigu and Their Potential Cancer Chemopreventive Activities. *J. Nat. Prod.* **2003**, *66*, 206–209. [CrossRef] [PubMed]
16. Pan, M.-H.; Chang, W.-L.; Lin-Shiau, S.-Y.; Ho, C.-T.; Lin, J.-K. Induction of Apoptosis by Garcinol and Curcumin through Cytochrome c Release and Activation of Caspases in Human Leukemia HL-60 Cells. *J. Agric. Food Chem.* **2001**, *49*, 1464–1474. [CrossRef] [PubMed]
17. De Meyts, P.; Whittaker, J. Structural Biology of Insulin and IGF1 Receptors: Implications for Drug Design. *Nat. Rev. Drug Discov.* **2002**, *1*, 769–783. [CrossRef] [PubMed]
18. Liao, C.-H.; Sang, S.; Liang, Y.-C.; Ho, C.-T.; Lin, J.-K. Suppression of Inducible Nitric Oxide Synthase and Cyclooxygenase-2 in Downregulating Nuclear Factor-Kappa B Pathway by Garcinol. *Mol. Carcinog.* **2004**, *41*, 140–149. [CrossRef]
19. Koeberle, A.; Northoff, H.; Werz, O. Identification of 5-Lipoxygenase and Microsomal Prostaglandin E2 Synthase-1 as Functional Targets of the Anti-Inflammatory and Anti-Carcinogenic Garcinol. *Biochem. Pharmacol.* **2009**, *77*, 1513–1521. [CrossRef] [PubMed]
20. Hong, J.; Sang, S.; Park, H.-J.; Kwon, S.J.; Suh, N.; Huang, M.-T.; Ho, C.-T.; Yang, C.S. Modulation of Arachidonic Acid Metabolism and Nitric Oxide Synthesis by Garcinol and Its Derivatives. *Carcinogenesis* **2006**, *27*, 278–286. [CrossRef] [PubMed]
21. Yamaguchi, F.; Ariga, T.; Yoshimura, Y.; Nakazawa, H. Antioxidative and Anti-Glycation Activity of Garcinol from *Garcinia Indica* Fruit Rind. *J. Agric. Food Chem.* **2000**, *48*, 180–185. [CrossRef] [PubMed]
22. Kolodziejczyk, J.; Masullo, M.; Olas, B.; Piacente, S.; Wachowicz, B. Effects of Garcinol and Guttiferone K Isolated from Garcinia Cambogia on Oxidative/Nitrative Modifications in Blood Platelets and Plasma. *Platelets* **2009**, *20*, 487–492. [CrossRef] [PubMed]
23. Balasubramanyam, K.; Altaf, M.; Varier, R.A.; Swaminathan, V.; Ravindran, A.; Sadhale, P.P.; Kundu, T.K. Polyisoprenylated Benzophenone, Garcinol, a Natural Histone Acetyltransferase Inhibitor, Represses Chromatin Transcription and Alters Global Gene Expression. *J. Biol. Chem.* **2004**, *279*, 33716–33726. [CrossRef] [PubMed]
24. Kopytko, P.; Piotrowska, K.; Janisiak, J.; Tarnowski, M. Garcinol-A Natural Histone Acetyltransferase Inhibitor and New Anti-Cancer Epigenetic Drug. *Int. J. Mol. Sci.* **2021**, *22*, 2828. [CrossRef]
25. Padhye, S.; Ahmad, A.; Oswal, N.; Sarkar, F.H. Emerging Role of Garcinol, the Antioxidant Chalcone from *Garcinia Indica* Choisy and Its Synthetic Analogs. *J. Hematol. Oncol.* **2009**, *2*, 38. [CrossRef] [PubMed]
26. Khare, C.P. *Indian Medicinal Plants: An Illustrated Dictionary*, 2nd ed.; Springer Science & Business Media: Berlin/Heidelberg, Germany, 2008; pp. 278–279.
27. Swami, S.B.; Thakor, N.J.; Patil, S.C. Kokum (*Garcinia Indica*) and Its Many Functional Components as Related to the Human Health: A Review. *J. Food Res. Technol.* **2014**, *2*, 130–142.
28. Tamil Selvi, A.; Joseph, G.S.; Jayaprakasha, G.K. Inhibition of Growth and Aflatoxin Production in Aspergillus Flavus by *Garcinia Indica* Extract and Its Antioxidant Activity. *Food Microbiol.* **2003**, *20*, 455–460. [CrossRef]
29. Khatib, N.A.; Kiran, P.; Patil, P.A. Evaluation of Anti Inflammatory Activity of *Garcinia Indica* Fruit Rind Extracts in Wistar Rats. *Int. J. Res. Ayurveda Pharm. IJRAP* **2010**, *1*, 449–454.
30. Varalakshmi, K.N.; Sangeetha, C.G.; Shabeena, A.N.; Sunitha, S.R.; Vapika, J. Antimicrobial and Cytotoxic Effects of *Garcinia Indica* Fruit Rind Extract. *Am.-Eurasian J. Agric. Environ. Sci.* **2010**, *7*, 652–656.
31. Ding, M.; Feng, R.; Wang, S.Y.; Bowman, L.; Lu, Y.; Qian, Y.; Castranova, V.; Jiang, B.-H.; Shi, X. Cyanidin-3-Glucoside, a Natural Product Derived from Blackberry, Exhibits Chemopreventive and Chemotherapeutic Activity. *J. Biol. Chem.* **2006**, *281*, 17359–17368. [CrossRef] [PubMed]
32. Tsuda, T.; Horio, F.; Uchida, K.; Aoki, H.; Osawa, T. Dietary Cyanidin 3-O-β-D-Glucoside-Rich Purple Corn Color Prevents Obesity and Ameliorates Hyperglycemia in Mice. *J. Nutr.* **2003**, *133*, 2125–2130. [CrossRef] [PubMed]
33. Baliga, M.S.; Bhat, H.P.; Pai, R.J.; Boloor, R.; Palatty, P.L. The Chemistry and Medicinal Uses of the Underutilized Indian Fruit Tree *Garcinia Indica* Choisy (Kokum): A Review. *Food Res. Int.* **2011**, *44*, 1790–1799. [CrossRef]
34. Parasharami, V.; Kunder, G.; Desai, N. Recent Pharmacological Advances of Endangered Species of South India: *Garcinia Indica* Choisy. *J. Sci. Res. Rep.* **2015**, *8*, 1–10. [CrossRef]
35. Jagtap, P.; Bhise, K.; Prakya, V. A Phytopharmacological Review on *Garcinia Indica*. *Int. J. Herb. Med.* **2015**, *3*, 2–7.
36. Panda, V.; Ashar, H.; Srinath, S. Antioxidant and Hepatoprotective Effect of *Garcinia Indica* Fruit Rind in Ethanol-Induced Hepatic Damage in Rodents. *Interdiscip. Toxicol.* **2012**, *5*, 207–213. [CrossRef] [PubMed]

37. Sangaonkar, G.M.; Pawar, K.D. *Garcinia Indica* Mediated Biogenic Synthesis of Silver Nanoparticles with Antibacterial and Antioxidant Activities. *Colloids Surf. B Biointerfaces* **2018**, *164*, 210–217. [CrossRef] [PubMed]
38. Barve, K. Garcinol Enriched Fraction from the Fruit Rind of *Garcinia Indica* Ameliorates Atherosclerotic Risk Factor in Diet Induced Hyperlipidemic C57BL/6 Mice. *J. Tradit. Complement. Med.* **2019**, *11*, 95–102. [CrossRef]
39. Patel, K.J.; Panchasara, A.K.; Barvaliya, M.J.; Purohit, B.M.; Baxi, S.N.; Vadgama, V.K.; Tripathi, C.B. Evaluation of Cardioprotective Effect of Aqueous Extract of *Garcinia Indica* Linn. Fruit Rinds on Isoprenaline-Induced Myocardial Injury in Wistar Albino Rats. *Res. Pharm. Sci.* **2015**, *10*, 388–396. [PubMed]
40. Dhamija, I.; Parle, M.; Kumar, S. Antidepressant and Anxiolytic Effects of *Garcinia Indica* Fruit Rind via Monoaminergic Pathway. *3 Biotech* **2017**, *7*, 131. [CrossRef] [PubMed]
41. Tung, Y.-C.; Shih, Y.-A.; Nagabhushanam, K.; Ho, C.-T.; Cheng, A.-C.; Pan, M.-H. Coleus Forskohlii and *Garcinia Indica* Extracts Attenuated Lipid Accumulation by Regulating Energy Metabolism and Modulating Gut Microbiota in Obese Mice. *Food Res. Int.* **2021**, *142*, 110143. [CrossRef] [PubMed]
42. Warrier, P.; Barve, K.; Prabhakar, B. Anti-Arthritic Effect of Garcinol Enriched Fraction Against Adjuvant Induced Arthritis. *Recent Pat. Inflamm. Allergy Drug Discov.* **2019**, *13*, 49–56. [CrossRef] [PubMed]
43. Ames, B.N.; Shigenaga, M.K.; Gold, L.S. DNA Lesions, Inducible DNA Repair, and Cell Division: Three Key Factors in Mutagenesis and Carcinogenesis. *Environ. Health Perspect.* **1993**, *101*, 35–44. [CrossRef] [PubMed]
44. Temple, N.J. Antioxidants and Disease: More Questions than Answers. *Nutr. Res.* **2000**, *20*, 449–459. [CrossRef]
45. Hur, S.J.; Lee, S.Y.; Kim, Y.-C.; Choi, I.; Kim, G.-B. Effect of Fermentation on the Antioxidant Activity in Plant-Based Foods. *Food Chem.* **2014**, *160*, 346–356. [CrossRef] [PubMed]
46. Deore, A.B.; Sapakal, V.D.; Naikwade, N.S. Antioxidant and Hepatoprotective Activity of *Garcinia Indica* Linn Fruit Rind. *Int. J Compr. Pharm.* **2011**, *2*, 1–5.
47. Singh, T.; Kasture, S.B.; Mohanty, P.K.; Jaliwala, Y.; Karchuli, M. In Vitro Antioxidative Activity of Phenolic and Flavonoid Compounds Extracted from Fruit of *Garcinia Indica*. *Int. J. Pharm. Life Sci.* **2011**, *2*, 613–616.
48. Mishra, A.; Bapat, M.M.; Tilak, J.C.; Devasagayam, T.P.A. Antioxidant Activity of *Garcinia Indica* (Kokam) and Its Syrup. *Curr. Sci.* **2006**, *91*, 90–93.
49. Rawri, R.K.; Bharathi, K.; Jayaveera, K.N.; Asdaq, S.M.B. In Vitro Antioxidant Properties of *Garcinia Indica* Linn Alcoholic Fruits Extracts. *J. Pharm. Sci. Innov.* **2013**, *2*, 9–12. [CrossRef]
50. Krishnamurthy, N.; Sampathu, S.R. Antioxydant Principles of Kokum Rind. *J. Food Sci. Technol. Mysore* **1988**, *25*, 44–45.
51. Ruch, R.J.; Cheng, S.J.; Klaunig, J.E. Prevention of Cytotoxicity and Inhibition of Intercellular Communication by Antioxidant Catechins Isolated from Chinese Green Tea. *Carcinogenesis* **1989**, *10*, 1003–1008. [CrossRef] [PubMed]
52. Darji, K.K.; Shetgiri, P.; D'mello, P.M. Evaluation of Antioxidant and Antihyperlipidemic Activity of Extract of *Garcinia Indica*. *Int. J. Pharm. Sci. Res.* **2010**, *1*, 175–181.
53. Sang, S.; Liao, C.-H.; Pan, M.-H.; Rosen, R.T.; Lin-Shiau, S.-Y.; Lin, J.-K.; Ho, C.-T. Chemical Studies on Antioxidant Mechanism of Garcinol: Analysis of Radical Reaction Products of Garcinol with Peroxyl Radicals and Their Antitumor Activities. *Tetrahedron* **2002**, *58*, 10095–10102. [CrossRef]
54. Astier, Y.; Bayley, H.; Howorka, S. Protein Components for Nanodevices. *Curr. Opin. Chem. Biol.* **2005**, *9*, 576–584. [CrossRef] [PubMed]
55. Bhakya, S.; Muthukrishnan, S.; Sukumaran, M.; Muthukumar, M. Biogenic Synthesis of Silver Nanoparticles and Their Antioxidant and Antibacterial Activity. *Appl. Nanosci.* **2016**, *6*, 755–766. [CrossRef]
56. Vo-Dinh, T. *Nanotechnology in Biology and Medicine: Methods, Devices, and Applications*, 1st ed.; CRC Press: Boca Raton, FL, USA, 2007; ISBN 978-0-429-12560-7.
57. Kulkarni, N.; Muddapur, U. Biosynthesis of Metal Nanoparticles: A Review. *J. Nanotechnol.* **2014**, *2014*, e510246. [CrossRef]
58. Apovian, C.M. Obesity: Definition, Comorbidities, Causes, and Burden. *Am. J. Manag. Care* **2016**, *22*, 10.
59. Williams, E.P.; Mesidor, M.; Winters, K.; Dubbert, P.M.; Wyatt, S.B. Overweight and Obesity: Prevalence, Consequences, and Causes of a Growing Public Health Problem. *Curr. Obes. Rep.* **2015**, *4*, 363–370. [CrossRef] [PubMed]
60. Lu, M.; Cao, Y.; Xiao, J.; Song, M.; Ho, C.-T. Molecular Mechanisms of the Anti-Obesity Effect of Bioactive Ingredients in Common Spices: A Review. *Food Funct.* **2018**, *9*, 4569–4581. [CrossRef]
61. Conforti, F.; Pan, M.-H. Natural Products in Anti-Obesity Therapy. *Molecules* **2016**, *21*, 1750. [CrossRef] [PubMed]
62. Lee, P.-S.; Teng, C.-Y.; Kalyanam, N.; Ho, C.-T.; Pan, M.-H. Garcinol Reduces Obesity in High-Fat-Diet-Fed Mice by Modulating Gut Microbiota Composition. *Mol. Nutr. Food Res.* **2019**, *63*, e1800390. [CrossRef] [PubMed]
63. Jena, B.S.; Jayaprakasha, G.K.; Singh, R.P.; Sakariah, K.K. Chemistry and Biochemistry of (−)-Hydroxycitric Acid from Garcinia. *J. Agric. Food Chem.* **2002**, *50*, 10–22. [CrossRef] [PubMed]
64. Tsuda, T.; Ueno, Y.; Aoki, H.; Koda, T.; Horio, F.; Takahashi, N.; Kawada, T.; Osawa, T. Anthocyanin Enhances Adipocytokine Secretion and Adipocyte-Specific Gene Expression in Isolated Rat Adipocytes. *Biochem. Biophys. Res. Commun.* **2004**, *316*, 149–157. [CrossRef] [PubMed]
65. Hong, J.-I.; Park, I.Y.; Kim, H.A. Understanding the Molecular Mechanisms Underlying the Pathogenesis of Arthritis Pain Using Animal Models. *Int. J. Mol. Sci.* **2020**, *21*, 533. [CrossRef] [PubMed]
66. Tang, C.-H. Research of Pathogenesis and Novel Therapeutics in Arthritis. *Int. J. Mol. Sci.* **2019**, *20*, 1646. [CrossRef] [PubMed]

67. Vogel, H. *Drug Discovery and Evaluation: Pharmacological Assays*, 2nd ed.; Springer Science & Business Media: Berlin/Heidelberg, Germany, 2007; pp. 902–942.
68. Zhu, F.; Du, B.; Xu, B. Anti-Inflammatory Effects of Phytochemicals from Fruits, Vegetables, and Food Legumes: A Review. *Crit. Rev. Food Sci. Nutr.* **2018**, *58*, 1260–1270. [CrossRef] [PubMed]
69. Dinarello, C.A. Anti-Inflammatory Agents: Present and Future. *Cell* **2010**, *140*, 935–950. [CrossRef] [PubMed]
70. Tanaka, T.; Narazaki, M.; Kishimoto, T. IL-6 in Inflammation, Immunity, and Disease. *Cold Spring Harb. Perspect. Biol.* **2014**, *6*, a016295. [CrossRef] [PubMed]
71. Edition, F. *Diagnostic and Statistical Manual of Mental Disorders: DSM-5*, 5th ed.; American Psychiatric Association: Washington, DC, USA, 2013; ISBN 978-0-89042-554-1.
72. Grundmann, O.; Nakajima, J.-I.; Kamata, K.; Seo, S.; Butterweck, V. Kaempferol from the Leaves of Apocynum Venetum Possesses Anxiolytic Activities in the Elevated plus Maze Test in Mice. *Phytomedicine* **2009**, *16*, 295–302. [CrossRef] [PubMed]
73. Abouhosseini Tabari, M.; Hajizadeh Moghaddam, A.; Maggi, F.; Benelli, G. Anxiolytic and Antidepressant Activities of Pelargonium Roseum Essential Oil on Swiss Albino Mice: Possible Involvement of Serotonergic Transmission. *Phytother. Res.* **2018**, *32*, 1014–1022. [CrossRef] [PubMed]
74. Benelli, G.; Maggi, F.; Nicoletti, M. Ethnopharmacology in the Fight against Plasmodium Parasites and Brain Disorders: In Memoriam of Philippe Rasoanaivo. *J. Ethnopharmacol.* **2016**, *193*, 726–728. [CrossRef] [PubMed]
75. Woolhouse, M.; Waugh, C.; Perry, M.R.; Nair, H. Global Disease Burden Due to Antibiotic Resistance—State of the Evidence. *J. Glob. Health* **2016**, *6*, 010306. [CrossRef]
76. Cattoir, V.; Felden, B. Future Antibacterial Strategies: From Basic Concepts to Clinical Challenges. *J. Infect. Dis.* **2019**, *220*, 350–360. [CrossRef] [PubMed]
77. Negi, P.S.; Jayaprakasha, G.K. Control of Foodborne Pathogenic and Spoilage Bacteria by Garcinol and *Garcinia Indica* extracts, and Their Antioxidant Activity. *J. Food Sci.* **2004**, *69*, FMS61–FMS65. [CrossRef]
78. Pasha, C.; Sayeed, S.; Ali, S.; Khan, Z. Antisalmonella Activity of Selected Medicinal Plants. *Turk. J. Biol.* **2009**, *33*, 59–64.
79. Kunder, G.; Parasharami, V. Evidence to Prove Why *Garcinia Indica* Choisy Leaves Does Not Respond to Hairy Root Induction by Agrobacterium Rhizogenes Mediated Transformation along with Positive Antimicrobial Activity. *Int. J. Curr. Microbiol. Appl. Sci.* **2014**, *3*, 720–730.
80. Ahmed, S.; Ahmad, M.; Swami, B.L.; Ikram, S. A Review on Plants Extract Mediated Synthesis of Silver Nanoparticles for Antimicrobial Applications: A Green Expertise. *J. Adv. Res.* **2016**, *7*, 17–28. [CrossRef]
81. Siddiq, A.M.; Parandhaman, T.; Begam, A.F.; Das, S.K.; Alam, M.S. Effect of Gemini Surfactant (16-6-16) on the Synthesis of Silver Nanoparticles: A Facile Approach for Antibacterial Application. *Enzym. Microb. Technol.* **2016**, *95*, 118–127. [CrossRef]
82. AESAN. Report of the Scientific Committee of the Spanish Agency for Food Safety and Nutrition (AESAN) on the Risk Associated with the Consumption of Food Supplements that Contain Garcinia Gummi-Gutta as an Ingredient. Available online: https://www.aesan.gob.es/AECOSAN/docs/documentos/seguridad_alimentaria/evaluacion_riesgos/informes_cc_ingles/GARCINIA_FOOD_SUPPLEMENTS.pdf (accessed on 15 December 2021).
83. Lunsford, K.E.; Bodzin, A.S.; Reino, D.C.; Wang, H.L.; Busuttil, R.W. Dangerous Dietary Supplements: *Garcinia Cambogia*-Associated Hepatic Failure Requiring Transplantation. *World J. Gastroenterol.* **2016**, *22*, 10071–10076. [CrossRef] [PubMed]
84. Crescioli, G.; Lombardi, N.; Bettiol, A.; Marconi, E.; Risaliti, F.; Bertoni, M.; Menniti Ippolito, F.; Maggini, V.; Gallo, E.; Firenzuoli, F.; et al. Acute Liver Injury Following Garcinia Cambogia Weight-Loss Supplementation: Case Series and Literature Review. *Intern. Emerg. Med.* **2018**, *13*, 857–872. [CrossRef] [PubMed]
85. Sharma, A.; Akagi, E.; Njie, A.; Goyal, S.; Arsene, C.; Krishnamoorthy, G.; Ehrinpreis, M. Acute Hepatitis Due to Garcinia Cambogia Extract, an Herbal Weight Loss Supplement. *Case Rep. Gastroint. Med.* **2018**, *2018*, 9606161. [CrossRef]
86. Liu, C.; Ho, P.C.-L.; Wong, F.C.; Sethi, G.; Wang, L.Z.; Goh, B.C. Garcinol: Current Status of Its Anti-Oxidative, Anti-Inflammatory and Anti-Cancer Effects. *Cancer Lett.* **2015**, *362*, 8–14. [CrossRef] [PubMed]
87. Aggarwal, V.; Tuli, H.S.; Kaur, J.; Aggarwal, D.; Parashar, G.; Chaturvedi Parashar, N.; Kulkarni, S.; Kaur, G.; Sak, K.; Kumar, M.; et al. Garcinol Exhibits Anti-Neoplastic Effects by Targeting Diverse Oncogenic Factors in Tumor Cells. *Biomedicines* **2020**, *8*, 103. [CrossRef] [PubMed]
88. Deb, S.; Phukan, B.C.; Mazumder, M.K.; Dutta, A.; Paul, R.; Bhattacharya, P.; Sandhir, R.; Borah, A. Garcinol, a Multifaceted Sword for the Treatment of Parkinson's Disease. *Neurochem. Int.* **2019**, *128*, 50–57. [CrossRef] [PubMed]

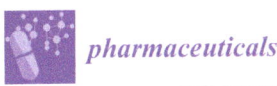

Review

Dietary Effects of Anthocyanins in Human Health: A Comprehensive Review

Ana C. Gonçalves [1], Ana R. Nunes [1], Amílcar Falcão [2,3], Gilberto Alves [1] and Luís R. Silva [1,*]

[1] CICS–UBI—Health Sciences Research Centre, University of Beira Interior, 6201-506 Covilhã, Portugal; anacarolinagoncalves@sapo.pt (A.C.G.); araqueln@gmail.pt (A.R.N.); gilberto@fcsaude.ubi.pt (G.A.)

[2] CIBIT—Coimbra Institute for Biomedical Imaging and Translational Research, University of Coimbra, Edifício do ICNAS, Pólo 3, Azinhaga de Santa Comba, 3000-548 Coimbra, Portugal; vr.amilcar.falcao@uc.pt

[3] Laboratory of Pharmacology, Faculty of Pharmacy, University of Coimbra, Pólo das Ciências da Saúde, Azinhaga de Santa Comba, 3000-548 Coimbra, Portugal

* Correspondence: luisfarmacognosia@gmail.com; Tel.: +351-275-329-077

Abstract: In recent years, the consumption of natural-based foods, including beans, fruits, legumes, nuts, oils, vegetables, spices, and whole grains, has been encouraged. This fact is essentially due to their content in bioactive phytochemicals, with the phenolic compounds standing out. Among them, anthocyanins have been a target of many studies due to the presence of catechol, pyrogallol, and methoxy groups in their chemical structure, which confer notable scavenging, anti-apoptotic, and anti-inflammatory activities, being already recommended as supplementation to mitigate or even attenuate certain disorders, such as diabetes, cancer, and cardiovascular and neurological pathologies. The most well-known anthocyanins are cyanidin 3-*O*-glucoside and cyanidin 3-*O*-rutinoside. They are widespread in nature, being present in considerable amounts in red fruits and red vegetables. Overall, the present review intends to discuss the most recent findings on the potential health benefits from the daily intake of anthocyanin-rich foods, as well as their possible pharmacological mechanisms of action. However, before that, some emphasis regarding their chemical structure, dietary sources, and bioavailability was done.

Keywords: anthocyanins; antioxidants; dietary source; bioavailability; biological activity; biosynthesis

Citation: Gonçalves, A.C.; Nunes, A.R.; Falcão, A.; Alves, G.; Silva, L.R. Dietary Effects of Anthocyanins in Human Health: A Comprehensive Review. *Pharmaceuticals* **2021**, *14*, 690. https://doi.org/10.3390/ph14070690

Academic Editor: Noelia Duarte

Received: 25 June 2021
Accepted: 16 July 2021
Published: 18 July 2021

Publisher's Note: MDPI stays neutral with regard to jurisdictional claims in published maps and institutional affiliations.

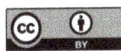

Copyright: © 2021 by the authors. Licensee MDPI, Basel, Switzerland. This article is an open access article distributed under the terms and conditions of the Creative Commons Attribution (CC BY) license (https://creativecommons.org/licenses/by/4.0/).

1. Introduction

In the past few years, it is widely accepted that the daily intake of medicinal herbs, fruits, and vegetables provides a wide array of benefits to human health [1]. This fact is essentially due to their composition, plentiful in several non-nutrient bioactive compounds, such as phenolics, whose abilities to modulate different processes and pathways in the human body, such as regulating glucose levels and boosting antioxidant, anti-inflammatory, anti-mutagenic, anticancer, and neuroprotective effects, are already well-known [2,3].

Considering that nature-based products have been used since ancient times to treat several disorders, such as colds, pain, gastrointestinal aches, and hypertension, among others, it is not surprising that this tendency continues to increase worldwide [4]. A clear example is their incorporation into pharmaceutical products used in cancer therapy [5,6]. According to the database of 2019, from the 247 anticancer drugs available in the market, about 81.0% are derived from natural products; the remaining ones are synthetic drugs (15.3%) or vaccines (3.65%) [3].

Among the phenolic compounds, anthocyanidins and their conjugated acyl-glycosylated or glycosylated forms, called anthocyanins, are both members of the flavonoids and an interesting class of water-soluble vacuolar pigments [7]. They are synthetized via the flavonoid path and considered the major contributors to the vivid red, orange, violet, and blue colours exhibited by various edible flowers, vegetables, fruits, some cereals, seeds and plant leaves, and their derivatives, such as juices, tea, and red wines [8]. They also have received much attention owing to their nutritional value, pharmacokinetic profile, pharmacological mechanisms, and health-promoting properties [9,10]. Indeed, recent human and animals surveys revealed that they are functional compounds able to increase antioxidant defences, diminish free radical damage, chronic inflammation and the risk of mutations, and attenuate, or even mitigate, the development and progression of many non-communicable and degenerative chronic disorders, namely, atherosclerosis, metabolic syndrome, eye and kidney complications, many cancer types, and also to control weight [6,11–19]. These biological activities are associated with their chemical structure, the presence of the catechol and pyrogallol groups standing out, allowing them to have the ability to chelate metal ions and neutralize free radicals and reactive species [4,20–22]. The predominant ones found in foodstuffs are cyanidin, delphinidin, pelargonidin, peonidin, petunidin, and malvidin glycosides [6,23,24].

This comprehensive review aimed to assess and elucidate the impact of anthocyanins and anthocyanin-rich foods on human health. For that, the first part of the manuscript focuses on a description regarding the chemical structure and function as well as main dietary sources of anthocyanins. Afterwards, the bioavailability and metabolism after intake are mentioned. Finally, we summarized and discussed the most recent literature regarding the main therapeutic effects of anthocyanins on different disorders.

2. Chemical Structure and Function of Anthocyanins

Phenolic compounds are secondary metabolites produced by plants to protect them against pathogens and predators, ultraviolet radiation, climate conditions, and acidified soils, acting also as attractants for pollinators, antifeedants, and phytoalexins [25,26]. They are also considered the main contributors to plants' colour, nutritional, and sensory characteristics [27]. Their structure presents at least one benzene ring coupled to one or more hydroxyl groups and can range from simple phenolic, low molecular weight and single-aromatic molecules to highly polymerized compounds [28]. In order to facilitate their distinction, phenolics are classified into two major groups: (i) non-flavonoid compounds (phenolic acids, tannins, lignans, coumarins, stilbenes, and curcuminoids) and (ii) flavonoid compounds (anthocyanidins, flavan-3-ols, and their oligomeric structures, recognized as proanthocyanidins, flavanones, flavanonols, flavones, flavonols, and isoflavones) [7,25,26]. Their biosynthesis, which is shown in Figure 1, comprises the shikimate, phenylpropanoid, and flavonoid pathways, and involves deamination, hydroxylation, and methylation reactions [25].

Concerning the flavonoids (Figure 2), they represent about two-thirds of the total dietary phenolics consumed, and currently, more than 9000 different flavonoids have been identified so far [29,30]. They all possess a common flavan nucleus, i.e., a 15 carbon-structure (C6 (A ring)-C3 (C ring)-C6 (B ring)), composed of 2 aromatic rings (A and B rings derived from the acetate/malonate and shikimate pathways, respectively), linked by a heterocyclic benzopyran 3-carbon ring that contains an oxygen atom (C ring) [26,31]. However, they differ in (i) the C ring unsaturation and oxidation state; (ii) A, B, and C ring substituents, such as the presence or absence of double bonds and carbonyl groups, and the possible occurrence of acylation, alkylation, glycosylation, oxygenation, and sulphonation processes; (iii) the position where the B ring is linked to the C ring; and (iv) location and number of hydroxy and methoxy groups on the B ring [26].

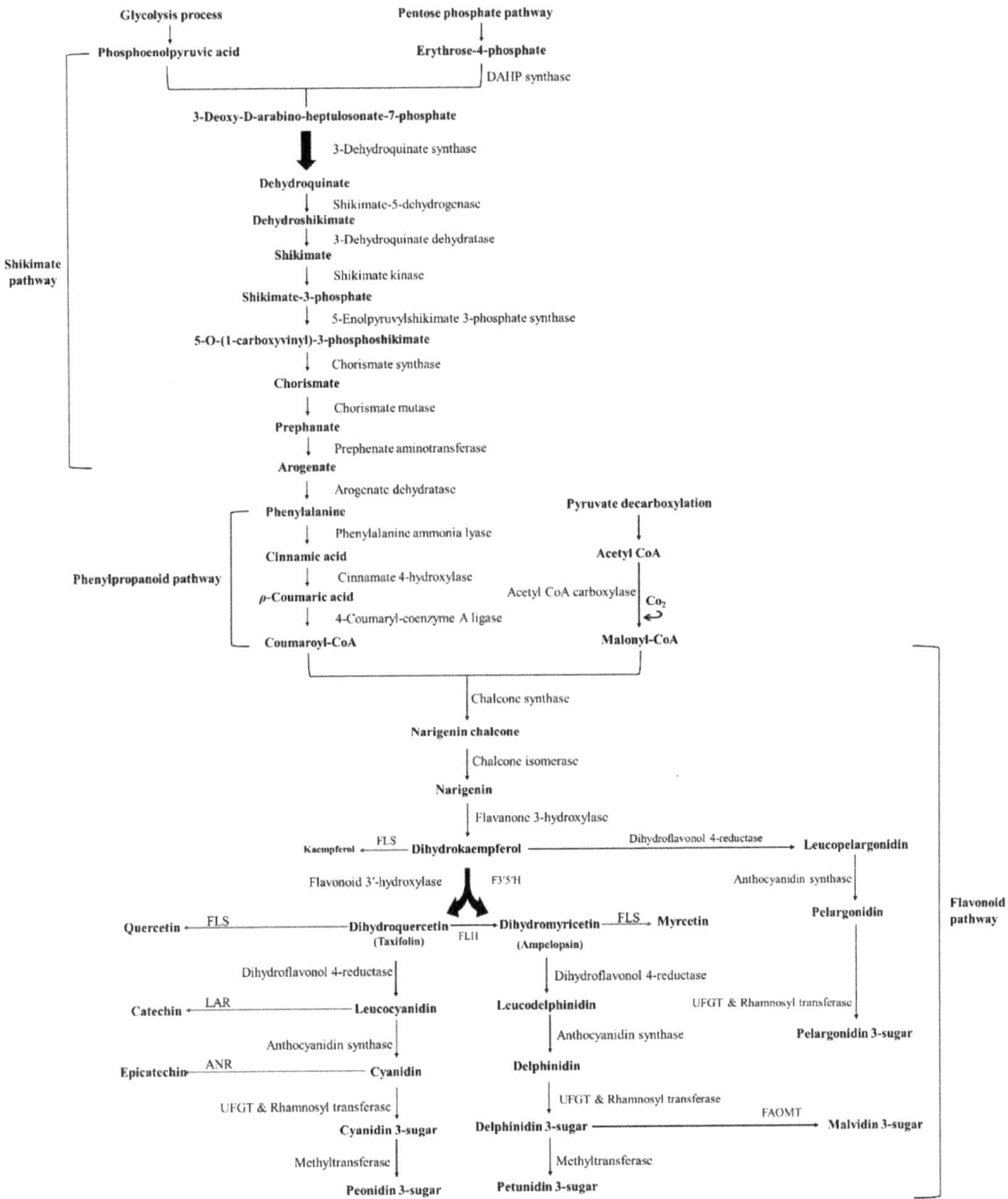

Figure 1. Biosynthesis pathways of the main anthocyanins found in foods. DAHP: 3-Deoxy-D-arabinoheptulosonate 7-phosphate; CoA: coenzyme A; F3′5′H: Flavonoid 3′, 5′-hydroxylase; FLH: Flavanone 3-hydroxylase; FLS: Flavonol synthase; LAR: Leucoanthocyanidin reductase; ANR: Anthocyanidin reductase; UFGT: UDP glucose flavonoid 3-O-glucosyltransferase; FAOMT: Flavonoid 3′, 5′-methyltransferase (adapted from [25]).

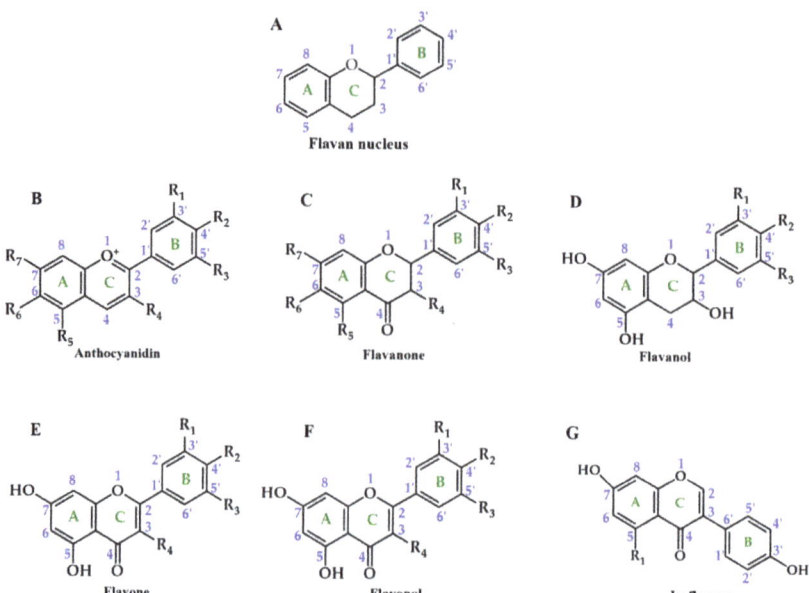

Figure 2. The basic structure of the flavonoids (**A**), which include anthocyanidins (e.g., cyanidin and pelargonidin) (**B**), flavanones (e.g., hesperidin and naringenin) (**C**), flavanols (e.g., catechin and epicatechin) (**D**), flavones (e.g., apigenin and luteolin) (**E**), flavonols (e.g., quercetin and kaempferol) (**F**), and isoflavones (e.g., daidzein and genistein) (**G**), differing in the level of oxidation and C ring saturation (adapted from [31]).

Focusing on anthocyanidins, their B ring is joined to the C ring through carbon 2 and the sugar residue of anthocyanins is typically found conjugated at carbon 3 [32,33] (Figure 3). Furthermore, their capacity to create flavylium cations makes them distinguishable from other flavonoid subclasses [22]. To date, about 27 different structural anthocyanin aglycones and 1000 anthocyanins are known [34,35]. In foods, the most commonly found are sugar moieties of cyanidin (50%), which is the most studied given their large distribution and number of hydroxyl groups, followed by pelargonidin, peonidin, and delphinidin (12%), and finally by petunidin and malvidin glycosides (7%) [8] (Figure 3). Together, they represent 90% of the total anthocyanins identified until now [36]. Their structure directly influences their biological potential, namely, the number of hydroxyl groups, the degree of glycosylation and acylation, the catechol residue on the B ring, and the oxonium ion on the C ring [37].

Therefore, the classification of anthocyanins is made according to (i) the number, position, and degree of methylation of the hydroxyl groups; (ii) the number and nature of the sugar moieties bonded to the aglycone; and (iii) the position of the aliphatic and/or aromatic carboxylate acids on the sugar molecule [38]. The stability of the anthocyanins is usually affected by the storage and processing conditions, temperature, and cooking, as well as by exposure to light and oxygen, the presence of enzymes, other phenolic compounds, metal ions, ascorbic acid, hydrogen peroxide (H_2O_2), water, and/or sulphites [37].

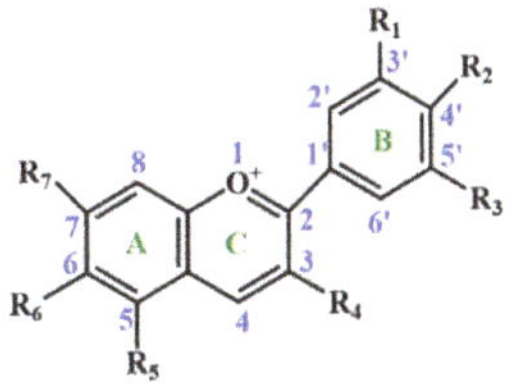

Anthocyanins	R_1	R_2	R_3	R_4	R_5	R_6	R_7	Colour
Cyanidin 3-O-sugar	OH	OH	H	Acgal, Acglu, Ara, Gal, Glu, Rut	OH	H	OH	Red
Delphinidin 3-O-sugar	OH	OH	OH	Acgal, Acglu, Ara, Gal, Glu, Rut	OH	H	OH	Pink
Malvidin 3-O-sugar	OCH$_3$	OH	OCH$_3$	Acgal, Acglu, Ara, Gal, Glu, Rut	OH	H	OH	Reddish purple
Pelargonidin 3-O-sugar	H	OH	H	Acgal, Acglu, Ara, Gal, Glu, Rut	OH	H	OH	Orange-Red
Peonidin 3-O-sugar	OCH$_3$	OH	H	Acgal, Acglu, Ara, Gal, Glu, Rut	OH	H	OH	Bluish purple
Petunidin 3-O-sugar	OCH$_3$	OH	OCH$_3$	Acgal, Acglu, Ara, Gal, Glu, Rut	OH	H	OH	Purple

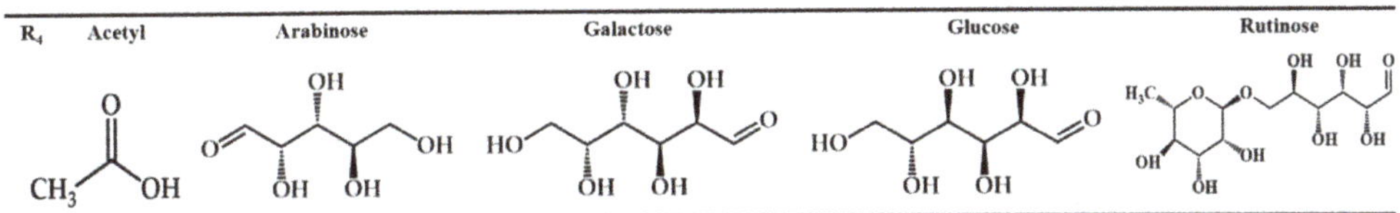

Figure 3. Representation of the main general chemical structure of anthocyanins. Acgal—acetylgalactose; Acglu—acetylglucose; Ara—arabinose; Gal—galactose; Glu—glucose; Rut—rutinoside (adapted from [35,37]).

3. Major Sources of Anthocyanins

Anthocyanins are widely spread in nature and are considered mainly responsible for the vibrant red, blue, and purple colours exhibited by vegetables, fruits, and their derivatives [37,39]. Their levels differ markedly among different species, being largely influenced by plant genotypes, and less by agricultural practices, growing area, climatic conditions, seasonal variability, temperature and light exposure, ripening stage, harvest time, and the adopted methods for processing and storage [9,40].

The daily average intake of anthocyanins is estimated to vary from several milligrams to hundreds of milligrams, although its evaluation is inaccurate and depends on the diet, gender, existence (or not) of food intolerances in individuals, and their quantities in foods [41]. Their intake by humans is higher in countries with a Mediterranean diet, plentiful in reddish berries and other red and blue-coloured fruits and vegetables, and red wine [23,42]. In Europe, the ingestion ranges from 19.8 mg per day (the Netherlands) to 64.9 mg per day (Italy) in men and 18.4 mg per day (Spain) to 44.1 mg per day (Italy) in women [24]. In the United States of America, Australia, and Asian countries, the intake is about 12.5, 24.2, and 37 mg per day per person, respectively [23,42,43]. Furthermore, and although it is not well established since they are non-essential nutrients, the recommended daily consumption of these coloured compounds has been evaluated, with China already recommending a daily intake of 50 mg per day/person in order to reduce oxidative stress levels and consequently the risk of cancer, metabolic syndrome, diabetes, degenerative diseases, and other pathologies [44].

In a general way, the primary sources of anthocyanins are berries (43% in Europe and 39% in the USA), red wine (22% in Europe and 18% in the USA), vegetables, and other fruits (19% in Europe and 9% in the USA) [45]. Table 1 presents the main sources of anthocyanins. A major amount of anthocyanins are found in berries, especially elderberries, chokeberries, blueberries, pomegranate, and açaí, presenting values superior to 282.5 mg cyanidin 3-glucoside equivalent per 100 g of fresh product [46,47]. Among the anthocyanins, cyanidin, malvidin, and delphinidin glycosides are the most found [47–50].

Table 1. Concentration of anthocyanins in fresh weight (FW) and dried weight (DW) in fruits, beverages, and vegetables.

Source	Maximum Anthocyanin Amount in FW (mg C3G/100 g)	Maximum Anthocyanin Amount in DW (mg C3G/100 g)	Dominant Anthocyanins	Reference
		Fruits		
Açaí	282.5–303.7		Cy 3,5-hexose pentose, Cy 3-O-glucoside, Cy 3-O-rutinoside, Pg 3-O-glucoside, Pn 3-O-glucoside, Pn 3-O-rutinoside, Cy 3-(acetyl)hexose	[51]
Acerola	6.5–8.4		Cy 3-rhamnoside, Pg 3-rhamnoside Cy, Pg	[51]
Apple	30.07–71.49 *		Cy 3-galactoside, Cy 3-O-glucoside, Cy 3-arabinoside, Pn 3-galactoside, Cy 7-arabinoside, Cy3-xyloside	[46,52]
Blackberries	70.3–201	909.3	Cy 3-O-glucoside, Cy 3-O-rutinoside, Cy 3-xyloside, Cy 3-malonylglucoside, Cy 3-dioxalylglucoside	[53,54]
Black currants	218.93	32,300 [1]	Dp 3-O-glucoside, Dp 3-O-rutinoside, Cy 3-O-glucoside, Cy 3-O-rutinoside	[55,56]
Blueberries	406.90	1160 [1]	Dp 3-O-galactoside, Dp 3-O-glucoside, Cy-3-O-galactoside, Dp 3-O-arabinoside, Cy-3-glucoside, Pt-3-galactoside, Cy 3-O-arabinoside, Pt 3-O-glucoside, Pn 3-O-arabinoside, Mv 3-O-galactoside, Mv 3-O-glucoside	[55,57]
Chokeberries	357.20		Cy 3-O-galactoside, Cy 3-arabinoside, Cy 3-O-glucoside, Cy xyloside	[55,58]
Cranberries	40.7–207.3 [1]		Cy 3-O-galactoside Cy 3-O-glucoside, Cy arabinoside, Pn galactoside, Pn 3-O-glucoside, Pn arabinoside	[59]
Elderberries	317.51	408.6–1066.6	Cy 3-O-glucoside, Cy 3-O-sambubioside	[55,60]
Fig	0.3–10.9	4.6–83	Cy 3-O-glucoside, Cy 3-O-rutinoside, Cy 3-sambubioside-5-glucoside, Cy 3,5-diglucoside	[61,62]
Grapes	38.70–186.02 [1]	135,960–533,630 [1]	Cy, Dp, Mv, Pn, Pt 3-O-glycosides; Mv, Pn, Pt 3-O-coumarylglucosides	[63,64]
Haskaps	449–697	2273	Cy 3,5-di-glucoside; Cy-3-galactoside, Cy 3-O-glucoside, Cy 3-O-rutinoside, Pg 3-O-glucoside; Pn 3-O-glucoside	[65,66]
Nectarine	0.22		Cy 3-O-glucoside, Cy 3-O-rutinoside	[46,67]
Plums	7.4–36.6 [1]		Cy 3-xyloside, Cy 3-O-glucoside, Cy 3-O-rutinoside, Pn 3-O-rutinoside, Pn 3-O-glucoside, Cy 3-galactoside, Cy 3-(6″-acetoyl)glucoside	[46,68]
Pomegranate	1500–2000		Dp 3,5-diglucoside, Cy 3-O-glucoside, Cy 3,5-diglucoside, Pg 3-O-glucoside, Pg 3,5-diglucoside	[69,70]
Peaches	0.27–2.50	0.28–15.34 [1]	Cy 3-O-rutinoside and glucoside	[71,72]

Table 1. Cont.

Source	Maximum Anthocyanin Amount in FW (mg C3G/100 g)	Maximum Anthocyanin Amount in DW (mg C3G/100 g)	Dominant Anthocyanins	Reference
Red cabbages	109–185	1111–1780	Cy 3-diglucoside-5-glucoside, Cy 3-(sinapoyl)(sinapoyl)-diglucoside-5-glucoside, Cy 3-(p-coumaroyl)-diglucoside-5-glucoside	[73,74]
Red currants	19.78	149.91 [1]	Cyanidin-3-O-sambusoside, Cy 3-O-glucoside, Cy 3-O-rutinoside	[55,75]
Red pears	1.2–12.0 [1]		Cy 3-O-galactoside, Cy 3-O-glucoside, Cy pentoside, Cy 3-O-arabinoside, Cy 3-O-rutinoside	[76]
Red raspberries	23.17–68.0	260.9–571.8	Cy 3-O-sophoroside, Cy 3-O-(2″-O-glucosyl)rutinoside, Cy 3-O-glucoside, Cy 3-O-rutinoside, Cy 3-O-(2″-O-xylosyl)rutinoside, Pg 3-O-sophoroside, Pg 3-O-glucoside, Cy 3,5-O-diglucoside	[53,55,77]
Strawberries	20–60 [1]	31.9–315.2 [2]	Pg 3-O-glucoside, Pg 3-O-glucoside, Cy 3-O-glucoside, Cy 3-O-rutinoside, Pg 3-O-glucoside, Pg 3-O-rutinoside, Pg 3-(malonoyl)glucoside, Pg 3-(6″-acetoyl)glucoside	[46,78,79]
Sweet cherries	2.06–462.77 [1]	107.70–218.36 [1]	Cy, Dp, Pg, Pn 3-O-rutinosides and glucosides, Cy 3-coumaroyl-diglucoside, Cy 3-O-sambubioside, Cy 3-5-diglucoside, Cy 3-sophoroside Cy 3-O-arabinoside Mv 3-O-glucoside-acetaldehyde	[40,80,81]
Tamarillo		29.70–486.84 [1]	Dp 3-O-rutinoside, Cy 3-O-rutinoside, Cy 3-O-glucoside, Pg 3-O-rutinoside	[82]
Tart cherries	65.06–82.40	114.59	Cy, Cy 3-O-sophoroside, Cy 3-glucosylrutinoside, Cy 3-O-glucoside, Cy 3-O-rutinoside, Pn 3-O-rutinoside	[55,83]
Tomato	7.1 [1]	5.48–29.86 [3]	Dp glycoside, Dp rutinoside, Dp p-coumaroyl-rutinoside Mv glycoside, Mv rutinoside, Mv p-coumaroyl-rutinoside-glycoside, Pt rutinoside, Pt p-coumaroyl-rutinoside, Pt p-coumaroyl-rutinoside-glycoside	[84,85]
Vegetables				
Black carrot	22.45 *	1.74–4.54 [1]	Cy 3-(p-coumaroyl)-diglucoside-5-glucoside	[47,86]
Eggplant	6.31	138 [4]	Dp 3-(p-coumaroylrutinoside)-5-glucoside, Dp 3-O-glucoside, Dp 3-glucosyl-rhamnoside, Pt -3-O-rutinoside, Cy -3-O-rutinoside	[49,50]

Table 1. Cont.

Source	Maximum Anthocyanin Amount in FW (mg C3G/100 g)	Maximum Anthocyanin Amount in DW (mg C3G/100 g)	Dominant Anthocyanins	Reference
Purple sweet potato	42.37 *		Pn 3-O-sophoroside-5-O-glucoside, Pn 3-O-glucoside, Cy 3-p-hydroxybenzoylsophoroside-5-glucoside, Pn 3-p-hydroxybenzoylsophoroside-5-glucoside, Cy 3-caffeoylsophoroside-5-glucoside, Pn 3-caffeoylsophoroside-5-glucoside, Cyanidin-3-caffeoyl-p-hydroxybenzoylsophoroside-5-glucoside, Pn 3-dicaffeoylsophoroside-5-glucoside, Pn 3-caffeoyl-p-hydroxybenzoylsophoroside-5-glucoside, Pn 3-caffeoy-feruloylsophoroside-5-glucosie	[47]
Red Chicory	39.20 *		Cy 3-O-glucoside, Cy 3-O-(6″-malonyl-glucoside)	[47]
Red onion	29.99		Cy 3-O-glucoside, Cy 3-O-laminaribioside, Cy 3-(6″-malonyl-glucoside), Cy 3-(6″-malonyl- laminaribioside), Cy 3-xylosylglucosylgalactoside, Dp 3,5-diglycosides	[47,87]
Beverages				
Blackberry juice	12.3–107		Cy 3-O-glycoside, Cy 3-O-rutinoside, Cy 3-xyloside, Cy malonylglucoside, Cy dioxalylglucoside	[54]
Pomegranate juice	7.2–20 [1]		Cy 3-O-glucoside, Cy 3,5-diglucoside, Dp 3,5-diglucoside, Cy 3,5-diglucoside, Pg 3,5-diglucoside, Dp 3-glucoside, Cy 3- O-glucoside; Pg 3-O-glucoside	[88]
Red wine	32.71–87.17 [1]		Cy, Dp, Mv, Pn, Pt 3-O-glycosides, Pn 3-O-acetylglucoside, Mv 3-O-acetylglucoside, Mv 3-O-coumarylglucoside, Pn 3-O-p-coumarylglucoside;	[48,89]
Tart cherry juice		72.2	Cy 3-sophoroside, Cy 3-glucosylrutinoside, Cy 3-O-glucoside, Cy 3-O-rutinoside, Cy, Pg, Pn 3-O-glucoside	[90]

FW, fresh weight; DW, dry weight; Cy, cyanidin; Dp, delphinidin; Mv, malvidin; Pg, pelargonidin; Pn, peonidin; Pt, petunidin. * mg cyanidin 3-galactoside equivalent per 100 g. [1] Total amount (weight) of anthocyanins identified by HPLC method. [2] mg pelargonidin 3-glucoside equivalent per 100 g. [3] mg malvidin 3-rutinoside equivalent per 100 g. [4] Delphinidin 3-glucoside equivalent per 100 g.

4. Anthocyanins' Bioavailability and Metabolism

Understanding the bioavailability of phenolics is crucial since, after consumption, their constituents undergo many modifications throughout the digestive tract (digestion, absorption, metabolization, and elimination), which have a great impact on their nutritional value and health-promoting properties [28,31].

Nowadays, it is established that the bioavailability of phenolics differs significantly between them, and therefore, the most abundant polyphenols in our dietary habits are not necessarily those that show the highest concentrations of active metabolites in organs and tissues [35]. Indeed, their bioavailability is highly dependent on the chemical structure of the phenolics, i.e., their molecular size, pattern of glycosylation and/or acylation (where acylation increases anthocyanin stability but declines their absorption), degree of polymerization, and conjugations and/or combinations with other compounds [36,91]. Furthermore, it is also influenced by the pH values observed along the gastrointestinal tract, facilitation of the compounds to cross membranes, digestibility, solubility, and absorption actions carried out by digestive enzymes, biliary acids, gut microbiota, and enterocytes. The food matrix maturity degree and cooking also influence the availability rates [35]. Although the thermal processing reduces anthocyanins' stability, at the same time, it damages the anthocyanin cell walls, increasing their body absorption [28].

It is also important to take into account that the bioavailability also varies among individuals—inter-individual variability—due to intrinsic aspects (e.g., age, sex, physiological and/or pathological states, and genetic factors), which induce marked differences regarding enzymes and microbiota activity [43].

Unlike other phenolics, anthocyanins are quickly metabolized and eliminated, and even in high amounts, they rarely reach concentration values considered active. In fact, the intake of 10 and 720 mg of anthocyanins only results in maximal plasma concentrations of 1.4 and 200 nanomolar, respectively, achieved between 30 min and 2 h [92–94].

Table 2 summarizes the principal human trials focused on the pharmacokinetic profile of anthocyanins observed after their ingestion in common foods and beverages. In a general way, less than 1.8% of consumed anthocyanins is normally absorbed. However, this percentage can decrease if they are ingested alone, with or after other compounds; i.e., if anthocyanins are consumed alone or after overnight fasting, their digestion happens in 1 hour [93,95], whereas if they are ingested accompanied by other foods and beverages, ingested with high-fat meals, or after a meal, it occurs only after 1.5 or 4 h, respectively [96]. They disappear from the blood circulatory system in less than 6 h [57].

Additionally, and considering that substitutions influence anthocyanin absorption, nowadays, it is well-described that pelargonidin derivatives are more readily absorbed than anthocyanins with more substituents on their B ring, such as peonidin-, delphinidin-, and cyanidin-based anthocyanins [46]. Furthermore, and comparing the sugar moieties, it was already verified that malvidin 3-O-arabinoside presents higher absorption rates than malvidin 3-O-glucoside [103].

Despite their low absorption and rapid metabolism, the regular consumption of anthocyanins is considered safe, and together with physical activity, it is encouraged as both can reduce the occurrence of several pathologies related to oxidative stress [36]. As far as we know, until now, no adverse effects regarding anthocyanin consumption have been reported. In fact, and focusing on human studies, most people who consumed 160 mg of anthocyanins twice a day for 2 months tolerated the extract; only 4% of the participants revealed side effects, namely at the gastrointestinal level and eczema [104,105].

Therefore, after being consumed, anthocyanins are metabolized in the mouth, where the action of oral microbiota removes the glycosidic groups and transforms them into their corresponding chalcones [106].

Table 2. Human studies considering the pharmacokinetic parameters of anthocyanins, after ingestion of common foods and beverages rich in this type of compound.

Intake	n [a]	Total Anthocyanins Intake	C_{max} [b]	t_{max} (h) [c]	AUC [d]	Urinary Excretion (%)	Reference
			Foods				
Blueberries (100 g)	5	1200 mg	13.1 ng/mL	4			[57]
Elderberries (12 g)	4	720 mg	97.4 nmol/L	1.2 h			[94]
Red raspberries (300 g)	9	292 μMol	0.1–180 nmol/L	1–1.5		0.007% (1–1.5 h)	[77]
			Beverages				
Red wine (300 mL)	6	218 mg		6		1.5–5.1% (12 h)	[89]
Red grape juice (400 mL)	9	Cy 3-O-glucoside	0.42 ng/mL	0.5	0.60 ng × h/mL (3 h)	0.09% (7 h)	[97]
		Dp 3-O-glucoside	6.12 ng/mL	0.5	11.9 ng × h/mL (3 h)	0.20% (7 h)	
		Mv 3-O-glucoside	48.8 ng/mL	0.5	71.7 ng × h/mL (3 h)	0.18% (7 h)	
		Pn 3-O-glucoside	27.3 ng/mL	0.5	49.7 ng × h/mL (3 h)	0.29% (7 h)	
		Pt 3-O-glucoside	16.1 ng/mL	0.5	31.5 ng × h/mL (3 h)	0.32% (7 h)	
		Σ = 283.5 mg	100.1 ng/mL	0.5	168.4 ng × h/mL		
Black currant juice (150 mL)	8	Cy 3-O-glucoside: 0.165 mg	5.0 nmol/L	1.34	11.0–19.6 ng × h/mL (4 h)	0.060% (8 h)	[96]
		Cy 3-O-rutinoside: 1.24 mg	46.3 nmol/L	3.45	19.6–24.9 ng × h/mL (4 h)	0.098% (8 h)	
		Dp 3-O-glucoside: 0.488 mg	22.7 nmol/L	4.19	11.0–16.3 ng × h/mL (4 h)	0.066 (8 h)	
		Dp 3-O-rutinoside: 1.68 mg	73.4 nmol/L	3.18	16.3–24.9 ng × h/mL (4 h)	0.11% (8 h)	
Açaí Juice (7 mL/kg of body weight)	12	165.9 mg/L	1138.51 ng/L	2	3314.04 ng × h/L (12 h)		[11]
Cranberry Juice (480 mL)	15	Cy 3-O-galactoside (18.7 mg)	1.38 nmol/L	1.27	3.91 nmol × h/L (4 h)	0.007% (4 h)	[98]
		Cy 3-O-glucoside (1.58 mg)	0.93 nmol/L	1.13	1.99 nmol × h/L (4 h)	0.007% (4 h)	
		Cy 3-O-arabinoside (16.47 mg)	3.61 nmol/L	1.47	9.16 nmol × h/L (4 h)	0.010% (4 h)	
		Mv 3-O-glucoside	0.56 nmol/L	0.93	1.25 nmol × h/L (4 h)		
		Pn 3-O-galactoside (30.83 mg)	4.64 nmol/L	1.47	12.00 nmol × h/L (4 h)	0.015% (4 h)	
		Pn 3-O-glucoside (5.85 mg)	0.71 nmol/L	1.40	1.85 nmol × h/L (4 h)	0.029% (4 h)	
		Pn 3-O-arabinose (21.03 mg)	1.78 nmol/L	1.27	4.13 nmol × h/L (4 h)	0.010% (4 h)	
		Σ = 94.47 mg					

Table 2. Cont.

Intake	n [a]	Total Anthocyanins Intake	C_{max} [b]	t_{max} (h) [c]	AUC [d]	Urinary Excretion (%)	Reference
Tart cherry juice (60 mL)	12	62.47 mg/L	2.75 μg × h/mL	1	106.4 μg × h/mL		[99]
Grape/blueberry juice (330 mL)	10	3,4-dihydroxybenzoic acid	7.6 nmol/L	1	568 nmol × min/L		[100]
		Cy 3-O-glucoside	0.10 nmol/L	1	6 nmol × min/L		
		Dp 3-O-glucoside	0.18 nmol/L	1.1	10 nmol × min/L		
		Mv 3-O-glucoside	1.5 nmol/L	1.1	103 nmol × min/L		
		Mv 3-O-glucuronide	1.1 nmol/L	2	114 nmol × min/L		
		Pn 3-O-glucuronide	1.1 nmol/L	1.8	114 nmol × min/L		
		Pn 3-O-glucoside	1.7 nmol/L	1	52 nmol × min/L		
		Pt 3-O-glucoside	0.8 nmol/L	1	12 nmol × min/L		
		Σ = 841 mg/L	1.21 nmol/L				
Orange juice	18	53.09 mg/L	0.63 nmol/L	0.96	8.99 nmol × h/L (8 h)	43–53% (2 h)	[101]
Chokeberry juice (0.8 mg/kg of body weight)	13		32.7 nmol/L	1.3	109.4 nmol × h/L (1 h)	0.25 (24 h)	[102]
Strawberry juice (34.7 mg)	14	Cy 3-O-glucoside: 7.8 μMol	0.6 nmol/L	2.1	1.7 nmol × h/L (10 h)		[95]
		Pg glucuronide	38.0 nmol/L	1.7	123.8 nmol × h/L (10 h)		
		Pg-3-O-glucoside: 58.8 μMol	5.2 nmol/L	1.3	15.0 nmol × h/L (10 h)		
		Pg 3-O-rutinoside: 9.7 μMol	0.4 nmol/L	1.9	1.4 nmol × h/L (10 h)		
		Σ = 76.6 μMol					

[a] Number of participants. [b] Maximum concentration in plasma. [c] Time to reach C_{max} in plasma. [d] Area under the curve, which describes the exposure of a compound over a set period of time.

After that, they pass along the gastrointestinal tract, starting in the stomach, where they do not suffer considerable changes, despite the acidic pH, and can be absorbed by bilitranslocase, becoming available for absorption (bioaccessibility) [106,107], or reach intestinal epithelial cells [108]. In fact, the literature suggests that it is possible that the gastric and intestinal bioavailability of anthocyanins are mainly done with the 3-monoglucosides, 3-monoglucoside acylated, and 3,5-diglucosides forms [106,107,109].

Therefore, anthocyanins can go through the portal vein to the liver and can be directed to the systemic circulation to be taken up by the target organs and tissues, or, if they are not absorbed, be discarded through urine and faeces (Figure 4) [41,110]. It is important to note that in intestines, liver, and kidneys, anthocyanins are metabolized by enzymes of phase I and phase II, being conjugated with additional hydroxyl, methyl, sulfuric, or glycoside groups in order to increase their availability [33,36,111].

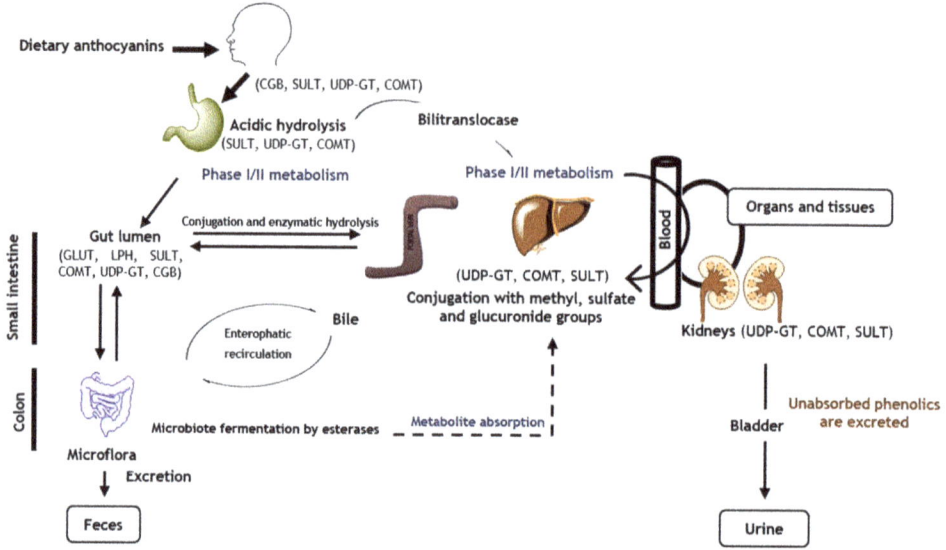

Figure 4. Anthocyanin absorption, distribution, metabolism, and excretion. CGB—cytosolic β-glucosidase; SULT—sulfotransferase; UDP-GT—glucuronosyltransferase; COMT—catechol-O-methyl transferase; GLUT—glucose transporters; LPH—lactase-phlorizin hydrolase.

In general, both native anthocyanidins and their conjugated forms are found in plasma and urine; nevertheless, the intact ones are more rapidly absorbed in the stomach (20–25%) and detected in plasma a few minutes after their ingestion [112]. This evidence is supported by previous studies based on the oral ingestion of red fruits, which revealed that anthocyanins are not metabolized into their aglycones, being directly absorbed and appearing in plasma 30 min after their consumption [92]. Their glycosylated forms are excreted in urine [8,93].

Notwithstanding, the major absorption rate is observed in the gut [33]. Therefore, in the gut, the lactase-phlorizin hydrolase (LPH) and β-glucosidase enzymes release the aglycone of the coloured compounds, increasing their hydrophobic character, thus facilitating their entrance by passive diffusion in epithelial cells [113]. Glycosides and acylated anthocyanins can also be absorbed by the small intestine due to the action of glucose transporters 1 and 3 (GLUT 1 and 3) [91,109,111,114]; however, the absorption of the acylated ones is four times lower than that of non-acylated anthocyanins [33]. Particularly, molecular docking studies revealed that smaller molecules interact with GLUT 1 and 3 by their glucose residue and AC rings, while larger compounds penetrate in both transporters by their C5 glucose, as well as B and coumaroyl rings [91,109].

Unabsorbed anthocyanins reach the colon and are hydrolysated within 20 min–2 h by colonic bacteria (e.g., α-galactosidase, β-D-glucuronidase, β-D-glucosidase, and α-rhamnosidase), which break down the glycosidic bonds and catalyse them into smaller phenolic compounds (e.g., benzaldehydes or hydroxytyrosol) or simple phenolic acids, such as ρ-hydroxybenzoic, homovanillic, phenylpropionic, protocatechuic, syringic, and vanillic acids, to simplify their absorption by colonic mucosa and consequently increase their availability [115]. This extensive metabolization is tremendously interesting and shows that the availability of anthocyanins is probably higher than we thought, and the reason why anthocyanins can be found in urine in amounts below 0.1% [91,116]. Indeed, a recent study indicates the intake of 300 g of red raspberries results in the identification of 18 different anthocyanin-derived metabolites [77]. Basically, delphinidin-based anthocyanins are transformed into 2,4,6-trihydroxybenzaldehyde, gallic, and syringic acids, while syringic, 4-hydroxybenzoic, and vanillic acids are the primary metabolites of malvidin, pelargonidin, and peonidin glucosides, respectively [111,117]. Cyanidin glycosides can produce around 35 metabolites, 31 being found in urine samples, 28 in faeces, and 17 in the circulatory system, where the main ones are 2,4,6-trihydroxybenzaldehyde, ρ-coumaric, protocatechuic and vanillic acids, and phenolic conjugates (e.g., hippuric, phenylacetic, and phenylpropenoic acids) [77,118].

Additionally, the cleavage of glycosidic bonds also enhances the beneficial effects exhibited by anthocyanins [33]. In fact, this modulation on colon microflora leads to the formation of short-chain fatty acids that together with phenolic acids induce a decrease in pH values, creating favourable conditions for the proliferation of probiotic bacteria, such as *Actinobacteria*, *Bifidobacteria*, and *Lactobacilli* [33,111]. These bacteria exert positive effects in the control of gastrointestinal and digestive disorders, allergies, eczema, and improvements in delicate cases of cardiac and mental illness [10,119].

5. Anthocyanin Encapsulation

Knowing that the incorporation of phenolic compounds into foods and pharmaceutical products is a challenge, due to their instability and susceptibility to degradation, during processing and storage, various delivery systems have been developed [4]. Among them, encapsulation is a good strategy. This technology allows entrapping an active agent, liquid, gas, or solid within a matrix or a polymeric wall in micro or nanoparticles, to protect the active compound from environmental conditions, undesirable interactions, and to control their transportation, release, and handling. The most common polymers used are carbohydrates (e.g., cellulose derivatives and maltodextrins), natural gums (e.g., alginates and gum arabic), lipids (e.g., emulsifiers and waxes), and/or proteins (e.g., dairy proteins, gelatine, and soy proteins) [33]. Additionally, their combination with other wall materials and some modifiers, such as antioxidants, chelate agents, and surfactants, can also increase the encapsulation benefits [4]. In a general way, the process of encapsulation is based on the formation of the wall around the compound of interest, ensuring that unwanted materials are kept outside, and preventing undesired leaks to happen. It is important to take into account, along with its cost, the particle size and physicochemical properties of the core and the origin of wall constituents, to favour capsule stability. To that end, several methods have been developed, and the best-known ones for anthocyanin encapsulation are emulsification, ionotropic gelation, thermal gelation, and spray-drying. This last one is the most applied technique (80–90% of encapsulated formulations are spray-dried) due to their cost and easy procedure [4]. Maltodextrins are the most used coating material given their ability to maintain anthocyanin stability [120].

Therefore, and in order to enhance their bioefficacy and stability, and thus prevent their rapid degradation, anthocyanins are mainly encapsulated with liposomes, nanocomplexes of alginate and chitosan, and gel emersions [34]. In fact, several studies already showed that anthocyanin nano-formulations, along with chemical modifications, favour their absorption and metabolization, and consequently increase their biological action [33]. Mueller et al. [112] conducted a human study and reported that the encapsulation of 2.4 g of blueberry anthocyanins with whey protein does not contribute to anthocyanin stabilization during intestinal passage given their ability to prolong their passage through the stomach, whereas the encapsulation with citrus pectin improves anthocyanin bioavailability and intestinal accessibility, thus increasing their concentrations in the bloodstream.

Furthermore, bioengineering-based, targeted drug delivery approaches using biodegradable PLGA@PEG nanoparticles revealed more notable results in both in vivo and in vitro Alzheimer's disease models than anthocyanins alone, namely, lower levels of oxidative stress and neuroinflammatory hallmarks [121,122]. Furthermore, 50 mg/mL of blueberry anthocyanins encapsulated in liposomal micelles also revealed higher anticancer activity than non-encapsulated anthocyanins on K562 human erythroleukemic cancer cells [123].

6. Putative Health Benefits

The low ingestion of fruits and vegetables causes around 1.7 million deaths worldwide, being related to 14% of gastrointestinal malignancies, 9% of stroke, and 11% of coronary artery disorders [36]. Therefore, it is undeniable the role of anthocyanins in promoting human health and welfare [105]. Several in vitro scavenging assays, animal and human cell lines studies, animal models, and human clinical trials already indicated that the consumption of foods, beverages, and supplements rich in anthocyanins brings numerous health benefits. In fact, this is due to the easy capacity of the anthocyanins to eliminate and/or neutralize free radicals and reactive species, chelate metals, control signalling pathways, diminish pro-inflammatory markers, and, thus, reduce the risk of cardiovascular pathologies, cancer, and neurodegeneration. Additionally, they also contribute to control weight and improve vision. The general health benefits resulting from the consumption of anthocyanins are shown in Figure 5.

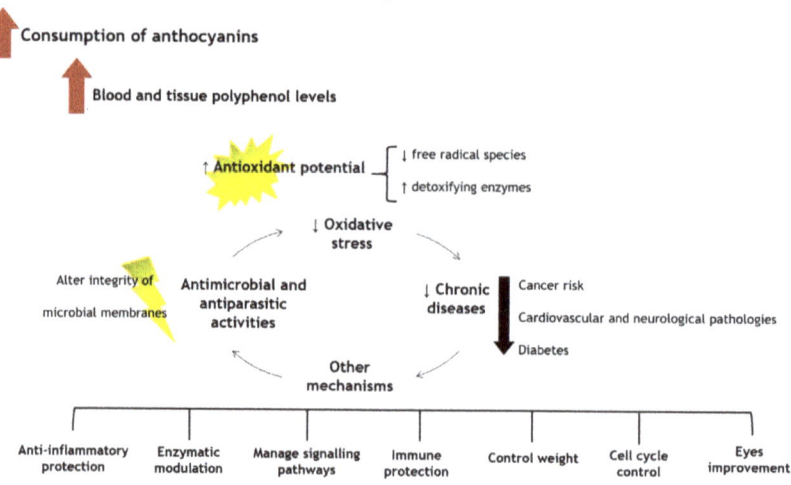

Figure 5. Health benefits of anthocyanins.

6.1. Antimicrobial Effects and Anti-Parasitic Activity

In order to attenuate the emerging resistance of microorganisms to antibiotics over time, natural products have gained much attention since they are rich in many metabolites with antimicrobial, antifungal, and anti-parasitic effects. In fact, these activities are part of the plants' defense mechanism against pathogens and infections during their development and growth. Among these phytochemicals, anthocyanins already showed capacity to reduce the replication and growth of some Gram-negative and Gram-positive bacteria and parasites [124,125].

Anthocyanins already revealed an ability to stop the replication of two common foodborne pathogens, *Escherichia coli* and *Salmonella*, exhibiting minimum inhibitory concentration (MIC) values varying from 10 to 400 mg/mL, and also to reduce the growth of *Desulfovibrio* spp. and *Enterococcus* pathogenic bacteria by increasing the abundance of probiotics, such as *Akkermansia* and *Bifidobacteria* [124]. These results are in accordance with those reported by Sun et al. [125], who also revealed that anthocyanin-rich extracts from blueberries can also destroy the cell membrane of *Listeria monocytogenes*, *Staphylococcus aureus*, and *Vibrio parahaemolyticus*, displaying MIC scores of 0.27, 0.21, and 0.030 mg/mL, respectively, after 24 h of exposure. Furthermore, it has also been reported that 100 μM cyanidin 3-*O*-glucoside can also inhibit the expression and secretion of *Helicobacter pylori* toxins by suppressing the SecA transcription pathway, thereby making the proteins' exportation difficult [126]. Even though delphinidin 3-*O*-rutinoside and cyanidin 3-*O*-rutinoside at 1% did not reveal any inhibitory effect, enriched fractions of berries at concentrations ranging from 0.1 to 1% showed capacity to inhibit the yeasts *Saccharomyces cerevisiae* and *Rhodotorula rubra*, and the bacteria *Bacillus cereus*, *Salmonella typhimurium*, and *Lactococcus lactis* cocci growth [127]. Mulberry anthocyanins also showed potential to interfere with the development of *Pseudomonas aeruginosa*, a microorganism associated with biofilm-mediated infections, exhibiting an MIC value of 2 mg/mL [128]. Similar results were observed concerning the anti-microbial effects of blackcurrants and cherries on suppressing the growth of *S. aureus*, *E. coli*, and *P. aeruginosa* bacteria [129]. More recently, Silva et al. reported that anthocyanin-rich blueberry extracts at concentrations superior to 1 mg/mL can also inhibit virulence factors, namely, the formation of biofilms and adhesion of *Acinetobacter baumannii* and *Proteus mirabilis* pathogenic microorganisms over 24 h of treatment [130].

A dose of 0.225 μg/mL of cornelian cherry fruits showed potential to stimulate murine immune response during *Trichinella spiralis* infection, a causative agent of human trichinellosis, by enhancing the $CD3^+$, $CD4^+$, and erythrocytes cells, promoting platelet aggregation and decreasing $CD8^+$ splenocyte cells when compared to *T. spiralis*-infected mice that did not receive the extract [131]. Besides, it has already been reported that Kenyan purple tea anthocyanins (200 mg/kg) can ameliorate post-treatment reactive encephalopathy associated with cerebral human trypanosomiasis, caused by *Trypanosoma brucei* parasites in a murine model, after 21 days of treatment, by delaying the establishment of the trypanosomes and increasing the glutathione and aconitase-1 levels in the brain compared to the untreated group [132]. Additionally, anthocyanins isolated from black soybean already revealed the potential to control chronic bacterial prostatitis, an infection from the lower genitourinary tract, in rat models, over 4 weeks of treatment at doses of 50 mg/kg administrated twice a day for 2 weeks compared to the control group, which did not receive anthocyanins [133].

In a general way, the antimicrobial, antifungal, and anti-parasitic activities of the anthocyanins are mainly due to their capacity to react with the DNA, proteins, and sulfhydryl groups and interfere with AKT, ATPase, and superoxide dismutase activities, which, in turn, decrease the citric acid cycle and microbial metabolism, and inhibit microbial enzymes [125,132]. These events deprive microorganisms of the substrate that they need, compromising their development and replication, the formation of biofilms and host ligand adhesion, and lead to cytoplasmatic membrane destabilization and consequent cell death.

6.2. Antioxidant Properties

Free radicals are a product of natural metabolism; however, their accumulation becomes toxic to cells and trigger many reactions, such as the oxidation of cellular components (nucleic acids, proteins, and fatty acids) and lipid peroxidation, accelerating aging processes, and eliciting the occurrence of many chronic diseases, such as neurodegenerative and cardiovascular disorders, cancer, atherosclerosis, and ulcerative colitis [4]. These reactive species can be derived from oxygen (e.g., hydroxyl, peroxyl, and superoxide) or nitrogen (e.g., nitric oxide and peroxynitrite). Besides, there are also even-numbered free radical species, such as H_2O_2 and lipid peroxide. Since synthetic antioxidants have various adverse effects on health, there is a trend towards relying on antioxidants from natural products. Currently, the notable antioxidant properties of anthocyanins are well-described, and it is mainly due to their conjugated rings and hydroxyl groups [41,134,135].

Many in vitro assays already demonstrated the antioxidant potential of anthocyanin derivatives and foods rich in them [136]. Focusing on individual anthocyanins, Rahman et al. [137] reported that delphinidin isolated from blueberry extracts shows the most considerable capacity to scavenge superoxide species, followed by petunidin > malvidin = cyanidin > peonidin > pelargonidin, at 1 µM. Similar results were obtained, regarding the capacity of these compounds, at the same concentration, to capture peroxynitrite radicals [133]. Moreover, cyanidin 3-O-glucoside at concentrations between 100 and 200 µM showed potential to protect human keratinocyte HaCaT cells against ultraviolet-A radiation, preventing DNA fragmentation and the release of hydrogen peroxide (H_2O_2) [138].

Regarding the anthocyanin-enriched fractions from natural products, extracts of blackberries, blueberries, strawberries, sweet cherries, and red raspberries at 10 µM displayed the potential to inhibit human LDL oxidation, having been two times more effective than an ascorbic acid control [139]. The coloured fraction of the sweet cherries also showed capacity to scavenge nitric oxide, in a concentration-dependent manner, displaying a half-maximal inhibitory concentration (IC_{50}) value of 47.44 µg/mL, being three times more active than ascorbic acid (IC_{50} = 179.69 µg/mL); it also protects human erythrocytes against haemoglobin oxidation and prevents haemolysis damage induced by peroxyl radicals, in a concentration-dependent manner (IC_{50} = 33.86 and 9.44 µg/mL, respectively). Positive correlations (r > 0.4) between anthocyanin content and antioxidant assays have been reported [134]. Additionally, the same extract also exhibited potential to capture superoxide species in a concentration-dependent manner (25% inhibitory concentration (IC_{25}) score of 16.58 µg/mL) and protect human adenocarcinoma Caco-2 cells against oxidative stress induced by tert-butyl hydroperoxide [130]. Blackberries extracts rich in anthocyanins revealed a ferric-reducing antioxidant power score of 191 µMol Fe^{2+}/L (extract concentrations between 10 and 200 µg/mL) [138] and also capacity to quench peroxyl radicals (4885 µMol Trolox equivalent/g) [140]. After 24 h of treatment, the same extract, at concentrations varying between 0.02 and 50 µg/mL, also showed an ability to protect human intestinal INT-407 normal cells against intracellular oxidation induced by 2,2'-azobis(2-amidinopropane) dihydrochloride (IC_{50} = 4.1 µg/mL) [140]. Blackberry and raspberry fruits also revealed lipid peroxidation inhibitory potential, displaying IC_{50} values lower than 50 µg/mL [141].

Concerning in vivo trials, delphinidin (1 mg/0.1 mL DMSO/mouse) showed capacity to protect mouse skin against UV-B radiation, preventing apoptosis after 8 h of exposure [142]. Additionally, rats that were fed during 35 days with anthocyanin extracts (4 mg/kg of body weight) from blackberries showed a meliorate antioxidant status compared to animals that did not receive these phenols in the diet, with lower levels of reactive species in the brain, liver, kidney, and plasma standing out (-35%, -44%, -17% and -8%, respectively), as well as higher catalase and glutathione peroxidase concentrations in the brain, kidney, and liver (+0.30, +0.65 and +0.05%, respectively) [143]. Anthocyanins from dabai fruits also showed potential to increase superoxide dismutase action (+10%) and to inhibit lipid peroxidation (-21%) in white rabbits that ingested 2000 mg/day of the extract for 8 weeks, compared to the control group. These benefits are attributed to the ability of anthocyanins to disrupt the activity of poly(ADP-ribose) polymerase 1 [144].

In humans, the ingestion of fresh strawberry fruits (300 g, possessing 9.57 mg of anthocyanins) by 13 healthy volunteers revealed the capacity to increase the plasma ferric-reducing antioxidant power (+3.1%), α-carotene (+7%), and vitamin C (+23%) levels [145]. Besides, 12 healthy participants who consumed açaí juice and pulp, composed of 165.9 mg/L and 303.8 mg/kg of anthocyanins, respectively, showed increments in plasma antioxidant capacity of 3- and 2.3-fold, respectively [11]. Furthermore, forty-seven healthy adults who consumed 30 mL of tart cherry concentrate diluted to a volume of 250 mL with water for 6 weeks showed higher levels of plasma ferric-reducing ability than the control group (+10%) [12]. A randomised cross-over study involving 30 healthy female participants who drank 330 mL of an anthocyanin-rich beverage over 14 days displayed increases in superoxide dismutase activity of about 6%, compared to the placebo group [146]. More recently, 300 g of blueberries ingested by ten young volunteers showed potential to protect human blood mononuclear cells against oxidative damage induced by H_2O_2 compared to the control, by reducing oxidative damage by 18% after 24 h of their consumption [147]. The same was verified after a 30-day-treatment with 500 g of strawberry fruits [148]. Anthocyanin-rich juices and nectars also showed potential to aid recovery after strenuous exercise by increasing the plasma total antioxidant capacity and diminishing lipid peroxidation and carbonyl species [149–151].

These considerable health-promoting properties are intimately linked to the capacity of anthocyanins to increase the glutathione levels by restoring or raising the activity of exogenous antioxidant enzymes and by activating the genes responsible for coding these enzymes. Besides, it is also due to their ability to inhibit NADPH and xanthine oxidases and modify arachidonic metabolism and mitochondrial respiration, and hence, reduce the formation of free radicals and reactive species, protecting cell components from damage [41]. Furthermore, anthocyanins can enter into cells and activate the Nrf2/HO-1 pathway, conferring resistance against oxidative damage and increasing antioxidant defence [152], and can interact with other natural antioxidants, such as other phenolic compounds, carotenoids, and vitamins, which also increase their ability to relieve oxidative stress [134]. Nevertheless, and although no study has revealed toxicity on humans, it is imperative to conduct further in vivo studies in order to reveal the safe dosage of phenolics intake, including of anthocyanins and anthocyanidins, as they can act as pro-oxidants in some conditions (e.g., a basic pH, high concentrations of transition metal ions, and the presence of oxygen, among others) [153].

6.3. Anti-Inflammatory Properties

Anthocyanins also possess anti-inflammatory capacity. Inflammatory conditions happen in response to pathogens that were not removed (e.g., autoimmunity) or due to an inadequate long-term response to stimuli (e.g., allergies). They are characterized by oedema, redness, pain, fever, function losses, and larger amounts of pro-inflammatory cytokines (e.g., tumour necrosis factor (TNF)-α, interleukin (IL)-6, and 1β) and nitric oxide radicals [154]. Therefore, it is important to be treated as soon as possible given their involvement in chronic disorders, such as asthma, obesity, gout, diabetes, cancer, atherosclerosis, and neurological pathologies.

Among the anthocyanins, cyanidin and delphinidin 3-O-glucosides already exhibited potential to reduce the C-reactive protein levels by 77% in human liver cancer HepG2 cells, and vascular cell adhesion molecule-1 secretion in endothelial cells by 47%, at concentrations of 50 µg/mL compared to the non-exposed cells group [13]. Additionally, delphinidin, petunidin, and malvidin 3,5-diglucosides also revealed capacity to inhibit nitric oxide release, and IL-6, IL-1β, and TNF-α in lipopolysaccharide (LPS)-induced RAW264.7 macrophages at concentrations of 80 µg/mL [152]. Anthocyanin extracts from raspberries (concentrations of 100, 150, and 200 µg/mL) also showed an ability to reduce the expression levels of cyclooxygenase-2 (COX-2), inducible nitric oxide synthase (iNOS), and IL 1β and IL-6, and to suppress AP-1 signalling and nuclear factor kappa B (NF-kB) pathways. Additionally, it was also verified that they can decrease IKK, IkBa, p65, and JNK phosphorylation, avoid p65 nuclear translocation in LPS/IFN-γ-stimulated RAW 264.7 macrophage cells [155], and inhibit lipoxygenase activity, at concentrations of 10, 25, and 50 µg/mL [154]. Similar results were obtained concerning the anthocyanins isolated from strawberries and blackberries at a concentration of 50 µg/mL [156], and purple sweet potato at 200 µg/mL [152]. Besides, anthocyanin-fractions extracted from berries also showed potential to reduce TNF-α, IL-8, and Regulated upon Activation, Normal T Cell Expressed and Presumably Secreted (RANTES) at doses between 10 and 25 µg/mL in human bronchial epithelial BEAS-2B normal cells treated with LPS [157]. These results are in line with those recently described by Chen et al., who proved that an anthocyanin-rich extract from mulberry fruits, at a concentration of 50 mg/mL, can reduce the IL-6, iNOS, phospho-p65, and phospho-IκBα pro-inflammatory markers, and increase the IL-10 concentration in RAW264.7 macrophage cells stimulated with LPS over 24 h of exposure [128].

Enriched fractions of anthocyanins from raspberries already showed anti-inflammatory effects in dextran sulphate sodium-induced acute colitis in mice. Animals ingested 20 mg/kg of the extract for 10 days. At the end of the study, blood samples were collected, and mice were sacrificed for histological assessment. The results were compared in the control group; i.e., rats only received a normal diet. The obtained data revealed that a diet rich in anthocyanins contributed to improve colitis damage, by enhancing pro-inflammatory markers reduction and controlling weight [155]. Similar data were observed by Pereira et al. [158], who's study was based on the administration of blueberries also in 2,4,6-trinitrobenzenesulfonic acid-induced colitis rat models, at concentrations of 10 mg/kg over 8 days of treatment, compared to an untreated group. This study proved the ability of anthocyanins to downregulate iNOS, inhibit COX-2 expression, decrease leukocyte infiltration, and increase antioxidant defence in the colon. Tart cherry anthocyanins (400 mg/kg) administered for 3 days also showed an ability to suppress inflammation-induced pain in rats, essentially due to their ability to inhibit cyclooxygenase-mediated synthesis of prostaglandins [159]. Furthermore, Kim et al. revealed that 5 mg of encapsulated anthocyanins per day can decrease COX-2, NOS3, IL-1β, and TNF-α inflammatory cytokines in mice brain [121]. Another study related to anthocyanins extracted from rice (at 25 μg/mL) proved that they can increase type I collagen gene expression and protect skin fibroblasts against H_2O_2 damage, essentially by inhibiting IκBα phosphorylation, NF-κB activation, and IL-6 production, over 24 h of exposure [160].

Regarding human studies, 150 hypercholesterolemic subjects who ingested 320 mg anthocyanin capsules, rich in cyanidin 3-O-glucoside and delphinidin 3-O-glucoside, daily for 24 weeks showed lower levels of C-reactive protein, vascular cell adhesion molecule-1, and plasma IL-1β levels (-20, -13 and -4%, respectively) when compared to the untreated group. No changes were detected regarding TNF-α concentrations, which indicate that the intervention was safe [13]. Jacob et al. reported that the consumption of 280 g of cherries (28 mg per 100 g of fresh weight) twice a day can also reduce the plasma C-reactive protein and nitric oxide levels by 29.4% and 16.8%, respectively, when compared with the baseline. A decrease in plasma urate (-14.5%) and increments in ascorbic acid ($+9$%) were also verified, highlighting the anti-gout effects of cherries. This trial was composed of ten healthy women who consumed cherries after an overnight fast [161]. These data are in accordance with Kelley et al., who conducted a study involving 18 healthy men and women that were subjected to the daily consumption of 280 g cherries for 28 days. The results revealed a decrease in C-reactive protein, nitric oxide, and RANTES at percentages of -25, -18 and -21%, respectively. No changes were observed in IL-6, neither in the high-, low-, and very-low-density lipoprotein cholesterols nor triglycerides, which can be considered evidence regarding the security of this supplementation dose [162]. Furthermore, ten healthy adult volunteers who drank 10 g of *Hibiscus sabdariffa* diluted in water showed lower monocyte chemoattractant protein-1 (-23.2%) levels, an important biomarker considering the evaluation of inflammatory disorders, after 3 h of their consumption compared to the placebo group [163]. Additionally, a pilot study, composed of 13 patients with mild to moderate ulcerative colitis, consumed 160 g of blueberries (4 trays per day), corresponding to 95 g dw (around 600 g of fresh fruit) during six weeks, revealed that 63.4% of patients achieved remission of the inflammatory bowel disease [164]. In another study, sixteen volunteers were subjected to the consumption of a 250 mL dose of anthocyanin-rich plum juice; the results obtained revealed a decrease in the C-protein reactive, IL-6, IL-1β, and TNF-α concentrations of -22, -7, -9 and -4%, respectively. These data were observed 4 h after the intake relative to the placebo group [165].

Besides the mentioned, anthocyanins also facilitate muscle recovery after intense exercise, attenuating its damage and inflammation [149–151]. Indeed, sixteen active students who drank 480 mL of blackcurrant nectar for eight consecutive days revealed lower levels of creatine kinase, a marker of muscle damage, and IL-6, 48 h post physical activity [149]. These results were similar as those obtained by Hurst et al. also based on the consumption of blackcurrant nectar (~240 mg total anthocyanins). In this work, a 5-week randomized placebo-controlled pilot trial composed of 36 volunteers revealed that the group who consumed this juice showed lower levels of pro-inflammatory TNF-α and IL-6 molecules and increments in anti-inflammatory IL-10 cytokines [151]. Furthermore, twenty runners who consumed 30 mL of tart cherry juice during 5 days before and 48 h after a marathon run also showed reduced levels of inflammatory markers (IL-6, uric acid, and C-protein reactive) compared to the placebo group [150].

These effects are closely linked to the ability of anthocyanins to prevent CD40 activation, a member of the tumour necrosis factor receptor superfamily [166]. Additionally, they also can inhibit the cyclooxygenase isoenzymes, COX-1 and COX-2, and interfere with the MAPK cascade [121]. Indeed, and through an in vitro cyclooxygenase inhibitory assay with enzymes from ram seminal vesicles, anthocyanins extracted from sweet cherries and raspberries, at a concentration-dose of 125 µg/mL, showed more potential to inhibit COX-1 activity (47.4 and 54.3%, respectively) than ibuprofen (39.8%) and naproxen (41.3%) at 10 µM [167].

6.4. Anticancer Properties

Cancer causes more deaths than strokes and coronary disorders and it is characterized by uncontrolled cell growth and proliferation [8]. Anthocyanins have demonstrated capacity to inhibit the initiation, promotion, and progression of types of cancer, such as human colon [134,168], liver and bladder [169,170], breast [171], brain [172], renal and skin [168], gastric [141], and thyroid [173] cancers, mainly due to their antioxidant properties and capacity to interfere with PI3K/Akt [174].

The capacity of anthocyanins to inhibit the growth of metastatic cells is not surprising. Indeed, the enriched fraction of anthocyanins from sweet cherries already showed an ability to inhibit human adenocarcinoma Caco-2 cells growth (inhibitory IC_{50} value of 667.84 µg/mL), causing necrosis at concentrations superior to 400 µg/mL, after 24 h of treatment [134]. Similar effects were verified using coloured phenolics from pollen, but at a higher concentration (10 mg/mL) [175]. Concentrations higher than 500 µg/mL of anthocyanin-rich extracts from the *Myrtaceae* family also showed an ability to reduce the proliferation of human colon adenocarcinoma HT-29 cells, mainly by arresting the G2/M phase, hence causing cell apoptosis in comparison with the control group over 24 h of treatment [176]. It was also already verified that anthocyanin-rich extracts from pomegranate at 50 µg/mL can reduce by 10% the growth of human bladder cancer T24 cells growth after 48 h of exposure, in comparison with untreated cells [170]. Additionally, and after 2 days of an incubation assay, anthocyanins from cherries also showed capacity to interfere with MDA-MB-453 and MDA-MB-231 breast cancer cell lines growth, revealing IC_{50} values of 45 and 149 µg/mL, respectively, without toxicity to MCF-10A normal breast cells [171]. Blackberry and raspberry fruits at 250 µg/mL also revealed effectiveness in stopping cancer cell growth, inhibiting human colon HCT-116, breast MCF-7, lung NCI-H460, and gastric AGS tumour cell lines by 50, 24, 54, and 37%, respectively, after 24 h of exposure [141]. Furthermore, 10 µg/µL of anthocyanins from mulberries revealed capacity to suppress thyroid SW1736 and HTh-7 cancer cell proliferation, by inducing apoptosis and autophagy-dependent cell death, and inhibiting protein kinase B and ribosomal protein S6 activation, after 72 h of treatment [173]. On the other hand, açaí extracts rich in anthocyanins showed the ability to suppress C-6 rat brain glioma cell growth, showing cell viability reductions of 62, 45, and 38% at concentrations of 50, 100, and 200 µg/mL, respectively, after 48 h of treatment [172]. More recently, Vilkickyte et al. reported that anthocyanins isolated from lingonberry fruits can suppress the viability of malignant melanoma IGR39 and renal CaKi-1 cancer cells, displaying IC_{50} values of 200 and 400 µg/mL, respectively [168].

Focusing on in vivo studies, the daily administration of berries (0.5 mg/kg body weight) in rats with induced oesophageal carcinoma showed an ability to reduce cancer growth by 22% over 20 weeks of treatment, when compared to the control group [177]. Adding 10% dietary freeze-dried berries to the standardized diet of rats also showed capacity to inhibit induced oesophagus cancer by 30–60% and colon cancer by up to 80% when compared to the control, over 25 weeks of treatment [178].

Furthermore, a recent study revealed that anthocyanins from blueberry extracts showed the capacity to prevent the formation and growth of colorectal cancer in azoxymethane/dextran sodium sulphate-treated Balb/c mice, which ingested a diet containing 10% of the extract during 9 weeks of treatment, compared with the control [179]. Anthocyanins from *Vitis coignetiae* Pulliat also showed the potential to inhibit the tumorigenicity in mice infected with Hep3B human hepatocellular carcinoma cells (5 μg/g of animal per day) [180].

On the other hand, berry anthocyanins displayed anticarcinogenic effects on lung cancer progression in rat xenograft models (reductions around 40%) treated with a diet supplemented with 7.5%, after 6 weeks of the intervention [181]. The supplementation during 1 month with 0.5% of cyanidin and peonidin 3-*O*-glucosides also exhibited the capacity to reduce Lewis lung carcinoma cells in mice [182].

In addition, the administration of delphinidin (2 mg, three times a week) in athymic nude mice implanted with PC3 cells resulted in significant inhibition of prostate tumour growth, essentially by reducing the expression of NF-κB/p65, Bcl2, Ki67, and PCNA after 8 weeks of treatment [183]. An anthocyanin mixture extracted from black soybean also inhibited xenograft growth of prostate cancer in mice treated with a daily oral anthocyanin (8 mg/kg) after 14 weeks of intervention [184].

Besides, the daily administration of anthocyanin-rich extracts from black rice (100 mg/kg, during 28 weeks) in mice xenografted with human tumour models showed the ability to reduce breast cancer growth, causing reductions around 41% [185], mainly due to their ability to inhibit growth factor receptor 2, a gene overexpressed in this type of cancer [186]. Blackthorn fruits at 0.2 mg daily (5 days a week, for one month) already showed potential to slow down tumour growth xenografts in immunodeficient mice injected with human colon HCT116 cancer cells [187]. Anthocyanins from black rice already showed potential to increase immune responses in murine leukaemia cells, at concentrations higher than 50 mg/kg over 3 weeks of treatment, promoting CD3 (T cell), CD19 (B cell), CD11b (monocyte), and macrophage phagocytosis, and decreasing the NK cell activity when compared to the untreated control group [188].

Regarding skin cancer, the administration of anthocyanins extracted from *Sorbus aucuparia* (5 mL/kg for 11 days) in rats showed potential to reduce melanoma [189]. Furthermore, Lee et al. reported that anthocyanins extracted from aronia conjugated with fucoidan, a natural polysaccharide extracted from seaweed, can prevent the development of induced skin tumour in mice when administered twice a week at a concentration of 900 mg/kg dose during 22 weeks [174].

Although there are no relevant studies regarding the anti-cancer effects on humans, it was already verified that the consumption of 20 g of black raspberry powder for between 2 and 4 weeks (three times per day) by Barrett's oesophagus patients, a precursor lesion for oesophageal tumour, can reduce the proliferation rates and CD 105-stained blood vessels, and increase apoptosis in colon tumours [190].

The ability of anthocyanins to inhibit the initiation and development of a tumour is closely associated with their ability to increase antioxidant defences, exert anti-inflammatory actions, and interfere with the ERK, JNK, PI3K/Akt, MAPK, and NF-κB pathways, as well as being associated with their regulated proteins and influence on the estrogenic/antiestrogenic levels [180,183]. Furthermore, these flavonoids compounds also showed apoptotic effects since they can activate the caspase cascade, reduce the mitochondria membrane potential, and modulate the cytochrome C and aromatase activities [185,191].

6.5. Neurological Properties

Knowing neurological pathologies are closely related to oxidative stress and inflammatory levels, it is not surprising that the consumption of secondary metabolites from plants, such as anthocyanins, can reduce their occurrence.

Anthocyanin-enriched fractions extracted from berries at 20 µg/mL already showed capacity to reduce nitric oxide, reactive oxygen, and carbonyl species, as well as the H_2O_2 levels and apoptotic protease caspase-3/7 activity in BV-2 microglia cells in about 20% relative to untreated cells. They also showed an ability to diminish anti-glycation and anti-Aβ A aggregation [192]. Furthermore, anthocyanin-rich extracts from blueberries at 0.01 µg/mL, together with cyanidin 3-*O*-glucoside, cyanidin 3-*O*-sophoroside, delphinidin 3-*O*-glucoside, and malvidin 3-*O*-glucoside at 1 µM, also revealed an ability to protect dopaminergic neurons from the primary cells of Parkinson's disease against rotenone toxicity, after 72 h of treatment, essentially by attenuating mitochondrial dysfunction [193].

Besides, it was already reported that anthocyanins (ingestion of 100 mg/kg for 10 months) can restore the ion pump activities in rats experimentally demyelinated with ethidium bromide, by diminishing the proinflammatory mediators' secretion and oxidative-stress levels and restoring the IL-10 levels [131]. Additionally, anthocyanins isolated from black bean at concentrations varying from 100 and 200 µg/mL (over 12 h of treatment) proved their ability to protect the hippocampal neurons of mice against toxicity induced by kainic acid, mainly thanks to their capacity to reduce the reactive oxygen species levels, caspase-3, AMPK activation, and mitochondrial cytochrome-c release into the cytoplasm, and in attenuating the Ca^{2+} perturbations, losses of mitochondrial integrity, and Bax accumulation [194]. Kim et al. revealed that 5 mg (administered during 14 days) of anthocyanins encapsulated in gold nanoparticles can cross the blood–brain barrier and reduce the amyloid-$β_{1-42}$ plaques and neuro-apoptotic markers (anti-Bax, anti-Bcl2, anti-caspase-3, anti-cytochrome c, and anti-P-JNK) by inhibiting the $ρ$-JNK/NF-$κ$B/$ρ$-GSK3$β$ pathway in mice brain [121].

Concerning human assays, a 12-week randomised study involving 49 older adults with mild-to-moderate dementia who drank 200 mL anthocyanin-rich cherry juice showed improvements in verbal fluency, learning, memory, and cognition when compared to the untreated group [14]. Similar neurological improvements were observed after 12 weeks of blueberry concentrate supplementation in healthy older adults, who drank 30 mL of blueberry juice compared to the placebo [15]. Whyte et al. also conducted a study involving one hundred and twenty-two older adults, which consumed 16 capsules per week over 3 months of blueberry-rich extracts. As expectable, better cognitive tasks regarding executive function, working memory, and episodic memory were registered in comparison to the placebo [195].

As mentioned before, the neuroprotective effects showed by anthocyanins are mainly due to their ability to cross the blood–brain barrier and protect neurons and glia cells from oxidative damage induced by reactive species and free radicals, reduce the inflammatory cytokines and β-amyloid concentrations, and to suppress NF-kB, the Nf E2-related factor-2 (Nrf-2) signalling pathway, COX, and caspase activities [119]. Furthermore, anthocyanins also can raise gene expression, GTPase activity, and detoxifying enzyme amounts, and therefore meliorate cerebrovascular and peripheral blood flow [196].

6.6. Anti-Diabetic and Anti-Obesity Effects

Diabetes mellitus, with type 2 standing out, affects several people worldwide, being associated with obesity, oxidative stress, inflammatory events, and cardiovascular risk [197]. Given the resistance developed to the current pharmaceutical drugs administrated, the ingestion of anthocyanin-rich products has been encouraged. In fact, anthocyanins already showed mechanisms capable to diminish insulin resistance, hyperglycaemia, proinflammatory cytokines, and radical species; inhibit gluconeogenesis and the action of the α-amylase and α-glucosidase carbohydrate-hydrolysing enzymes; and, consequently, restore the glucose levels, incentive insulin secretion, and pancreatic β-cells proliferation [198,199].

Among the anthocyanins, cyanidin 3-O-glucoside already showed potential to inhibit pancreatic α-amylase activity, revealing an IC_{50} value of 24.4 µM [200]. Anthocyanin-enriched fractions from sweet cherries also showed the capacity to inhibit the α-glucoside action, showing to be three times more efficient than the acarbose control, which is the current pharmaceutical drug used to treat type 2 diabetes, but whose intake cause several gastrointestinal side effects [134]. Besides, anthocyanins from *Cornus kousa* displayed anti-angiogenic effects in the pre-adipocyte cell line 3T3-L1s, suppressing lipogenesis and adipogenesis in comparison with untreated cells after 8 days of exposure [201].

The oral administration of acarbose combined with cyanidin 3-O-rutinoside (30 mg/kg) also revealed an ability to alleviate postprandial hyperglycaemia and inhibit intestinal α-glucosidase in normal rats over three hours of intervention, as compared with the control group [202]. Besides, it was already documented that the glucoside of cyanidin can also meliorate diabetes-related endothelial dysfunction in mice that received a 6 mg/kg diet for 8 weeks, by stimulating adiponectin expression and improving flow-mediated dilation [203]. On the other hand, black currant anthocyanins showed the ability to reduce body weight gain and glucose levels and improve insulin sensitivity in mice that were fed with 8 mg/day of anthocyanins for 8 weeks. Converted into human equivalent doses, these ones are estimated to be 1.5 g/day of total anthocyanins for an average adult [56]. Furthermore, the daily administration of anthocyanins from *Hibiscus sabdariffa* L. (300 mg/kg) in obese-hypercholesterolemic rats revealed the capacity to reduce their weight, as well as to improve their lipid profile and liver enzymes action over 3 weeks of treatment in comparison to the group that did not receive the diet [198]. Blueberry anthocyanins also showed anti-obesity effects. Indeed, their administration at doses of 200 mg/kg during one month showed the ability to reduce the body weight of obese C57BL/6 mice by 19.4% and also diminish the glucose and pro-inflammatory levels, improve the lipid profile, and suppress the peroxisome proliferator-activated receptor-γ, FAS genes, and fatty acid synthesis over a 16-week treatment in contrast to the untreated group [204]. These results were similar as those reported by Kwon et al. and Wu et al. regarding the oral ingestion of anthocyanins from black soybean, black rice, and purple corn by obese rats [16,205].

Regarding human studies, it was already reported that twenty dyslipidaemic children and adolescents who daily ingested 50 g of cornelian cherry fruits, during 6 weeks, showed better lipid, apolipoprotein and vascular inflammation profiles and lower levels of LDL and triglycerides, intracellular adhesion molecule-1 and vascular cell adhesion molecule-1 (-10, -13, -30 and -25%, respectively). Higher levels regarding apolipoprotein A (+11.6%) and a diminished content of apolipoprotein B (-13.6%) were also verified [197].

The anthocyanins potential to be used as novel therapeutic agents against diabetes and obesity is fundamentally attributed to their chemical structure, which gives them inhibitory effects on the carbohydrate-hydrolysing enzymes' action and capacity to interact in a competitive and/or non-competitive mode with the enzymes' substrate and create hydrophobic bonds with these enzymes, thereby discontinuing their act and retard carbohydrate absorption [134,200]. Furthermore, anthocyanins also revealed the capacity to raise GLUT 4 membrane translocation expression and upregulate the signalling pathway of the peroxisome proliferator-activated receptors, encouraging adipocyte glucose uptake and improving the lipid profile [10].

6.7. Cardiovascular Properties

Cardiovascular pathologies are the principal cause of morbidity and mortality worldwide. They are intimately associated with the adoption of unhealthy behaviours, such as smoking, excessive alcohol intake, and other risk factors, including metabolic syndrome [33]. Several studies indicate that the daily intake of anthocyanin-rich fruits, vegetables and beverages can attenuate, or even prevent, the occurrence of coronary events, since they can modulate lipid metabolism, fat deposition, and endothelial function, as well as reduce blood pressure and vascular adhesion molecules expression. These activities are intimately associated with their antioxidant and anti-inflammatory characteristics [206].

Particularly, cyanidin 3-O-glucoside and delphinidin 3-O-glucoside at concentrations of 50 µM showed the ability to reduce in vitro platelet aggregation and lysosome secretion, essentially by reducing β-thromboglobulin, serotonin ATP, platelet factor 4, CD63, and transforming growth factor β1 secretion after 40 min of exposure [207]. Moreover, it was already documented that cyanidin 3-O-glucoside can stimulate adiponectin expression and improve flow-mediated dilation in human adipose tissues and human aortic endothelial cells treated with 50 µM of cyanidin 3-O-glucoside after 24 h of exposure [203]. Blueberry anthocyanidins (cyanidin, delphinidin, and malvidin) are also reported to inhibit human umbilical vein endothelial cell-induced tube formation in a co-culture with fibroblasts at concentrations ranging from 0.3 and 10 µM [208].

Moreover, 50 µg/mL of anthocyanin-enriched fractions from strawberries already showed capacity to reduce the triglycerides and low-density lipoprotein (LDL) contents around 17% and 23%, respectively, in HepG2 cells after 24 h of treatment [169]. Additionally, 50 mg/mL of encapsulated anthocyanins extracted from blueberries and black currants already showed the potential to inhibit platelet aggregation by suppressing P-selectin expression and stimulate the thromboxane A2 pathway [209].

Concerning in vivo trials, it was already reported that blueberry anthocyanin-enriched extracts can attenuate cyclophosphamide-induced cardiac damage in rats, treated with 80 mg/kg during four weeks by ameliorating the arterial blood pressure, heart rate, and activities of the heart enzymes, and improving cardiac dysfunction, left ventricular hypertrophy, and fibrosis. Additionally, they also showed the potential to prevent cardiomyocyte apoptosis [206].

Furthermore, 31 pre-hypertensive men who ingested a single dose of 640 mg anthocyanins daily for 4 weeks revealed higher levels of high-density lipoprotein (HDL) concentrations and lower concentrations of triglycerides [210]. Moreover, the consumption of two capsules (80 mg each per day during 28 days) rich in anthocyanins already showed the ability to reduce monocyte-platelet aggregate formation (-39%), procaspase activating compound-1 (-10%), P-selectin (-14%), and inhibit platelet endothelial cell adhesion molecule-1 expression (-14%) [17]. In another work, the authors reported that the consumption of 250 g per day of blueberry powder, for 6 weeks, by 13 volunteers showed an ability to increase natural killer cells and reduce arterial stiffness in sedentary males and females, mainly by diminishing diastolic pressure [211]. This fact is in accordance with Whyte et al. [195]. These authors conducted a study involving 122 volunteers who consumed 16 capsules per week of blueberry-rich extracts (100 mg of anthocyanins/capsule) over six months. Habanova et al. reported a study of 36 volunteers who consumed 150 g of frozen blueberries 3 times a week, for 6 weeks. The obtained results revealed lower levels of LDL glucose albumin, aminotransferase, alkaline phosphatase, and γ-glutamyltransferase, accompanied by higher levels of HDL when compared to the baseline [212]. These data are in line with that reported by Arevström et al., who conducted a study based on the daily ingestion of 40 g of blueberries powder (equivalent to 480 g fresh blueberries) over 8 weeks of treatment [213]. Additionally, reductions around 5% in systolic and diastolic blood pressures were also observed in older adults with mild-to-moderate dementia who drank 200 mL anthocyanin-rich cherry juice for 12 weeks [156]. Similar results were reported by Draijer et al., who conducted a human trial involving 60 subjects who consumed 6 grape-wine extract capsules (~247.3 mg anthocyanins per capsule) every day over ten weeks. Additionally, a reduction in endothelin-1 by 10% was also found compared to the control group [214]. The obtained results are in line in those obtained by Igwe et al., who conducted a pilot cross-over study involving 24 adults, but who focused on the intake of 100 mL of anthocyanin-rich plum juice three times a day [215]. Besides, the dietary supplementation of 500 mg of aronia extracts over 12 weeks also revealed the capacity to modulate the lipid profile by diminishing the fasting plasma total cholesterol (-8%), LDL, (-11%) and LDL receptor protein in peripheral blood mononuclear cells (-31.9%), as compared to placebo group. Significant correlations between the obtained results and cyanidin 3-O-galactoside and peonidin 3-O-galactoside contents were found [216]. Similar results were reported by Bakkar et al., who conducted a study involving twelve overweight middle-aged men that consumed 226 mg of encapsulated anthocyanins from tart cherries daily for 28 days [217]. Furthermore, blueberries also showed the potential to reduce the peak postprandial glucose levels and extend the postprandial glucose response in 17 healthy young adults who consumed a range of doses varying from 310 and 724 mg of freeze-dried wild blueberry powder, 2 h following their consumption [218]. Beyond that, the oral ingestion of 320 mg of anthocyanins isolated from berries, over 12 weeks, by hypercholesterolemic individuals also showed the potential to increase brachial artery flow-mediated dilation (+10%) and HDL amounts (+12.8%), and diminish serum soluble vascular adhesion molecule-1, triglycerides, and LDL concentrations (−11.6, −4.1 and −10.0%, respectively) [219], and also glycated haemoglobin (HbA1c) (−0.14%) [118]. Additionally, it has also been mentioned that the intake of four anthocyanins capsules per day (total of 320 mg/day) can reduce plasma β-thromboglobulin, soluble P-selectin, platelet factor 4, and transforming growth factor β1 levels in hypercholesterolaemic patients for 24 weeks of treatment as compared with the baseline [207]. These positive effects are correlated with the delphinidin 3-O-glucoside and cyanidin 3-O-glucoside concentrations [219]. Similar effects were reported in adults overweight and obese who drank 200 mL blood orange juice twice a day for 2 weeks [19]. The consumption of one 350 mg capsule every 8 h for 2 months also showed the potential to meliorate the lipid profile of hyperlipidaemic patients, by reducing the total cholesterol, triglyceride, and LDL by −27.6, −19.2%, and −26.3%, respectively, and raising HDL by +37.5% when compared with the baseline [220]. On the other hand, seven days' intake of 600 mg per day of blackcurrant extracts containing 210 mg of anthocyanins showed the potential to increase vasodilation, total haemoglobin, and cardiac output, and decrease the muscle oxygen saturation, which is beneficial in improving exercise performance [221].

Therefore, the regular consumption of anthocyanin-rich foods and beverages can contribute to reduce the risk of cardiomyopathies, coronary problems, and ischemia [8,33]. These effects are due to the antioxidant and anti-inflammatory effects of anthocyanins, given that nitric oxide radicals and pro-inflammatory cytokines are critical factors in cardiovascular diseases. In fact, these compounds can inhibit p38 mitogen-activated protein kinases, c-Jun N-terminal kinase activation, and the PI3K/Akt signalling pathways, consequently attenuating eNOS phosphorylation and cGMP production, interrupt MAPK activation, and the recruitment of TNF-receptor-associated factors-2 in lipids, in the way of protecting endothelial cells from CD-40 proinflammatory effects [166].

6.8. Eye Improvement

In vivo and in vitro evidence also revealed that anthocyanins can improve the eyes and thus vision, owing to their ability to increase blood circulation in retina capillaries and the production of retinal pigments, which, in turn, improve night vision and protect eyes from oxidative damage, diabetic retinopathy, and molecular degeneration [8].

Anthocyanins isolated from blackberries at 100 µg/mL showed potential to protect human adult retinal pigment epithelial ARPE-19 cells against oxidative stress induced by H_2O_2, by increasing the activity of heme-oxygenase-1 and glutathione S-transferase-pi antioxidant enzymes after 24 h of exposure [222]. Similar data were reported by Sundalius [223] regarding blueberry anthocyanins, over 7 days of treatment.

Concerning in vivo studies, delphinidin 3-O-rutinoside at 10 µM already showed an ability to relax the bovine ciliary smooth muscle through activation of the endothelin-1 receptor and NO/cGMP pathway, inhibiting myosin light chain phosphorylation, hence causing relaxation [224]. Additionally, anthocyanins extracted from black currants showed the potential to inhibit vitreous-chamber depth enlargement, and the axial and ocular lengths of chicks when compared to the controls, over 3 days of treatment at a dose concentration of 200 mg/kg [225].

Focusing on human assays, a double-blind, placebo-controlled, crossover study involving healthy volunteers revealed that the daily intake of six capsules rich in blackcurrant anthocyanins at a concentration of 50 mg can improve dark adaptation, video display terminal work-induced transient refractive alteration, and asthenopia symptoms (visual fatigue) in comparison to the placebo [226]. In another study based on the ingestion of anthocyanins from blueberry, the results revealed that the patients with normal-tension glaucoma presented vision improvement, not only due to anthocyanins' oxidative properties but also owing to their ability to increase the blood circulation [18].

Given that, it was already reported that intact anthocyanins can pass through the blood-aqueous barrier and blood-retinal barrier in rats and rabbits, being widely distributed in ocular tissues [224]. This evidence, together with their antioxidative effects and blood circulation improvements, suggests that anthocyanins can be considered a potential drug therapy for treating ophthalmological diseases, such as myopia and glaucoma [8,18].

7. Conclusions

Anthocyanins are the coloured compounds largely found in nature, for which evidence indicates that their regular consumption offers several health benefits to human health, mainly due to their ability to reduce free radicals, reactive species, and pro-inflammatory markers. These abilities can counteract oxidative stress levels, avoid the development of inflammatory processes, and protect human organs and cell components against damage, and thus confer protection at distinct levels. Thus, anthocyanins' structure, biochemistry, and encapsulation have been deeply studied in order to increase their use, stability, and consequent bioavailability and action. Until now, and although more in vivo and clinical trials are needed, evidence suggests that anthocyanins are promising candidates for the engineering of new pharmaceutical drugs, and can be used as an alternative or as an adjuvant therapy capable to attenuate or prevent the occurrence of many disorders, including diabetes, cancer, and cardiovascular and neurological pathologies. In fact, their use in pharmaceutical products, nutraceuticals, foods, and as food colourants is increasing worldwide.

Author Contributions: Conceptualization, A.C.G., A.F., G.A. and L.R.S.; methodology, A.C.G.; formal analysis, A.C.G.; investigation, A.C.G.; data curation, A.C.G. and A.R.N.; writing, A.C.G.; revising and visualization, A.R.N., G.A., A.F. and L.R.S.; supervision, A.F., G.A. and L.R.S., project administration, G.A. All authors have read and agreed to the published version of the manuscript.

Funding: This research was supported by FCT (Portugal), MCTES (Portugal), EFS (European Social Fund through the Regional Operational Program Centro) and EU (European Union).

Institutional Review Board Statement: Not applicable.

Informed Consent Statement: Not applicable.

Data Availability Statement: Data sharing not applicable.

Acknowledgments: A.C.G. and A.R.N. thank FCT—Foundation for Science and Technology (Lisbon, Portugal) and EFS—European Social Fund through the Regional Operational Program Centro for their PhD fellowship (2020.04947.BD and SFRH/BD/139137/2018, respectively). Figures 2 and 3 were created with ChemDraw Professional 16.0 (CambridgeSoft, Perkin Elmer Inc., Waltham, MA, USA).

Conflicts of Interest: All authors declare no conflict of interest.

References

1. Mannino, G.; Perrone, A.; Campobenedetto, C.; Schittone, A. Phytochemical profile and antioxidative properties of *Plinia trunciflora* fruits: A new source of nutraceuticals. *Food Chem.* **2020**, *307*, 125515. [CrossRef] [PubMed]
2. Ożarowski, M.; Karpiński, T.M.; Szulc, M.; Wielgus, K.; Kujawski, R.; Wolski, H.; Seremak-Mrozikiewicz, A. Plant phenolics and extracts in animal models of preeclampsia and clinical trials—Review of perspectives for novel therapies. *Pharmaceuticals* **2021**, *14*, 269. [CrossRef] [PubMed]
3. Newman, D.J.; Cragg, G.M. Natural products as sources of new drugs over the nearly four decades from 01/1981 to 09/2019. *J. Nat. Prod.* **2020**, *83*, 770–803. [CrossRef] [PubMed]
4. Martín, J.; Kuskoski, E.M.; Navas, M.J.; Asuero, A.G. Antioxidant capacity of anthocyanin pigments. In *Flavonoids-From Biosynthesis to Human Health*; Justino, G.C., Ed.; IntechOpen: London, UK, 2017; pp. 205–255.

5. Aziz, M.A.; Sarwar, M.S.; Akter, T.; Uddin, M.S.; Xun, S.; Zhu, Y.; Islam, M.S.; Hongjie, Z. Polyphenolic molecules targeting STAT3 pathway for the treatment of cancer. *Life Sci.* **2021**, *268*, 118999. [CrossRef] [PubMed]
6. Grosso, G.; Stepaniak, U.; Topor-Madry, R.; Szafraniec, K.; Pajak, A. Estimated dietary intake and major food sources of polyphenols in the Polish arm of the HAPIEE study. *Nutrition* **2014**, *30*, 1398–1403. [CrossRef] [PubMed]
7. Alappat, B.; Alappat, J. Anthocyanin pigments: Beyond aesthetics. *Molecules* **2020**, *25*, 5500. [CrossRef]
8. Khoo, H.E.; Azlan, A.; Tang, S.T.; Lim, S.M. Anthocyanidins and anthocyanins: Colored pigments as food, pharmaceutical ingredients, and the potential health benefits. *Food Nutr. Res.* **2017**, *61*, 1361779. [CrossRef]
9. Bendokas, V.; Skemiene, K.; Trumbeckaite, S.; Passamonti, S.; Borutaite, V.; Liobikas, J. Anthocyanins: From plant pigments to health benefits at mitochondrial level. *Crit. Rev. Food Sci. Nutr.* **2020**, *60*, 3352–3365. [CrossRef] [PubMed]
10. Sivamaruthi, B.S.; Kesika, P.; Chaiyasut, C. The influence of supplementation of anthocyanins on obesity-associated comorbidities: A concise review. *Foods* **2020**, *9*, 687. [CrossRef] [PubMed]
11. Mertens-Talcott, S.U.; Rios, J.; Jilma-Stohlawetz, P.; Pacheco-Palencia, L.A.; Meibohm, B.; Talcott, S.T.; Derendorf, H. Pharmacokinetics of anthocyanins and antioxidant effects after the consumption of anthocyanin-rich açai juice and pulp (*Euterpe oleracea* Mart.) in human healthy volunteers. *J. Agric. Food Chem.* **2008**, *56*, 7796–7802. [CrossRef]
12. Lynn, A.; Mathew, S.; Moore, C.T.; Russell, J.; Robinson, E.; Soumpasi, V.; Barker, M.E. Effect of a tart cherry juice supplement on arterial stiffness and inflammation in healthy adults: A randomised controlled trial. *Plant Foods Hum. Nutr.* **2014**, *69*, 122–127. [CrossRef]
13. Zhu, Y.; Ling, W.; Guo, H.; Song, F.; Ye, Q.; Zou, T.; Li, D.; Zhang, Y.; Li, G.; Xiao, Y.; et al. Anti-inflammatory effect of purified dietary anthocyanin in adults with hypercholesterolemia: A randomized controlled trial. *Nutr. Metab. Cardiovasc. Dis.* **2013**, *23*, 843–849. [CrossRef]
14. Kent, K.; Charlton, K.; Roodenrys, S.; Batterham, M.; Potter, J.; Traynor, V.; Gilbert, H.; Morgan, O.; Richards, R. Consumption of anthocyanin-rich cherry juice for 12 weeks improves memory and cognition in older adults with mild-to-moderate dementia. *Eur. J. Nutr.* **2017**, *56*, 333–341. [CrossRef]
15. Bowtell, J.L.; Aboo-Bakkar, Z.; Conway, M.; Adlam, A.-L.R.; Fulford, J. Enhanced task related brain activation and resting perfusion in healthy older adults after chronic blueberry supplementation. *Appl. Physiol. Nutr. Metab.* **2017**, *42*, 773–779. [CrossRef]
16. Kwon, S.H.; Ahn, I.S.; Kim, S.-O.; Kong, C.S.; Chung, H.Y.; Do, M.S.; Park, K.Y. Anti-obesity and hypolipidemic effects of black soybean anthocyanins. *J. Med. Food* **2007**, *10*, 552–556. [CrossRef] [PubMed]
17. Thompson, K.; Hosking, H.; Pederick, W.; Singh, I.; Santhakumar, A.B. The effect of anthocyanin supplementation in modulating platelet function in sedentary population: A randomised, double-blind, placebo-controlled, cross-over trial. *Br. J. Nutr.* **2017**, *118*, 368–374. [CrossRef]
18. Shim, S.H.; Kim, J.M.; Choi, C.Y.; Kim, C.Y.; Park, K.H. Ginkgo biloba extract and bilberry anthocyanins improve visual function in patients with normal tension glaucoma. *J. Med. Food* **2012**, *15*, 818–823. [CrossRef] [PubMed]
19. Li, L.; Lyall, G.K.; Martinez-blazquez, J.A.; Vallejo, F.; Tomas-barberan, F.A.; Birch, K.M.; Boesch, C. Blood orange juice consumption increases flow-mediated dilation in adults with overweight and obesity: A randomized controlled trial. *J. Nutr.* **2020**, *150*, 2287–2294. [CrossRef] [PubMed]
20. Tang, P.; Monica Giusti, M. Metal chelates of petunidin derivatives exhibit enhanced color and stability. *Foods* **2020**, *9*, 11–15. [CrossRef] [PubMed]
21. Mladěnka, P.; Říha, M.; Martin, J.; Gorová, B.; Matějíček, A.; Spilková, J. Fruit extracts of 10 varieties of elderberry (*Sambucus nigra* L.) interact differently with iron and copper. *Phytochem. Lett.* **2016**, *18*, 232–238. [CrossRef]
22. Sinopoli, A.; Calogero, G.; Bartolotta, A. Computational aspects of anthocyanidins and anthocyanins: A review. *Food Chem.* **2019**, *297*, 124898. [CrossRef]
23. Wu, X.; Beecher, G.R.; Holden, J.M.; Haytowitz, D.B.; Gebhardt, S.E.; Prior, R.L. Concentrations of anthocyanins in common foods in the United States and estimation of normal consumption. *J. Agric. Food Chem.* **2006**, *54*, 4069–4075. [CrossRef] [PubMed]
24. Zamora-Ros, R.; Knaze, V.; Luján-Barroso, L.; Slimani, N.; Romieu, I.; Fedirko, V.; Magistris, M.S.; Ericson, U.; Amiano, P.; Trichopoulou, A.; et al. Estimated dietary intakes of flavonols, flavanones and flavones in the European Prospective Investigation into Cancer and Nutrition (EPIC) 24 hour dietary recall cohort. *Br. J. Nutr.* **2011**, *106*, 1915–1925. [CrossRef]
25. Rienth, M.; Vigneron, N.; Darriet, P.; Sweetman, C.; Burbidge, C.; Bonghi, C.; Walker, R.P.; Famiani, F.; Castellarin, S.D. Grape berry secondary metabolites and their modulation by abiotic factors in a climate change scenario—A review. *Front. Plant Sci.* **2021**, *12*, 1–26. [CrossRef]
26. Šamec, D.; Karalija, E.; Šola, I.; Vujčić Bok, V.; Salopek-Sondi, B. The role of polyphenols in abiotic stress response: The influence of molecular structure. *Plants* **2021**, *10*, 118. [CrossRef] [PubMed]
27. Legua, P.; Domenech, A.; Martinez, J.J.; Sánchez-Rodríguez, L.; Hernández, F.; Carbonell-Barrachina, A.A.; Melgarejo, P. Bioactive and volatile compounds in sweet cherry cultivars. *J. Food Nutr. Res.* **2017**, *5*, 844–851. [CrossRef]
28. Bresciani, L.; Martini, D.; Mena, P.; Tassotti, M.; Calani, L.; Brigati, G.; Brighenti, F.; Holasek, S.; Malliga, D.E.; Lamprecht, M.; et al. Absorption profile of (poly)phenolic compounds after consumption of three food supplements containing 36 different fruits, vegetables, and berries. *Nutrients* **2017**, *9*, 194. [CrossRef] [PubMed]
29. Wang, T.-Y.; Li, Q.; Bi, K.-S. Bioactive flavonoids in medicinal plants: Structure, activity and biological fate. *Asian J. Pharm. Sci.* **2018**, *13*, 12–23. [CrossRef]

30. Landete, J.M. Dietary intake of natural antioxidants: Vitamins and polyphenols. *Crit. Rev. Food Sci. Nutr.* **2013**, *53*, 706–721. [CrossRef]
31. Cosme, P.; Rodríguez, A.B.; Espino, J.; Garrido, M. Plant phenolics: Bioavailability as a key determinant of their potential health-promoting applications. *Antioxidants* **2020**, *9*, 1263. [CrossRef]
32. Diaconeasa, Z.; Ioana, S.; Xiao, J.; Leopold, N.; Ayvaz, Z.; Danciu, C.; Ayvaz, H.; Sttănilă, A.; Nistor, M.; Socaciu, C. Anthocyanins, vibrant color pigments, and their role in skin cancer prevention. *Biomedicines* **2020**, *8*, 336. [CrossRef]
33. Mattioli, R.; Francioso, A.; Mosca, L.; Silva, P. Anthocyanins: A comprehensive review of their chemical properties and health effects on cardiovascular and neurodegenerative diseases. *Molecules* **2020**, *25*, 3809. [CrossRef] [PubMed]
34. Ullah, R.; Khan, M.; Shah, S.A.; Saeed, K.; Kim, M.O. Natural antioxidant anthocyanins—A hidden therapeutic candidate in metabolic disorders with major focus in neurodegeneration. *Nutrients* **2019**, *11*, 1195. [CrossRef]
35. Ribnickya, D.M.; Roopchand, D.E.; Oren, A.; Grace, M.; Poulev, A.; Lila, M.A.; Havenaar, R.; Raskin, I. Effects of a high fat meal matrix and protein complexation on the bioaccessibility of blueberry anthocyanins using the TNO gastrointestinal model (TIM-1). *Food Chem.* **2014**, *142*, 349–357. [CrossRef]
36. Wallace, T.C.; Giusti, M.M. Anthocyanins. *Adv. Nutr.* **2015**, *6*, 620–622. [CrossRef] [PubMed]
37. Prior, R.L.; Wu, X. Anthocyanins: Structural characteristics that result in unique metabolic patterns and biological activities. *Free Radic. Res.* **2006**, *40*, 1014–1028. [CrossRef] [PubMed]
38. Tena, N.; Martín, J.; Asuero, A.G. State of the art of anthocyanins: Antioxidant activity, sources, bioavailability, and therapeutic effect in human health. *Antioxidants* **2020**, *9*, 451. [CrossRef] [PubMed]
39. White, B.L.; Howard, L.R.; Prior, R.L. Proximate and polyphenolic characterization of cranberry pomace. *J. Agric. Food Chem.* **2010**, *58*, 4030–4036. [CrossRef] [PubMed]
40. Gonçalves, A.C.; Campos, G.; Alves, G.; Garcia-Viguera, C.; Moreno, D.A.; Silva, L.R. Physical and phytochemical composition of 23 Portuguese sweet cherries as conditioned by variety (or genotype). *Food Chem.* **2021**, *335*, 127637. [CrossRef] [PubMed]
41. Pojer, E.; Mattivi, F.; Johnson, D.; Stockley, C.S. The case for anthocyanin consumption to promote human health: A review. *Compr. Rev. Food Sci. Food Saf.* **2013**, *12*, 483–508. [CrossRef] [PubMed]
42. Escobar-Cévoli, R.; Castro-Espín, C.; Béraud, V.; Buckland, G.; Zamora-Ros, R. An overview of global flavonoid intake and its food sources. In *Flavonoids—From Biosynthesis to Human Health*; Justino, G.C., Ed.; InTech: London, UK, 2017; pp. 371–391.
43. Igwe, E.O.; Charlton, K.E.; Probst, Y.C. Usual dietary anthocyanin intake, sources and their association with blood pressure in a representative sample of Australian adults. *J. Hum. Nutr. Diet.* **2019**, *32*, 578–590. [CrossRef]
44. Chinese Nutrition Society. *Chinese DRIs Handbook*; Standards Press of China: Beijing, China, 2013.
45. Kim, K.; Vance, T.M.; Chun, O.K. Estimated intake and major food sources of flavonoids among US adults: Changes between 1999–2002 and 2007–2010 in NHANES. *Eur. J. Nutr.* **2016**, *55*, 833–843. [CrossRef]
46. Wu, X.; Prior, R.L. Identification and characterization of anthocyanins by HPLC-ESI-MS/MS in common foods in the United States: Fruits and berries. *J. Agric. Food Chem.* **2005**, *53*, 2589–2599. [CrossRef]
47. Frond, A.D.; Iuhas, C.I.; Stirbu, I.; Leopold, L.; Socaci, S.; Andreea, S.; Ayvaz, H.; Andreea, S.; Mihai, S.; Zorita, D.; et al. Phytochemical characterization of five edible purple-reddish vegetables: Anthocyanins, flavonoids, and phenolic acid derivatives. *Molecules* **2019**, *24*, 1536. [CrossRef] [PubMed]
48. Kharadze, M.; Japaridze, I.; Kalandia, A.; Vanidze, M. Anthocyanins and antioxidant activity of red wines made from endemic grape varieties. *Ann. Agrar. Sci.* **2018**, *16*, 181–184. [CrossRef]
49. Horincar, G.; Enachi, E.; Bolea, C.; Râpeanu, G.; Aprodu, I. Value-added lager beer enriched with eggplant (*Solanum melongena* L.) peel extract. *Molecules* **2020**, *25*, 731. [CrossRef]
50. Zambrano-Moreno, E.L.; Chávez-Jáuregui, R.N.; Plaza, M.d.L.; Wessel-Beaver, L. Phenolic content and antioxidant capacity in organically and conventionally grown eggplant (*Solanum melongena*) fruits following thermal processing. *Food Sci. Technol.* **2015**, *35*, 414–420. [CrossRef]
51. de Rosso, V.V.; Hillebrand, S.; Montilla, E.C.; Bobbio, F.O.; Winterhalter, P.; Mercadante, A.Z. Determination of anthocyanins from acerola (*Malpighia emarginata* DC.) and açai (*Euterpe oleracea* Mart.) by HPLC–PDA–MS/MS. *J. Food Compos. Anal.* **2008**, *21*, 291–299. [CrossRef]
52. Polat, M.; Okatan, V.; Güçlü, S.F.; Çolak, A.M. Determination of some chemical characteristics and total antioxidant capacity in apple varieties grown in Posof/Ardahan region. *Int. J. Agric. Environ. Food Sci.* **2018**, *2*, 131–134. [CrossRef]
53. Wang, S.Y.; HsinShan, L. Antioxidant activity in fruits and leaves of blackberry, raspberry, and strawberry varies with cultivar and developmental stage. *J. Agric. Food Chem.* **2000**, *48*, 140–146. [CrossRef] [PubMed]
54. Fan-Chiang, H.-J.; Wrolstad, R.E. Anthocyanin pigment composition of blackberries. *JFS C Food Chem. Toxicol.* **2005**, *70*, 198–202. [CrossRef]
55. Jakobek, L.; Seruga, M.; Novak, I.; Medvidovic-Kosanovic, M. Flavonols, phenolic acids and antioxidant activity of some red fruits. *Dtsch. Leb.* **2007**, *103*, 369–378.
56. Esposito, D.; Damsud, T.; Wilson, M.; Grace, M.H.; Strauch, R.; Li, X.; Lila, M.A.; Komarnytsky, S. Black currant anthocyanins attenuate weight gain and improve glucose metabolism in diet-induced obese mice with intact, but not disrupted, gut microbiome. *J. Agric. Food Chem.* **2015**, *63*, 6172–6180. [CrossRef] [PubMed]
57. Mazza, G.; Kay, C.D.; Cottrell, T.; Holub, B.J. Absorption of anthocyanins from blueberries and serum antioxidant status in human subjects. *J. Agric. Food Chem.* **2002**, *50*, 45–48. [CrossRef] [PubMed]

58. Zielińska, A.; Siudem, P.; Paradowska, K.; Gralec, M.; Kaźmierski, S.; Wawer, I. Aronia melanocarpa fruits as a rich dietary source of chlorogenic acids and anthocyanins: 1H-NMR, HPLC-DAD, and chemometric studies. *Molecules* **2020**, *25*, 3234. [CrossRef] [PubMed]
59. Jasutiene, L.; Cesonienė, I.; Sarkinas, A. Phenolics and anthocyanins in berries of European cranberry and their antimicrobial activity. *Medicina* **2009**, *45*, 992–999.
60. Duymuş, H.G.; Göger, F.; Başer, K.H.C. In vitro antioxidant properties and anthocyanin compositions of elderberry extracts. *Food Chem.* **2014**, *155*, 112–119. [CrossRef]
61. Solomon, A.; Golubowicz, S.; Yablowicz, Z.; Grossman, S.; Bergman, M.; Gottlieb, H.E.; Altman, A.; Kerem, Z.; Flaishman, M.A. Antioxidant activities and anthocyanin content of fresh fruits of common fig (*Ficus carica* L.). *J. Agric. Food Chem.* **2006**, *54*, 7717–7723. [CrossRef]
62. Kamiloglu, S.; Capanoglu, E. Polyphenol content in figs (Ficus carica L.): Effect of sun-drying. *Int. J. Food Prop.* **2015**, *18*, 521–535. [CrossRef]
63. Silva, L.R.; Queiroz, M. Bioactive compounds of red grapes from Dão region (Portugal): Evaluation of phenolic and organic profile. *Asian Pac. J. Trop. Biomed.* **2016**, *6*, 315–321. [CrossRef]
64. Kallithraka, S.; Aliaj, L.; Makris, D.P.; Kefalas, P. Anthocyanin profiles of major red grape (*Vitis vinifera* L.) varieties cultivated in Greece and their relationship with in vitro antioxidant characteristics. *Int. J. Food Sci. Technol.* **2009**, *44*, 2385–2393. [CrossRef]
65. Khattab, R.; Brooks, M.S.-L.; Ghanem, A. Phenolic analyses of haskap berries (*Lonicera caerulea* L.): Spectrophotometry versus high performance liquid chromatography. *Int. J. Food Prop.* **2016**, *19*, 1708–1725. [CrossRef]
66. Celli, G.B.; Ghanem, A.; Brooks, M.S.L. Optimization of ultrasound-assisted extraction of anthocyanins from haskap berries (*Lonicera caerulea* L.) using Response Surface Methodology. *Ultrason. Sonochem.* **2015**, *27*, 449–455. [CrossRef] [PubMed]
67. Cantín, C.M.; Moreno, M.A.; Gogorcena, Y. Evaluation of the antioxidant capacity, phenolic compounds, and vitamin C content of different peach and nectarine [*Prunus persica* (L.) batsch] breeding progenies. *J. Agric. Food Chem.* **2009**, *57*, 4586–4592. [CrossRef]
68. Usenik, V.; Štampar, F.; Veberič, R. Anthocyanins and fruit colour in plums (*Prunus domestica* L.) during ripening. *Food Chem.* **2009**, *114*, 529–534. [CrossRef]
69. Passafiume, R.; Perrone, A.; Sortino, G.; Gianguzzi, G.; Saletta, F.; Gentile, C.; Farina, V. Chemical-physical characteristics, polyphenolic content and total antioxidant activity of three Italian-grown pomegranate cultivars. *NFS J.* **2019**, *16*, 9–14. [CrossRef]
70. Zhu, F.; Yuan, Z.; Zhao, X.; Yin, Y.; Feng, L. Composition and contents of anthocyanins in different pomegranate cultivars. *Acta Hortic.* **2015**, *1089*, 35–41.
71. Mihaylova, D.; Popova, A.; Desseva, I.; Petkova, N.; Stoyanova, M.; Vrancheva, R.; Slavov, A.; Slavchev, A.; Lante, A. Comparative study of early- and mid-ripening peach (*Prunus persica* L.) varieties: Biological activity, macro-, and micro- nutrient profile. *Foods* **2021**, *10*, 164. [CrossRef]
72. Bento, C.; Gonçalves, A.C.; Silva, B.; Silva, L.R. Assessing the phenolic profile, antioxidant, antidiabetic and protective effects against oxidative damage in human erythrocytes of peaches from Fundão. *J. Funct. Foods* **2018**, *43*, 224–233. [CrossRef]
73. Wiczkowski, W.; Szawara-Nowak, D.; Topolska, J. Red cabbage anthocyanins: Profile, isolation, identification, and antioxidant activity. *Food Res. Int.* **2013**, *51*, 303–309. [CrossRef]
74. Ahmadiani, N.; Robbins, R.J.; Collins, T.M.; Giusti, M.M. Anthocyanins contents, profiles, and color characteristics of red cabbage extracts from different cultivars and maturity stages. *J. Agric. Food Chem.* **2014**, *62*, 7524–7531. [CrossRef]
75. Jara-Palacios, M.J.; Santisteban, A.; Gordillo, B.; Hernanz, D.; Heredia, F.J.; Escudero-Gilete, M.L. Comparative study of red berry pomaces (blueberry, red raspberry, red currant and blackberry) as source of antioxidants and pigments. *Eur. Food Res. Technol.* **2019**, *245*, 1–9. [CrossRef]
76. Galvis Sánchez, A.C.; Gil-Izquierdo, A.; Gil, M.I. Comparative study of six pear cultivars in terms of their phenolic and vitamin C contents and antioxidant capacity. *J. Sci. Food Agric.* **2003**, *83*, 995–1003. [CrossRef]
77. Ludwig, I.A.; Mena, P.; Calani, L.; Borges, G.; Pereira-Caro, G.; Bresciani, L.; Del Rio, D.; Lean, M.E.J.; Crozier, A. New insights into the bioavailability of red raspberry anthocyanins and ellagitannins. *Free Radic. Biol. Med.* **2015**, *89*, 758–769. [CrossRef] [PubMed]
78. Wang, H.; Nair, M.G.; Strasburg, G.M.; Booren, M.; Gray, J.; Dewitt, D.L. Cyclooxygenase active bioflavonoids from Balaton tart cherry and their structure activity relationships. *Phytomedicine* **2000**, *7*, 15–19. [CrossRef]
79. Silva, F.L.; Escribano-Bailón, M.T.; Pérez Alonso, J.J.; Rivas-Gonzalo, J.C.; Santos-Buelga, C. Anthocyanin pigments in strawberry. *LWT-Food Sci. Technol.* **2007**, *40*, 374–382. [CrossRef]
80. Gonçalves, A.C.; Bento, C.; Silva, B.M.; Silva, L.R. Sweet cherries from Fundão possess antidiabetic potential and protect human erythrocytes against oxidative damage. *Food Res. Int.* **2017**, *95*, 91–100. [CrossRef] [PubMed]
81. Martini, S.; Conte, A.; Tagliazucchi, D. Phenolic compounds profile and antioxidant properties of six sweet cherry (Prunus avium) cultivars. *Food Res. Int.* **2017**, *97*, 15–26. [CrossRef]
82. Diep, T.; Pook, C.; Yoo, M. Phenolic and anthocyanin compounds and antioxidant activity of Tamarillo (*Solanum betaceum* Cav.). *Antioxidants* **2020**, *9*, 169. [CrossRef]
83. Cao, J.; Jiang, Q.; Lin, J.; Li, X.; Sun, C.; Chen, K. Physicochemical characterisation of four cherry species (*Prunus* spp.) grown in China. *Food Chem.* **2015**, *173*, 855–863. [CrossRef]
84. Borghesi, E.; González-Miret, M.L.; Escudero-Gilete, M.L.; Malorgio, F.; Heredia, F.J.; Meléndez-Martínez, A.J. Effects of salinity stress on carotenoids, anthocyanins, and color of diverse tomato genotypes. *J. Agric. Food Chem.* **2011**, *59*, 11676–11682. [CrossRef]

85. Blando, F.; Berland, H.; Maiorano, G.; Durante, M.; Mazzucato, A.; Picarella, M.E.; Nicoletti, I.; Gerardi, C.; Mita, G.; Andersen, Ø.M. Nutraceutical characterization of anthocyanin-rich fruits produced by "Sun Black" tomato line. *Front. Nutr.* **2019**, *6*, 133. [CrossRef] [PubMed]
86. Kammerer, D.; Carle, R.; Schieber, A. Quantification of anthocyanins in black carrot extracts (*Daucus carota* ssp. sativus var. atrorubens Alef.) and evaluation of their color properties. *Eur. Food Res. Technol.* **2004**, *219*, 479–486. [CrossRef]
87. Shi-Lin, Z.; Peng, D.; Yu-Chao, X.; Jian-Jun, W. Quantification and analysis of anthocyanin and flavonoids compositions, and antioxidant activities in onions with three different colors. *J. Integr. Agric.* **2016**, *15*, 2175–2181.
88. Legua, P.; Melgarejo, P.; Martínez, J.J.; Martínez, R.; Hernández, F. Evaluation of Spanish pomegranate juices: Organic acids, sugars, and anthocyanins. *Int. J. Food Prop.* **2012**, *15*, 481–494. [CrossRef]
89. Lapidot, T.; Harel, S.; Granit, R.; Kanner, J. Bioavailability of red wine anthocyanins as detected in human urine. *J. Agric. Food Chem.* **1998**, *46*, 4297–4302. [CrossRef]
90. Kirakosyan, A.; Seymour, E.M.; Llanes, D.E.U.; Kaufman, P.B.; Bolling, S.F. Chemical profile and antioxidant capacities of tart cherry products. *Food Chem.* **2009**, *115*, 20–25. [CrossRef]
91. Oliveira, H.; Roma-Rodrigues, C.; Santos, A.; Veigas, B.; Brás, N.; Faria, A.; Calhau, C.; De Freitas, V.; Baptista, P.V.; Mateus, N.; et al. GLUT1 and GLUT3 involvement in anthocyanin gastric transport- Nanobased targeted approach. *Sci. Rep.* **2019**, *789*, 1–14. [CrossRef]
92. European Food Safety Authority. Scientific opinion on the re-evaluation of anthocyanins (E 163) as a food additive. *EFSA J.* **2013**, *11*, 3145.
93. Matsumoto, H.; Inaba, H.; Kishi, M.; Tominaga, S.; Hirayama, M.; Tsuda, T. Orally administered delphinidin 3-rutinoside and cyanidin 3-rutinoside are directly absorbed in rats and humans and appear in the blood as the intact forms. *J. Agric. Food Chem.* **2001**, *49*, 1546–1551. [CrossRef]
94. Cao, G.; Muccitelli, H.U.; Sánchez-Moreno, C.; Prior, R.L. Anthocyanins are absorbed in glycated forms in elderly women: A pharmacokinetic study. *Am. J. Clin. Nutr.* **2001**, *73*, 920–926. [CrossRef]
95. Sandhu, A.K.; Huang, Y.; Xiao, D.; Park, E.; Edirisinghe, I.; Burton-Freeman, B. Pharmacokinetic characterization and bioavailability of strawberry anthocyanins relative to meal intake. *J. Agric. Food Chem.* **2016**, *64*, 4891–4899. [CrossRef]
96. Nielsen, I.L.F.; Dragsted, L.O.; Ravn-haren, G.; Freese, R.; Rasmussen, S.E. Absorption and excretion of black currant anthocyanins in humans and watanabe heritable hyperlipidemic rabbits. *J. Agric. Food Chem.* **2003**, *51*, 2813–2820. [CrossRef]
97. Bitsch, R.; Netzel, M.; Frank, T.; Strass, G.; Bitsch, I. Bioavailability and biokinetics of anthocyanins from red grape juice and red wine. *J. Biomed. Biotechnol.* **2004**, *2004*, 293–298. [CrossRef]
98. Milbury, P.E.; Vita, J.A.; Blumberg, J.B. Anthocyanins are bioavailable in humans following an acute dose of cranberry juice. *J. Nutr.* **2010**, *140*, 1099–1104. [CrossRef] [PubMed]
99. Keane, K.M.; Bell, P.G.; Lodge, J.K.; Constantinou, C.L.; Jenkinson, S.E.; Bass, R.; Howatson, G. Phytochemical uptake following human consumption of Montmorency tart cherry (*L. Prunus cerasus*) and influence of phenolic acids on vascular smooth muscle cells in vitro. *Eur. J. Nutr.* **2016**, *55*, 1695–1705. [CrossRef]
100. Kuntz, S.; Rudloff, S.; Asseburg, H.; Borsch, C.; Fröhling, B.; Unger, F.; Dold, S.; Spengler, B.; Römpp, A.; Kunz, C. Uptake and bioavailability of anthocyanins and phenolic acids from grape/blueberry juice and smoothie in vitro and in vivo. *Br. J. Nutr.* **2015**, *113*, 1044–1055. [CrossRef] [PubMed]
101. Giordano, L.; Coletta, V.; Tamburrelli, C.; D'Imperio, M.; Crescente, M.; Silvestri, C.; Rapisarda, P.; Reforgiato Recupero, G.; De Curtis, A.; Iacoviello, L.; et al. Four-week ingestion of blood orange juice results in measurable anthocyanin urinary levels but does not affect cellular markers related to cardiovascular risk: A randomized cross-over study in healthy volunteers. *Eur. J. Nutr.* **2012**, *51*, 541–548. [CrossRef] [PubMed]
102. Wiczkowski, W.; Romaszko, E.; Piskula, M.K. Bioavailability of cyanidin glycosides from natural chokeberry (*Aronia melanocarpa*) juice with dietary-relevant dose of anthocyanins in humans. *J. Agric. Food Chem.* **2010**, *58*, 12130–12136. [CrossRef] [PubMed]
103. McGhie, T.K.; Ainge, G.D.; Barnett, L.E.; Cooney, J.M.; Jensen, D.J. Anthocyanin glycosides from berry fruit are absorbed and excreted unmetabolized by both humans and rats. *J. Agric. Food Chem.* **2003**, *51*, 4539–4548. [CrossRef]
104. Morazzoni, P.; Bombardelli, E. *Vaccinium myrtillus* L. *Fitoterapia* **1996**, *67*, 3–29.
105. He, J.; Giusti, M.M. Anthocyanins: Natural colorants with health-promoting properties. *Annu. Rev. Food Sci. Technol.* **2010**, *1*, 163–187. [CrossRef]
106. Oliveira, H.; Perez-Gregório, R.; Freitas, V.; Mateus, N.; Fernandes, I. Comparison of the in vitro gastrointestinal bioavailability of acylated and non-acylated anthocyanins: Purple-fleshed sweet potato vs red wine. *Food Chem.* **2018**, *276*, 410–418. [CrossRef] [PubMed]
107. Passamonti, S.; Vrhovsek, U.; Mattivi, F. The interaction of anthocyanins with bilitranslocase. *Biochem. Biophys. Res. Commun.* **2002**, *296*, 631–636. [CrossRef]
108. Velderrain-Rodríguez, G.R.; Palafox-Carlos, H.; Wall-Medrano, A.; Ayala-Zavala, J.F.; Chen, C.Y.O.; Robles-Sánchez, M.; Astiazaran-García, H.; Alvarez-Parrilla, E.; González-Aguilar, G.A. Phenolic compounds: Their journey after intake. *Food Funct.* **2014**, *5*, 189–197. [CrossRef]
109. Han, F.; Oliveira, H.; Brás, N.F.; Fernandes, I.; Cruz, L.; de Freitas, V.; Mateus, N. In vitro gastrointestinal absorption of red wine anthocyanins–Impact of structural complexity and phase II metabolization. *Food Chem.* **2020**, *317*, 126398. [CrossRef] [PubMed]

110. Ramos, P.; Herrera, R.; Moya-león, M.A. Anthocyanins: Food sources and benefits to consumer's health. In *Handbook of Anthocyanins*; Warner, L.M., Ed.; Nova Science Publishers, Inc.: New York, NY, USA, 2014; pp. 363–384.
111. Eker, M.E.; Aaby, K.; Budic-Leto, I.; Brncic, S.R.; El, S.N.; Karakaya, S.; Simsek, S.; Manach, C.; Wiczkowski, W.; De Pascual-Teresa, S. A review of factors affecting anthocyanin bioavailability: Possible implications for the inter-individual variability. *Foods* **2020**, *9*, 2. [CrossRef] [PubMed]
112. Mueller, D.; Jung, K.; Winter, M.; Rogoll, D.; Melcher, R.; Kulozik, U.; Schwarz, K.; Richling, E. Encapsulation of anthocyanins from bilberries–Effects on bioavailability and intestinal accessibility in humans. *Food Chem.* **2018**, *248*, 217–224. [CrossRef] [PubMed]
113. Rodriguez-Mateos, A.; Vauzour, D.; Krueger, C.G.; Shanmuganayagam, D.; Reed, J.; Calani, L.; Mena, P.; Del Rio, D.; Crozier, A. Bioavailability, bioactivity and impact on health of dietary flavonoids and related compounds: An update. *Arch. Toxicol.* **2014**, *88*, 1803–1853. [CrossRef] [PubMed]
114. Norberto, S.; Silva, S.; Meireles, M.; Faria, A.; Pintado, M.; Calhau, C. Blueberry anthocyanins in health promotion: A metabolic overview. *J. Funct. Foods* **2013**, *5*, 1518–1528. [CrossRef]
115. Azzini, E.; Bugianesi, R.; Romano, F.; Di Venere, D.; Miccadei, S.; Durazzo, A.; Foddai, M.S.; Catasta, G.; Linsalata, V.; Maiani, G. Absorption and metabolism of bioactive molecules after oral consumption of cooked edible heads of *Cynara scolymus* L. (cultivar Violetto di Provenza) in human subjects: A pilot study. *Br. J. Nutr.* **2007**, *97*, 963–969. [CrossRef]
116. Martini, S.; Conte, A.; Tagliazucchi, D. Bioactivity and cell metabolism of *in vitro* digested sweet cherry (*Prunus avium*) phenolic compounds. *Int. J. Food Sci. Nutr.* **2018**, *70*, 335–348. [CrossRef]
117. Dharmawansa, K.V.S.; Hoskin, D.W.; Rupasinghe, H.P. Chemopreventive effect of dietary anthocyanins against gastrointestinal cancers: A review of recent advances and perspectives. *Int. J. Mol. Sci.* **2020**, *21*, 6555. [CrossRef] [PubMed]
118. Mueller, D.; Jung, K.; Winter, M.; Rogoll, D.; Melcher, R.; Richling, E. Human intervention study to investigate the intestinal accessibility and bioavailability of anthocyanins from bilberries. *Food Chem.* **2017**, *231*, 275–286. [CrossRef] [PubMed]
119. Lin, S.; Wang, Z.; Lam, K.L.; Zeng, S.; Tan, B.K.; Hu, J. Role of intestinal microecology in the regulation of energy metabolism by dietary polyphenols and their metabolites. *Food Nutr. Res.* **2019**, *63*, 1–12. [CrossRef] [PubMed]
120. Yang, L.; Ling, W.; Yang, Y.; Chen, Y.; Tian, Z.; Du, Z.; Chen, J.; Xie, Y.; Liu, Z.; Yang, L. Role of purified anthocyanins in improving cardiometabolic risk factors in chinese men and women with prediabetes or early untreated diabetes—A randomized controlled trial. *Nutrients* **2017**, *9*, 1104. [CrossRef]
121. Kim, M.J.; Rehman, S.U.; Amin, F.U.; Kim, M.O. Enhanced neuroprotection of anthocyanin-loaded PEG-gold nanoparticles against Aβ1-42-induced neuroinflammation and neurodegeneration via the NF-KB /JNK/GSK3β signaling pathway. *Nanomed. Nanotechnol. Biol. Med.* **2017**, *13*, 2533–2544. [CrossRef]
122. Amin, F.U.; Shah, S.A.; Badshah, H.; Khan, M.; Kim, M.O. Anthocyanins encapsulated by PLGA@PEG nanoparticles potentially improved its free radical scavenging capabilities via p38/JNK pathway against Aβ1-42-induced oxidative stress. *J. Nanobiotechnol.* **2017**, *15*, 12. [CrossRef]
123. Thibado, S.; Thornthwaite, J.; Ballard, T.; Goodman, B. Anticancer effects of bilberry anthocyanins compared with Nu-traNanoSphere encapsulated bilberry anthocyanins. *Mol. Clin. Oncol.* **2017**, *8*, 330–335. [CrossRef]
124. Ma, Y.; Ding, S.; Fei, Y.; Liu, G.; Jang, H.; Fang, J. Antimicrobial activity of anthocyanins and catechins against foodborne pathogens Escherichia coli and Salmonella. *Food Control* **2019**, *106*, 106712. [CrossRef]
125. Sun, X.; Zhou, T.; Wei, C.; Lan, W.; Zhao, Y.; Pan, Y.; Wu, V.C.H. Antibacterial effect and mechanism of anthocyanin rich Chinese wild blueberry extract on various foodborne pathogens. *Food Control* **2018**, *94*, 155–161. [CrossRef]
126. Kim, S.H.; Park, M.; Woo, H.; Tharmalingam, N.; Lee, G.; Rhee, K.J.; Eom, Y. Bin; Han, S.I.; Seo, W.D.; Kim, J.B. Inhibitory effects of anthocyanins on secretion of *Helicobacter pylori* CagA and VacA toxins. *Int. J. Med. Sci.* **2012**, *9*, 838–842. [CrossRef] [PubMed]
127. Bendokas, V.; Šarkinas, A.; Jasinauskienė, D.; Anisimovienė, N.; Morkūnaitė-Haimi, Š.; Stanys, V.; Šikšnianas, T. Antimicrobial activity of berries extracts of four Ribes species, their phenolic content and anthocyanin composition. *Folia Hortic.* **2018**, *30*, 249–257. [CrossRef]
128. Chen, H.; Yu, W.; Chen, G.; Meng, S.; Xiang, Z.; He, N. Antinociceptive and antibacterial properties of anthocyanins and flavonols from fruits of black and non-black mulberries. *Molecules* **2018**, *23*, 4. [CrossRef]
129. Majiene, D.; Liobikas, J.; Trumbeckaite, S.; Kopustinskiene, D.M.; Bendokas, V.; Sasnauskas, A.; Šikšnianas, T.; Liegiute, S.; Anisimoviene, N. Antioxidative and antimicrobial activity of anthocyanin-rich extracts from fruits of blackcurrant and cherry. *Acta Hortic.* **2014**, *1040*, 173–178. [CrossRef]
130. Silva, S.; Costa, E.M.; Mendes, M.; Morais, R.M.; Calhau, C.; Pintado, M.M. Antimicrobial, antiadhesive and antibiofilm activity of an ethanolic, anthocyanin-rich blueberry extract purified by solid phase extraction. *J. Appl. Microbiol.* **2016**, *121*, 693–703. [CrossRef]
131. Carvalho, F.B.; Gutierres, J.M.; Bohnert, C.; Zago, A.M.; Abdalla, F.H.; Vieira, J.M.; Palma, H.E.; Oliveira, S.M.; Spanevello, R.M.; Duarte, M.M.; et al. Anthocyanins suppress the secretion of proinflammatory mediators and oxidative stress, and restore ion pump activities in demyelination. *J. Nutr. Biochem.* **2015**, *26*, 378–390. [CrossRef]
132. Rashid, K.; Wachira, F.N.; Nyariki, J.N.; Isaac, A.O. Kenyan purple tea anthocyanins and coenzyme-Q10 ameliorate post treatment reactive encephalopathy associated with cerebral human African trypanosomiasis in murine model. *Parasitol. Int.* **2014**, *63*, 417–426. [CrossRef]

133. Yoon, B.I.; Bae, W.J.; Choi, Y.S.; Kim, S.J.; Ha, U.S.; Hong, S.H.; Sohn, D.W.; Kim, S.W. Anti-inflammatory and antimicrobial effects of anthocyanin extracted from black soybean on chronic bacterial prostatitis rat model. *Chin. J. Integr. Med.* **2018**, *24*, 621–626. [CrossRef]
134. Gonçalves, A.C.; Rodrigues, M.; Santos, A.O.; Alves, G.; Silva, L.R. Antioxidant status, antidiabetic properties and effects on Caco-2 cells of colored and non-colored enriched extracts of sweet cherry fruits. *Nutrients* **2018**, *10*, 1688. [CrossRef]
135. Kähkönen, M.P.; Heinonen, M. Antioxidant activity of anthocyanins and their aglycons. *J. Agric. Food Chem.* **2003**, *51*, 628–633. [CrossRef]
136. Sadeer, N.B.; Montesano, D.; Albrizio, S.; Zengin, G.; Mahomoodally, M.F. The versatility of antioxidant assays in food science and safety-Chemistry, applications, strengths, and limitations. *Antioxidants* **2020**, *9*, 709. [CrossRef]
137. Rahman, M.M.; Ichiyanagi, T.; Komiyama, T.; Hatano, Y.; Konishi, T. Superoxide radical- and peroxynitrite-scavenging activity of anthocyanins; structure-activity relationship and their synergism. *Free Radic. Res.* **2006**, *40*, 993–1002. [CrossRef]
138. Tarozzi, A.; Marchesi, A.; Hrelia, S.; Angeloni, C.; Andrisano, V.; Fiori, J.; Cantelli-Forti, G.; Hrelia, P. Protective effects of Cyanidin-3-O-β-glucopyranoside against UVA-Induced Oxidative Stress in Human Keratinocytes. *Photochem. Photobiol.* **2005**, *81*, 623–629. [CrossRef]
139. Heinonen, I.M.; Meyer, A.S.; Frankel, E.N. Antioxidant activity of berry phenolics on human low-density lipoprotein and liposome oxidation. *J. Agric. Food Chem.* **1998**, *46*, 4107–4112. [CrossRef]
140. Elisia, I.; Hu, C.; Popovich, D.G.; Kitts, D.D. Antioxidant assessment of an anthocyanin-enriched blackberry extract. *Food Chem.* **2007**, *101*, 1052–1058. [CrossRef]
141. Bowen-Forbes, C.S.; Zhang, Y.; Nair, M.G. Anthocyanin content, antioxidant, anti-inflammatory and anticancer properties of blackberry and raspberry fruits. *J. Food Compos. Anal.* **2010**, *23*, 554–560. [CrossRef]
142. Afaq, F.; Syed, D.N.; Malik, A.; Hadi, N.; Sarfaraz, S.; Kweon, M.H.; Khan, N.; Zaid, M.A.; Mukhtar, H. Delphinidin, an anthocyanidin in pigmented fruits and vegetables, protects human HaCaT keratinocytes and mouse skin against UVB-mediated oxidative stress and apoptosis. *J. Investig. Dermatol.* **2007**, *127*, 222–232. [CrossRef]
143. Hassimotto, N.M.A.; Lajolo, F.M. Antioxidant status in rats after long-term intake of anthocyanins and ellagitannins from blackberries. *J. Sci. Food Agric.* **2011**, *91*, 523–531. [CrossRef] [PubMed]
144. Khoo, H.E.; Azlan, A.; Nurulhuda, M.H.; Ismail, A.; Abas, F.; Hamid, M.; Roowi, S. Antioxidative and cardioprotective properties of anthocyanins from defatted Dabai extracts. *Evid. Based Complement. Altern. Med.* **2013**, *2013*, 434057. [CrossRef]
145. Azzini, E.; Intorre, F.; Vitaglione, P.; Napolitano, A.; Foddai, M.S.; Durazzo, A.; Fumagalli, A.; Catasta, G.; Rossi, L.; Venneria, E.; et al. Absorption of strawberry phytochemicals and antioxidant status changes in humans. *J. Berry Res.* **2010**, *1*, 81–89. [CrossRef]
146. Kuntz, S.; Kunz, C.; Herrmann, J.; Borsch, C.H.; Abel, G.; Fröhling, B.; Dietrich, H.; Rudloff, S. Anthocyanins from fruit juices improve the antioxidant status of healthy young female volunteers without affecting anti-inflammatory parameters: Results from the randomised, double-blind, placebo-controlled, cross-over ANTHONIA (ANTHOcyanins in Nutrition) study. *Br. J. Nutr.* **2014**, *112*, 925–936. [CrossRef]
147. Del Bo', C.; Riso, P.; Campolo, J.; Møller, P.; Loft, S.; Klimis-Zacas, D.; Brambilla, A.; Rizzolo, A.; Porrini, M. A single portion of blueberry (*Vaccinium corymbosum* L) improves protection against DNA damage but not vascular function in healthy male volunteers. *Nutr. Res.* **2013**, *33*, 220–227. [CrossRef] [PubMed]
148. Bialasiewicz, P.; Prymont-Przyminska, A.; Zwolinska, A.; Sarniak, A.; Wlodarczyk, A.; Krol, M.; Glusac, J.; Nowak, P.; Markowski, J.; Rutkowski, K.P.; et al. Addition of strawberries to the usual diet decreases resting chemiluminescence of fasting blood in healthy subjects—possible health-promoting effect of these fruits Consumption. *J. Am. Coll. Nutr.* **2013**, *4*, 274–287. [CrossRef]
149. Hutchison, A.T.; Flieller, E.B.; Dillon, K.J.; Leverett, B.D. Black currant nectar reduces muscle damage and inflammation following a bout of high-intensity eccentric contractions. *J. Diet. Suppl.* **2014**, *13*, 1–15. [CrossRef] [PubMed]
150. Howatson, G.; McHugh, M.P.; Hill, J.A.; Brouner, J.; Jewell, A.P.; Van Someren, K.A.; Shave, R.E.; Howatson, S.A. Influence of tart cherry juice on indices of recovery following marathon running. *Scand. J. Med. Sci. Sport.* **2010**, *20*, 843–852. [CrossRef] [PubMed]
151. Hurst, R.D.; Lyall, K.A.; Wells, R.W.; Sawyer, G.M.; Lomiwes, D.; Ngametua, N.; Hurst, S.M. Daily consumption of an anthocyanin-rich extract made from New Zealand blackcurrants for 5 weeks supports exercise recovery through the management of oxidative stress and inflammation: A randomized placebo controlled pilot study. *Front. Nutr.* **2020**, *7*, 1–15. [CrossRef] [PubMed]
152. Jiang, T.; Zhou, J.; Liu, W.; Tao, W.; He, J.; Jin, W.; Guo, H.; Yang, N.; Li, Y. The anti-inflammatory potential of protein-bound anthocyanin compounds from purple sweet potato in LPS-induced RAW264.7 macrophages. *Food Res. Int.* **2020**, *137*, 109647. [CrossRef]
153. Fernandez-Panchon, M.S.; Villano, D.; Troncoso, A.M.; Garcia-Parrilla, M.C. Antioxidant activity of phenolic compounds: From in vitro results to in vivo evidence. *Crit. Rev. Food Sci. Nutr.* **2008**, *48*, 649–671. [CrossRef] [PubMed]
154. Szymanowska, U.; Baraniak, B. Antioxidant and potentially anti-inflammatory activity of anthocyanin fractions from pomace obtained from enzymatically treated raspberries. *Antioxidants* **2019**, *8*, 299. [CrossRef]
155. Li, L.; Wang, L.; Wu, Z.; Yao, L.; Wu, Y.; Huang, L.; Liu, K.; Zhou, X.; Gou, D. Anthocyanin-rich fractions from red raspberries attenuate inflammation in both RAW264.7 macrophages and a mouse model of colitis. *Sci. Rep.* **2014**, *4*, 6234. [CrossRef] [PubMed]
156. Van de Velde, F.; Esposito, D.; Grace, M.H.; Pirovani, M.E.; Lila, M.A. Anti-inflammatory and wound healing properties of polyphenolic extracts from strawberry and blackberry fruits. *Food Res. Int.* **2019**, *121*, 453–462. [CrossRef] [PubMed]
157. Jang, B.K.; Lee, J.W.; Choi, H.; Yim, S.V. Aronia melanocarpa fruit bioactive fraction attenuates lps-induced inflammatory response in human bronchial epithelial cells. *Antioxidants* **2020**, *9*, 816. [CrossRef] [PubMed]

158. Pereira, S.R.; Pereira, R.; Figueiredo, I.; Freitas, V.; Dinis, T.C.P.; Almeida, L.M. Comparison of anti-inflammatory activities of an anthocyanin-rich fraction from Portuguese blueberries (*Vaccinium corymbosum* L.) and 5-aminosalicylic acid in a TNBS-induced colitis rat model. *PLoS ONE* **2017**, *12*, e0174116. [CrossRef] [PubMed]
159. Tall, J.M.; Seeram, N.P.; Zhao, C.; Nair, M.G.; Meyer, R.A.; Raja, S.N. Tart cherry anthocyanins suppress inflammation-induced pain behavior in rat. *Behav. Brain Res.* **2004**, *153*, 181–188. [CrossRef]
160. Palungwachira, P.; Tancharoen, S.; Phruksaniyom, C.; Klungsaeng, S.; Srichan, R.; Kikuchi, K.; Nararatwanchai, T. Antioxidant and anti-inflammatory properties of anthocyanins extracted from *Oryza sativa* L. in primary dermal fibroblasts. *Oxid. Med. Cell. Longev.* **2019**, *2019*, 2089817. [CrossRef]
161. Jacob, R.A.; Spinozzi, G.M.; Vicky, A.; Kelley, D.S.; Prior, R.L.; Hess-Pierce, B.; Kader, A.A. Consumption of cherries lowers plasma urate in healthy women. *J. Nutr.* **2003**, *133*, 1826–1829. [CrossRef] [PubMed]
162. Kelley, D.S.; Rasooly, R.; Jacob, R.A.; Kader, A.A.; Mackey, B.E. Consumption of Bing sweet cherries lowers circulating concentrations of inflammation markers in healthy men and women. *J. Nutr.* **2006**, *136*, 981–986. [CrossRef]
163. Beltrán-Debón, R.; Alonso-Villaverde, C.; Aragonès, G.; Rodríguez-Medina, I.; Rull, A.; Micol, V.; Segura-Carretero, A.; Fernández-Gutiérrez, A.; Camps, J.; Joven, J. The aqueous extract of *Hibiscus sabdariffa* calices modulates the production of monocyte chemoattractant protein-1 in humans. *Phytomedicine* **2010**, *17*, 186–191. [CrossRef]
164. Biedermann, L.; Mwinyi, J.; Scharl, M.; Frei, P.; Zeitz, J.; Kullak-Ublick, G.A.; Vavricka, S.R.; Fried, M.; Weber, A.; Humpf, H.U.; et al. Bilberry ingestion improves disease activity in mild to moderate ulcerative colitis-An open pilot study. *J. Crohn's Colitis* **2013**, *7*, 271–279. [CrossRef]
165. do Rosario, V.A.; Chang, C.; Spencer, J.; Alahakone, T.; Roodenrys, S.; Francois, M.; Weston-Green, K.; Hölzel, N.; Nichols, D.S.; Kent, K.; et al. Anthocyanins attenuate vascular and inflammatory responses to a high fat high energy meal challenge in overweight older adults: A cross-over, randomized, double-blind clinical trial. *Clin. Nutr.* **2020**, *40*, 879–889. [CrossRef]
166. Xia, M.; Ling, W.; Zhu, H.; Wang, Q.; Ma, J.; Hou, M.; Tang, Z.; Li, L.; Ye, Q. Anthocyanin prevents CD40-activated proinflammatory signaling in endothelial cells by regulating cholesterol distribution. *Arterioscler. Thromb. Vasc. Biol.* **2007**, *27*, 519–524. [CrossRef] [PubMed]
167. Seeram, N.P.; Momin, R.; Nair, M.G.; Bourquin, L.D. Cyclooxygenase inhibitory and antioxidant cyanidin glycosides in cherries and berries. *Phytomedicine* **2001**, *8*, 362–369. [CrossRef] [PubMed]
168. Vilkickyte, G.; Raudone, L.; Petrikaite, V. Phenolic fractions from *Vaccinium vitis-idaea* L. and their antioxidant and anticancer activities assessment. *Antioxidants* **2020**, *9*, 1261. [CrossRef]
169. Forbes-Hernández, T.Y.; Gasparrini, M.; Afrin, S.; Cianciosi, D.; González-Paramás, A.M.; Santos-Buelga, C.; Mezzetti, B.; Quiles, J.L.; Battino, M.; Giampieri, F.; et al. Strawberry (cv. Romina) methanolic extract and anthocyanin-enriched fraction improve lipid profile and antioxidant status in HepG2 cells. *Int. J. Mol. Sci.* **2017**, *18*, 1149. [CrossRef]
170. Masci, A.; Coccia, A.; Lendaro, E.; Mosca, L.; Paolicelli, P.; Cesa, S. Evaluation of different extraction methods from pomegranate whole fruit or peels and the antioxidant and antiproliferative activity of the polyphenolic fraction. *Food Chem.* **2016**, *202*, 59–69. [CrossRef]
171. Lage, N.N.; Anne, M.; Layosa, A.; Arbizu, S.; Chew, B.P.; Pedrosa, M.L.; Mertens-Talcott, S.; Talcott, S.; Noratto, G.D. Dark sweet cherry (*Prunus avium*) phenolics enriched in anthocyanins exhibit enhanced activity against the most aggressive breast cancer subtypes without toxicity to normal breast cells. *J. Funct. Foods* **2020**, *64*, 103710. [CrossRef]
172. Hogan, S.; Chung, H.; Zhang, L.; Li, J.; Lee, Y.; Dai, Y.; Zhou, K. Antiproliferative and antioxidant properties of anthocyanin-rich extract from açai. *Food Chem.* **2010**, *118*, 208–214. [CrossRef]
173. Long, H.L.; Zhang, F.F.; Wang, H.L.; Yang, W.S.; Hou, H.T.; Yu, J.K.; Liu, B. Mulberry anthocyanins improves thyroid cancer progression mainly by inducing apoptosis and autophagy cell death. *Kaohsiung J. Med. Sci.* **2018**, *34*, 255–262. [CrossRef]
174. Lee, J.Y.; Jo, Y.; Shin, H.; Lee, J.; Chae, S.U.; Bae, S.K.; Na, K. Anthocyanin-fucoidan nanocomplex for preventing carcinogen induced cancer: Enhanced absorption and stability. *Int. J. Pharm.* **2020**, *586*, 119597. [CrossRef]
175. Sousa, C.; Moita, E.; Valentão, P.; Fernandes, F.; Monteiro, P.; Andrade, P.B. Effects of colored and noncolored phenolics of Echium plantagineum L. bee pollen in Caco-2 cells under oxidative stress induced by tert-butyl hydroperoxide. *J. Agric. Food Chem.* **2015**, *63*, 2083–2091. [CrossRef]
176. Simas Frauches, N.; Montenegro, J.; Amaral, T.; Abreu, J.P.; Laiber, G.; Junior, J.; Borguini, R.; Santiago, M.; Pacheco, S.; Nakajima, V.M.; et al. Antiproliferative activity on human colon adenocarcinoma cells and in vitro antioxidant effect of anthocyanin-rich extracts from peels of species of the Myrtaceae family. *Molecules* **2021**, *26*, 564. [CrossRef]
177. Stoner, G.D.; Wang, L.-S. Chemoprevention of esophageal squamous cell carcinoma with berries. *Top. Curr. Chem.* **2013**, *329*, 1–20. [PubMed]
178. Stonera, G.D.; Wanga, L.-S.; Zikrib, N.; Chenc, T.; Hechtd, S.S.; Huang, C.; Sardoc, C.; Lechner, J.F. Cancer prevention with freeze-dried berries and berry components. *Semin. Cancer Biol.* **2008**, *17*, 403–410. [CrossRef] [PubMed]
179. Lippert, E.; Ruemmele, P.; Obermeier, F.; Goelder, S.; Kunst, C.; Rogler, G.; Dunger, N.; Messmann, H.; Hartmann, A.; Endlicher, E. Anthocyanins prevent colorectal cancer development in a mouse model. *Digestion* **2017**, *95*, 275–280. [CrossRef]
180. Kim, M.J.; Paramanantham, A.; Lee, W.S.; Yun, J.W.; Chang, S.H.; Kim, D.C.; Park, H.S.; Choi, Y.H.; Kim, G.S.; Ryu, C.H.; et al. Anthocyanins derived from Vitis coignetiae Pulliat contributes anti-cancer effects by suppressing NF-κB pathways in Hep3B human hepatocellular carcinoma cells and In Vivo. *Molecules* **2020**, *25*, 5445. [CrossRef]

181. Aqil, F.; Jeyabalan, J.; Kausar, H.; Munagala, R.; Singh, I.P.; Gupta, R. Lung cancer inhibitory activity of dietary berries and berry polyphenolics. *J. Berry Res.* **2016**, *6*, 105–114. [CrossRef]
182. Chen, P.-N.; Chu, S.-C.; Chiou, H.-L.; Chiang, C.-L.; Yang, S.-F.; Hsieh, Y.-S. Cyanidin 3-glucoside and peonidin 3-glucoside inhibit tumor cell growth and induce apoptosis in vitro and suppress tumor growth in vivo. *Nutr. Cancer* **2005**, *53*, 232–243. [CrossRef]
183. Hafeez, B.; Siddiqui, I.A.; Asim, M.; Malik, A.; Afaq, F.; Adhami, V.M.; Saleem, M.; Din, M.; Mukhtar, H. A dietary anthocyanidin delphinidin induces apoptosis of human prostate cancer PC3 cells in vitro and in vivo: Involvement of nuclear factor-κB signaling. *Cancer Res.* **2008**, *68*, 8564–8572. [CrossRef]
184. Ha, U.S.; Bae, W.J.; Kim, S.J.; Yoon, B.I.; Hong, S.H.; Lee, J.Y.; Hwang, T.K.; Hwang, S.Y.; Wang, Z.; Kim, S.W. Anthocyanin induces apoptosis of du-145 cells in vitro and inhibits xenograft growth of prostate cancer. *Yonsei Med. J.* **2015**, *56*, 16–23. [CrossRef] [PubMed]
185. Hui, C.; Bin, Y.; Xiaoping, Y.; Long, Y.; Chunye, C.; Mantian, M.; Wenhua, L. Anticancer activities of an anthocyanin-rich extract from black rice against breast cancer cells in vitro and in vivo. *Nutr. Cancer* **2010**, *62*, 1128–1136. [CrossRef]
186. Liu, W.; Xu, J.; Liu, Y.; Yu, X.; Tang, X.I.; Wang, Z.H.I.; Li, X.I.N. Anthocyanins potentiate the activity of trastuzumab in human epidermal growth factor receptor 2-positive breast cancer cells in vitro and in vivo. *Mol. Med. Rep.* **2014**, *10*, 1921–1926. [CrossRef] [PubMed]
187. Condello, M.; Pellegrini, E.; Spugnini, E.P.; Baldi, A.; Amadio, B.; Vincenzi, B.; Occhionero, G.; Delfine, S.; Mastrodonato, F.; Meschini, S. Anticancer activity of "Trigno M", extract of *Prunus spinosa* drupes, against in vitro 3D and in vivo colon cancer models. *Biomed. Pharmacother.* **2019**, *118*, 109281. [CrossRef] [PubMed]
188. Fan, M.J.; Yeh, P.H.; Lin, J.P.; Huang, A.C.; Lien, J.C.; Lin, H.Y.; Chung, J.G. Anthocyanins from black rice (Oryza sativa) promote immune responses in leukemia through enhancing phagocytosis of macrophages in vivo. *Exp. Ther. Med.* **2017**, *14*, 59–64. [CrossRef]
189. Razina, T.G.; Zueva, E.P.; Ulrich, A.V.; Rybalkina, O.Y.; Chaikovskii, A.V.; Isaikina, N.V.; Kalinkina, G.I.; Zhdanov, V.V.; Zyuz'Kov, G.N. Antitumor effects of *Sorbus aucuparia* L. extract highly saturated with anthocyans and their mechanisms. *Bull. Exp. Biol. Med.* **2016**, *162*, 93–97. [CrossRef]
190. Kresty, L.A.; Mallery, S.R.; Stoner, G.D. Black raspberries in cancer clinical trials: Past, present and future. *J. Berry Res.* **2016**, *6*, 251–261. [CrossRef] [PubMed]
191. Lazzè, M.C.; Savio, M.; Pizzala, R.; Cazzalini, O.; Perucca, P.; Scovassi, A.I.; Stivala, L.A.; Bianchi, L. Anthocyanins induce cell cycle perturbations and apoptosis in different human cell lines. *Carcinogenesis* **2004**, *25*, 1427–1433. [CrossRef]
192. Ma, H.; Johnson, S.L.; Liu, W.; Dasilva, N.A.; Meschwitz, S.; Dain, J.A.; Seeram, N.P. Evaluation of polyphenol anthocyanin-enriched extracts of blackberry, black raspberry, blueberry, cranberry, red raspberry, and strawberry for free radical scavenging, reactive carbonyl species trapping, anti-glycation, anti-β-amyloid aggregation, and mic. *Int. J. Mol. Sci.* **2018**, *19*, 461. [CrossRef]
193. Strathearn, K.E.; Yousef, G.G.; Grace, M.H.; Roy, S.L.; Tambe, M.A.; Ferruzzi, M.G.; Wu, Q.; Simon, J.E.; Ann, M.; Rochet, J.-C. Neuroprotective effects of anthocyanin- and proanthocyanidin-rich extracts in cellular models of Parkinson's disease. *Brain Res.* **2014**, *1555*, 60–77. [CrossRef]
194. Ullah, I.; Park, H.Y.; Kim, M.O. Anthocyanins protect against kainic acid-induced excitotoxicity and apoptosis via ROS-activated AMPK pathway in hippocampal neurons. *CNS Neurosci. Ther.* **2014**, *20*, 327–338. [CrossRef]
195. Whyte, A.R.; Cheng, N.; Fromentin, E.; Williams, C.M. A randomized, double-blinded, placebo-controlled study to compare the safety and efficacy of low dose enhanced wild blueberry powder and wild blueberry extract (ThinkBlue™) in maintenance of episodic and working memory in older adults. *Nutrients* **2018**, *10*, 660. [CrossRef] [PubMed]
196. Bendokas, V.; Stanys, V.; Mažeikienė, I.; Trumbeckaite, S.; Baniene, R.; Liobikas, J. Anthocyanins: From the field to the antioxidants in the body. *Antioxidants* **2020**, *9*, 819. [CrossRef] [PubMed]
197. Asgary, S.; Kelishadi, R.; Rafieian-Kopaei, M.; Najafi, S.; Najafi, M.; Sahebkar, A. Investigation of the lipid-modifying and antiinflammatory effects of Cornus mas L. supplementation on dyslipidemic children and adolescents. *Pediatr. Cardiol.* **2013**, *34*, 1729–1735. [CrossRef]
198. Noordin, L.; Wan Mohamad Noor, W.N.I.; Safuan, S.; Wan Ahmad, W.A.N. Therapeutic effects of anthocyanin-rich *Hibiscus sabdariffa* L. extract on body mass index, lipid profile and fatty liver in obese-hypercholesterolaemic rat model. *Int. J. Basic Clin. Pharmacol.* **2019**, *9*, 1. [CrossRef]
199. Güder, A.; Gür, M.; Engin, M.S. Antidiabetic and antioxidant properties of bilberry (*Vaccinium myrtillus* Linn.) fruit and their chemical composition. *J. Agric. Sci. Technol.* **2015**, *17*, 401–414.
200. Akkarachiyasit, S.; Yibchok-Anun, S.; Wacharasindhu, S.; Adisakwattana, S. In vitro inhibitory effects of cyanidin-3-rutinoside on pancreatic α-amylase and its combined effect with acarbose. *Molecules* **2011**, *16*, 2075–2083. [CrossRef]
201. Khan, M.I.; Shin, J.H.; Shin, T.S.; Kim, M.Y.; Cho, N.J.; Kim, J.D. Anthocyanins from Cornus kousa ethanolic extract attenuate obesity in association with anti-angiogenic activities in 3T3-L1 cells by down-regulating adipogeneses and lipogenesis. *PLoS ONE* **2018**, *13*, e0208556. [CrossRef]
202. Adisakwattana, S.; Yibchok-Anun, S.; Charoenlertkul, P.; Wongsasiripat, N. Cyanidin-3-rutinoside alleviates postprandial hyperglycemia and its synergism with acarbose by inhibition of intestinal α-glucosidase. *J. Clin. Biochem. Nutr.* **2011**, *49*, 36–41. [CrossRef] [PubMed]
203. Liu, Y.; Li, D.; Zhang, Y.; Sun, R.; Xia, M. Anthocyanin increases adiponectin secretion and protects against diabetes-related endothelial dysfunction. *Am. J. Physiol. Endocrinol. Metab.* **2014**, *306*, 975–988. [CrossRef]

204. Wu, T.; Jiang, Z.; Yin, J.; Long, H.; Zheng, X. Anti-obesity effects of artificial planting blueberry (*Vaccinium ashei*) anthocyanin in high-fat diet- treated mice. *Int. J. Food Sci. Nutr.* **2016**, *67*, 257–264. [CrossRef]
205. Wu, T.; Liu, R. Anthocyanins in black rice, soybean and purple corn increase fecal butyric acid and prevent liver inflammation in high fat diet-induced obese mice. *Food Funct.* **2017**, *8*, 3178–3186. [CrossRef]
206. Liu, Y.; Tan, D.; Shi, L.; Liu, X.; Zhang, Y.; Tong, C.; Song, D.; Hou, M. Blueberry anthocyanins-enriched extracts attenuate cyclophosphamide-induced cardiac injury. *PLoS ONE* **2015**, *10*, 1–18. [CrossRef]
207. Song, F.; Zhu, Y.; Shi, Z.; Tian, J.; Deng, X.; Ren, J.; Andrews, M.C.; Ni, H.; Ling, W.; Yang, Y. Plant food anthocyanins inhibit platelet granule secretion in hypercholesterolaemia: Involving the signalling pathway of PI3K–Akt. *Thromb. Haemost.* **2014**, *112*, 981–991. [CrossRef] [PubMed]
208. Matsunaga, N.; Tsuruma, K.; Shimazawa, M.; Yokota, S.; Hara, H. Inhibitory actions of bilberry anthocyanidins on angiogenesis. *Phyther. Res.* **2009**, *24*, S42–S47. [CrossRef] [PubMed]
209. Gaiz, A.; Kundur, A.R.; Colson, N.; Shibeeb, S.; Singh, I. Assessment of in vitro effects of anthocyanins on platelet function. *Altern. Ther. Health Med.* **2020**, *26*, 12–17. [PubMed]
210. Hassellund, S.S.; Flaa, A.; Kjeldsen, S.E.; Seljeflot, I.; Karlsen, A.; Erlund, I.; Rostrup, M. Effects of anthocyanins on cardiovascular risk factors and inflammation in pre-hypertensive men: A double-blind randomized placebo-controlled crossover study. *J. Hum. Hypertens.* **2013**, *27*, 100–106. [CrossRef]
211. McAnulty, L.S.; Collier, S.R.; Landram, M.J.; Whittaker, D.S.; Isaacs, S.E.; Klemka, J.M.; Cheek, S.L.; Arms, J.C.; McAnulty, S.R. Six weeks daily ingestion of whole blueberry powder increases natural killer cell counts and reduces arterial stiffness in sedentary males and females. *Nutr. Res.* **2014**, *34*, 577–584. [CrossRef]
212. Habanova, M.; Saraiva, J.A.; Haban, M.; Schwarzova, M.; Chlebo, P.; Predna, L.; Gažo, J.; Wyka, J. Intake of bilberries (*Vaccinium myrtillus* L.) reduced risk factors for cardiovascular disease by inducing favorable changes in lipoprotein profiles. *Nutr. Res.* **2016**, *36*, 1415–1422. [CrossRef]
213. Arevström, L.; Bergh, C.; Landberg, R.; Wu, H.; Rodriguez-Mateos, A.; Waldenborg, M.; Magnuson, A.; Blanc, S.; Fröbert, O. Freeze-dried bilberry (*Vaccinium myrtillus*) dietary supplement improves walking distance and lipids after myocardial infarction: An open-label randomized clinical trial. *Nutr. Res.* **2019**, *62*, 13–22. [CrossRef]
214. Draijer, R.; de Graaf, Y.; Slettenaar, M.; de Groot, E.; Wright, C.I. Consumption of a polyphenol-rich grape-wine extract lowers ambulatory blood pressure in mildly hypertensive subjects. *Nutrients* **2015**, *7*, 3138–3153. [CrossRef]
215. Igwe, E.O.; Charlton, K.E.; Roodenrys, S.; Kent, K.; Fanning, K.; Netzel, M.E. Anthocyanin-rich plum juice reduces ambulatory blood pressure but not acute cognitive function in younger and older adults: A pilot crossover dose-timing study. *Nutr. Res.* **2017**, *47*, 28–43. [CrossRef]
216. Xie, L.; Vance, T.; Kim, B.; Lee, S.G.; Caceres, C.; Wang, Y.; Hubert, P.A.; Lee, J.Y.; Chun, O.K.; Bolling, B.W. Aronia berry polyphenol consumption reduces plasma total and low-density lipoprotein cholesterol in former smokers without lowering biomarkers of inflammation and oxidative stress: A randomized controlled trial. *Nutr. Res.* **2017**, *37*, 67–77. [CrossRef] [PubMed]
217. Bakkar, Z.A.; Fulford, J.; Gates, P.E.; Jackman, S.R.; Jones, A.M.; Bond, B.; Bowtell, J.L. Montmorency cherry supplementation attenuates vascular dysfunction induced by prolonged forearm occlusion in overweight, middle-aged men. *J. Appl. Physiol.* **2019**, *126*, 246–254. [CrossRef] [PubMed]
218. Bell, L.; Lamport, D.J.; Butler, L.T.; Williams, C.M. A study of glycaemic effects following acute anthocyanin-rich blueberry supplementation in healthy young adults. *Food Funct.* **2017**, *8*, 3104–3110. [CrossRef] [PubMed]
219. Zhu, Y.; Xia, M.; Yang, Y.; Liu, F.; Li, Z.; Hao, Y.; Mi, M.; Jin, T.; Ling, W. Purified anthocyanin supplementation improves endothelial function via NO-cGMP activation in hypercholesterolemic individuals. *Clin. Chem.* **2011**, *57*, 1524–1533. [CrossRef]
220. Kianbakht, S.; Abasi, B.; Hashem Dabaghian, F. Improved lipid profile in hyperlipidemic patients taking vaccinium arctostaphylos fruit hydroalcoholic extract: A randomized double-blind placebo-controlled clinical trial. *Phyther. Res.* **2014**, *28*, 432–436. [CrossRef]
221. Cook, M.D.; Myers, S.D.; Gault, M.L.; Willems, M.E.T. Blackcurrant alters physiological responses and femoral artery diameter during sustained isometric contraction. *Nutrients* **2017**, *9*, 556. [CrossRef] [PubMed]
222. Milbury, P.E.; Graf, B.; Curran-Celentano, J.M.; Blumberg, J.B. Bilberry (*Vaccinium myrtillus*) anthocyanins modulate heme oxygenase-1 and glutathione S-transferase-pi expression in ARPE-19 cells. *Investig. Ophthalmol. Vis. Sci.* **2007**, *48*, 2343–2349. [CrossRef] [PubMed]
223. Sundalius, N.M. *Examination of Blueberry Anthocyanins in Prevention of Age-Related Macular Degeneration through Retinal Pigment Epithelial Cell Culture Study*; Louisiana State University and Agricultural and Mechanical College: Baton Rouge, LA, USA, 2008.
224. Matsumoto, H.; Kamm, K.E.; Stull, J.T.; Azuma, H. Delphinidin-3-rutinoside relaxes the bovine ciliary smooth muscle through activation of ETB receptor and NO/cGMP pathway. *Exp. Eye Res.* **2005**, *80*, 313–322. [CrossRef]
225. Iida, H.; Nakamura, Y.; Matsumoto, H.; Takeuchi, Y.; Harano, S.; Ishihara, M.; Katsumi, O. Effect of black-currant extract on negative lens-induced ocular growth in chicks. *Ophthalmic Res.* **2010**, *44*, 242–250. [CrossRef] [PubMed]
226. Nakaishi, H.; Matsumoto, H.; Tominaga, S.; Hirayama, M. Effects of black currant anthocyanoside intake on dark adaptation and VDT work-induced transient refractive alteration in healthy humans. *Altern. Med. Rev.* **2000**, *5*, 553–562. [PubMed]

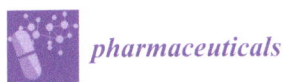

Review

Mycosporine-Like Amino Acids (MAAs): Biology, Chemistry and Identification Features

Vanessa Geraldes [1,2] and Ernani Pinto [2,*]

1. School of Pharmaceutical Sciences, University of São Paulo, Avenida Prof. Lineu Prestes, 580, Butantã, São Paulo-SP CEP 05508-000, Brazil; vanessa.geraldes@usp.br
2. Centre for Nuclear Energy in Agriculture, University of São Paulo, Piracicaba, Piracicaba-SP CEP 13400-970, Brazil
* Correspondence: ernani@usp.br

Abstract: Mycosporines and mycosporine-like amino acids are ultra-violet-absorbing compounds produced by several organisms such as lichens, fungi, algae and cyanobacteria, especially upon exposure to solar ultraviolet radiation. These compounds have photoprotective and antioxidant functions. Mycosporine-like amino acids have been used as a natural bioactive ingredient in cosmetic products. Several reviews have already been developed on these photoprotective compounds, but they focus on specific features. Herein, an extremely complete database on mycosporines and mycosporine-like amino acids, covering the whole class of these natural sunscreen compounds known to date, is presented. Currently, this database has 74 compounds and provides information about the chemistry, absorption maxima, protonated mass, fragments and molecular structure of these UV-absorbing compounds as well as their presence in organisms. This platform completes the previous reviews and is available online for free and in the public domain. This database is a useful tool for natural product data mining, dereplication studies, research working in the field of UV-absorbing compounds mycosporines and being integrated in mass spectrometry library software.

Keywords: mycosporines; mycosporine-like amino acids (MAAs); mass spectrometry; database; photoprotective compounds; UV-absorbing compounds

1. Ultraviolet Radiation and Natural UV-Absorbing Compounds

The solar radiation reaching Earth is composed of infrared radiation (>800 nm), visible (photosynthetically active radiation, PAR, 400-750 nm) and ultraviolet radiation (UVR, 200–400 nm). UVR is divided into ultraviolet A (UVA, 320–400 nm), ultraviolet B (UVB, 280–320 nm) and ultraviolet C (UVC, 200–280 nm). Very small proportions of UVR contribute to the total irradiation on the Earth's surface: 0% of UVC (which is completely absorbed by the ozone layer), less than 1% of UVB and less than 7% of UVA. However, this part of the solar spectrum is highly energetic [1]. Photosynthetic organisms harness PAR to convert light into chemical energy. An obligate requirement for PAR results in prolonged exposure to UVR, which is detrimental for most sun-exposed organisms. Furthermore, due to the ozone depletion, the amount of UV reaching Earth tends to increase [2]. In order to circumvent the photodamage, several organisms have evolved biochemical and mechanical defenses [3]. Among these is the ability to synthesize UV-screening compounds such as phenylpropanoids and flavonoids (in higher plants), melanin (in animals), mycosporines, mycosporine-like amino acids (in cyanobacteria, fungi, algae and animals) and several other photoprotective compounds [4]. As well as providing protection against ambient UV radiation, these substances have other physiological roles. In previous studies, the characteristics of a wide diversity of UV-absorbing compounds are explored [4].

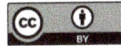

2. Mycosporine-Like Amino Acids

Mycosporines and mycosporine-like amino acids (MAAs) are a large family of natural UV-absorbing sunscreens [5–9], having evolved for protection against chronic UVR exposure in a wide variety of organisms such as cyanobacteria, microalgae, fungi, seaweeds, corals, lichens, as well as in freshwater and marine animals [5,8]. Their presence is evidence not only of their importance as natural UV-screening compounds but also of their early phylogenetic innovation [4]. MAAs were first reported in the 1960s [10–12]. Since then, many studies have been carried out and several MAAs have been identified as well as information on their structure, distribution, properties and functions.

2.1. Physico-Chemical Characteristics of MAAs

MAAs are low-molecular-weight (generally < 400 Da), colorless and water-soluble compounds. They are highly stable molecules under environmental conditions. They are composed of either an aminocyclohexenone or an aminocyclohexenimine ring, carrying nitrogen substituents. Aminocyclohexenone derivatives contain a cyclohexenone conjugated with an amino acid, such as mycosporine-glycine and mycosporine-taurine. Aminocyclohexenimine possesses a cyclohexenimine conjugated with a glycine or a methylamine attached to the third carbon atom and an amino acid or amino alcohol or enaminone chromophore to the first carbon atom (Figure 1) [13]. Glycosidic bonds or sulfate esters may occur within the imine group [14]. This group includes palythine, shinorine, porphyra-334, catenelline, hexose-bound porphyra-334, etc. MAA absorption maxima are between 268 and 362 nm, depending on their molecular structure, namely in the type of ring and substituents [15]. MAAs also have high molecular absorptivities (ε = 12.400–58.800 $M^{-1} \cdot cm^{-1}$), and due to these characteristics, they are the strongest UVA-absorbing compounds in nature, and they are also effective against UVB radiations, which explains their potential role in photoprotection. MAAs are predominantly cytoplasmatic due to their high water solubility that enables MAAs to be easily dispersed in the cytoplasm [9]. Previous studies reviewed the physico-chemical properties of several MAAs [16].

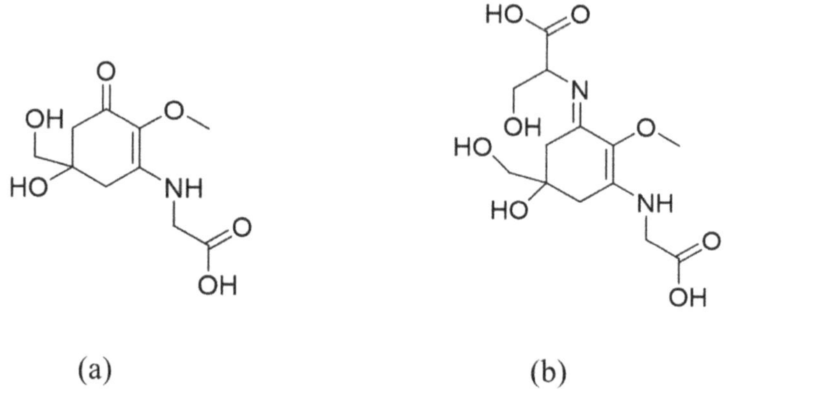

(a) (b)

Figure 1. Examples of mycosporine-like amino-acids (MAAs) structures: (**a**) mycosporine-glycine (oxo-mycosporine); (**b**) shinorine (imino-mycosporine).

2.2. Occurrence and Distribution in the Environment

Wittenberg et al. (1960) isolated, for the first time, compounds with high UV absorption from a siphonophore, *Physalia physalis* [10]. In 1965, mycosporines were discovered in fungal sporulating mycelia [12]. A few years later, MAAs have also been detected in corals and cyanobacteria from the Great Barrier Reef [11]. Since then, MAAs have been identified in a wide variety of organisms, such as heterotrophic bacteria [17], fungi [18], cyanobacteria [5,19], microalgae [20–22], macroalgae [23], lichens [6], invertebrates (e.g., dinoflagellates, sponges, corals, sea urchins and crustaceans) [2,24,25] and vertebrates (e.g., fishes) [26,27]. Several studies reported that animals can acquire MAAs from their food or through symbiosis and then subsequently accumulate them [28,29]. MAAs are not found in higher plants, in which UVR protection is provided by flavonoids, nor in higher vertebrates, in which the protective function is assumed by melanin [4]. MAAs are present especially in organisms that live in environments with high levels of UVR. Their composition varies according to the taxonomic group with the frequent coexistence of several MAAs with different absorption maxima allowing a more effective protective filter [8]. Several environmental factors, such as light, temperature, salinity and nutrients, influence the concentration of MAAs. Enhanced MAA contents, for example, were found in environments with a basic pH, a high ultraviolet radiation and high concentrations of phosphate and nitrate. Salinity, dissolved oxygen and variations of sea surface temperature also influence, in a secondary way, MAA content [30]. UV radiation is one of the most important factors that influences the accumulation of MAA and results in changes in the MAA profile of organisms. MAA synthesis is also affected by spectral variability and intensity [31,32]. Other factors, such as changes in salinity and nutrient availability, stimulate the production of MAAs. The content and composition of UV-absorbing MAAs are also affected by seasonal fluctuations [33,34]. These changes are mainly controlled by the solar radiation regime and nitrate regime. Guihéneuf et al. (2018) studies the temporal and spatial variability of mycosporine-like amino acids in seaweeds. An increase in total MAA contents in all species was induced by increasing daily light doses and irradiance levels, from winter to spring, but without clear significant correlations with light and/or temperature. Nutrient concentrations, in particular nitrate, appear to be a limiting factor for seaweed to accumulate MAAs when exposed to extreme light/irradiance stress [34].

2.3. MAA Biosynthesis

Cyanobacteria must have been the original MAA producer with the genes involved in MAA biosynthesis being transferred to other organisms, and MAAs may have been an early evolution to deal with cellular stress caused by UVR exposure [4]. Multiple lines of evidence support that MAAs are derived from conversion of the shikimate pathway [35], which is known for the synthesis of aromatic amino acids. The precursor of the six-membered carbon ring common to all MAAs is 3-dehydroquinate (3-DHQ). Three-DHQ transforms into gadusol and then 4-deoxygadusol (4-DG). However, contrasting evidence suggests that 4-DG is derived from conversion of the pentose phosphate pathway intermediate sedoheptulose-7-phosphate (SH-7P) [35–37]. Despite experimental data that support the pentose phosphate pathway, the use of the shikimate route inhibitors, such as glyphosate and tyrosine, has demonstrated the ability to abolish MAA biosynthesis in cyanobacteria [13] and corals [38]. Furthermore, the deletion of the gene encoding the enzyme cyclase-2-*epi*-5-*epi*-valiolone synthase (EVS) in cyanobacterium *Anabaena variabillis* ATCC 29413 still produced shinorine [39]. These results suggested that the shikimate pathway is the most predominant route for MAA synthesis in sufficient amounts to provide photoprotection, and the quantities of MAAs produced by the pentose phosphate pathway should have other biological functions [39]. However, there are clear links between the pentose phosphate and shikimate pathways. In both routes, 4-DG is the parent core structure of MAAs and the addition of glycine yielding mycosporine-glycine. This simple mono-substituted cyclohexenone-type MAA is a common intermediate in the production of di-substituted (aminocyclohexenimine-type) MAAs through the addition of a single amino acid residue (serine, threonine, etc.) yielding some common MAAs such as porphyra-334 and shinorine. This step encodes a nonribosomal peptide synthase (NRPS)-like protein or a D-alanyl-D-alanine ligase (D-ala-D-ala ligase) [13,36]. Figure 2 presents a proposed biosynthetic pathway of MAAs. Other MAAs are synthesized by modification in the attached side groups and nitrogen substituents (e.g., esterification, amidation, dehydration, decarboxylation, hydroxylation, sulfonation and glycosylation). The variations of amino acid side-chains are responsible for the difference in the absorption spectra of MAAs [15,40].

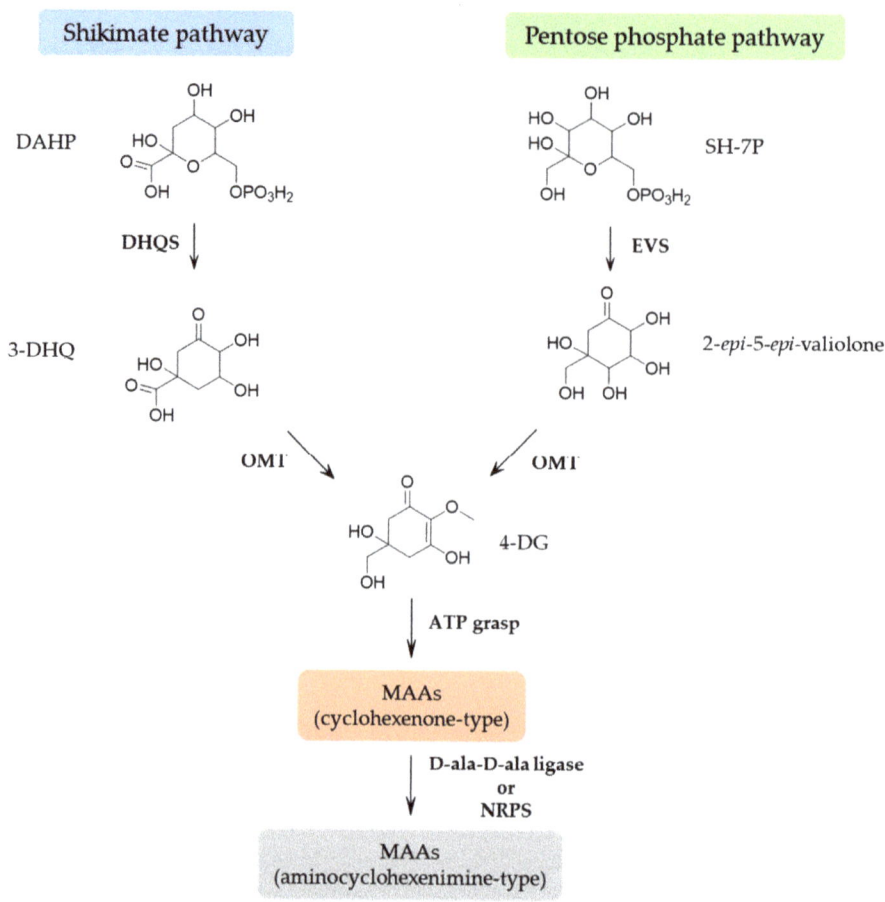

Figure 2. Proposed biosynthetic pathway of mycosporine-like amino acids. DAHP: 3-deoxy-D-arabino-heptulosonate phosphate, DHQS: 3-dehydroquinate synthase, 3-DHQ: 3-dehydroquinate, SH-7P: sedoheptulose-7-phosphate, EVS: cyclase-2-*epi*-5-*epi*-valiolone synthase, OMT: *O*-methyltransferase, 4DG: 4-deoxygadusol, ATP: adenosine triphosphate, NRPS: nonribosomal peptide synthase, D-ala-D-ala-ligase: D-alanyl-D-alanine ligase.

2.4. Heterologous Expression

The poor understanding of the biosynthesis pathways involved in the production of specific MAA is one of the reasons for the lack of widespread use of MAA in the industry in an economically viable way. Further understanding of these biosynthetic pathways can lead to easier large-scale production, for example, in a heterologous bacterial host [15,37]. Balskus et al. (2010) elucidated the biosynthesis of shinorine via heterologous expression in *Escherichia coli* [36]. The heterologous expression of MAAs in *Escherichia coli* also resulted in the production of 4-deoxygadusol, mycosporine-glycine, mycosporine-lysine and mycosporine-ornithine [36,37]. Shinorine and mycosporine-glycine-alanine have artificially been produced by heterologous expression in Actinomycetales [41]. Nowadays, most efforts are focused on the production of MAAs by genetically modified microorganisms as an alternative production of natural MAAs [9,37]. The heterologous expression of MAAs is significant from a biotechnological perspective, as MAAs are the active ingredient in next-generation sunscreens [37].

2.5. Chemical Synthesis and Analogs

The chemical synthesis of MAAs was motivated due to the low extraction yield from MAA-producing organisms and the need for large scale production. Several synthesized chemical structures were developed with interesting photoprotective and antioxidant properties [42–45]. The synthetic analogue of mycosporine-glycine, tetrahydropyridine, was considered hydrolytically and oxidatively stable for commercial application in sunscreens [46]. An efficient and environmentally friendly procedure by ultrasound and microwave for preparing MAA analogs was described by Andreguetti et al. (2013). These analogs showed high antioxidant effect [47]. Analogs with a high absorbance intensity in UVA and UVB regions, without in vitro cytotoxicity, were prepared by Nguyen et al. (2013) [48]. Recently, Losantos et al. (2017) developed a series of potential UV sunscreens with easy synthetic routes, providing a suitable source for their use in commercial products [42]. Bedoux et al. (2020) published a complete review of these chemical syntheses [49].

2.6. MAA Extraction, Identification and Quantification

2.6.1. Extraction

Since MAAs are potential compounds to be used as sunscreens in cosmetic products, the extraction protocol must be optimized taking into account their physicochemical and absorption properties and must use environmentally friendly and inexpensive solvents [9,50]. Traditional extraction method is usually performed by a solid/liquid extraction from the raw material and is carried out on fresh or lyophilized samples with different temperature ranges [51,52]. Due to its high solubility in aqueous solution, extraction generally uses polar solvents, as aqueous ethanol or methanol. Chaves-Peña et al. (2020) compared the extraction in 20% aqueous methanol and in distilled water, and no significant differences were observed. According to their results, the drying and subsequent re-dissolution of the pellets declined total MAA concentrations [50]. Geraldes et al. (2020) developed a fast and efficient extraction protocol, without the need for pre-concentration procedures. This protocol uses only water and volatile additives as the extractor solvents, and the extracts were directly injected to a high-performance liquid chromatograph (HPLC). This extraction protocol is not only easy-to-handle but also uses solvents without certified toxic effects [32].

2.6.2. Identification

HPLC was the most common method to separate and identify MAAs by using retention times and UV spectra. Although UV detection is sensitive because of high attenuation coefficients (ε) for MAAs, this method is poor in selectivity, since biosynthetic congeners can easily influence MAA identification [32]. Moreover, no commercial sources for standard compounds exist and few laboratories worldwide have the capacity to provide reference material against which structural elucidation of MAAs can be verified. In this sense, LC-MS is a good alternative to provide high sensitivity and selectivity for analysis of MAAs. A method for MAA identification was developed using an ultrahigh-performance liquid chromatography with diode array detection coupled to quadrupole time-of-flight mass spectrometry (UHPLC-DAD-QTOFMS) with an electrospray ionization source (ESI) and showed to be fast, reliable and a powerful tool for identification and screening of MAAs in several organisms, such as cyanobacteria, dinoflagellates, macroalgae and microalgae [42]. Regarding MAA purification, HPLC is the most used method. Geraldes et al. (2020) published a protocol using a semi-preparative HPLC-DAD fitted to a Luna C18 (2) column and 0.2% (v/v) formic acid solution as buffer A [32].

2.6.3. Quantification

MAAs were often quantified based on molar attenuation coefficients using HPLC techniques. However, nowadays, liquid chromatography coupled with mass spectrometry (LC-MS) is the most common technique, because this method provides high sensitivity and selectivity for analysis of MAAs [32,51]. Whitehead and Hedges (2002) published a quantitative method that allowed the quantification of MAAs based on molecular weights, individual retention time and UV absorption maxima [53]. An LC-MS method using hydrophilic interaction chromatography (HILIC) was published by Hartmann et al. (2015) [54]. Although this method afforded good linear correlation coefficients, it did not account for some important validation parameters such as recovery and matrix effects. Geraldes et al. (2020) described a rapid quantitative method for LC-MS/MS analysis of MAAs that allowed the quantification of MAAs based on individual retention times, molecular weights and specific mass transitions using multiple reaction monitoring (MRM) experiments instead of a full scan [32]. This method has been thoroughly validated taking into account the ICH and EURACHEM guidelines for the following parameters: specificity, linearity, precision (repeatability and reproducibility within the laboratory), accuracy, extraction recovery, matrix effects and stability. In addition, the working range, as well as the limits of detection and quantification, were evaluated [32]. This technique improved the selectivity and sensitivity of the method, allowing mass distinction of isomeric compounds [16].

2.7. MAA Structural Elucidation

The structural elucidation of new derivatives of mycosporine-like amino acids is usually established by tandem mass spectrometry (MS/MS) and 1D and 2D nuclear magnetic resonance (NMR) spectroscopy [9,55]. Previous studies focusing on the fragmentation patterns of MAAs showed a loss of mass 15 when analyzed by positive mode ESI–MS/MS. This highly characteristic loss is due to elimination of a methyl radical CH_3 [56,57]. The detection of the production $[M + H - 59]^+$ related to the elimination of the methyl radical and subsequently CO_2 is also common in MAAs [56]. Thus, the screening of these eliminations could be a suitable tool to assign the presence of novel MAAs in different samples by neutral loss or product ion scans in mass spectrometry analyzers. For aminocyclohexenimines, the elimination of the remaining lateral chain can produce the product ion m/z 186. This ion can undergo a fragmentation process to produce the ion m/z 155. Then, this product ion loses either NH_3 or H_2O by neutral elimination to produce the ions m/z 138 and 137, respectively [57]. These product ions could provide additional information concerning the occurrence of new MAAs in a crude extract. However, the presence of some product ions may be reduced or not occur in certain MAA fragmentation processes [58]. Thus, the selection of the product ions should be carried out carefully in analytical methods for the analysis of extracts containing potential novel MAAs. Regarding NMR spectroscopic data, they show characteristic patterns allowing them to be comparable. For example, oxo-mycosporines and imino-mycosporines can be distinguished through the chemical shift of C-1 in ^{13}C NMR experiments, which is more around 180 ppm for oxo-mycosporines and 160 ppm for imino-mycosporines. The ^1H NMR data usually revealed the presence of the coupling of the pairs of duplets from the diasterotopic methylenes, with a geminal coupling constant around 17 Hz, corresponding to the four protons on C-4 and C-6 that show chemical shifts around 30–40 ppm between them. The hydroxymethyl group at C-5 and the methoxyl group at C-2 usually appear very close around 3.60 ppm as two singlets [9,13,59] (Figure 3).

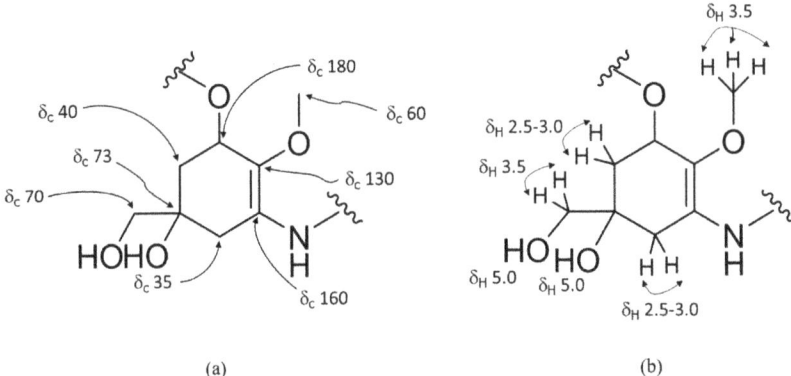

Figure 3. Structure of an oxomycosporine with NMR results for (**a**) ^{13}C (125 MHz, D$_2$O) and (**b**) ^{1}H (500 MHz, D$_2$O). For iminomycosporine ^{13}C NMR (125 MHz, D$_2$O) δ_C = 160 (C-1).

2.8. MAA Photoprotective Role

The MAA photoprotective role against UVR is due to their absorption spectra and molar attenuation coefficients. Their absorption gradient (268–362 nm) cover most of the UVR spectrum (~295–400 nm) that reaches the Earth's surface, while their high molar attenuation coefficients demonstrate how strongly MAAs absorb light at this wavelength range. The concentration of MAAs in organisms is directly related to their level of UVR exposure, which depends on latitude and altitude, seasonality and water depth [15,33,60,61]. They preferentially accumulate in tissues that receive the highest UVR exposure [62]. Photoprotection of MAAs has been demonstrated in a wide variety of species and prevents UVB-induced damage [63,64]. MAAs have been found in the cytoplasm of several cyanobacteria; however, in *Nostoc commune*, MAAs accumulate extracellularly, resulting in a more effective protection against ultraviolet radiation [65]. The presence of MAAs in animals supports their photoprotective role not only to producers but also to herbivores and even carnivores [8]. MAAs are also found in fossils that confirm their protective function against the UVR harmful effects in the early geological eras [66].

2.9. MAA Additional Protective Roles

Generally, MAA production is induced when organisms are exposed to UVR [67,68]. The photoprotective function is the most important role that MAAs play in nature. This is verified by the abundance of MAAs in organisms exposed to high UVR intensities [69]. However, MAAs can be produced constitutively in some species [5,13], and functionality could be linked to their individual structures [70]. Thus, MAAs may have additional protective roles in many other biological processes beyond their well-known UV sunscreen role. These compounds have convincingly demonstrated to possess physiologically relevant antioxidant properties [8,40]. Furthermore, MAAs are involved in osmotic regulation, desiccation and many other cellular functions [15,69]. An extensive review about these additional roles of MAAs has been carried out by Oren et al. (2007). However, the significance of these additional functions and the effects of different forms of stress on MAA synthesis are still poorly understood [69].

2.9.1. Antioxidant and ROS Scavenging Function

UVR exposure generates oxidative stress and can produce reactive oxygen species (ROS) and DNA damage. This oxidative DNA damage can lead to mutations and inhibit DNA repair [71]. Antioxidants can reduce the harmful effects of ROS and can, thus, help to prevent oxidative stress [72]. Some MAAs may protect the cell not only by absorbing UVR and dissipating the energy as heat before it could reach the critical cellular targets but also as scavengers of free radicals due to their antioxidant role [31,73]. This function has been demonstrated in several MAAs from a wide variety of organisms [74–79]. MAAs have also been shown to prevent lipid peroxidation and superoxide radicals, blocking the aftereffect of oxidative damage [80]. Several assays demonstrated that MAAs have antioxidant properties and efficiently prevent oxidative stress through filtering and direct and indirect quenching mechanisms [81,82]. The antioxidant abilities of MAAs (ORAC values, lipid peroxidation inhibition, DPPH and ABTS radical extinction, singlet oxygen quenching, superoxide anion radical scavenging, hydrogen peroxide extinction activities and physiological activities) have been provided in recent reviews [40,83]. However, the exact mechanism is yet to be elucidated.

2.9.2. Osmotic Stress

The concentrations of intracellular solute are directly related to the concentration of salt in which the cell lives [69]. Thus, osmotic stress is one of the stressors MAAs seem to have an action against. In hypersaline environments, cyanobacteria usually contain high concentrations of MAAs suggesting that these compounds may have an osmotic function helping the cells to cope with the high salinity. In these environments, cell dehydration and reactive oxygen species (ROS) production can occur, leading to oxidative stress. Through the synthesis of MAAs, osmotic balance can be restored [31]. Oren (1997) reported that a halotolerant cyanobacterium, inhabiting a gypsum crust, has an extremely high concentration of MAA ($\geq$98 mM), being responsible for about 3% of the cells' wet weight. It was observed that a reduction in the salt concentrations of its surroundings was accompanied with a rapid expulsion of MAAs [84]. Thus, MAAs may be involved in the adaptation of sea ice algae to osmotic variations. MAA production could be induced specifically either by exposure to UVB radiation or by osmotic stress, and a significant synergistic enhancement of MAA production was observed when both stress factors were combined. Although osmotic stress could induce MAA synthesis, MAAs play no significant role in attaining osmotic homeostasis [85]. Singh et al. (2008) proposed that salt treatment resulted in an increase in MAA content in the absence of UV radiation and had synergistic effects with UV stress [86]. Waditee-Sirisattha et al. (2013) recently demonstrated that the accumulation of MAAs, in a halotolerant cyanobacterium, was stimulated more under high salinity rather than under UVB radiation [87].

2.9.3. Desiccation Stress

Desiccation is responsible for cell damage by affecting cytoplasmic components (such as DNA and proteins) and cell membrane fluidity. The production of polysaccharides and antioxidant compounds are some of the techniques to overcome the consequences of drying [64,88]. Few studies have been carried out to assess the effects on MAA concentration in microorganisms exposed to desiccation stress [63,64,89,90]. Desiccation stress leads to an increase in total MAA content. This group of compounds may be acting by modifying the structure of the extracellular matrix. Expulsion of the MAA is observed after rehydration. The combination of desiccation and irradiation stimulate MAA production. Colonies of fungi exposed to desiccation, UV radiation and nutrient scarcity contain high concentrations of mycosporine-glutaminol-glucoside. The survival and longevity potential of the vegetative hyphae of these fungi may be associated with the presence of these compounds [90]. Olsson-Francis et al. (2003) stated that cyanobacteria stressed experimentally by desiccation increased their MAA concentration. In this study, they suggest that the formation of an extracellular sheath may be related to desiccation [63]. Joshi et al. (2018) also proposed that desiccation together with UVB radiation led to an increase in the concentration of MAAs preventing and protecting cells from the harmful effects of these factors [64].

2.9.4. Thermal Stress

There are a few reports of thermal stress protection by an increase in MAA induction in a range of organisms. Michalek-Wagner (2001) stated that MAA content was upregulated under heat stress, and their concentrations were further enhanced during simultaneous exposure to UV [91]. In contrast, some authors suggested that thermal stress had no effect on MAA production with or without UVR [85,86].

2.9.5. Photosynthesis Accessory Pigments

An early study reported that MAAs may act as a photosynthetic accessory pigment due to its UVA absorption and subsequent production of small amounts of fluorescence at wavelengths close to the absorbance of chlorophyll-a. This result suggested that MAAs may increase photosynthetic efficiency. However, MAAs are only weakly fluorescent and are generally produced in environments of high irradiance, in which photosynthetic wavelengths are not the limiting factor for photosynthesis [92]. So far, this study has never been substantiated [69].

2.9.6. Nitrogen Storage

MAAs are nitrogenous compounds that contain at least one nitrogen atom per molecule that can be released when required. Thus, MAAs may serve as an intracellular nitrogen storage [93]. A synergistic effect between ammonium ions and UVR was observed and resulted in an increase in MAA content [93]. If MAAs are accumulated as intracellular nitrogen storage compounds, nitrogen mobilization should occur whenever other suitable forms of nitrogen are absent. However, there is no evidence about the intracellular degradation of MAAs and the release of nitrogen atoms that support the proposal that MAAs may be nitrogen storage molecules [69].

2.9.7. Reproductive Regulation

There is evidence that mycosporines and MAAs are involved in reproduction in fungi and marine invertebrates [69]. Mycosporines have been related to sporulating mycelia and were considered as biochemical markers for reproductive states of fungi or as reproduction markers [69,90]. Several studies reported that most MAAs reach their maximum concentration in ovaries and eggs at the time of ovarian reproductive maturity and spawning, which may be near the seasonal minima and maxima of solar irradiation [94,95]. Although a protective role is clearly demonstrated in marine invertebrate embryos, the exact function of MAAs in ovaries and eggs has not been determined [62].

2.9.8. Ecological Interactions

Some MAAs play a role in ecological connectivity between organisms, as intraspecific alarm cues or cell-cell interaction tools, suggesting that MAAs can function as compounds of fundamental importance in marine ecosystems. The alarm cues are released in the ink secretion of sea hares and cause avoidance behaviors in neighboring conspecifics. The highest concentration of MAAs was concentrated in the defensive secretions and in the skin of these organisms [96]. In *M. aeruginosa* PCC 7806, shinorine was found to accumulate in an extracellular matrix, and this compound could be synthesized for its role in extracellular matrix formation and cell–cell interaction [97].

2.10. Cosmetical Application of MAAs as Sunscreen

As with other organisms, human exposure to ultraviolet radiation can cause damage, such as erythema or "sunburn" over the short term and premature skin aging and skin cancer over the long term [98]. Thus, protection against ultraviolet radiation is extremely important through the use of appropriate clothing and sunscreen, which are part of an overall prevention strategy [98,99]. Several photoprotective products are available on the market. They contain synthetic organic filters (e.g., oxybenzone, avobenzone, aminobenzoic acid), inorganic filters (e.g., titanium dioxide, zinc oxide) or a combination of both [100].

The frequent use of synthetic sunscreens can affect human health, causing allergic reactions, phototoxicity and endocrine disorders [101–103]. In addition, synthetic UVR filters are not environmentally friendly causing a negative impact in the marine life, including bioaccumulation in several species, hormonal changes and endocrine disruption in fish, hydrogen peroxide production and bleaching of corals [102,104–106]. This fact led Hawaii to ban some types of sunscreens, such as oxybenzone [107]. Subsequently, the Western Pacific Nation of Palau, the city of Key West, Florida and the US Virgin Islands have also passed similar bans [108]. Thus, there was a change in consumer trends with a strong demand in the cosmetics market for more natural products, since they are seen as safer and better and may be able to replace the existing ones. MAAs have been widely studied as natural alternatives to potentially toxic synthetic sunscreens and anti-aging products [8,15,83]. Several studies suggested that MAA have potential for the protection of human skin from a diverse range of adverse effects of solar UVR. Kageyama et al. (2019) provide an overview of MAAs, as potential anti-aging ingredients, which includes the molecular and cellular mechanisms through which MAAs might protect the skin. In addition to their UV-absorbing properties, these compounds have the potential to protect against skin aging, including antioxidative activity, anti-inflammatory activity, inhibition of protein-glycation and inhibition of collagenase activity [83]. MAAs are also highly stable over a wide range of temperature and pH [32,102]. These characteristics make them excellent cosmeceutical ingredients for skincare, cosmetics and pharmaceutical products [109,110]. However, only a few MAA products are currently available, and they still need to be exploited on a large scale. Mibelle AG Biochemistry developed a natural active compound, called Helioguard 365®, which contains MAA porphyra-334 and shinorine from the red seaweed *Porphyra umbilicalis*. Another MAA extract, named Helionori®, is also marketed by Gelyma [111]. Although these ingredients protect in UVA region, they provide minimal protection in the more damaging UVB range. Moreover, the MAA content in the formulation is usually very low when compared to the concentration of UVR filters in most sunscreen products. Thus, this ingredient ends up having a negligible influence on the SPF claims of the product [15]. Some MAA-based skin products have been marketed, such as Aethic Sôvée, a sunscreen with an environmentally friendly appeal. However, it is important to invest efforts to speed up the technological advancement of MAA application as an organic sunscreens [31].

2.11. Other Biotechnological Applications of MAAs

UV exposure alters the properties and durability of non-biological materials and affects their lifetime. MAAs have also nonmedical applications, as additives to protect plastics, paints and varnishes against UVR that exclusively consist of natural compounds [112]. These materials are biocompatible, photoresistant and thermoresistant and provide an efficient protection against UVA and UVB [112]. Figure 4 summarizes the main applications of MAAs including in cosmetics, biological functions and sources.

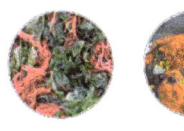
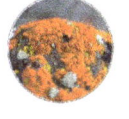
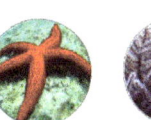
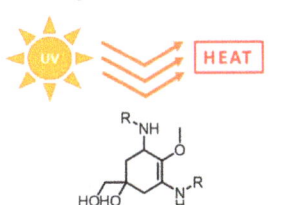
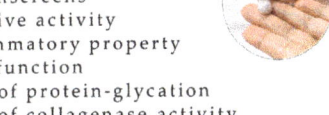

Figure 4. Mycosporine-like amino acids sources, biological functions and applications.

2.12. Patents on MAAs

Currently, there are already a large number of patents in international databases for several products and methods with MAAs. A list of patents on MAAs was obtained from patent databases such as the World Intellectual Property Organization, WIPO (http://www.wipo.int/patentscope/search/en/search.jsf), European Patent Office (http://www.epo.org/searching/free/espacenet.html) and United States Patents and Trademark Office (http://www.uspto.gov/patents/process/search/index.jsp). The search yielded a total of 48 patents on MAAs products and methods that are summarized in Supplementary Materials (Table S1).

2.13. MAA Database—MYCAS

There are several software for searching for commercial natural products. However, they do not cover most mycosporine-like amino acids, and they are not in the public domain. Over time, some MAA databases have been developed [22,23,40]. Although, none of them contains complete and detailed information on all mycosporines and mycosporine-like amino acids identified in the bibliography. Sinha et al. (2007) constructed an excellent database that provides information on various mycosporines and MAAs reported in several organisms. However, this database is now out of date [22]. Wada et al. (2015) published a study focused on MAAs with radical scavenging activities. This work resumed the structures and the physical and chemical properties of these MAAs. Nevertheless, this database did not include all MAAs known to date [40]. Sun et al. (2020) developed a database that summarized the studies related to MAAs in marine macroalgae. However, this work does not contain information on MAAs present in organisms other than macroalgae [23]. Thus, the purpose of this work is to cover this gap, so we present a database on mycosporines and mycosporine-like amino acids, called MYCAS. Our study covers the whole class of these natural sunscreen compounds known to date. This platform will be available online for free and will be in the public domain. It may also be incorporated into databases and search software of mass spectrometry for metabolomic and genomic studies. This platform provides information about their corresponding absorption maxima (λmax), molar attenuation (ε), molecular formula, exact mass, molecular structure, fragments and the organisms in which these compounds were found. Thus, MYCAS facilitate the search for mycosporine-like amino acids in different species and in dereplication studies. Our results are summarized in Supplementary Materials (Table S2).

2.14. Main Tasks for Future Research and Perspectives

The optimization of MAA production on an industrial scale is essential to enable the use of these photoprotective compounds in cosmetical field. Thus, it is extremely important that resources are invested to optimize the production of MAAs and to increase the concentration in organisms, including GMO. At the same time, alternatives should be researched, such as heterologous expression or organic synthesis of analogues. The isolation and purification methods of MAAs are other processes that require further research. These techniques should be as simple and sustainable as possible to allow their application on a large scale. The commercial applicability of these compounds, as well as their impact on the environment and human health, should also be investigated to confirm the feasibility of using these photoprotective compounds on an industrial scale and warranty their safety.

3. Conclusions

Mycosporines and mycosporine-like amino acids are a large family of natural UV-absorbing compounds. To date, more than 70 molecules have been identified in several organisms from different phyla (Arthropoda, Cnidaria, Chordata, Cyanobacteria, Echinodermata, Fungi, Lichen, Macroalgae—Chlorophyta, Phaeophyta and Rhodophyta, Microalgae—Bacillariophyta, Charophyta, Chlorophyta, Dinoflagellata, Miozoa, Ochrophyta and Mollusca). Although there are several reviews on these photoprotective compounds, none include all of the MAAs known to date. In addition, the information is dispersed, and there is no review that summarizes all the information, namely the structural information, spectrometric data and presence in organisms. Here, we present an extremely complete database on mycosporines and mycosporine-like amino acids, called MYCAS, that covers the whole class of these natural sunscreen compounds. Currently, MYCAS has 74 compounds, with structural information and spectrometric data and will be updated annually. This platform is available online (http://www.cena.usp.br/ernani-pinto-mycas), for free and in the public domain. MYCAS allows users to access to all MAAs already described in nature. Our database may also be incorporated into in-house libraries, as well as mass spectrometry software for metabolomic and genomic studies. Thus, MYCAS is a useful tool for scientists working with MAAs and researchers in the field of developing UV-protecting cosmetics from natural sources.

Supplementary Materials: The following are available online at https://www.mdpi.com/1424-8247/14/1/63/s1, Table S1: Patents on mycosporines and mycosporine-like amino acids, Table S2: Mycosporines and mycosporine-like amino acids (MAAs) with their corresponding absorption maxima (λmax), molar absorptivities (ε), molecular formula, exact mass, molecular structure, fragments (underline font represents [M + H]$^+$) and phylum.

Author Contributions: V.G. and E.P. have worked in the conception and design of this review. V.G. searched the data on mycosporine-like amino acids and summarized the database. V.G. analyzed the data and drafted the article. E.P. have made substantial contributions to conception of this manuscript and approve the final version for submission. Both authors have read and agreed to the published version of the manuscript.

Funding: This research was funded by the Fundação de Amparo à Pesquisa do Estado de São Paulo-FAPESP (FAPESP 2019/27707-3 and 2013/07914-8), University of São Paulo Foundation (FUSP) (Project#1979), the Coordination for the Improvement of Higher Education Personnel—

CAPES (Project # 23038.001401/2018-92) and the National Council for Scientific and Technological Development—CNPq (311048/2016-1 and 439065/2018-6).

Conflicts of Interest: The authors declare no conflict of interest.

References

1. Neale, P.J.; Whitehead, R.F.; Díaz, S.B.; Morrow, J.H.; Booth, C.R.; Mopper, K.; Kieber, D.J.; Vincent, W.F.; Roy, S.; Jeffrey, W.H.; et al. *Spectral Weighting Functions for Quantifying Effects of UV Radiation in Marine Ecosystems*; Cambridge University Press (CUP): Cambridge, UK, 2000; pp. 72–100.
2. Carreto, J.I.; Carignan, M.O.; Montoya, N.G.; Cozzolino, E.; Akselman, R. Mycosporine-like amino acids and xanthophyll-cycle pigments favour a massive spring bloom development of the dinoflagellate Prorocentrum minimum in Grande Bay (Argentina), an ozone hole affected area. *J. Mar. Syst.* **2018**, *178*, 15–28. [CrossRef]
3. Rastogi, R.P.; Madamwar, D.; Nakamoto, H.; Incharoensakdi, A. Resilience and self-regulation processes of microalgae under UV radiation stress. *J. Photochem. Photobiol. C Photochem. Rev.* **2019**, *43*, 100322. [CrossRef]
4. Cockell, C.S.; Knowland, J. Ultraviolet radiation screening compounds. *Biol. Rev. Camb. Philos. Soc.* **1999**, *74*, 311–345. [CrossRef]
5. Geraldes, V.; Jacinavicius, F.R.; Genuário, D.B.; Pinto, E. Identification and distribution of mycosporine-like amino acids in Brazilian cyanobacteria using ultrahigh-performance liquid chromatography with diode array detection coupled to quadrupole time-of-flight mass spectrometry. *Rapid Commun. Mass Spectrom.* **2020**, e8634. [CrossRef] [PubMed]
6. Shukla, V.; Kumari, R.; Patel, D.K.; Upreti, D.K. Characterization of the diversity of mycosporine-like amino acids in lichens from high altitude region of Himalaya. *Amino Acids* **2015**, *48*, 129–136. [CrossRef] [PubMed]
7. D'Agostino, P.M.; Javalkote, V.S.; Mazmouz, R.; Pickford, R.; Puranik, P.R.; Neilan, B.A. Comparative Profiling and Discovery of Novel Glycosylated Mycosporine-Like Amino Acids in Two Strains of the Cyanobacterium Scytonema cf. crispum. *Appl. Environ. Microbiol.* **2016**, *82*, 5951–5959. [CrossRef] [PubMed]
8. Chrapusta, E.; Kaminski, A.; Duchnik, K.; Bober, B.; Adamski, M.; Bialczyk, J. Mycosporine-Like Amino Acids: Potential Health and Beauty Ingredients. *Mar. Drugs* **2017**, *15*, 326. [CrossRef] [PubMed]
9. La Barre, S.; Roullier, C.; Boustie, J. Mycosporine-Like Amino Acids (MAAs) in Biological Photosystems. In *Outstanding Marine Molecules*; Wiley: Hoboken, NJ, USA, 2014; pp. 333–360.
10. Wittenberg, J.B. The source of carbon monoxide in the float of the Portuguese man-of-war. *Physalia physalis* L. *J. Exp. Biol.* **1960**, *37*, 698–705.
11. Shibata, K. Pigments and a UV-absorbing substance in corals and a blue-green alga living in the Great Barrier Reef1. *Plant Cell Physiol.* **1969**, *10*, 325–335. [CrossRef]
12. Leach, C.M. Ultraviolet-Absorbing Substances Associated with Light-Induced Sporulation in Fungi. *Can. J. Bot.* **2008**, *43*, 185–200. [CrossRef]
13. Geraldes, V.; De Medeiros, L.S.; Lima, S.T.; Alvarenga, D.O.; Gacesa, R.; Long, P.F.; Fiore, M.F.; Pinto, E. Genetic and biochemical evidence for redundant pathways leading to mycosporine-like amino acid biosynthesis in the cyanobacterium Sphaerospermopsis torques-reginae ITEP-024. *ALGAE* **2020**, *35*, 177–187. [CrossRef]
14. Ishihara, K.; Watanabe, M.; Uchida, H.; Suzuki, T.; Yamashita, M.; Takenaka, H.; Nazifi, E.; Matsugo, S.; Yamaba, M.; Sakamoto, T. Novel glycosylated mycosporine-like amino acid, 13-O-(β-galactosyl)-porphyra-334, from the edible cyanobacterium Nostoc sphaericum -protective activity on human keratinocytes from UV light. *J. Photochem. Photobiol. B Biol.* **2017**, *172*, 102–108. [CrossRef] [PubMed]
15. Lawrence, K.P.; Long, P.F.; Young, A.R. Mycosporine-Like Amino Acids for Skin Photoprotection. *Curr. Med. Chem.* **2019**, *25*, 5512–5527. [CrossRef]
16. Carreto, J.I.; Carignan, M.O. Mycosporine-Like Amino Acids: Relevant Secondary Metabolites. Chemical and Ecological Aspects. *Mar. Drugs* **2011**, *9*, 387–446. [CrossRef]
17. Arai, T.; Nishijima, M.; Adachi, K.; Sano, H. Isolation and structure of a UV absorbing substance from the marine bacterium *Micrococcus* sp. AK-334. *Mar. Biotechnol. Institute* **1992**, 2-35-10, 88–94.
18. Libkind, D.; Sommaruga, R.; Zagarese, H.; Van Broock, M. Mycosporines in carotenogenic yeasts. *Syst. Appl. Microbiol.* **2005**, *28*, 749–754. [CrossRef] [PubMed]
19. Jain, S.; Prajapat, G.; Abrar, M.; Ledwani, L.; Singh, A.; Agrawal, A. Cyanobacteria as efficient producers of mycosporine-like amino acids. *J. Basic Microbiol.* **2017**, *57*, 715–727. [CrossRef]
20. Llewellyn, C.A.; Airs, R. Distribution and Abundance of MAAs in 33 Species of Microalgae across 13 Classes. *Mar. Drugs* **2010**, *8*, 1273–1291. [CrossRef]
21. Gröniger, A.; Sinha, R.; Klisch, M.; Häder, D.-P. Photoprotective compounds in cyanobacteria, phytoplankton and macroalgae—A database. *J. Photochem. Photobiol. B Biol.* **2000**, *58*, 115–122. [CrossRef]
22. Sinha, R.P.; Singh, S.P.; Häder, D.-P. Database on mycosporines and mycosporine-like amino acids (MAAs) in fungi, cyanobacteria, macroalgae, phytoplankton and animals. *J. Photochem. Photobiol. B: Biol.* **2007**, *89*, 29–35. [CrossRef]
23. Sun, Y.; Zhang, N.; Zhou, J.; Dong, S.; Zhang, X.; Guo, L.; Guo, G. Distribution, Contents, and Types of Mycosporine-Like Amino Acids (MAAs) in Marine Macroalgae and a Database for MAAs Based on These Characteristics. *Mar. Drugs* **2020**, *18*, 43. [CrossRef] [PubMed]

24. Rosic, N.; Dove, S. Mycosporine-Like Amino Acids from Coral Dinoflagellates. *Appl. Environ. Microbiol.* **2011**, *77*, 8478–8486. [CrossRef] [PubMed]
25. Oda, Y.; Zhang, Q.; Matsunaga, S.; Fujita, M.J.; Sakai, R. Two New Mycosporine-like Amino Acids LC-343 and Mycosporine-ethanolamine from the Micronesian Marine Sponge Lendenfeldia chondrodes. *Chem. Lett.* **2017**, *46*, 1272–1274. [CrossRef]
26. Chioccara, F.; Gala, A.D.; De Rosa, M.; Novellino, E.; Prota, G. Mycosporine aminoacids and related compounds from the eggs of fishes. *Bulletin des Sociétés Chimiques Belges* **2010**, *89*, 1101–1106. [CrossRef]
27. Osborn, A.R.; Almabruk, K.H.; Holzwarth, G.; Asamizu, S.; Ladu, J.; Kean, K.M.; Karplus, P.A.; Tanguay, R.L.; Bakalinsky, A.T.; Mahmud, T. De novo synthesis of a sunscreen compound in vertebrates. *eLife* **2015**, *4*, e05919. [CrossRef]
28. Newman, S.; Dunlap, W.C.; Nicol, S.; Ritz, D. Antarctic krill (Euphausia superba) acquire a UV-absorbing mycosporine-like amino acid from dietary algae. *J. Exp. Mar. Biol. Ecol.* **2000**, *255*, 93–110. [CrossRef]
29. Helbling, E.W.; Menchi, C.F.; Villafañe, V.E. Bioaccumulation and role of UV-absorbing compounds in two marine crustacean species from Patagonia, Argentina. *Photochem. Photobiol. Sci.* **2002**, *1*, 820–825. [CrossRef]
30. Briani, B.; Sissini, M.N.; Lucena, L.A.; Batista, M.B.; Costa, I.O.; Nunes, J.M.C.; Schmitz, C.; Ramlov, F.; Maraschin, M.; Korbee, N.; et al. The influence of environmental features in the content of mycosporine-like amino acids in red marine algae along the Brazilian coast. *J. Phycol.* **2018**, *54*, 380–390. [CrossRef]
31. Rosic, N. Mycosporine-Like Amino Acids: Making the Foundation for Organic Personalised Sunscreens. *Mar. Drugs* **2019**, *17*, 638. [CrossRef]
32. Geraldes, V.; De Medeiros, L.S.; Jacinavicius, F.R.; Long, P.F.; Pinto, E. Development and validation of a rapid LC-MS/MS method for the quantification of mycosporines and mycosporine-like amino acids (MAAs) from cyanobacteria. *Algal Res.* **2020**, *46*, 101796. [CrossRef]
33. Jofre, J.; Celis-Plá, P.S.M.; Figueroa, F.L.; Navarro, N.P. Seasonal Variation of Mycosporine-Like Amino Acids in Three Subantarctic Red Seaweeds. *Mar. Drugs* **2020**, *18*, 75. [CrossRef] [PubMed]
34. Guihéneuf, F.; Gietl, A.; Stengel, D.B. Temporal and spatial variability of mycosporine-like amino acids and pigments in three edible red seaweeds from western Ireland. *Environ. Boil. Fishes* **2018**, *30*, 2573–2586. [CrossRef]
35. Pope, M.A.; Spence, E.; Seralvo, V.; Gacesa, R.; Heidelberger, S.; Weston, A.J.; Dunlap, W.C.; Shick, J.M.; Long, P.F. O-Methyltransferase Is Shared between the Pentose Phosphate and Shikimate Pathways and Is Essential for Mycosporine-Like Amino Acid Biosynthesis inAnabaena variabilisATCC 29413. *ChemBioChem* **2014**, *16*, 320–327. [CrossRef] [PubMed]
36. Balskus, E.P.; Walsh, C.T. The Genetic and Molecular Basis for Sunscreen Biosynthesis in Cyanobacteria. *Sciences* **2010**, *329*, 1653–1656. [CrossRef] [PubMed]
37. Katoch, M.; Mazmouz, R.; Chau, R.; Pearson, L.A.; Pickford, R.; Neilan, B.A. Heterologous Production of Cyanobacterial Mycosporine-Like Amino Acids Mycosporine-Ornithine and Mycosporine-Lysine in Escherichia coli. *Appl. Environ. Microbiol.* **2016**, *82*, 6167–6173. [CrossRef]
38. Shick, J.M.; Romaine-Lioud, S.; Ferrier-Pagès, C.; Gattuso, J.-P. Ultraviolet-B radiation stimulates shikimate pathway-dependent accumulation of mycosporine-like amino acids in the coral Stylophora pistillata despite decreases in its population of symbiotic dinoflagellates. *Limnol. Oceanogr.* **1999**, *44*, 1667–1682. [CrossRef]
39. Spence, E.; Dunlap, W.C.; Shick, J.M.; Long, P.F. Redundant Pathways of Sunscreen Biosynthesis in a Cyanobacterium. *ChemBioChem* **2012**, *13*, 531–533. [CrossRef]
40. Wada, N.; Sakamoto, T.; Matsugo, S. Mycosporine-Like Amino Acids and Their Derivatives as Natural Antioxidants. *Antioxidants* **2015**, *4*, 603–646. [CrossRef]
41. Miyamoto, K.T.; Komatsu, M.; Ikeda, H. Discovery of Gene Cluster for Mycosporine-Like Amino Acid Biosynthesis from Actinomycetales Microorganisms and Production of a Novel Mycosporine-Like Amino Acid by Heterologous Expression. *Appl. Environ. Microbiol.* **2014**, *80*, 5028–5036. [CrossRef]
42. Losantos, R.; Funes-Ardoiz, I.; Aguilera, J.; Herrera-Ceballos, E.; García-Iriepa, C.; Campos, P.J.; Sampedro, D. Rational Design and Synthesis of Efficient Sunscreens to Boost the Solar Protection Factor. *Angew. Chem.* **2017**, *129*, 2676–2679. [CrossRef]
43. Gouault, N.; Nguyen, K.H.; Tomasi, S.; Costuas, K. Photoprotective Compounds, Compositions Including Same and Uses Thereof. U.S. Patent Application No. 14/782925, 3 October 2016.
44. Abou-Khalil, E.; Raeppel, S.; Raeppel, F. Imino Compounds as Protecting Agents against Ultraviolet Radiations. U.S. Patent No. 9487474B2, 8 November 2016.
45. York, M.; Ryan, J.H.; Savage, G.P.; Meyer, A.G.; Jarvis, K. UV Absorbing Compounds, Compositions Comprising Same and Uses Thereof. U.S. Patent No. 10519111, 31 December 2019.
46. Chalmers, P.J.; Fitzmaurice, N.; Rigg, D.J.; Thang, S.H.; Bird, G. UV-Absorbing Compounds and Compositions. International Patent Application PCT/AU90/00078; Publication No. WO90/09995. Australian Patent 653495, 23 February 1990.
47. Andreguetti, D.; Stein, E.M.; Pereira, C.M.P.; Pinto, E.; Colepicolo, P. Antioxidant properties and UV absorbance pattern of mycosporine-like amino acids analogs synthesized in an environmentally friendly manner. *J. Biochem. Mol. Toxicol.* **2013**, *27*, 305–312. [CrossRef] [PubMed]
48. Nguyen, K.H.; Tomasi, S.; Le Roch, M.; Toupet, L.; Renault, J.; Uriac, P.; Gouault, N. Gold-Mediated Synthesis and Functionalization of Chiral Halopyridones. *J. Org. Chem.* **2013**, *78*, 7809–7815. [CrossRef] [PubMed]
49. Bedoux, G.; Pliego-Cortés, H.; Dufau, C.; Hardouin, K.; Boulho, R.; Freile-Pelegrín, Y.; Robledo, D.; Bourgougnon, N. Production and properties of mycosporine-like amino acids isolated from seaweeds. *Adv. Bot. Res.* **2020**, 213–245. [CrossRef]

50. Chaves-Peña, P.; De La Coba, F.; Figueroa, F.L.; Korbee, N. Quantitative and Qualitative HPLC Analysis of Mycosporine-Like Amino Acids Extracted in Distilled Water for Cosmetical Uses in Four Rhodophyta. *Mar. Drugs* **2019**, *18*, 27. [CrossRef] [PubMed]
51. Hartmann, A.; Murauer, A.; Ganzera, M. Quantitative analysis of mycosporine-like amino acids in marine algae by capillary electrophoresis with diode-array detection. *J. Pharm. Biomed. Anal.* **2017**, *138*, 153–157. [CrossRef]
52. Rosic, N.N.; Braun, C.; Kvaskoff, D. Extraction and Analysis of Mycosporine-Like Amino Acids in Marine Algae. *Nat. Prod. From Mar. Algae* **2015**, 119–129. [CrossRef]
53. Whitehead, K.; Hedges, J.I. Analysis of mycosporine-like amino acids in plankton by liquid chromatography electrospray ionization mass spectrometry. *Mar. Chem.* **2002**, *80*, 27–39. [CrossRef]
54. Hartmann, A.; Becker, K.; Karsten, U.; Remias, D.; Ganzera, M. Analysis of Mycosporine-Like Amino Acids in Selected Algae and Cyanobacteria by Hydrophilic Interaction Liquid Chromatography and a Novel MAA from the Red Alga Catenella repens. *Mar. Drugs* **2015**, *13*, 6291–6305. [CrossRef]
55. Orfanoudaki, M.; Hartmann, A.; Miladinovic, H.; Nguyen-Ngoc, H.; Karsten, U.; Ganzera, M. Bostrychines A–F, Six Novel Mycosporine-Like Amino-Acids and a Novel Betaine from the Red Alga Bostrychia scorpioides. *Mar. Drugs* **2019**, *17*, 356. [CrossRef]
56. Cardozo, K.H.M.; Carvalho, V.M.; Pinto, E.; Colepicolo, P. Fragmentation of mycosporine-like amino acids by hydrogen/deuterium exchange and electrospray ionisation tandem mass spectrometry. *Rapid Commun. Mass Spectrom.* **2005**, *20*, 253–258. [CrossRef]
57. Cardozo, K.H.; Vessecchi, R.; Carvalho, V.M.; Pinto, E.; Gates, P.J.; Colepicolo, P.; Galembeck, S.E.; Lopes, N.P. A theoretical and mass spectrometry study of the fragmentation of mycosporine-like amino acids. *Int. J. Mass Spectrom.* **2008**, *273*, 11–19. [CrossRef]
58. Cardozo, K.H.M.; Vessecchi, R.; Galembeck, S.E.; Guaratini, T.; Gates, P.J.; Pinto, E.; Lopes, N.P.; Colepicolo, P. A Fragmentation study of di-acidic mycosporine-like amino acids in electrospray and nanospray mass spectrometry. *J. Braz. Chem. Soc.* **2009**, *20*, 1625–1631. [CrossRef]
59. Orfanoudaki, M.; Hartmann, A.; Karsten, U.; Ganzera, M. Chemical profiling of mycosporine-like amino acids in twenty-three red algal species. *J. Phycol.* **2019**, *55*, 393–403. [CrossRef] [PubMed]
60. Lalegerie, F.; Stiger-Pouvreau, V.; Connan, S. Temporal variation in pigment and mycosporine-like amino acid composition of the red macroalga Palmaria palmata from Brittany (France): Hypothesis on the MAA biosynthesis pathway under high irradiance. *Environ. Boil. Fishes* **2020**, *32*, 2641–2656. [CrossRef]
61. Lalegerie, F.; Lajili, S.; Bedoux, G.; Taupin, L.; Stiger-Pouvreau, V.; Connan, S. Photo-protective compounds in red macroalgae from Brittany: Considerable diversity in mycosporine-like amino acids (MAAs). *Mar. Environ. Res.* **2019**, *147*, 37–48. [CrossRef] [PubMed]
62. Shick, J.M.; Dunlap, W.C. Mycosporine-Like Amino Acids and Related Gadusols: Biosynthesis, Accumulation, and UV-Protective Functions in Aquatic Organisms. *Annu. Rev. Physiol.* **2002**, *64*, 223–262. [CrossRef] [PubMed]
63. Olsson-Francis, K.; Watson, J.S.; Cockell, C.S. Cyanobacteria isolated from the high-intertidal zone: A model for studying the physiological prerequisites for survival in low Earth orbit. *Int. J. Astrobiol.* **2013**, *12*, 292–303. [CrossRef]
64. Joshi, D.; Mohandass, C.; Mohandass, C. Effect of UV-B Radiation and Desiccation Stress on Photoprotective Compounds Accumulation in Marine Leptolyngbya sp. *Appl. Biochem. Biotechnol.* **2017**, *184*, 35–47. [CrossRef]
65. Ehling-Schulz, M.; Bilger, W.; Scherer, S. UV-B-induced synthesis of photoprotective pigments and extracellular polysaccharides in the terrestrial cyanobacterium Nostoc commune. *J. Bacteriol.* **1997**, *179*, 1940–1945. [CrossRef]
66. Suganya, T.; Varman, M.; Masjuki, H.; Renganathan, S. Macroalgae and microalgae as a potential source for commercial applications along with biofuels production: A biorefinery approach. *Renew. Sustain. Energy Rev.* **2016**, *55*, 909–941. [CrossRef]
67. Rastogi, R.P.; Incharoensakdi, A. UV radiation-induced biosynthesis, stability and antioxidant activity of mycosporine-like amino acids (MAAs) in a unicellular cyanobacterium Gloeocapsa sp. CU2556. *J. Photochem. Photobiol. B Biol.* **2014**, *130*, 287–292. [CrossRef] [PubMed]
68. Shang, J.-L.; Zhang, Z.-C.; Yin, X.-Y.; Chen, M.; Yan-Chao, Y.; Wang, K.; Feng, J.-L.; Xu, H.-F.; Yin, Y.-C.; Tang, H.; et al. UV-B induced biosynthesis of a novel sunscreen compound in solar radiation and desiccation tolerant cyanobacteria. *Environ. Microbiol.* **2017**, *20*, 200–213. [CrossRef] [PubMed]
69. Oren, A.; Gunde-Cimerman, N. Mycosporines and mycosporine-like amino acids: UV protectants or multipurpose secondary metabolites? *FEMS Microbiol. Lett.* **2007**, *269*, 1–10. [CrossRef] [PubMed]
70. Woolley, J.M.; Staniforth, M.; Horbury, M.D.; Richings, G.W.; Wills, M.; Stavros, V.G. Unravelling the Photoprotection Properties of Mycosporine Amino Acid Motifs. *J. Phys. Chem. Lett.* **2018**, *9*, 3043–3048. [CrossRef]
71. McAdam, E.; Brem, R.; Karran, P. Oxidative Stress–Induced Protein Damage Inhibits DNA Repair and Determines Mutation Risk and Therapeutic Efficacy. *Mol. Cancer Res.* **2016**, *14*, 612–622. [CrossRef]
72. Hossain, F.; Ratnayake, R.; Meerajini, K.; Kumara, K.L.W. Antioxidant properties in some selected cyanobacteria isolated from fresh water bodies of Sri Lanka. *Food Sci. Nutr.* **2016**, *4*, 753–758. [CrossRef]
73. Fuentes-Tristan, S.; Parra-Saldívar, R.; Iqbal, H.M.; Carrillo-Nieves, D. Bioinspired biomolecules: Mycosporine-like amino acids and scytonemin from Lyngbya sp. with UV-protection potentialities. *J. Photochem. Photobiol. B Biol.* **2019**, *201*, 111684. [CrossRef]
74. Korteerakul, C.; Honda, M.; Ngoennet, S.; Hibino, T.; Waditee-Sirisattha, R.; Kageyama, H. Antioxidative and Antiglycative Properties of Mycosporine-Like Amino Acids-Containing Aqueous Extracts Derived from Edible Terrestrial Cyanobacteria. *J. Nutr. Sci. Vitaminol.* **2020**, *66*, 339–346. [CrossRef]

75. Gacesa, R.; Lawrence, K.P.; Georgakopoulos, N.D.; Yabe, K.; Dunlap, W.C.; Barlow, D.J.; Wells, G.; Young, A.R.; Long, P.F. The mycosporine-like amino acids porphyra-334 and shinorine are antioxidants and direct antagonists of Keap1-Nrf2 binding. *Biochimie* **2018**, *154*, 35–44. [CrossRef]
76. Torres, P.; Santos, J.P.; Chow, F.; Ferreira, M.J.P.; Dos Santos, D.Y. Comparative analysis of in vitro antioxidant capacities of mycosporine-like amino acids (MAAs). *Algal Res.* **2018**, *34*, 57–67. [CrossRef]
77. Cheewinthamrongrod, V.; Kageyama, H.; Palaga, T.; Takabe, T.; Waditee-Sirisattha, R. DNA damage protecting and free radical scavenging properties of mycosporine-2-glycine from the Dead Sea cyanobacterium in A375 human melanoma cell lines. *J. Photochem. Photobiol. B Biol.* **2016**, *164*, 289–295. [CrossRef] [PubMed]
78. Panich, U.; Sittithumcharee, G.; Rathviboon, N.; Jirawatnotai, S. Ultraviolet Radiation-Induced Skin Aging: The Role of DNA Damage and Oxidative Stress in Epidermal Stem Cell Damage Mediated Skin Aging. *Stem Cells Int.* **2016**, *2016*, 1–14. [CrossRef] [PubMed]
79. Tarasuntisuk, S.; Palaga, T.; Kageyama, H.; Waditee-Sirisattha, R. Mycosporine-2-glycine exerts anti-inflammatory and antioxidant effects in lipopolysaccharide (LPS)-stimulated RAW 264.7 macrophages. *Arch. Biochem. Biophys.* **2019**, *662*, 33–39. [CrossRef] [PubMed]
80. De La Coba, F.; Aguilera, J.; Figueroa, F.L.; De Gálvez, M.V.; Herrera, E. Antioxidant activity of mycosporine-like amino acids isolated from three red macroalgae and one marine lichen. *Environ. Boil. Fishes* **2009**, *21*, 161–169. [CrossRef]
81. Lawrence, K.P.; Gacesa, R.; Long, P.F.; Young, A.R. Molecular photoprotection of human keratinocytes in vitro by the naturally occurring mycosporine-like amino acid palythine. *Br. J. Dermatol.* **2018**, *178*, 1353–1363. [CrossRef] [PubMed]
82. Rastogi, R.P.; Sonani, R.R.; Madamwar, D.; Incharoensakdi, A. Characterization and antioxidant functions of mycosporine-like amino acids in the cyanobacterium Nostoc sp. R76DM. *Algal Res.* **2016**, *16*, 110–118. [CrossRef]
83. Kageyama, H.; Waditee-Sirisattha, R. Antioxidative, Anti-Inflammatory, and Anti-Aging Properties of Mycosporine-Like Amino Acids: Molecular and Cellular Mechanisms in the Protection of Skin-Aging. *Mar. Drugs* **2019**, *17*, 222. [CrossRef]
84. Oren, A. Mycosporine-like amino acids as osmotic solutes in a community of halophilic cyanobacteria. *Geomicrobiol. J.* **1997**, *14*, 231–240. [CrossRef]
85. Portwich, A.; Garcia-Pichel, F. Ultraviolet and osmotic stresses induce and regulate the synthesis of mycosporines in the cyanobacterium Chlorogloeopsis PCC 6912. *Arch. Microbiol.* **1999**, *172*, 187–192. [CrossRef]
86. Singh, S.P.; Klisch, M.; Sinha, R.P.; Häder, D.-P. Effects of Abiotic Stressors on Synthesis of the Mycosporine-like Amino Acid Shinorine in the CyanobacteriumAnabaena variabilisPCC 7937. *Photochem. Photobiol.* **2008**, *84*, 1500–1505. [CrossRef]
87. Waditee-Sirisattha, R.; Kageyama, H.; Sopun, W.; Tanaka, Y.; Takabe, T. Identification and Upregulation of Biosynthetic Genes Required for Accumulation of Mycosporine-2-Glycine under Salt Stress Conditions in the Halotolerant Cyanobacterium Aphanothece halophytica. *Appl. Environ. Microbiol.* **2014**, *80*, 1763–1769. [CrossRef] [PubMed]
88. Abed, R.M.M.; Polerecky, L.; Al-Habsi, A.; Oetjen, J.; Strous, M.; De Beer, D. Rapid Recovery of Cyanobacterial Pigments in Desiccated Biological Soil Crusts following Addition of Water. *PLoS ONE* **2014**, *9*, e112372. [CrossRef] [PubMed]
89. Gorbushina, A.; Kotlova, E.R.; Sherstneva, O.A. Cellular responses of microcolonial rock fungi to long-term desiccation and subsequent rehydration. *Stud. Mycol.* **2008**, *61*, 91–97. [CrossRef] [PubMed]
90. Gorbushina, A.; Whitehead, K.; Dornieden, T.; Niesse, A.; Schulte, A.; Hedges, J.I. Black fungal colonies as units of survival: Hyphal mycosporines synthesized by rock-dwelling microcolonial fungi. *Can. J. Bot.* **2003**, *81*, 131–138. [CrossRef]
91. Michalek-Wagner, K. Seasonal and sex-specific variations in levels of photo-protecting mycosporine-like amino acids (MAAs) in soft corals. *Mar. Biol.* **2001**, *139*, 651–660. [CrossRef]
92. Sivalingam, P.M.; Ikawa, T.; Nisizawa, K. Physiological Roles of a Substance 334 in Algae. *Bot. Mar.* **1976**, *19*, 9–22. [CrossRef]
93. Peinado, N.K.; Díaz, R.T.A.; Figueroa, F.L.; Helbling, E.W. Ammonium and UV Radiation Stimulate the Accumulation of Mycosporine-Like Amino Acids in *Porphyra columbina* (Rhodophyta) from Patagonia, Argentina. *J. Phycol.* **2004**, *40*, 248–259. [CrossRef]
94. Carroll, A.K.; Shick, J.M. Dietary accumulation of UV-absorbing mycosporine-like amino acids (MAAs) by the green sea urchin (*Strongylocentrotus droebachiensis*). *Mar. Biol.* **1996**, *124*, 561–569. [CrossRef]
95. Bandaranayake, W.M.; Bourne, D.J.; Sim, R.G. Chemical Composition during Maturing and Spawning of the Sponge Dysidea herbacea (Porifera: Demospongiae). *Comp. Biochem. Physiol. Part B Biochem. Mol. Biol.* **1997**, *118*, 851–859. [CrossRef]
96. Kicklighter, C.E.; Kamio, M.; Nguyen, L.; Germann, M.W.; Derby, C.D. Mycosporine-like amino acids are multifunctional molecules in sea hares and their marine community. *Proc. Natl. Acad. Sci.* **2011**, *108*, 11494–11499. [CrossRef]
97. Hu, C.; Völler, G.; Süßmuth, R.; Dittmann, E.; Kehr, J.-C. Functional assessment of mycosporine-like amino acids inMicrocystis aeruginosastrain PCC 7806. *Environ. Microbiol.* **2015**, *17*, 1548–1559. [CrossRef] [PubMed]
98. Couteau, C.; Coiffard, L. Phycocosmetics and Other Marine Cosmetics, Specific Cosmetics Formulated Using Marine Resources. *Mar. Drugs* **2020**, *18*, 322. [CrossRef] [PubMed]
99. Mancuso, J.B.; Maruthi, R.; Wang, S.Q.; Lim, H.W. Sunscreens: An Update. *Am. J. Clin. Dermatol.* **2017**, *18*, 643–650. [CrossRef] [PubMed]
100. Stoddard, M.; Lyons, A.; Moy, R. Skin Cancer Prevention: A Review of Current Oral Options Complementary to Sunscreens. *J. Drugs Dermatol. JDD* **2018**, *17*, 1266–1271. [PubMed]
101. Ruszkiewicz, J.A.; Pinkas, A.; Ferrer, B.; Peres, T.V.; Tsatsakis, A.; Aschner, M. Neurotoxic effect of active ingredients in sunscreen products, a contemporary review. *Toxicol. Rep.* **2017**, *4*, 245–259. [CrossRef]

102. De La Coba, F.; Aguilera, J.; Korbee, N.; Gálvez, M.N.-D.; Herrera-Ceballos, E.; Álvarez-Gómez, F.; Figueroa, F.L. UVA and UVB Photoprotective Capabilities of Topical Formulations Containing Mycosporine-like Amino Acids (MAAs) through Different Biological Effective Protection Factors (BEPFs). *Mar. Drugs* **2019**, *17*, 55. [CrossRef]
103. Wang, J.; Pan, L.; Wu, S.; Lu, L.; Xu, Y.; Zhu, Y.; Guo, M.; Zhuang, S. Recent Advances on Endocrine Disrupting Effects of UV Filters. *Int. J. Environ. Res. Public Health* **2016**, *13*, 782. [CrossRef]
104. Galamgam, J.; Linou, N.; Linos, E. Sunscreens, cancer, and protecting our planet. *Lancet Planet. Health* **2018**, *2*, e465–e466. [CrossRef]
105. Schneider, S.L.; Lim, H.W. Review of environmental effects of oxybenzone and other sunscreen active ingredients. *J. Am. Acad. Dermatol.* **2019**, *80*, 266–271. [CrossRef]
106. Dinardo, J.C.; A Downs, C. Dermatological and environmental toxicological impact of the sunscreen ingredient oxybenzone/benzophenone-3. *J. Cosmet. Dermatol.* **2017**, *17*, 15–19. [CrossRef]
107. Ouchene, L.; Litvinov, I.V.; Netchiporouk, E. Hawaii and Other Jurisdictions Ban Oxybenzone or Octinoxate Sunscreens Based on the Confirmed Adverse Environmental Effects of Sunscreen Ingredients on Aquatic Environments. *J. Cutan. Med. Surg.* **2019**, *23*, 648–649. [CrossRef] [PubMed]
108. Narla, S.; Lim, H.W. Sunscreen: FDA regulation, and environmental and health impact. *Photochem. Photobiol. Sci.* **2020**, *19*, 66–70. [CrossRef] [PubMed]
109. Pangestuti, R.; Siahaan, E.A.; Kim, S.-K. Photoprotective Substances Derived from Marine Algae. *Mar. Drugs* **2018**, *16*, 399. [CrossRef]
110. Pathak, J.; Pandey, A.; Maurya, P.K.; Rajneesh, R.; Sinha, R.P.; Singh, S.P. Cyanobacterial Secondary Metabolite Scytonemin: A Potential Photoprotective and Pharmaceutical Compound. *Proc. Natl. Acad. Sci. India Sect. B Boil. Sci.* **2020**, *90*, 467–481. [CrossRef]
111. Thiyagarasaiyar, K.; Goh, B.H.; Jeon, Y.-J.; Yow, Y.-Y. Algae Metabolites in Cosmeceutical: An Overview of Current Applications and Challenges. *Mar. Drugs* **2020**, *18*, 323. [CrossRef] [PubMed]
112. Fernandes, S.C.M.; Alonso-Varona, A.; Palomares, T.; Zubillaga, V.; Labidi, J.; Bulone, V. Exploiting Mycosporines as Natural Molecular Sunscreens for the Fabrication of UV-Absorbing Green Materials. *ACS Appl. Mater. Interfaces* **2015**, *7*, 16558–16564. [CrossRef]

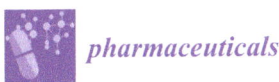

Review

Plant Terpenoids as Hit Compounds against Trypanosomiasis

Raquel Durão [1,†], Cátia Ramalhete [1,2,†], Ana Margarida Madureira [1], Eduarda Mendes [1] and Noélia Duarte [1,*]

1. Research Institute for Medicines (iMED.Ulisboa), Faculdade de Farmácia, Universidade de Lisboa, Av. Prof. Gama Pinto, 1649-003 Lisboa, Portugal; raquel-durao@campus.ul.pt (R.D.); catiar@uatlantica.pt (C.R.); afernand@ff.ulisboa.pt (A.M.M.); ermendes@ff.ulisboa.pt (E.M.)
2. ATLANTICA—Instituto Universitário, Fábrica da Pólvora de Barcarena, 2730-036 Barcarena, Portugal
* Correspondence: mduarte@ff.ulisboa.pt
† These authors contributed equally to this work.

Abstract: Human African trypanosomiasis (sleeping sickness) and American trypanosomiasis (Chagas disease) are vector-borne neglected tropical diseases, caused by the protozoan parasites *Trypanosoma brucei* and *Trypanosoma cruzi*, respectively. These diseases were circumscribed to South American and African countries in the past. However, human migration, military interventions, and climate changes have had an important effect on their worldwide propagation, particularly Chagas disease. Currently, the treatment of trypanosomiasis is not ideal, becoming a challenge in poor populations with limited resources. Exploring natural products from higher plants remains a valuable approach to find new hits and enlarge the pipeline of new drugs against protozoal human infections. This review covers the recent studies (2016–2021) on plant terpenoids, and their semi-synthetic derivatives, which have shown promising in vitro and in vivo activities against Trypanosoma parasites.

Keywords: terpenoids; Trypanosoma; human African trypanosomiasis; sleeping disease; human American trypanosomiasis; Chagas disease

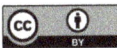

1. Introduction

Human African trypanosomiasis (sleeping sickness) and American trypanosomiasis (Chagas disease) are among the twenty Neglected Tropical Diseases (NTDs) defined as such by the World Health Organization (WHO). NTDs are a heterogeneous group of diseases including, among others, several parasitic, viral, and bacterial infections, responsible for high morbidity and mortality, and affecting more than one billion people globally [1–3]. Sometimes, the impact of NTDs on health can be underestimated because many infections are asymptomatic and associated with long incubation periods. Nevertheless, NTDs are recognized as a public health problem, particularly for people living in rural and conflict areas in developing countries [1]. These diseases are considered neglected due to the general lack of attention in developed countries and almost non-existent financial investment in the research and development of new drugs and vaccines [4]. In addition to all these problems, the COVID-19 pandemic has been affecting the programs of mass drug administration and other NTD control measures [5,6]. Currently, the pharmacological therapy of NTDs is not ideal, as it has some limitations that include severe side effects, unfavorable toxicity profiles, prolonged treatment duration, difficult administration procedures, and development of drug resistance [7–9]. The investment in these therapeutic areas by large pharmaceutical companies is not financially attractive due to the poor prospect of financial returns. Thus, the research of drugs against these diseases is not motivated by commercial reasons. Additionally, many pharmaceutical companies take an opportunistic approach to drug repositioning, using drugs that were previously developed and registered for other therapeutic indications and applying them in the treatment of NTDs. This strategy has obvious advantages, namely reduced development costs. However, the major disadvantage is the non-introduction of new specific drugs used in the treatment of these diseases [7].

Therefore, the discovery and development of new drugs is essential and urgent and should embrace the development of new therapeutic classes, the reduction in toxicity in the host, better administration processes, and the development of combined therapies [10]. One of the main strategies includes the phytochemical study of plants and other natural sources (marine organisms, animals, microorganisms, and fungi). Natural products have played an important role in the drug discovery and development processes [11]. However, in recent decades, most pharmaceutical companies have reduced their drug discovery and development programs from natural sources, largely due to the development of combinatorial chemistry programs [7]. Nevertheless, despite the large number of drugs derived from total synthesis, natural products and/or synthetic derivatives using their novel structures, contribute to the global number of new chemical entities that continue to be introduced on the market [12].

Over the last decade, several reviews have reported the bioactivity of natural products against protozoan neglected diseases [7,13–21]. However, natural products described in these reviews were obtained from different sources, including microbial [19], endophytes [20] and other fungi [21], marine [22], or animal origins [23,24]. Some reviews also present a mix of natural compounds origins [7,17]. Regarding natural products from plants, since 2016, there have been some reviews focusing exclusively on compounds from higher plants [16,18,25–30]. Nevertheless, the information is scattered amongst the diverse antiprotozoal diseases, compound families, and sources. To the best of our knowledge, a comprehensive review gathering the data concerning the most recent studies on terpenic compounds with antitrypanosomal activities is still missing. Therefore, in this work, a compilation of terpenes obtained from plants and evaluated for their activity against *T. brucei* and *T. cruzi*, covering the period from 2016 to 2021, will be presented and discussed. When available, data regarding in vivo activity and considerations about possible mechanisms of action will be also addressed.

The literature search was performed from June to December 2021 using Web of Science, ScienceDirect, PubMed, and some official websites (WHO, DNDi, CDC). An appropriate combination of keywords and truncation was selected and adapted for each database (for example, combinations of terpenoids or terpenes with Trypanosoma, Human African trypanosomiasis, and Chagas disease). Only peer-reviewed research articles or reviews in a six-year timespan (2016–2021) and in English language were considered. No restriction geographical origin of authors was applied. In particular cases, important reviews older than six years were also included. The literature was individually screened, applying as exclusion criteria, poor quality, inaccurate data, not considered relevant to the aim of the review, and articles reporting antitrypanosomal activity of extracts. Mendeley Reference Manager Software (2020) was used to manage the references and eliminate duplicates.

2. Trypanosomiasis

2.1. Human African Trypanosomiasis (HAT)

HAT is endemic in 36 African countries, with approximately 60 million people at risk, and approximately 10.8 million people living in areas of moderate to high risk of infection. In 1995, about 25,000 cases were detected and about 300,000 cases remained undetected. However, in 2001, the WHO launched an initiative to strengthen control and surveillance, and HAT declined in the following years. In 2019, less than 1000 cases were reported. It is noteworthy that this reduction is not due to a lack of control efforts as active and passive screening have been maintained at similar levels (about 2.5 million people screened per year) [31]. HAT is essentially present in poorer and rural areas, affecting populations dedicated to agriculture, fishing, livestock, and hunting, who are more exposed to the vector of transmission. Furthermore, their access to adequate health services is limited, thus lacking medical surveillance, also associated with difficulties in diagnosis and treatment [32]. This parasitic disease is transmitted mostly by the bite of the tsetse fly (*Glossina palpalis*), but other routes of transmission are possible, such as congenital transmission, blood transfusion, and transplants, despite being poorly documented [33]. The life cycle of *Trypanosoma brucei* sp. is illustrated in Figure 1 and reviewed elsewhere [10,34].

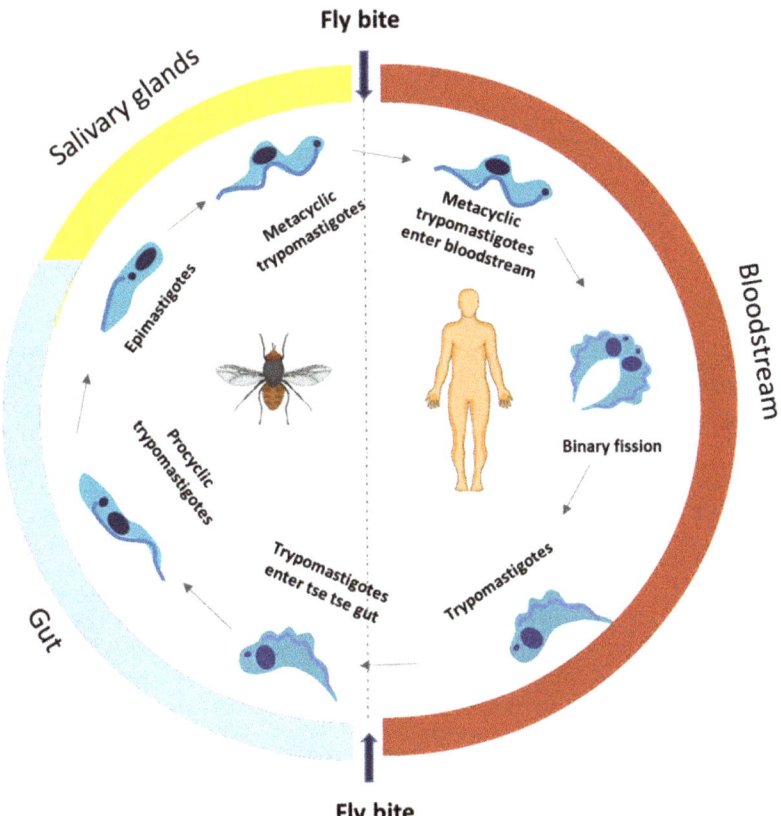

Figure 1. The life cycle of *T. brucei*.

There are two subspecies of *Trypanosoma brucei* (*T. b.*), *T. b. gambiense*, and *T. b. rhodesiense*, with different geographic distributions. *T. b. gambiense* is found in 24 countries in West and Central Africa, accounting for more than 98% of reported cases. *T. b. rhodesiense* is present in 13 countries in East Africa, representing less than 3% of reported cases [32]. The two subspecies have different rates of progression and clinical characteristics. Infections by *T. b. gambiense* are characterized by a low parasitemia, with slow progression leading to the development of the chronic form of the disease, while *T. b. rhodesiense* progresses rapidly with high parasitemia, being characterized by the acute form. Both infections, if not diagnosed and treated, lead to death [34]. The clinical evolution of HAT has two phases. In the first phase, also known as the hemolymphatic phase, the parasite is found in the host's blood and lymphatic stream. This initial phase includes non-specific symptoms such as pyrexia, headache, muscle and joint pain, weight loss and even enlarged lymph nodes, usually in the neck area. The second or neurologic phase (meningoencephalitis) occurs when the parasite crosses the blood–brain barrier and reaches the central nervous system. The clinical manifestations are usually behavioral changes, such as anxiety and irritability, sensory, motor, and sleep cycle disorders [32,33].

2.1.1. Antitrypanosomal Chemotherapy Targets and Current Drugs against HAT

Trypanosome-specific metabolic and cellular pathways represent excellent molecular targets. The ability to synthesize polyamines, putrescine, and spermidine, is of vital importance for the proliferation of bloodstream forms in trypanosomes. In this process, ornithine decarboxylase has a crucial function. This enzyme is considered the best-validated drug target in *T. brucei*, which is the target of eflornithine, a drug that is used clinically for the treatment of HAT [10,35]. In addition, the enzyme N-myristoyltransferase (NMT) has been well validated as a molecular target for HAT since its inhibition may lead to the death of the parasites. NMT catalyzes the covalent attachment of myristate, a 14-carbon saturated fatty acid, via amide bond to the N-terminal glycine residue of several proteins. NMT is also present in humans, but *T. brucei* is extremely sensitive to NMT inhibition, probably because endocytosis occurs at a very high rate in *T. brucei* [36]. Recently, significant progress in targeting the ubiquitin-proteasome system was reported [37]. The ubiquitin-proteasome system (UPS) is a crucial protein degradation system in eukaryotes and is essential for the survival of eukaryotes including trypanosomatids. There are promising inhibitors of this, but the overall success of clinical trials is low and therefore more drug candidates are needed. The bloodstream forms of *T. brucei* produce energy exclusively through glycolysis. Thus, inhibition of glycolytic enzymes, such as glyceraldehyde 3-phosphate dehydrogenase, phosphoglycerate mutase, phosphofructokinase and pyruvate kinase, could be a potential therapeutic approach. However, there is little prospect of killing trypanosomes by suppressing glycolysis unless inhibition is irreversible or uncompetitive, owing to the enormous glycolytic flux through the system [10,35]. Regarding redox metabolism, a fundamental metabolic difference between host and parasite is the existence of trypanothione reductase in trypanosomes instead of glutathione reductase, which is essential for the parasite's survival. The inhibition of trypanothione reductase compromises the parasite's oxidative defenses, sometimes leading to its death. Unfortunately, until now, compounds suitable for clinical development have not been discovered [10].

Currently, there is no vaccination or chemoprophylaxis for HAT, and its combat is mainly conducted through prophylactic measures aimed at reducing the reservoir of the disease and controlling the vector. The latter is the main strategy in use, which aims to minimize human contact with the fly. The recommended measures in the most affected areas are the use of clothes with neutral colors, and the use of insecticide repellents [34]. Recently, rapid diagnostic tests have been also developed in order to detect the presence of the antigen, offering accurate and sensitive results [38]. The treatment of HAT depends essentially on the stage of the disease and the causative agent. Until recently, five drugs have been used to treat sleeping sickness, donated by manufacturers to WHO for free distribution [38]. For the first phase, suramin (Naganinum®, Naganol®) and pentamidine (Nebupent®, Pentam®) are the first line drugs. For the final stage of sleeping sickness, the treatment includes the use of melarsoprol (Arsobal®), eflornithine (Vaniqa®) and the nifurtimox (Lampit®) -eflornithine combination therapy (NECT) [39]. Recently, fexinidazole was approved by the European Medicine Agency (EMA) and the United States Food and Drug Administration (USFDA) as the first all-oral therapy for the treatment of phase-1 and phase-2 HAT [39]. Additionally, acoziborole a recently developed benzoxaborole, is currently in advanced clinical trials, for treatment of phase-1 and phase-2 caused by both *T.b. gambiense* and *T.b. rhodesiense*. Acoziborole is orally bioavailable, and importantly, curative with one dose [40].

2.2. Human American Trypanosomiasis (Chagas Disease, CD)

Human American trypanosomiasis, commonly known as Chagas disease (CD), is endemic in 21 countries in Latin America. However, human migrations have turned it into a global disease with a significant number of cases in non-endemic regions such as Canada or Europe, among others. CD is present in rural areas and affects populations living in poverty. The WHO estimates that about 6 to 7 million people worldwide are infected and there are approximately 70 million people at risk [41,42]. CD is caused by the protozoan parasite *Trypanosoma cruzi* (*T. cruzi*), and it is generally transmitted by vectors, such as the triatomine hematophagous insects of the *Reduviidae* family, usually known as "barbers". The other transmission routes are blood transfusions, transplantation, congenital transmission, and oral transmission (breast milk), and also by ingestion of contaminated food. The life cycle of *Trypanosoma cruzi* is illustrated in Figure 2 and reviewed elsewhere [41–43].

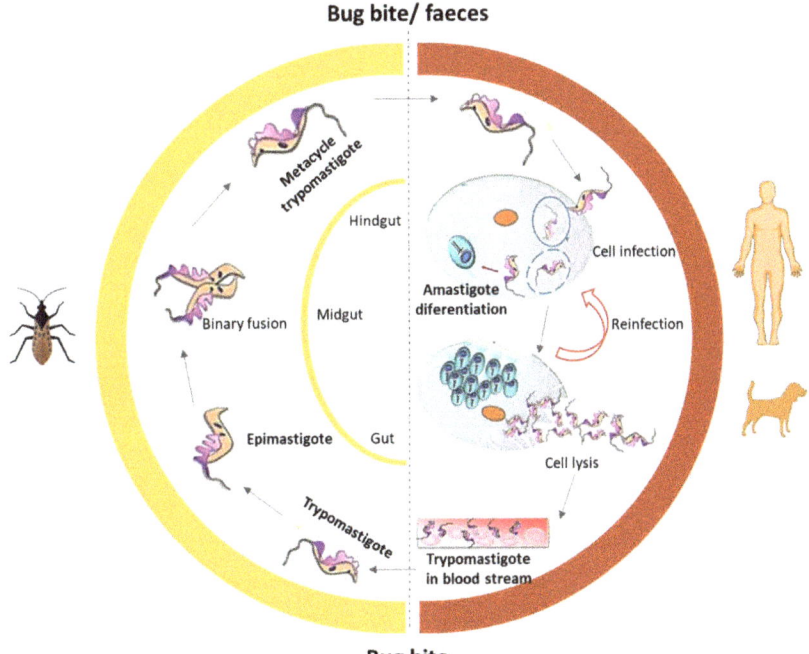

Figure 2. The life cycle of *T. cruzi*.

CD has two successive clinical phases, an acute phase, and a chronic phase. The acute phase can be symptomatic or, most frequently asymptomatic. The initial acute phase occurs immediately after the infection, which can last for weeks or months. It is characterized by local manifestations such as the Romaña Sign, when the parasite penetrates the conjunctiva, or the skin, causing a skin lesion or a purplish swelling of the lids of one eye called Chagoma. After a period of 4 to 8 weeks, the parasitemia decreases and the clinical manifestations spontaneously disappear in 90% of the cases, when the disease enters the chronic phase [41,43]. During the chronic phase, the parasites are in the heart and gastrointestinal tract. Despite the long-lasting nature of the infection in which most individuals do not develop overt pathology, there are about 30% of people who can achieve the chronic phase, characterized by progressive heart and/or digestive disease. In most of these cases, it takes decades to become apparent. Cardiomyopathy is the most serious result of *T. cruzi* infection, and in many areas of South America, it is a major cause of heart disease. Digestive symptoms, including megaesophagus and megacolon, also have serious consequences and may require surgery [43–47]

2.2.1. Antitrypanosomal Chemotherapy Targets and Current Drugs against CD

Infective trypomastigotes and intracellular replicative amastigotes are the clinically relevant life-cycle stages of *T. cruzi* that are potential targets for drug intervention [4,48]. *T. cruzi* requires specific sterols for cell viability and proliferation at all stages of the life cycle. The main sterol component of the parasite is ergosterol, while in the mammalian hosts it is cholesterol. Inhibitors of sterol biosynthesis have been shown antitrypanosomal in vitro activity [48]. Other trypanosomal targets are related to cysteine proteases that are involved in many crucial processes, including host cell invasion, cell division, and differentiation. *T.*

cruzi contains a cysteine protease, cruzipain, which is responsible for proteolytic activity at all stages of the parasite's life. Although no inhibitors of this family of enzymes have progressed to clinical trials, the parasite cysteine proteases remain a promising area of research [47,48]. In addition, the trypanothione reductases and synthetases have also been considered key enzymes in the oxidative metabolism of the parasite. Although several potential inhibitors of the trypanothione reductase possess potent in vitro anti-*T. cruzi* activity, to date, none have achieved parasitological cure in animal models [47].

Only two old nitroheterocyclic drugs, benznidazole (Rochagan® or Rodanil®) and nifurtimox (Lampit®) have been available for the treatment of CD, as reviewed elsewhere [41,49]. They are effective for the acute phase of infection, but they have variable efficacy in the chronic phase of the disease, besides requiring prolonged treatment (60–90 days). In addition, significant problems of resistance have emerged with both drugs. In this context, there is an urgent need for more efficacious and safer drugs or drugs regimens, in particular for the treatment of the chronic stage of the infection. Presently, new benznidazole monotherapy regimens with reduced exposure to improve tolerability while maintaining efficacy, and combination regimens of benznidazole with fosravuconazole to improve efficacy are being developed [50].

3. Terpenic Compounds with Antitrypanosomal Activity

Herein, 150 terpenic compounds with antitrypanosomal activity, isolated from plants or obtained by derivatization, and reported in the literature from 2016 to 2021, are presented (Figures 3–15 and Tables 1 and 2). For clarity reasons, the terpenes are divided into four classes: monoterpenes and iridoids (C10, Figure 3), sesquiterpenes (C15, Figures 4–9), diterpenes (C20, Figures 10–12), and triterpenes (C30, Figures 13–15). The selected compounds were tested for their in vitro activity against *T. brucei* (*T. b. brucei*, and *T. b. rhodesiense*), and *T. cruzi*. Additionally, the in vivo results of some compounds were also described.

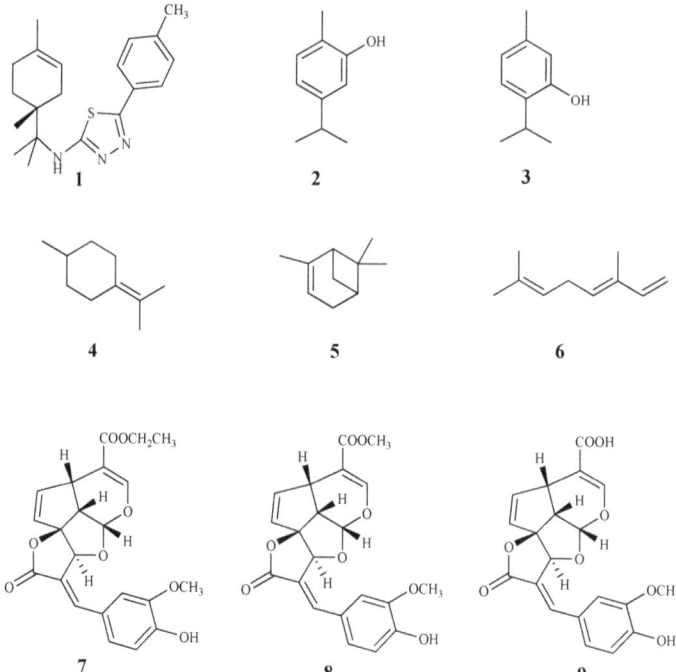

Figure 3. Structures of monoterpenes (1–6) and iridoids (7–9).

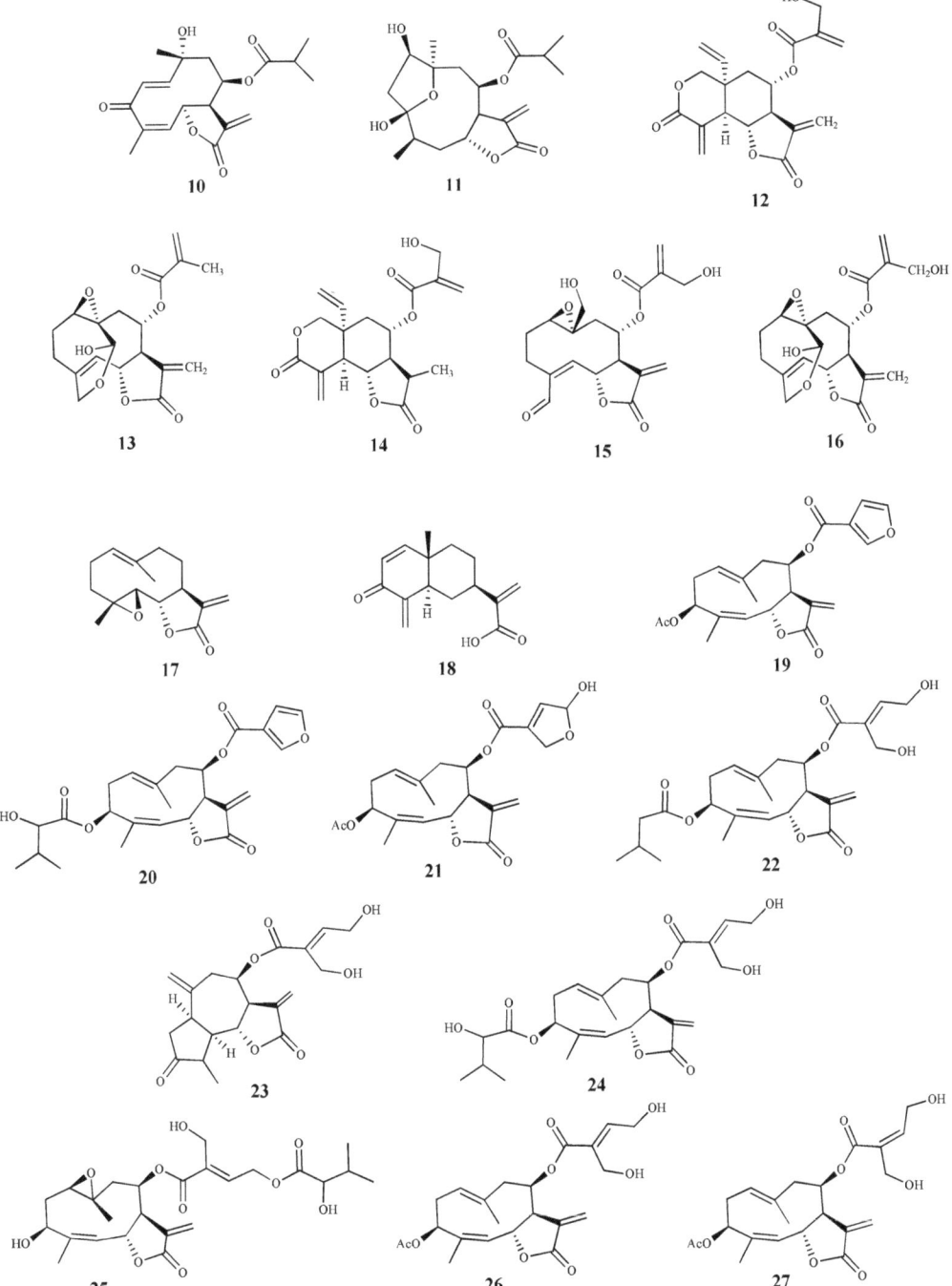

Figure 4. Structures of sesquiterpenes **10–27**.

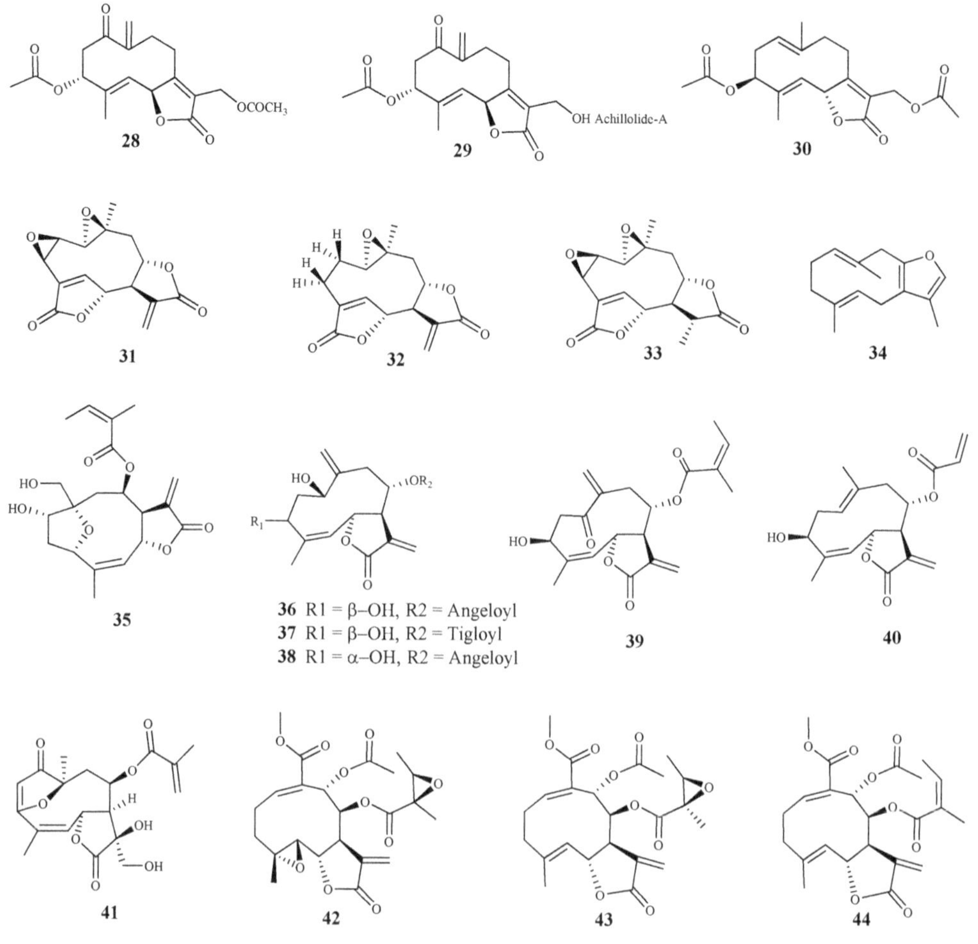

Figure 5. Structures of sesquiterpenes 28–44.

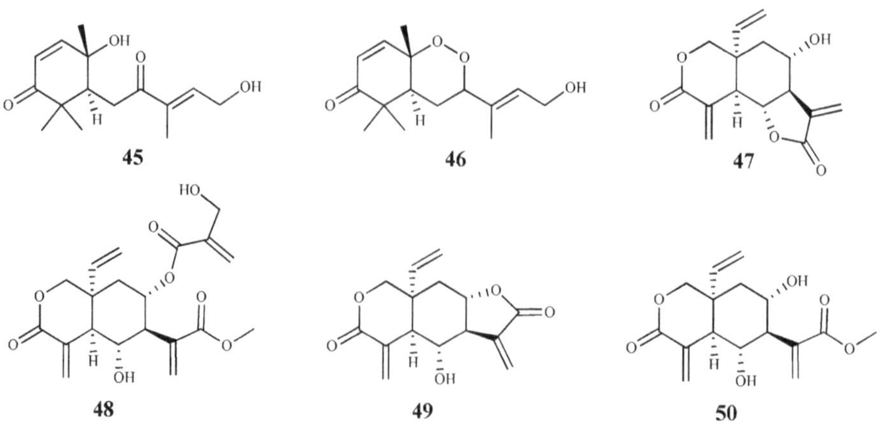

Figure 6. Structures of sesquiterpenes 45–50.

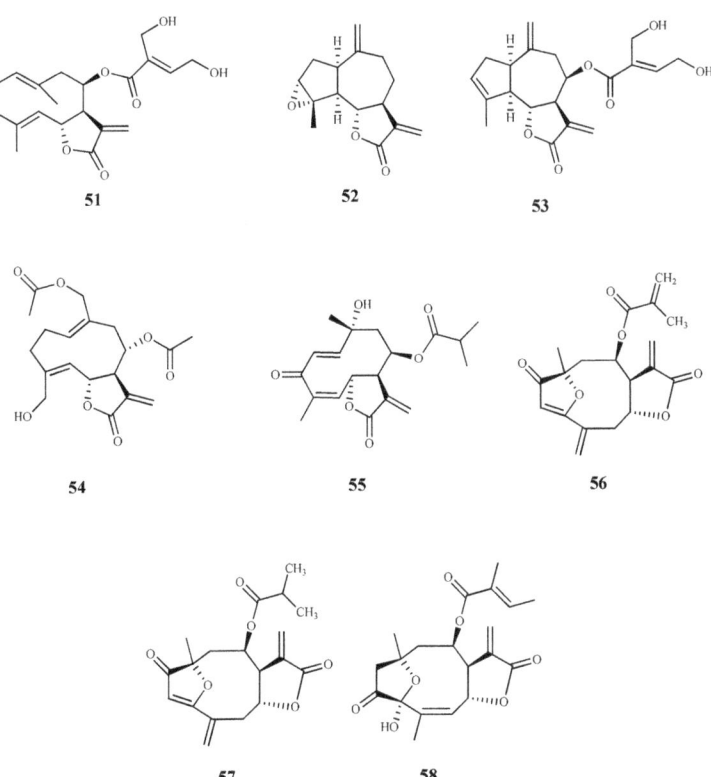

Figure 7. Structures of sesquiterpenes 51–58.

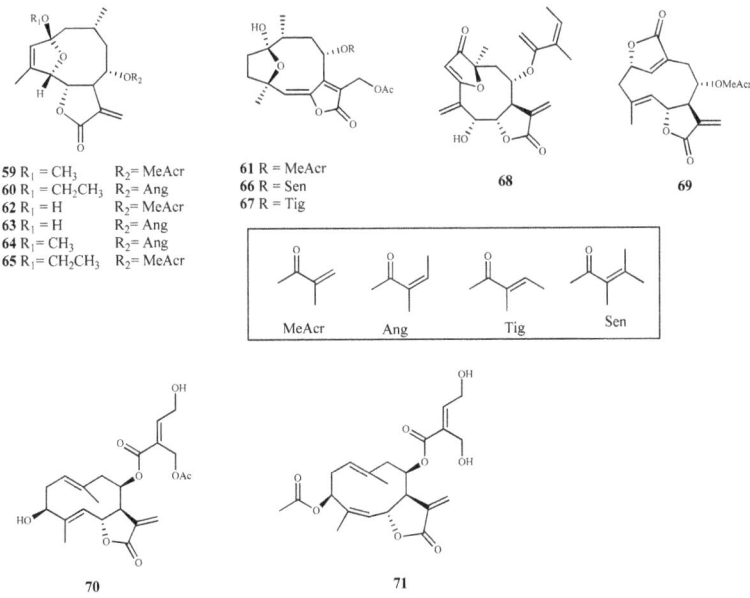

Figure 8. Structures of sesquiterpenes 59–71.

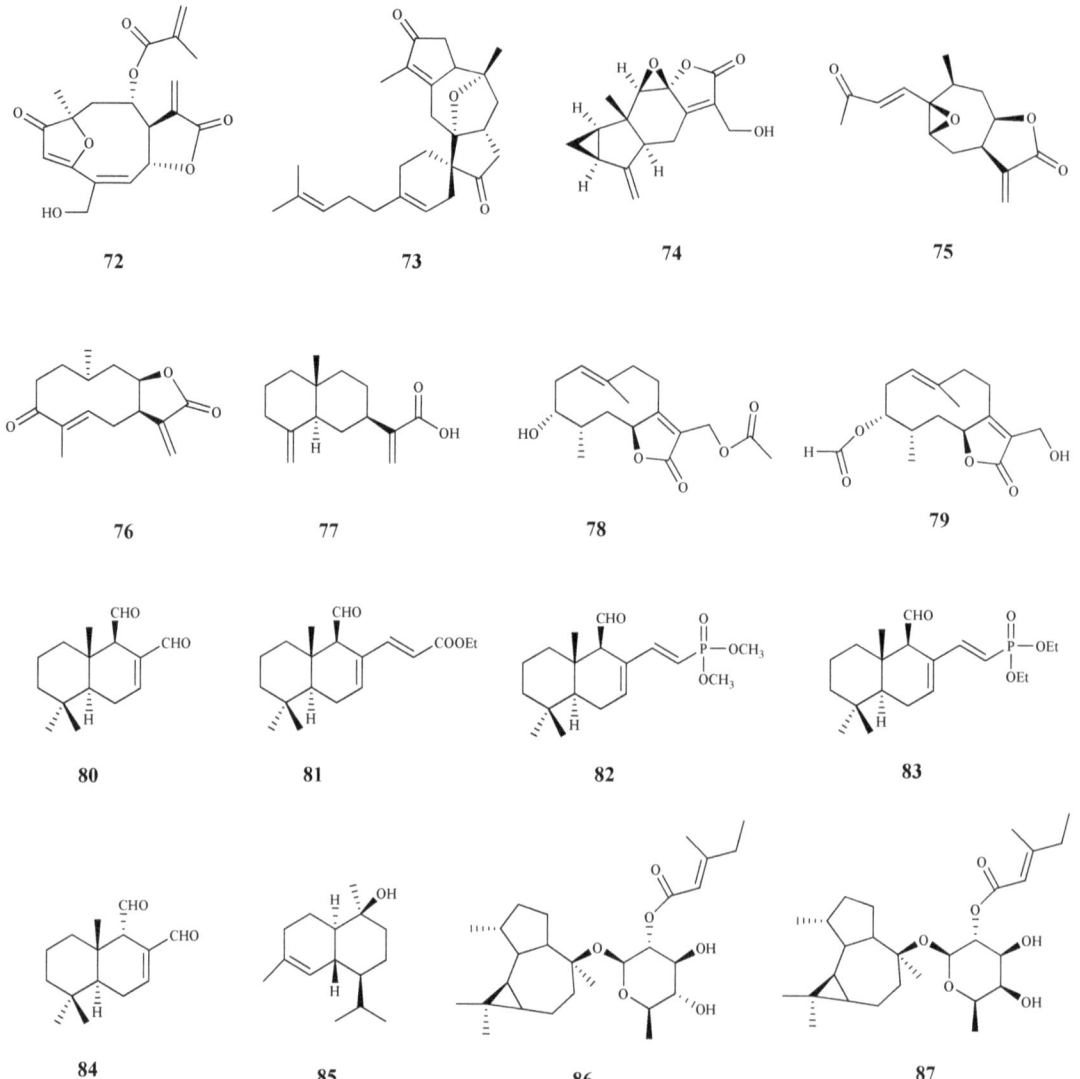

Figure 9. Structures of sesquiterpenes **72–87**.

The in vitro antitrypanosomal activities are expressed in micromolar concentrations (μM) and some were transformed into this unit to allow an accurate comparison. Furthermore, the in vitro cytotoxicity of these compounds on mammalian cells lines is also indicated, when evaluated simultaneously, allowing the assessment of the selectivity index (SI). SI is defined as the ratio between the half-maximal cytotoxic concentration against the mammalian cell line (CC_{50}) and the half-maximal inhibitory concentration against the parasite (IC_{50}) [51,52]. Although the SI values do not allow extrapolation to the in vivo condition, this parameter is valuable for the selection of compounds with selective activity against trypanosomes.

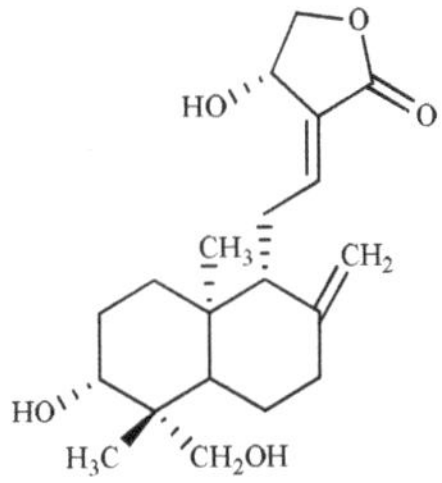

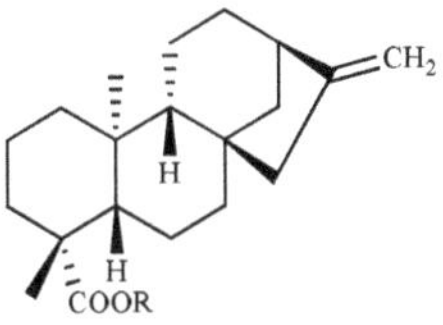

90 R = H
92 R = CH$_3$
93 R = 4-BrPhCH$_2$

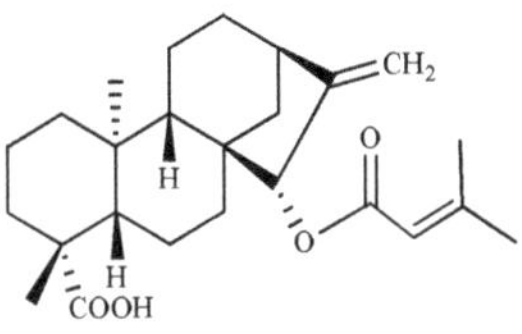

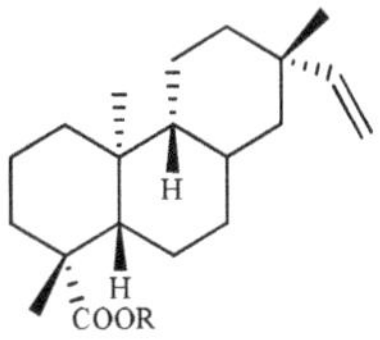

91 R = H
94 R = CH$_3$

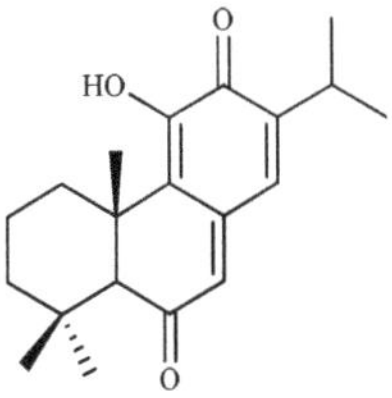

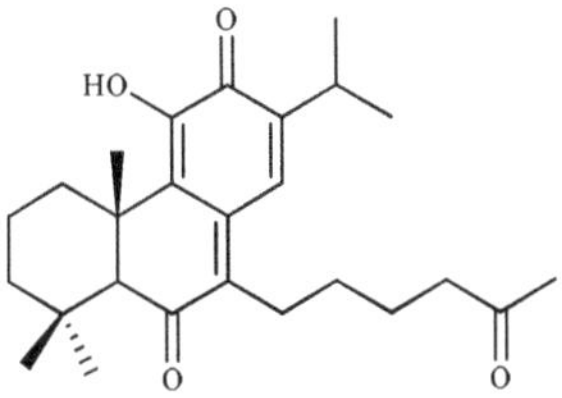

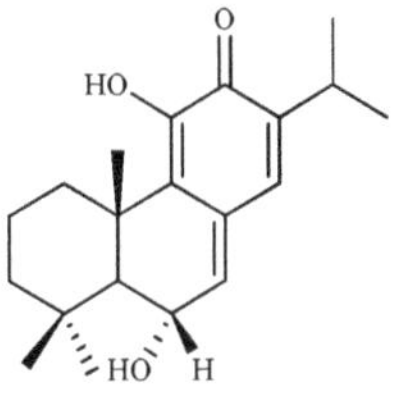

Figure 10. Structures of diterpenes **88–97**.

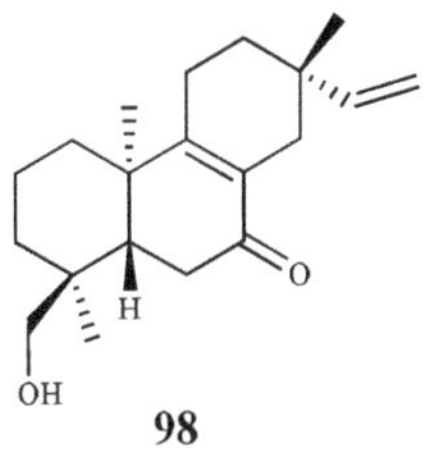

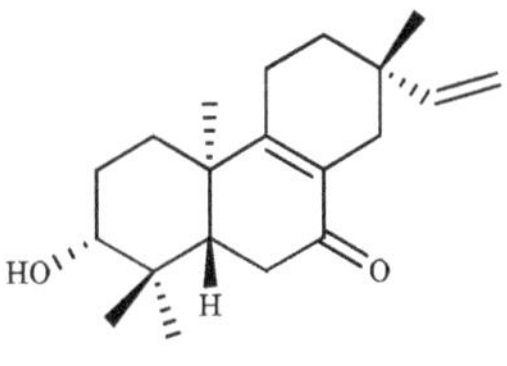

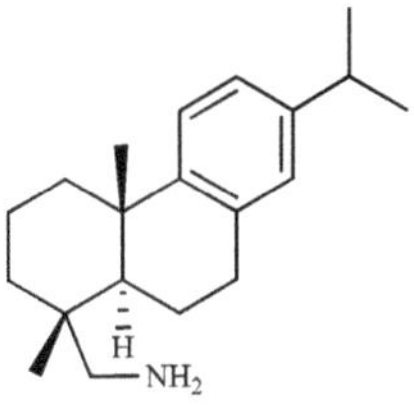

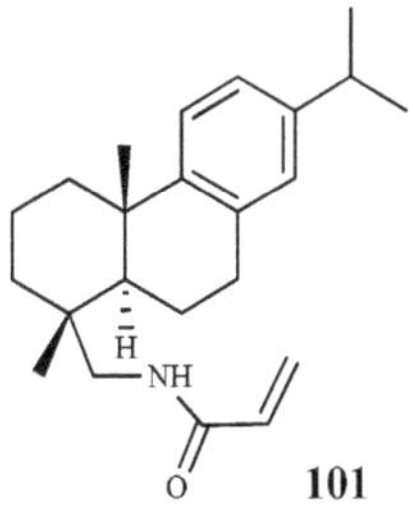

Figure 11. Structures of diterpenes **98–104**.

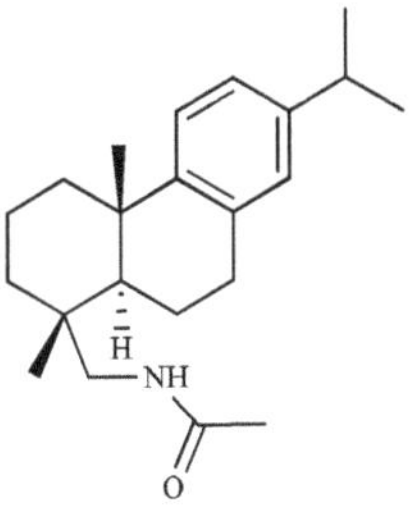

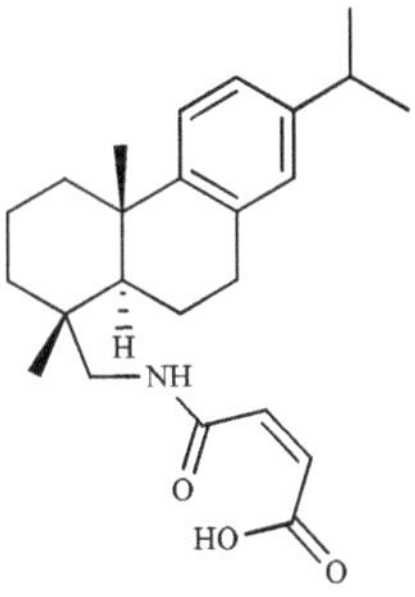

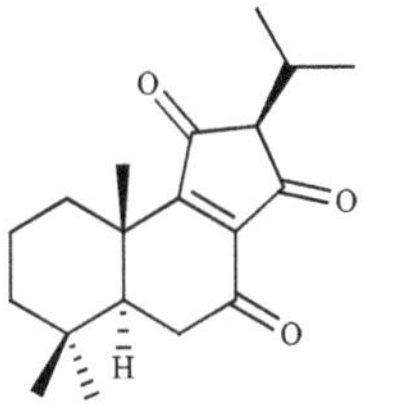

105
106
107
108
109
110
111
112
113
114
115

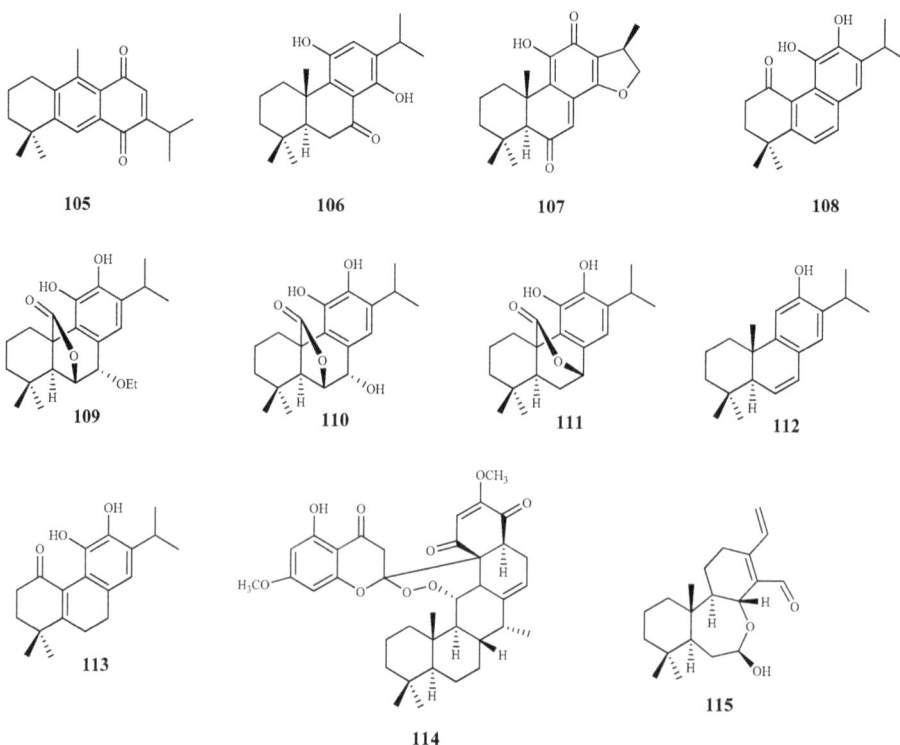

Figure 12. Structures of diterpenes **105–115**.

116
117 R= Xyl (2->1)Rha
118
119
120
121

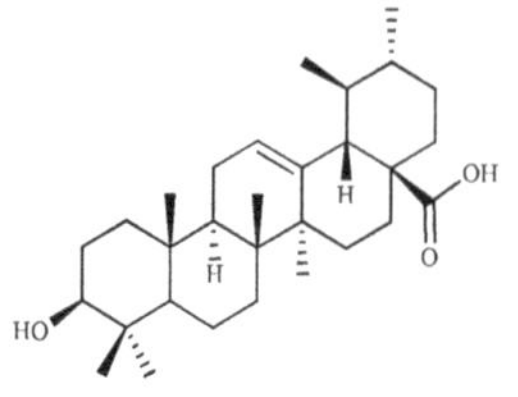

Figure 13. Structures of triterpenes **116–121**.

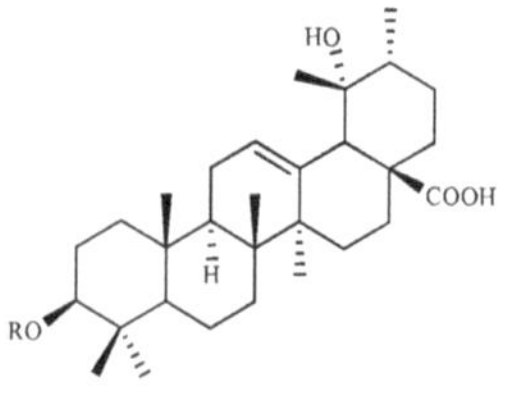

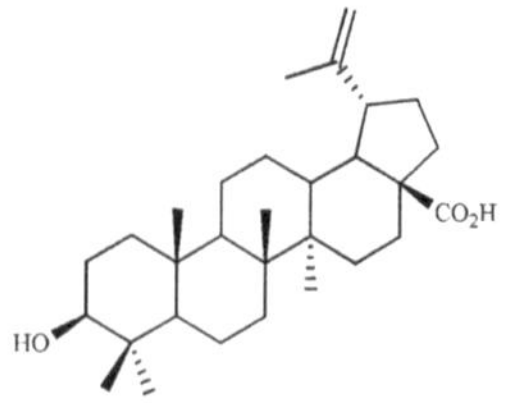

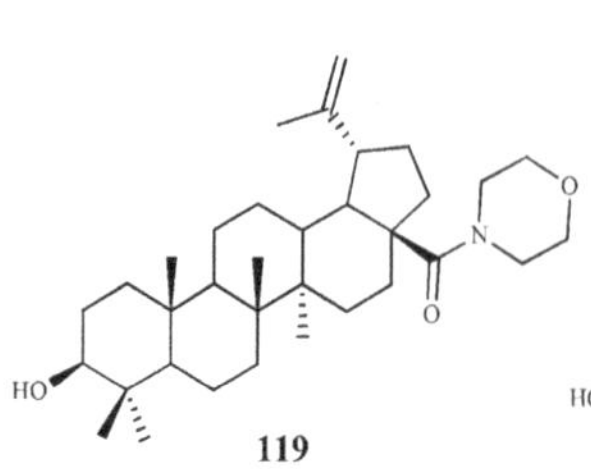

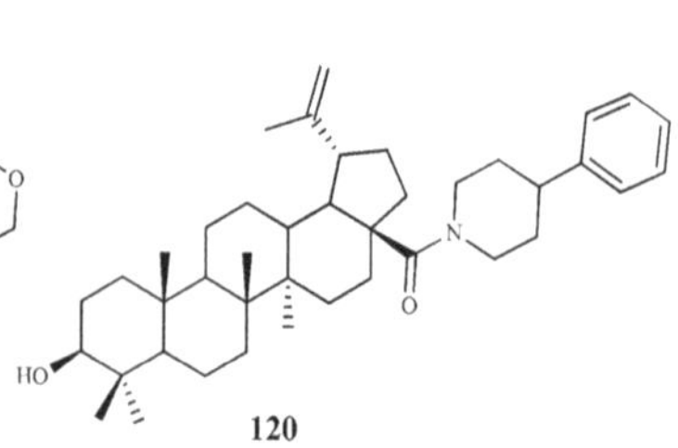

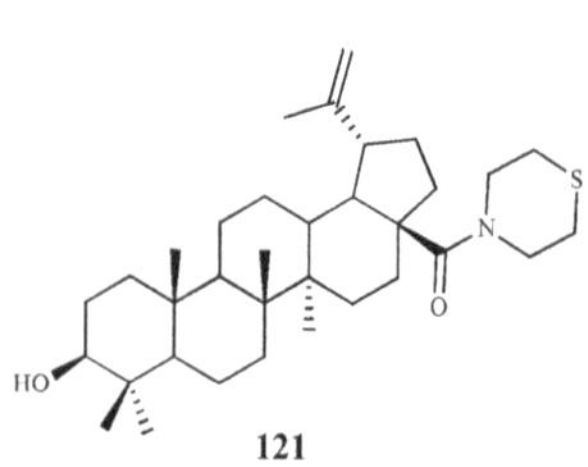

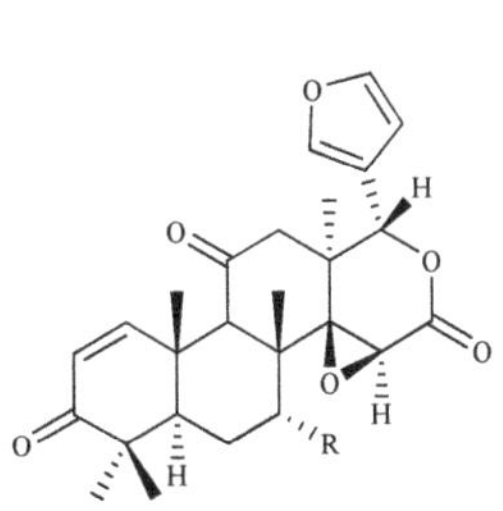

Figure 14. Structures of triterpenes **122–135**.

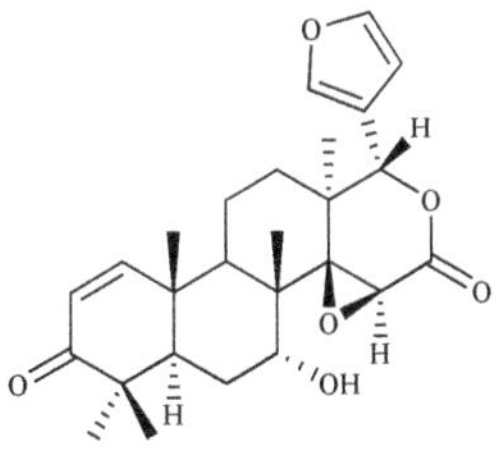

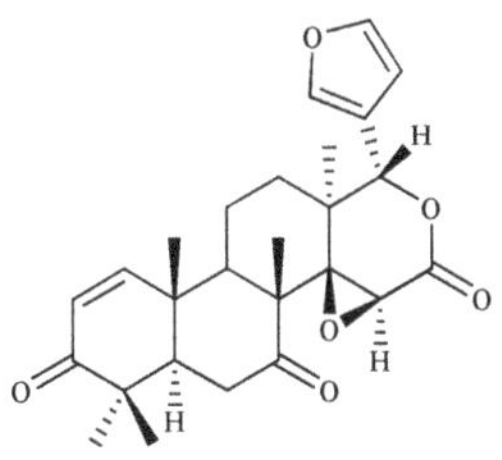

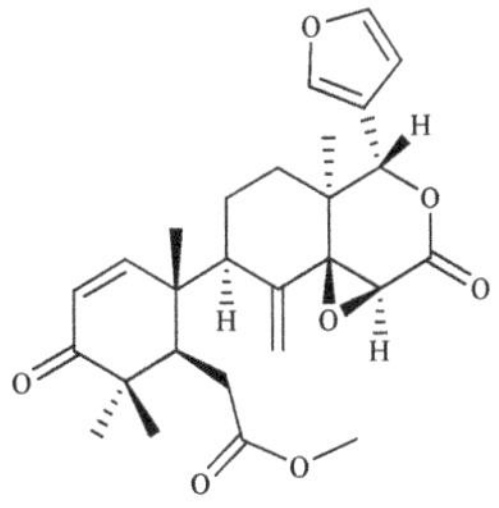

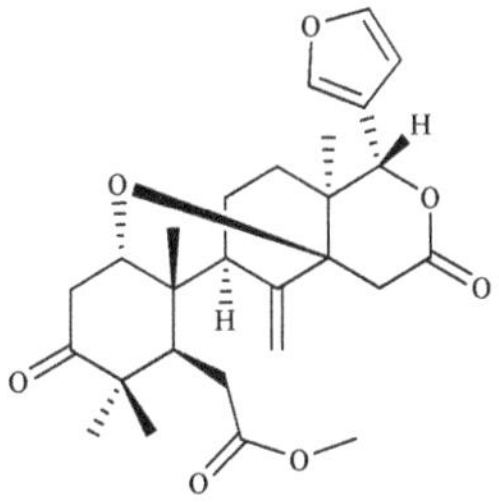

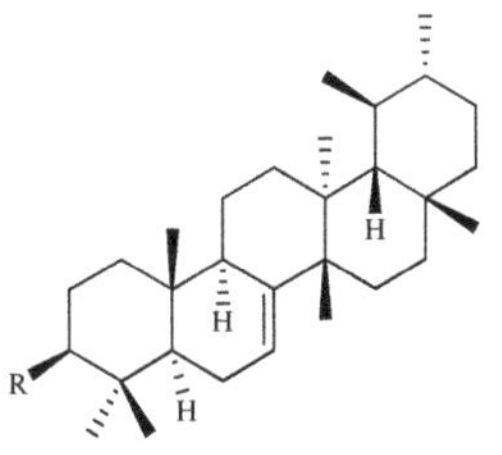

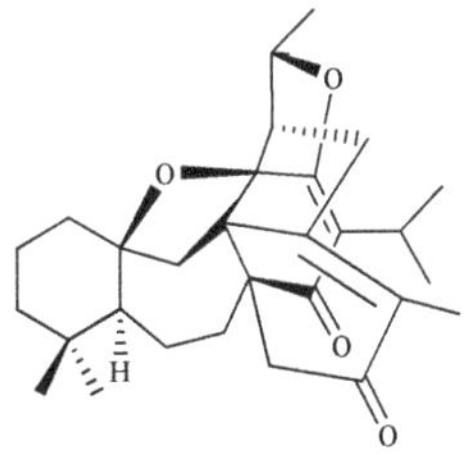

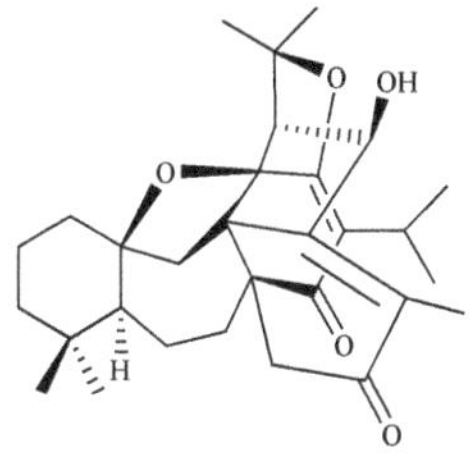

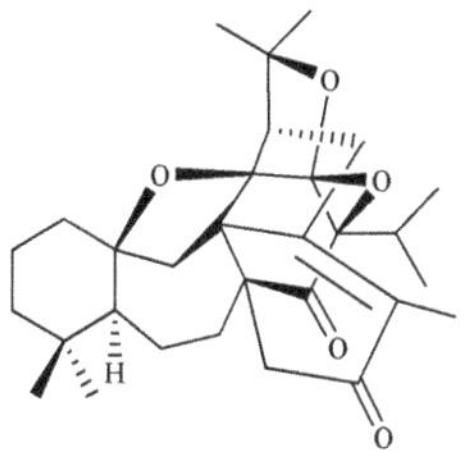

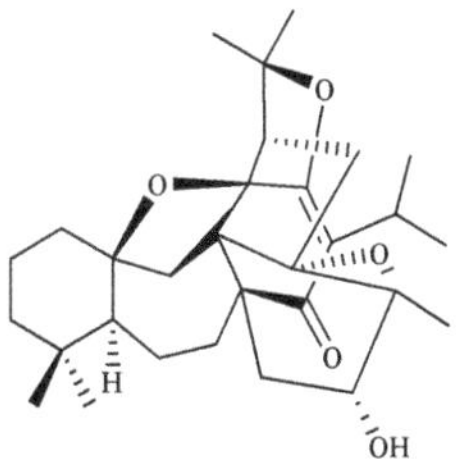

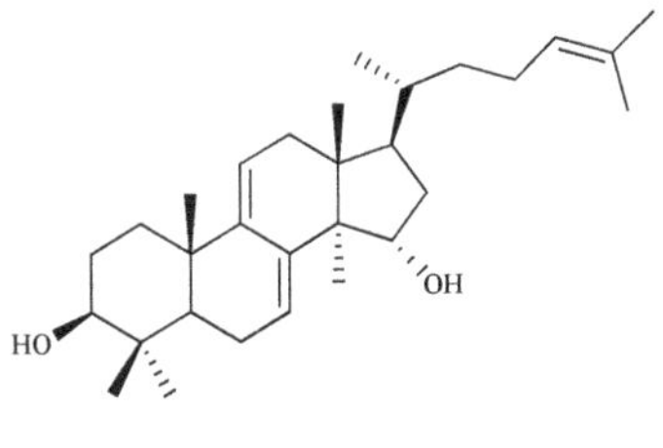

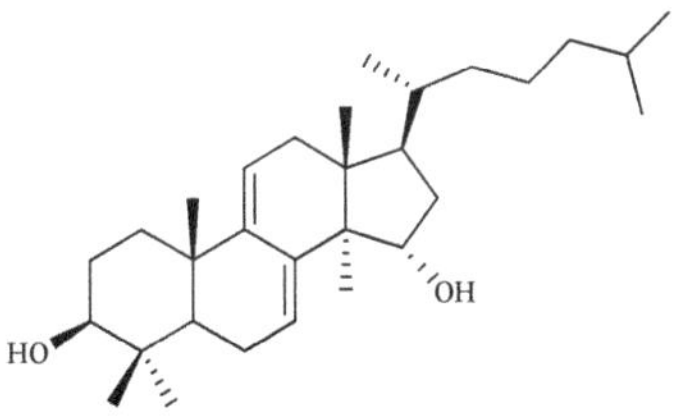

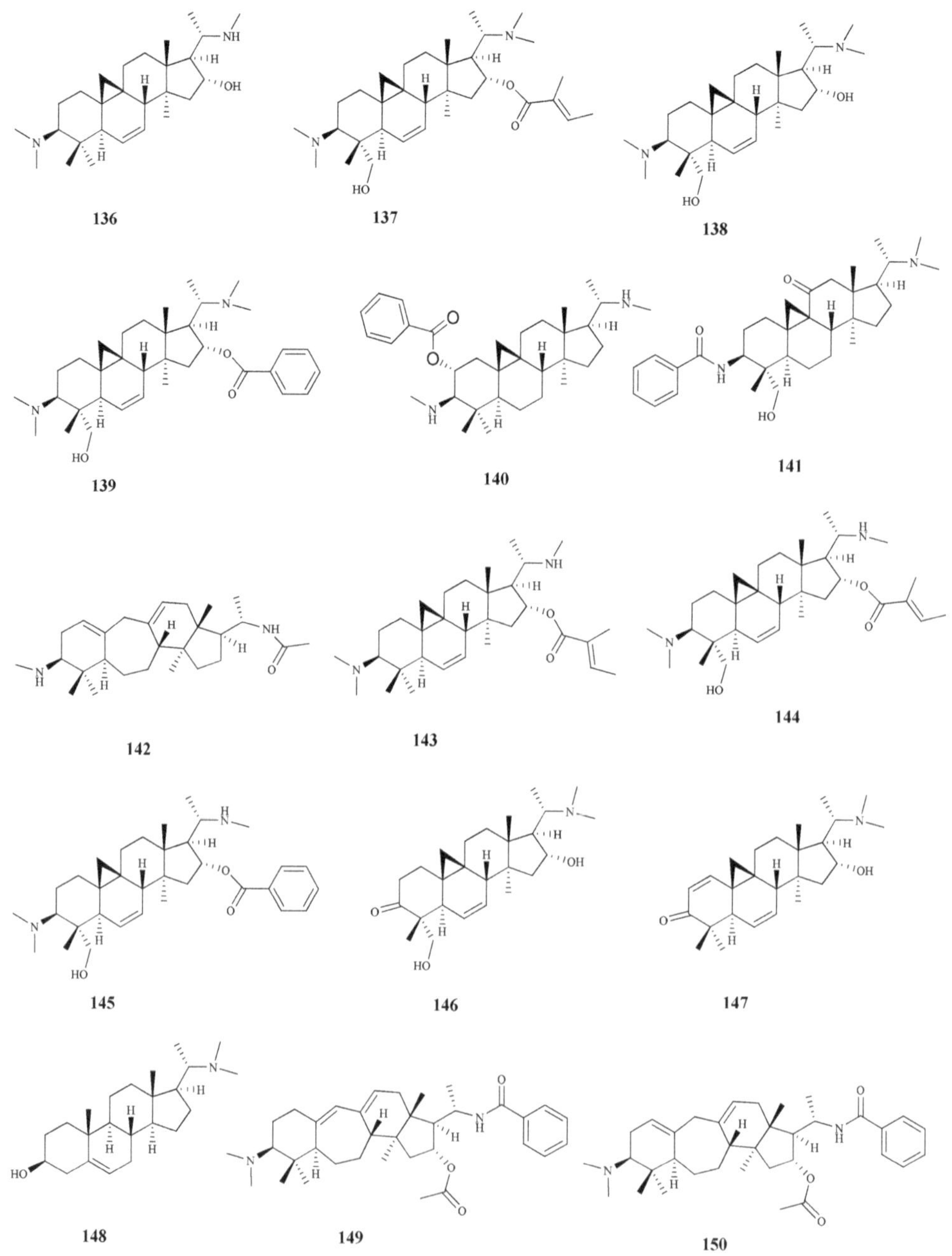

Figure 15. Structures of triterpenes **136–150**.

Presently, there are general and specific criteria proposed by DNDi aiming at identifying hit and lead compounds for further development of drugs against trypanosomiasis, and other infectious diseases. Although these criteria are not strictly applied, they are very important to guide the development of hit and lead series, taking into account their potency, selectivity, toxicity, and chemical profile, among other requirements [51]. For a hit definition, the criteria are divided into two main sets: the disease-specific criteria that focus on potency, efficacy, pathogenicity, and the compound-specific criteria that evaluate the chemical profile of the compounds, in silico pharmacokinetics and pharmacodynamics (DMPK), as well as the physical properties that are predictive of oral therapy [52]. Accordingly, a compound is considered active if it has an $IC_{50} \leq 10$ µM in the in vitro assay against the bloodstream forms of *T. b. brucei* subspecies, and against the *T. cruzi* intracellular amastigote forms (TcVI (Tulahuen) or TcII/Y strain) [51,52]. The selectivity of the promising hit compound should be 10-fold higher for the parasite than for the mammalian cell line tested. On the other hand, a lead compound for a future drug against HAT or CD should display an IC_{50} value more than 10–20-fold higher than the IC_{50} value of the hit compound, and ideally, its selectivity should be ≥ 50 times higher for the parasite than for the mammalian cell line. Moreover, a significant reduction in parasitemia and/or increase in life-span should be observed in the acute mouse model of HAT at the end of the treatment with up to 4 doses at 50 mg/kg (*i.p* or *p.o*). Concerning CD, the lead selection criteria include a hit that causes an 80% parasitemia reduction in organs or tissues, or no parasites detected at the end of treatment and an increase in lifespan with up to 10 doses at 50 mg/kg (*p.o*) in a mouse model [51,52].

3.1. Monoterpenes and Iridoids

Compound **1** is a limonene benzaldehyde-thiosemicarbazone derivative that showed in vitro antitrypanosomal activity and high selectivity against *T. cruzi* amastigotes (IC_{50} 1.3 µM, CC_{50} 795 µM, mammalian LLCMK2; SI = 611.2). It is believed that this compound act by inhibiting the proliferation of *T. cruzi* and inducing morphological changes that lead to the cell death of the parasite. In addition, a reduction in cell volume, depolarization of the mitochondrial membrane and an increase in production of reactive oxygen species (ROS) were also observed. Due to promising in vitro results, an in vivo study was performed on a murine model of acute Chagas disease, and a significant reduction in parasitemia in animals treated with **1** alone (100 mg/kg/day) or combined with benznidazole (5 mg/kg/day each) was found, when compared to the untreated animals. Moreover, it was observed that the survival rate of the animals treated with both compounds during the period of infection was the same that the group treated just with benznidazole, however, with only 5% of the dose used [53].

The essential oil of *Origanum onites* L. and its major components carvacrol (**2**) and thymol (**3**) were evaluated for their antitrypanosomal activity against *T. b. rhodesiense* trypomastigote forms (mammalian stage), and *T. cruzi* amastigotes. Good results were only observed against *T. b. rhodesiense*, and both compounds showed IC_{50} values of 1.0 µM and 0.73 µM, respectively, and a high selectivity for the parasite (SI = 327.5 and 454.4, respectively, L6 mammalian cell line). Additionally, in the in vivo *T. b. brucei* mouse model, only compound **3** extended the mean survival of animals, while none cured the infected animals when compared to the reference drug pentamidine [54].

The essential oils of some Apiaceae plants (*Echinophora spinosa* L., *Sison amomum* L., *Crithmum maritimum* L., *Helosciadium nodiflorum* (L.) W.D.J.Koch) were studied against *T. brucei* bloodstream forms (TC221 BSFs strain), showing IC_{50} values in the range of 2.7–10.7 µg/mL. From those, only the essential oil of *C. maritimum* had a good selectivity (SI = 13, mouse Balb3T3 fibroblasts cell line). Additionally, using the same parasite, the trypanocidal activity of the major compounds (**4–6**) of *C. maritimum* was also tested. Terpinolene (**4**) was the most potent showing an IC_{50} value of 0.26 µM with a SI = 180. Two other compounds displayed promising activities on the same model namely α-pinene (**5**, IC_{50} = 7.4 µM, SI > 100) and β-ocimene (**6**, IC_{50} = 8 µM, SI > 91) [55].

Three tetracyclic iridoids (**7–9**) were isolated from *Morinda lucida* Benth., a plant traditionally used to treat parasitic diseases in West Africa. Iridoids were evaluated for their in vitro activity against the bloodstream forms of *T. b. brucei*. Compound **7** was the most active (IC_{50} 0.43 µM) and less toxic than **8** (IC_{50} 1.27 µM), displaying CC_{50} values of 14.24 µM (SI = 33.1) and 4.74 µM (SI = 3.7), respectively [56]. The activity of compound **9** is lower than **7** and **8** (IC$_{50}$ 3.75 µM), but it did not show cytotoxicity (CC$_{50}$ ≤ 50 µM) [56]. The main structural differences between compounds **7–9** are the functional groups at C-4 on the side chain. Compound **9** has a carboxylic acid, while compound **7** and **8** have ethyl ester and methyl functional groups, respectively [56]. SI values of the three compounds showed that **7** and **9** are more specific against the parasite than compound **8**. Compound **7** was tested in vivo, and a complete clearance of parasitemia, with 100% cure for 20 days post infection, was observed, when 5 consecutive daily shots of 30 mg/kg of compound **7** were taken. It was concluded that compounds **7** and **9** suppressed the expression of paraflagellum rod protein subunit 2, and caused cell cycle alteration, which can preceded apoptosis induction in the bloodstream form of the parasite [56].

3.2. Sesquiterpenes

Two sesquiterpene lactones (**10** and **11**) were isolated from the methanolic extract of *Tithonia diversifolia* (Hemsl) A. Grey, and their activities were evaluated against the blood forms of T. brucei [57]. Compound **10** was the most active, exhibiting a very low IC$_{50}$ value (0.012 µM), but displaying a high cytotoxicity on the mammalian fibroblasts cells (CC$_{50}$ 0.036 µM, SI = 3). Likewise, compound **11** showed antitrypanosomal activity (IC$_{50}$ 0.97 µM) and high cytotoxicity (CC$_{50}$ 1.27 µM, SI = 1.3) [57]. Some considerations can be made regarding the mechanism of action of these sesquiterpene lactones in the parasite cells. Due to the characteristic α,β-unsaturated lactone function present in these structures, which can act as a Michael acceptor, these compounds react with nucleophiles, such as thiol groups in proteins, leading to macromolecular dysfunction, oxidative stress and genetic mutations [57]. The presence of an extra carbonyl group conjugated with two double bonds in **10** can explain the higher antitrypanosomal activity of **10** when compared with **11**. In fact, the mechanism of action of these compounds against trypanosomes may be related with formation of thiol adducts with components found in the intracellular medium (namely trypanothione, glutathione and thiol groups in proteins). The parasite's cells become more vulnerable to oxidative stress with reduction in trypanothione [57].

Several sesquiterpene lactones were isolated from the dichloromethane extract of *Vernonia cinerascens* Sch.Bip., and evaluated for their in vitro activity against the blood forms of T. b. rhodesiense and for cytotoxicity on the L6 mammalian cell line [58]. Lactone **12** was the most active and selective exhibiting an IC$_{50}$ value of 0.16 µM and SI = 35. Compounds **13** and **14** also showed activity against T. b rhodesiense (IC$_{50}$ values of 0.5 µM and 1.1 µM, SI = 13 and 4.2, respectively), being lactone **13** the most selective [58]. Compounds **15** and **16** exhibited similar activities; however, compound **15** showed a higher selectivity (IC$_{50}$ values of 4.8 µM and 5.0 µM, SI = 27 and 4.3, respectively). Moreover, lactones **12–16** displayed the lowest cytotoxicity in the cells tested [CC$_{50}$ 5.6 µM (**12**), CC$_{50}$ 6.9 µM (**13**), CC$_{50}$ 4.7 µM (**14**), CC$_{50}$ 128 µM (**15**), CC$_{50}$ 22 µM (**16**)] [58,59].

Two sesquiterpene lactones (**17** and **18**) isolated from the dichloromethane extract of *Tarchonanthus camphoratus* L. aerial parts, and twenty sesquiterpene lactones, including compounds **19–27** obtained from *Schkuhria pinnata* (Lam.) Kuntze ex Thell. were studied for their in vitro antitrypanosomal activity and cytotoxicity on mammalian L6 cell lines [60]. Lactones **17** and **18** were active against *T. b. rhodesiense* with IC$_{50}$ values of 0.39 µM and 2.8 µM, respectively. Furthermore, **17** (SI = 18.6, CC$_{50}$ 7.2 µM) proved to be more selective although it was more cytotoxic than **18** (SI = 6.2, CC$_{50}$ 17.3 µM) [60]. Regarding compounds isolated from *S. pinnata*, most of them displayed antitrypanosomal activity with IC$_{50}$ values ranging from 0.10 to 7.30 µM, Compounds **19** and **20** stood out for their high activities against the trypomastigotes, with IC$_{50}$ values of 0.10 and 0.13 µM, respectively. However, they exhibited cytotoxicity on the cells tested (CC$_{50}$ values of 2.10 and 3.90 µM, respectively) despite exhibiting some selectivity (SI = 20.5 and 29.7, respectively). Compounds **21** (IC$_{50}$ 0.35 µM, SI = 11.5) and **22** (IC$_{50}$ 0.52 µM, SI = 13) were particularly active, but cytotoxic against the mammalian cell lines assayed (CC$_{50}$ values of 4.10 and 6.80 µM, respectively). Moreover, compounds **23** (IC$_{50}$ 0.60 µM, SI = 19.2), **24** (IC$_{50}$ 0.82 µM, SI = 13.4), **25** (IC$_{50}$ 0.91 µM, SI = 15.8) and **26** (IC$_{50}$ 0.92 µM, SI = 15.8) also showed very good activities. Finally, sesquiterpene **27** display an IC_{50} value of 1.7 µM, and was the most selective and least cytotoxic in this group of compounds (SI = 31.1 and CC_{50} 54.6 µM) [60].

Three sesquiterpene lactones (**28–30**) were isolated from the dichloromethane extract of *Achillea fragrantissima* (Forssk.) Sch.Bip. and tested against trypomastigote forms of *T. b. brucei* [61]. Lactone **28** was the most active (IC_{50} 3.03 µM), while lactones **29** and **30** showed the same activity against the parasite with IC_{50} value of 10.97 µM. The authors did not assess the cytotoxicity of these compounds on mammalian cells [61].

Four sesquiterpene lactones were isolated by bioassay-guided fractionation from extracts of *Mikania variifolia* Hieron. and *Mikania micrantha* Kunth, and evaluated against the epimastigote, trypomastigote and amastigote forms of *T. cruzi*. Compounds **31** and **32** were found in both extracts (2.2% and 0.4% for *M. variifolia*, and 21.0% and 6.4% for *M. micrantha*, respectively, calculated based on the dry extract) [62]. Three of the isolated lactones (**31**, **32**, and **33**) showed trypanocidal activity, being active against the epimastigote form with IC_{50} values of 2.41 (SI = 31.9), 0.29 (SI = 992.5) and 8.55 (SI = 5.2) µM, respectively [62]. Compounds **31**, **32** and **33** also displayed activity against the trypomastigote form of the parasite with IC_{50} values of 7.24 (SI = 10.6), 5.43 (SI = 54.0) and 1.03 (SI = 49.0) µM, respectively. Finally, the activities of **31**, **32** and **33** against the amastigote forms were lower than those observed for the two previous forms of the parasite (IC_{50} 15.5, 22.8 and 29.1 µM, and SI = 4.3, 12.5, and 1.5, respectively). From those compounds, **32** was the most selective for the human infective parasite, showing a SI of 54 when assayed on human monocyte leukemia THP1 cells. Due to its good selectivity, **32** was also tested in an in vivo model of *T. cruzi* infection, and was able to decrease the parasitemia and the weight loss associated with the acute phase of the parasite infection. Additionally, 70% of treated mice (1 mg/kg of body weight/day) survived, while all of the control mice died by day 22 after the infection. The authors also observed that this compound increased the production of TNF-α and IL-12 by macrophages [62].

The essential oils from different parts of *Smyrnium olusatrum* L. were evaluated against the bloodstream forms of *T. b. brucei*. All oils effectively inhibited the growth of the parasite [63]. From the main constituents of essential oils, sesquiterpene **34** exhibited a significant and selective inhibitory activity against the tested parasite (IC_{50} 3.0 µM, SI = 30, mouse Balb/3T3 fibroblast)) [63].

From *Anthemis nobilis* L. dichlorometane extract, 19 sesquiterpene lactones, including 15 germacranolides, 2 seco-sesquiterpenes, 1 guaianolide sesquiterpene lactone, and 1 cadinane acid were obtained [64]. Among these compounds, thirteen were tested for their in vitro activity against the bloodstream forms of *T. b rhodesiense*, with compound **35** being the most potent and selective (IC_{50} 0.08 µM, SI = 63.1). Compounds **36–38** exhibited also a significant anti-trypanosomal activity, but with lower selectivity (**36**, IC_{50} 0.61 µM, SI = 8.3; **37**, IC_{50} 0.36 µM, SI = 14.1; **38**, IC_{50} 0.88 µM, SI = 8.3). Moreover, the compounds were assessed against *T. cruzi* intracellular amastigotes, and the best result was observed for compound **39** (IC_{50} 2.8 µM), but a very low selectivity index was also observed (SI = 0.5). Compound **39** also exhibited a good activity against *T. b rhodesiense* (IC_{50} 0.4 µM), but with a low selectivity due to its cytotoxicity on mammalian L6 cells (CC_{50} 1.5 µM, SI = 3.8). Compound **40** was considered the one with higher selectivity for *T. cruzi* (IC_{50} 4.2 µM, SI = 6.1) [64].

Calea pinnatifida (R. Br.) Less. is used in folk medicine as giardicidal, amoebicidal and to treat digestive disorders. Its phytochemical study led to the isolation of a furanoheliangolide sesquiterpene lactone (11,13-dihydroxy-calaxin, **41**) which showed a promising trypanocidal activity, displaying an IC_{50} value of 8.30 µM against *T. cruzi* amastigotes, and inhibiting the parasite growth in 94.3%. However, compound **41** presented a low selectivity for the parasite cells (CC_{50} < 15.60 µM on THP-1 cells) [65].

Three sesquiterpene lactones (**42–44**) were isolated from *Smallanthus sonchifolius* (Poepp.) H. Rob. and evaluated against *T. cruzi* epimastigotes, using benzonidazole as positive control [66]. Compounds **42** and **43** showed identical activities with IC_{50} values of 0.78 and 0.79 µM, respectively. Lactone **44** was also active exhibiting an IC_{50} value of 1.38 µM. All compounds were more effective than benzonidazole (IC$_{50}$ 10.6 µM). The authors did not assess the cytotoxicity of these compounds on mammalian cells. Due to the high in vitro activity, compounds **42** and **43** were also tested on mice inoculated with *T. cruzi* trypomastigotes. A significant decrease in circulating parasites (50–71%) was observed, with no signs of toxicity in the dose administrated (1 mg/kg/day). Complementary studies showed marked ultrastructural alteration in trypanosome parasites when treated with these compounds [66].

Several sesquiterpenes isolated from the Cameroonian spice *Scleria striatinux* De Wild. were studied for their in vitro and in silico antiparasitic activity [67]. From those, sesquiterpene **45** exhibited the best activity against *T. cruzi* and *T. b. rhodesiense* bloodstreams forms, with IC$_{50}$ values of 0.025 µM (SI = 0.74) and 0.002 µM (SI = 8.3), respectively, but the compounds were cytotoxic on HT-29 (human bladder carcinoma) cells. On the other hand, compound **46** showed better activity against *T. b. rhodesiense* than *T. cruzi*, with IC$_{50}$ values of 0.025 µM (SI = 3.4) and 0.085 µM (SI = 1), respectively [67]. The in silico drug metabolism and pharmacokinetic parameters of these two sesquiterpene isomers were also studied, showing compound **46** a good solubility profile, moderate partition coefficient and acceptable in silico pharmacokinetic properties. Similar characteristics were observed for compound **45**, but with less optimal parameters, namely for the partition coefficient [67]. Nevertheless, despite the good pharmacokinetic features and the low IC$_{50}$ values observed, SI values were very small, and compounds also showed a considerable cytotoxicity against HT-29 cell line, which reduces its possible application as a hit compound.

Vernonia lasiopus (O.Hoffm.) H.Rob. extracts were obtained with solvents of different polarities and evaluated in vitro for antiprotozoal activity [59]. The dichloromethane extract was shown to be particularly active against *T. b. rhodesiense*, and its phytochemical study led to the isolation and identification of six sesquiterpene lactones. These compounds were tested for their in vitro antitrypanosomal activity and cytotoxicity on L6 mammalian cells [59]. Compound **47**, the main component of the extract, was the most potent against *T. b. rhodesiense* trypomastigotes (IC$_{50}$ 0.185 µM); however, it displayed some cytotoxicity (CC$_{50}$ 2.68 µM and SI = 14.5). Moreover, compound **48** presented very similar values (IC$_{50}$ 0.26 µM, CC$_{50}$ 3.67 µM, SI = 14.4). Lactone **49** was the least selective (SI = 4.5) and displayed some cytotoxicity (CC$_{50}$ 2.26 µM), despite showing a considerable antitrypanosomal activity (IC$_{50}$ 0.51 µM). Compound **50** was the least cytotoxic compound in this group (CC$_{50}$ 34.6 µM, SI = 13.7) still showing a good activity against trypomastigotes (IC$_{50}$ 2.53 µM) [59].

On a recent work, the sesquiterpene lactones eupatoriopicrin (**51**), estafietin (**52**), eupahakonenin B (**53**) and minimolide (**54**) isolated from Argentinean Astearaceae species, which had previously showed activity against *T. cruzi* epimastigotes, were tested against other forms of the parasite [68]. On the bloodstream forms of *T. cruzi* the IC$_{50}$ values obtained were 19.9 µM (**51**, SI = 12.9), 33.0 µM (**53**, SI = 10.4), and 21.0 µM (**54**, SI = 12.8). On the intracellular *T. cruzi* amastigotes the most active compound was **51** with an IC$_{50}$ value of 6.3 µM (SI = 40.6). Moderate activities were observed for compound **54** (IC$_{50}$ = 25.1 µM; SI = 10.7), and **53** (IC$_{50}$ = 89.3 µM; SI = 3.8) against the same form of the parasite. The majority of compounds showed a significant selectivity for the parasite forms tested compared to Vero cells. The in vivo administration of eupatoriopicrin (**51**, 1 mg/kg/day) to mice infected with *T. cruzi* trypomastigotes, for five consecutive days, produced a significant reduction in the parasitemia levels in comparison with non-treated animals (area under parasitemia curves 4.48 vs. 30.47, respectively), being this reduction similar to that achieved with the reference drug, benznidazole. Authors also presented some information regarding the prevention of tissue damage during the chronic phase of the parasite infection, showing beneficial effects on skeletal and cardiac muscular tissues of infected mice treated with the sesquiterpenoid compound. Compound **52** was inactive [68].

The sesquiterpene lactone **55** (tagitinin C) isolated from leaves of *Tithonia diversifolia* (Hemsl.) A. Gray showed a high inhibition activity against the epimastigote forms of *T. cruzi*, with IC$_{50}$ of 1.15 µM, being more active than benznidazole (35.81 µM). However, the cytotoxic concentration (6.54 µM) and the selectivity index (5.69) of compound **55** did not show to be favorable. In an in vivo combination assay, it was observed a complete suppression of parasitemia and parasitological cure in all infected mice (100%) compared to those receiving benznidazole alone (70%). Moreover, despite its lower in vitro selectivity index, compound **55** was well tolerated during the in vivo assays. Interestingly, it was also found that tagitinin C was able to reduce myocarditis, especially when combined with benznidazole [69].

The antitrypanosomal potential of three sesquiterpene lactones (**56–58**) isolated from *Helianthus tuberosus* L. (Asteraceae) was evaluated against *T. b. rhodesiense* trypamastigote bloodstream form (**56**, IC_{50} 0.077 µM; **57**, 0.26 µM; **58**, 0.92 µM) and *T. cruzi* trypomastigotes (**56**, IC_{50} 1.6 µM; **57**, 3.1 µM; **58**, 5.7 µM); however, the selectivity index was not promising (CC_{50} between 0.52 and 3.9 µM, on L6 rat skeletal myoblasts) [70].

Seventeen sesquiterpene lactones were isolated from five plant species of Vernonieae tribe and assessed against *T. cruzi* epimastigotes [71]. The best trypanocidal effect was observed by elephantopus-type sesquiterpene lactones **59** (IC_{50} 1.5 µM) and **60** (IC_{50} 2.1 µM), obtained from *Vernonanthura nebularum* (Cabrera) H. Rob., and hirsutinolide **61** (IC_{50} 2.0 µM), isolated from *Vernonanthura pinguis* (Griseb.) H.Rob. Furthermore, these compounds showed a high selectivity for the parasite (SI > 14) when compared to their cytotoxic effect against the mammalian Hela cells. Compounds **62–65**, also isolated from *V. nebularum*, showed a good antitrypanosomal activity on the same strain with IC_{50} values ranging from 3.7 to 9.7 µM, being compound **62** the most selective (IC_{50} = 3.7 µM and SI = 14.3). From *V. pinguis*, besides compound **61**, compounds **66** (IC_{50} 10.7 µM; SI = 9.0) and **67** (IC_{50} 8.1 µM; SI = 13.9) were also isolated and displayed a significant activity; however, it was lower than the observed to hirsutinolide (**61**). From the remaining species, compound **68** (IC_{50} 6.8 µM; SI = 1.6) isolated from *Centratherum puctatum* ssp. Punctatum Cass. and compound **69** (IC_{50} 4.7 µM; SI = 11.5) isolated from *Elephantopus mollis* Kunth also showed antitrypanosomal activity [71].

The sesquiterpene lactones eucannabinolide (**70**) and santhemoidin C (**71**), isolated from the dewaxed dichloromethane extract of *Urolepis hecatantha* (DC.) R.King & H.Rob., were active on *T. cruzi* epimastigotes with IC_{50} values of 10 µM and 18 µM, respectively. Both compounds showed low SI values (CC_{50} > 15 µM for **70** and CC_{50} = 15 µM for **71**) [72].

Goyazensolide (**72**) is a sesquiterpene lactone isolated from *Lychnophora passerina* (Mart ex DC) Gardn. that displayed promising results against the intracellular amastigote form of *T. cruzi* (IC_{50} = 0.181 µM/24 h, and IC_{50} = 0.020 µM/48 h), showing a higher selectivity index than the positive control benznidazol (SI = 52.82 and 915.0 for **72**, at 24 h and 48 h, respectively, and SI = 4.85 and 41.0 for benznidazol, at 24 h and 48 h, respectively). Further in vivo assays were performed and **72** showed an important therapeutic activity in mice infected with *T. cruzi*, which was demonstrated by the high percentage of negative parasitological tests employed by the authors in the successive post-treatment evaluations [73].

From the leaves of *Hedyosmum brasiliense* Mart. Ex Miq., five sesquiterpene lactones together with a sesterpene were isolated and tested against the amastigote and trypomastigote forms of *T. cruzi*. Among the assessed compounds, compound **73**, with a rare terpenoid structure, was the most active displaying an IC_{50} value of 21.6 µM and SI > 9 for the amastigote form, and an IC_{50} value of 28.1 µM and SI > 7 for the trypomastigote. The remaining compounds were inactive, excepting compound **74** that exhibited a very weak activity against both parasite forms tested, and a decrease in selectivity for the parasite when compared with selectivity of compound **73** [74].

The bio-guided fractionation of ethanolic extract of leaves of *Inula viscosa* (L.) Greuter (Asteraceae) led to the isolation of two sesquiterpenoids (**75** and **76**), which were tested against *T. cruzi* epimastigotes with IC_{50} values of 4.99 µM and 15.52 µM, respectively. Both compounds showed modest SI (3.67 and 3.38, respectively), when compared to murine macrophages cells [75]. A preliminary structure-activity study of these compounds demonstrated the importance of the lactone ring to the antiparasitic activity. Regarding the mechanism of action, authors suggested that compounds induced programmed cell death in the tested parasite [75].

Costic acid (**77**), a eudesmane sesquiterpenoid isolated from the bio-guided fractionation of the n-hexane extract of *Nectandra barbellata* Coe-Teix. Twigs (Lauraceae) induced a trypanocidal effect with high selectivity for the intracellular amastigote form of *T. cruzi* (IC$_{50}$ 7.9 µM). A modest activity against *T. cruzi* trypomastigotes was also observed (IC$_{50}$ 37.8 µM). No cytotoxicity was observed on L929 human cells, revealing its selectivity for both forms of the parasite (CC$_{50}$ > 200 µM, SI > 25 on amastigote forms and SI > 5 on trypomastigote forms). The authors suggested that costic acid (**77**) has a key action on the mitochondria activity of the parasite [76].

Some germacranolide sesquiterpene lactones were isolated from the aerial parts and flowers of *Tanacetum sonbolii* Mozaff. Compounds **78** and **79** were the most active showing an IC$_{50}$ of 5.1 and 10.2 µM, respectively, against *T. b. rhodesiense* bloodstream forms, and SI values of 3.9 (**78**) and 4.0 (**79**) when compared with rat myoblast (L6) cells [77].

The bicyclic drimane-type sesquiterpene polygodial (**80**), firstly isolated from *Polygonum hydropiper* L. (Polygonaceae), and some natural and synthetic compounds of the same family were evaluated for growth inhibition against the amastigote, trypomastigote, and epimastigote forms of *T. cruzi*. The parent drug **80** exhibited a moderate inhibitory activity (GI$_{50}$ = 34.4 µM amastigotes; GI$_{50}$ = 68.2 µM trypomastigotes; GI$_{50}$ = 51.0 µM epimastigotes). The best inhibition growth activities were observed for its synthetic derivatives, namely compound **81** (GI$_{50}$ = 9.9 µM amastigotes; GI$_{50}$ = 8.4 µM trypomastigotes; GI$_{50}$ = 13.0 µM epimastigotes), **82** (GI$_{50}$ = 6.7 µM amastigotes; GI$_{50}$ = 6.4 µM trypomastigotes; GI$_{50}$ = 12.3 µM epimastigotes), and **83** (GI$_{50}$ = 8.3 µM amastigotes; GI$_{50}$ = 6.9 µM trypomastigotes; GI$_{50}$ = 7.2 µM epimastigotes). Selectivity index values were not determined. The synthetic α,β-unsaturated phosphonate (**83**) was favorably compared with the clinically approved drugs benznidazole and nifurtimox during a competition assay, being even effective against trypomastigotes, contrarily to benznidazole that showed no activity against this trypanosomal form. The effect of polygodial derivative **81** on the growth of the parasite in infected human retinal pigment epithelial (ARPE) cells was studied using confocal microscopy. A significant reduction in the intracellular parasites was observed, with no alterations of replication or viability of the cells [78]. Compound **80** was also previously isolated from the Chilean species *Drimys winteri*, and was tested on the same parasite forms with weak comparable results. On this work, the authors associated the trypanosomal activity of this compound with intracellular effects occurring in the parasite, namely, mitochondrial dysfunctions, ROS production and autophagic phenotype [79].

Epi-polygodial (**84**), isolated from the Brazilian plant *Drimys brasiliensis* Miers (Winteraceae), exhibited a high parasite selectivity towards *T. cruzi* trypomastigotes (IC$_{50}$ = 5.01 µM, SI > 40 to NCTC cells). Authors correlated the antitrypanosomal activity of this compound with its effects on cellular membranes by the interaction of **84** with DPPE-monolayers (the Langmuir monolayers of dipalmitoylphosphoethanolamine) at the air–water interface, which affects the physical chemical properties of the mixed film [80].

The sesquiterpene (-)-T-cadinol (**85**) isolated from *Casearia sylvestris* Sw. displayed a moderate activity against amastigotes and trypomastigotes forms of *T. cruzi* with IC$_{50}$ values of 15.8 and 18.2 µM, respectively, and no toxic effect on the mammalian cells was observed (CC$_{50}$ 200 µM, SI > 15). The mechanism of action was studied using different techniques, and it was observed that **85** affected the parasite mitochondria. However, additional studies are necessary in order to confirm this organelle as a candidate target [81].

A sesquiterpene glycoside ester (**86**) isolated from the flowers of *Calendula officinalis* L. have shown a moderate activity against *T. brucei* (IC$_{50}$ 16.9 µM). A closely similar compound (**87**), only differing in the type of sugar residue, did not display antitrypanosomal activity, suggesting the importance of sugar moiety conformation to the activity [82].

3.3. Diterpenes

Andrographolide (**88**) is a labdane-type diterpene, isolated from *Andrographis paniculate* (Burm. F.) Wall. Ex Nees, with reported anticancer, anti-inflammatory, antioxidant, cardioprotective and hepatoprotective properties [83]. To determine its effect on the viability of *T. brucei* procyclic trypomastigotes (the form of the parasite that differentiate in the insect gut), the parasites were incubated at different concentrations (0–200 µM) for 72 h. Compound **88** inhibited the growth of the parasite, exhibiting an IC_{50} = 8.3 µM and SI = 8.5. At this concentration, no cytotoxic effect was observed (CC_{50} 70.5 µM) [83]. Giemsa staining of parasites treated with **88** allowed the observation of morphological changes, in particular, loss of integrity, damage to the cell membrane, general rounding, and loss of cells' flagella. Ultimately, the authors concluded that the trypanocidal activity of **88** is mediated by inducing the oxidative stress together with the depolarization of the mitochondrial membrane potential, generating an apoptosis-like programmed cell death [83].

The phytochemical study of aerial parts of *Baccharis retusa* DC., a medicinal plant used in Brazilian folk medicine to treat parasitic diseases, allowed the isolation and identification of the kaurane-type diterpene **89**. This compound was active against *T. cruzi* trypomastigotes (IC_{50} 3.8 µM) with a high selectivity (SI = 50.0) due to its reduced cytotoxicity (CC_{50} 189.7 µM) on NCTC cells [84].

Ent-kaurenoic acid (**90**) and *ent*-pimaradienoic acid (**91**) were used as starting material to obtain several derivatives. From those, the *ent*-kaurane derivatives **92** (IC_{50} < 12.5 µM) and **93** (IC_{50} 26.1 µM) showed the highest antitrypanosomal activity when compared to compound **90** (IC_{50} 225.8 µM). Regarding the ent-pimaradienoic acid (**91**, IC_{50} 68.7 µM) set, compound **94** (IC_{50} 3.8 µM) was the most active against trypomastigotes forms of *T. cruzi*. However, due to the lack of cytotoxicity data it is not possible to determine the selectivity index of these compounds [85].

Three quinone methide-type diterpenes (**95**–**97**) were isolated from the roots of *Salvia austriaca* Jacq. and tested for their in vitro activity against *T. b. rhodesiense* and *T. cruzi*. Cytotoxicity was determined on L6 cells [86]. The diterpene **95** was the most active and selective against *T. b. rhodesiense* trypomastigotes (IC_{50} 0.05 µM and SI = 38). However, despite exhibiting an IC_{50} value of 7.11 µM against *T. cruzi* amastigotes, its selectivity was very low (SI = 0.27). Compounds **96** and **97** also showed activity against both parasites, being more active against *T. b. rhodesiense* with IC_{50} values of 0.62 µM (SI = 5.0) and 1.67 µM (SI = 2.4), respectively. Regarding their activity against *T. cruzi*, an IC_{50} value of 7.76 µM (SI = 0.4), and 7.63 µM (SI = 0.5) was observed for compound **96** and **97**, respectively [86], but the compounds were not selective to the parasite.

The phytochemical study of dichloromethane extract of *Aldama discolors* (Baker) E.E.Schill. & Panero leaves led to the isolation of four structurally and biosynthetically related diterpenes. These were evaluated for in vitro activity against *T. b. rhodesiense* trypomastigotes and *T. cruzi* amastigotes [87]. Among the isolated diterpenes, compound **98** showed a moderate in vitro activity with an IC_{50} value of 15.4 µM against *T. cruzi*, and an IC_{50} 24.3 µM for *T. b. rhodesiense*. On the other hand, compound **99**, structurally similar to **98**, showed less activity against the amastigote forms of *T. cruzi* (IC_{50} 19.4 µM), and no activity against the trypomastigote forms of *T. b. rhodesiense*. The selectivity of these compounds was very low, with SI values ranging from 2 to 4 [87].

The commercially available dehydroabietylamine (**100**), an abietane-type diterpenoid isolated in large amount from *Plectranthus* genus, was used as a starting material to produce a set of amides derivatives. Among these compounds, **100**–**103** were tested against *T. cruzi* amastigotes, showing compound **103** the highest antitrypanosomal activity and selectivity (IC_{50} 0.6 µM; SI = 58). The remaining compounds, including **100**, in spite of displaying antitrypanosomal activity (IC_{50} values between 3.7 and 7.4 µM) were not very selective to the parasite, showing CC_{50} values ranging from 6.5 to 33.5 µM when tested on the human cell line (SI values between 1 and 6, L6 rat myoblasts) [88].

Leriifolione (**104**), isolated from the lipophilic extract of the roots of *Salvia leriifolia* Benth., showed high activity against *T. b. rhodesiense* (IC$_{50}$ 1.0 µM) and *T. cruzi* (IC$_{50}$ 4.6 µM), but an undesirable cytotoxicity on L6 cells (SI = 2.6 and 0.6, respectively) [89].

From the *n*-hexane extract of the roots of *Zhumeria majdae* Rech. F., eight abietane-type diterpenes were isolated. The antitrypanosomal activity was investigated for compounds **105**, **106**, and **107** against *T. b. rhodesiense* and *T. cruzi*. All the compounds showed a high activity against *T. b. rhodesiense*, (IC$_{50}$ = 3.6 µM, 1.8 µM, and 0.1 µM to **105**, **106**, and **107**, respectively), being compound **106** the most selective for the parasite when compared with L6 cell line tested (**105**, SI = 1.7; **106**, SI = 21.9; **107**, SI = 15.4). None of the compounds were active against *T. cruzi* [90].

Seventeen diterpenes were isolated from the aerial parts of *Perovskia abrotanoides* Kar. These compounds were evaluated for antiprotozoal activity (*T. cruzi* amastigotes, and *T. b rhodesiense* trypomastigotes), and cytotoxicity was also assessed on rat skeletal myoblast L6 cell line. Most of the diterpenes were less active against *T. cruzi* than against *T. b rhodesiense* [91]. Compound **108** showed the best activity against *T. b. rhodesiense* (IC$_{50}$ 0.5 µM, SI = 10.5). However, it was inactive against *T. cruzi*, showing a lack of selectivity (IC$_{50}$ 58.7 µM; SI = 0.1, CC$_{50}$ 5.2 µM). With similar activity, but less cytotoxic (CC$_{50}$ 12.1 µM) than **108**, compound **109** displayed an IC$_{50}$ value of 0.8 µM (SI = 14.9) against *T. b. rhodesiense* and an IC$_{50}$ of 34.7 µM (SI = 0.3) against *T. cruzi*. Compounds **110–113** were particularly active against *T. b. rhodesiense*, displaying IC$_{50}$ values ranging from 3.8 to 12 µM but low SI values (SI = 1.5–12.5) [91].

Bokkosin (**114**), a new cassane diterpene isolated from the Nigerian species *Calliandra portoricensis* Hassk. used in traditional medicine to treat tuberculosis, and helmintic diseases, showed a strong trypanocidal activity against the bloodstream forms of *T. b. brucei*, sensitive (IC$_{50}$ = 1.1. µM) and resistant to pentamidine (IC$_{50}$ = 0.5 µM). A highly favorable selectivity for the parasite strains was also observed, when compared with its cytotoxic effect on two mammalian cell lines (CC$_{50}$ = 269 µM; SI = 246, on U937; CC$_{50}$ = 230 µM; SI = 215, on RAW 246.7) [92].

From the *n*-hexane and ethylacetate extracts of the roots of *Acacia nilotica* L. several diterpenes were isolated. Among them, the cassane-type diterpenoid **115** was tested against the *T. b brucei* bloodstream form, exhibiting a high activity a (IC$_{50}$ 1.4 µM). Additionally, **115** was tested for its cytotoxic effect on human HEK cells (CC$_{50}$ = 29.5 µM; SI = 21.1) displaying a significant selectivity for the parasite [93].

3.4. Triterpenes

Ursolic acid (**116**) was tested for antitrypanosomal activity against *T. brucei* trypomastigotes displaying an IC$_{50}$ value of 3.35 µM. Similar IC$_{50}$ values were also obtained by Catteau et al. (IC$_{50}$ 2.4 µM, CC$_{50}$ > 11.1 µM). However, it is important to note that the compound showed a lack of selectivity for the trypanosoma parasite due to its cytotoxic effect against the mammalian WI38 cells used [94]. In order two find out a possible mode of action, in silico molecular modelling studies were also performed using the parasitic enzymes of the trypanosome, namely trypanothione reductase, methionyl-tRNA synthetase, and inosine-adenosine-guanosine nucleoside hydrolase [95]. Ursolic acid showed a good binding affinity for trypanothione reductase and methionyl-tRNA synthetase, which was higher than that obtain for the reference drug difluoromethylornithine. On the other hand, no inhibition was observed for inosine–adenosine–guanosine. These data may suggest that the inhibition of the two former enzymes may be responsible for the antitrypanosomal activity of compound **116** [95].

A new ursane-type triterpenoid glycoside (**117**) isolated from the dried roots of *Vangueria agrestis* (Schweinf. ex Hiern) Lantz exhibited a considerable growth suppressing effect against *T. brucei* trypomastigotes (IC$_{50}$ 11.1 µM and IC$_{90}$ 12.3 µM). However, no cytotoxicity studies on mammalian cell lines were performed [96].

Betulin acid (**118**), a lupane-type pentacyclic triterpene, and some semysynthetic amide derivatives were tested against *T. cruzi* trypomastigotes. Compound **118** showed a moderate activity (IC$_{50}$ 19.5 µM and SI = 18.8), while an increasing activity was observed in derivatives **119** (IC$_{50}$ 1.8 µM, SI = 17.3), **120** (IC$_{50}$ 5.0 µM, SI = 10.7), and **121** (IC$_{50}$ 5.4 µM, SI = 5.3). The mechanism of action of compound **119** in trypomastigotes was studied and seemed to be associated with the death of the parasite by necrosis, characterized by the rupture of the membrane, flagellar retraction, and appearance of atypical cytoplasmic vacuoles and dilation of the Golgi cisterns. Furthermore, the amide derivatives of compound **118** act by reduction in the invasion process, as well as the development of the intracellular parasite in host cells [97]. Sousa et al. corroborated those mechanistic results, showing that betulinic acid was able to inhibit all the development forms of *T. cruzi* (namely epimastigotes, trypomastigotes and amastigotes) not only by using necrotic processes but also due to modifications on the parasite mitochondrial membrane potential and the increase in reactive oxygen species [98].

Six limonoids (**122–127**) obtained from the roots of *Pseudocedrela kotschyi* (Schweinf.) Harms were investigated for their trypanocidal activity using bloodstream forms of *T. brucei*, showing GI$_{50}$ values ranging from 2.5 to 14.5 µM. The most active compound was **122** (GI$_{50}$ 2.5 µM) but showed some cytotoxicity on human HL-60 cells (GI$_{50}$ 31.5 µM). On the other hand, limonoid **125** exhibited a similar activity (GI$_{50}$ 3.18 µM) with no cytotoxic effect on the mammalian cell line (GI$_{50}$ > 100 µM) [99].

From *Tabernaemontana longipes* Donn.Sm., baurenol acetate (**128**) was isolated and tested for its ability to inhibit the growth of *T. brucei* bloodstream forms, showing an IC$_{50}$ value of 3.1 µM. Baurenol (**129**) displayed a higher activity against the same parasite (IC$_{50}$ = 2.7 µM). Both compounds showed a low effect on cellular viability on Hep G2 cells (IC$_{50}$ > 80 µM) [100].

Four new triterpenoids (**130–133**), with a rare scaffold, isolated from *Salvia hydrangea* DC. ex Benth. showed antitrypanosomal activity against *T. cruzi* amastigotes with IC$_{50}$ values ranging from 3.5 to 19.8 µM, with no significant activity against *T. b. rhodesiense* trypomastigotes All the compounds showed a modest selectivity (SI ranging from 2.4 to 10.7; L6 cell line) [101].

Two lanostane-type triterpenoids, polycarpol (**134**) and dihydropolycarpol (**135**) were isolated from *Greenwayodendron suaveolens* (Engl. & Diels) Verdc., a plant traditional used in Congo to treat malaria. Both compounds were tested against *T. b. brucei* (IC$_{50}$ = 8.1 µM; SI < 1.0, **134**; IC$_{50}$ = 8.1 µM; SI = 2.4, **135**), and *T. cruzi* (IC$_{50}$ = 1.4 µM; SI = 2.0, **134**; IC$_{50}$ = 2.4 µM; SI = 8.1, **135**), showing good activities but very low selectivity [102].

From *Buxus sempervirens* L. leaf extract, several triterpenic-alkaloid derivatives were isolated, being the majority tested for their activity against *T. b. rhodesiense*. Cytotoxicity assays were performed on mammalian L6 cells. Compounds **136–142** displayed high activities with IC$_{50}$ values < 3 µM. The highest activities and selectivities for the parasite strain tested were obtained for compounds **136** (IC$_{50}$ = 1.5 µM; SI = 25), **138** (IC$_{50}$ = 2.3 µM; SI = 42), **141** (IC$_{50}$ = 2.4 µM; SI = 30), and **142** (IC$_{50}$ = 1.3 µM; SI = 33). In spite of its promising activity against the parasite (IC$_{50}$ = 1.1 µM), compound **146** showed a lower selectivity (SI = 12). The remaining compounds **143–150** displayed a significant activity with IC$_{50}$ values ranging from 3.1 µM (compound **149**) to 9.0 µM (compound **144**), but a modest selectivity to the parasite (SI < 9) [103].

Table 1. Plant terpenoids with anti-*T. brucei* activity (2016–2021).

Compound [a]	Plant	Parasite (Form) [b]	IC$_{50}$ (µM)	SI	Refs.
Monoterpenes and Iridoids					
carvacrol (2)	*Origanum onites* L.	*T. b. rhodesiense* (tryp.)	1.0	327.5	[54]
thymol (3)	*Origanum onites* L.	*T. b. rhodesiense* (tryp.)	0.73	454.4	[54]
terpinolene (4)	*Crithmum martimum* L.	*T. brucei* (tryp.)	0.26	180.0	[55]
α-pinene (5)	*Crithmum martimum* L.	*T. brucei* (tryp.)	7.4	>100	[55]
β-ocimene (6)	*Crithmum martimum* L.	*T. brucei* (tryp.)	8.0	>91	[55]
ML-F52 (7)	*Morinda lucida* Benth.	*T. b. brucei* (tryp.)	0.43	33.1	[56]
molucidin (8)	*Morinda lucida* Benth.	*T. b. brucei* (tryp.)	1.27	3.7	[56]
ML-2-3 (9)	*Morinda lucida* Benth.	*T. b. brucei* (tryp.)	3.75	>13.3	[56]
Sesquiterpenes					
tagitinin C (10)	*Tithonia diversifolia* (Hemsl) A. Grey	*T. brucei* (tryp.)	0.012	3.0	[57]
tagitinin A (11)	*Tithonia diversifolia* (Hemsl) A. Grey	*T. brucei* (tryp.)	0.97	1.3	[57]
vernodalin (12)	*Vernonia cinerascens* Sch.Bip.	*T. b. rhodesiense* (tryp.)	0.16	35.0	[58,59]
11β, 13-dihydrovernolide (13)	*Vernonia cinerascens* Sch.Bip.	*T. b. rhodesiense* (tryp.)	0.5	13.0	[58,59]
11β, 13-dihydrovernodaline (14)	*Vernonia cinerascens* Sch.Bip.	*T. b. rhodesiense* (tryp.)	1.1	4.2	[58,59]
vernocinerascolide (15)	*Vernonia cinerascens* Sch.Bip.	*T. b. rhodesiense* (tryp.)	4.8	27.0	[58,59]
11β, 13-dihydrohydroxtvernolide (16)	*Vernonia cinerascens* Sch.Bip.	*T. b. rhodesiense* (tryp.)	5.0	4.3	[58,59]
parthenolide (17)	*Tarchonanthus camphoratus* L.	*T. b. rhodesiense* (tryp.)	0.39	18.6	[60]
3-oxo-1,2-dehydrocostic acid (18)	*Tarchonanthus camphoratus* L.	*T. b. rhodesiense* (tryp.)	2.8	6.2	[60]
santhemoidin A (19)	*Schkuhria pinnata* (Lam.) Kuntze ex Thell.	*T. b. rhodesiense* (tryp.)	0.10	20.5	[60]
3β-(2″-hydroxyisovaleroyloxy)-8β-(3-furoyloxy)costunolide (20)	*Schkuhria pinnata* (Lam.) Kuntze ex Thell.	*T. b. rhodesiense* (tryp.)	0.13	29.7	[60]
2″-dehydroeucannabinolidesemiacetal (21)	*Schkuhria pinnata* (Lam.) Kuntze ex Thell.	*T. b. rhodesiense* (tryp.)	0.35	11.5	[60]
3-desacetyl-3-isovaleroyleucannabinolide (22)	*Schkuhria pinnata* (Lam.) Kuntze ex Thell.	*T. b. rhodesiense* (tryp.)	0.52	13.0	[60]
3-oxo-4β,15-dihydroliquistrin-[4′,5′-dihydroxytigloyloxy] (23)	*Schkuhria pinnata* (Lam.) Kuntze ex Thell.	*T. b. rhodesiense* (tryp.)	0.60	19.2	[60]
schkuhrin II (24)	*Schkuhria pinnata* (Lam.) Kuntze ex Thell.	*T. b. rhodesiense* (tryp.)	0.82	13.4	[60]
1(10)-epoxy-3β-hydroxy-8β-[5′-hydroxy-4′-(2″-hydroxyisovaleroyloxy)tigloyloxy]costunolide (25)	*Schkuhria pinnata* (Lam.) Kuntze ex Thell.	*T. b. rhodesiense* (tryp.)	0.91	15.8	[60]
eucannabinolide (26)	*Schkuhria pinnata* (Lam.) Kuntze ex Thell.	*T. b. rhodesiense* (tryp.)	0.92	15.8	[60]

Table 1. Cont.

Compound [a]	Plant	Parasite (Form) [b]	IC$_{50}$ (µM)	SI	Refs.
28	*Achillea fragrantissima* (Forssk.) Sch.Bip.	*T. b. brucei* (tryp.)	3.03	n.d	[61]
29	*Achillea fragrantissima* (Forssk.) Sch.Bip.	*T. b. brucei* (tryp.)	10.97	n.d	[61]
30	*Achillea fragrantissima* (Forssk.) Sch.Bip.	*T. b. brucei* (tryp.)	10.97	n.d	[61]
isofuranodiene (34)	*Smyrnium olusatrum* L.	*T. brucei* (tryp.)	3.0	30.0	[63]
furanonobilin (35)	*Anthemis nobilis* L.	*T. b. rhodesiense* (tryp.)	0.08	63.1	[64]
hydroxyisonobilin (36)	*Anthemis nobilis* L.	*T. b. rhodesiense* (tryp.)	0.61	8.3	[64]
8-tigloylhydroxyisonobilin (37)	*Anthemis nobilis* L.	*T. b. rhodesiense* (tryp.)	0.36	14.1	[64]
3-*epi*-hydroxyisonobilin (38)	*Anthemis nobilis* L.	*T. b. rhodesiense* (tryp.)	0.88	8.3	[64]
nobilinon A (39)	*Anthemis nobilis* L.	*T. b. rhodesiense* (tryp.)	0.4	3.8	[64]
45	*Scleria striatinux* De Wild.	*T. b. rhodesiense* (tryp.)	0.002	8.3	[67]
46	*Scleria striatinux* De Wild.	*T. b. rhodesiense* (tryp.)	0.025	3.4	[67]
vernolepin (47)	*Vernonia lasiopus* (O.Hoffm.) H.Rob.	*T. b. rhodesiense* (tryp.)	0.185	14.5	[59]
vernodalol (48)	*Vernonia lasiopus* (O.Hoffm.) H.Rob.	*T. b. rhodesiense* (tryp.)	0.26	14.4	[59]
vernomenin (49)	*Vernonia lasiopus* (O.Hoffm.) H.Rob.	*T. b. rhodesiense* (tryp.)	0.51	4.5	[59]
8-desacylvernodalol (50)	*Vernonia lasiopus* (O.Hoffm.) H.Rob.	*T. b. rhodesiense* (tryp.)	2.53	13.7	[59]
4,15-*iso*-atriplicolide methacrylate (56)	*Helianthus tuberosus* L.	*T. b. rhodesiense* (tryp.)	0.077	6.7	[70]
4,15-*iso*-atriplicolide isobutryrate (57)	*Helianthus tuberosus* L.	*T. b. rhodesiense* (tryp.)	0.26	3.38	[70]
heliantuberolide-8-O-tiglate is (58)	*Helianthus tuberosus* L.	*T. b. rhodesiense* (tryp.)	0.92	4.24	[70]
78	*Tanacetum sonbolii* Mozaff.	*T. b. rhodesiense* (tryp.)	5.1	3.9	[77]
79	*Tanacetum sonbolii* Mozaff.	*T. b. rhodesiense* (tryp.)	10.2	4.0	[77]
Diterpenes					
andrographolide (88)	*Andrographis paniculate* (Burm. F.) Wall. Ex Nees	*T. brucei* procyclic trypomastigotes	8.3	8.5	[83]
taxodione (95)	*Salvia austriaca* Jacq.	*T. b. rhodesiense* (tryp.)	0.05	38.0	[86]
7-(20-oxohexyl)-taxodione (96)	*Salvia austriaca* Jacq.	*T. b. rhodesiense* (tryp.)	0.62	5.0	[86]
taxodone (97)	*Salvia austriaca* Jacq.	*T. b. rhodesiense* (tryp.)	1.67	2.4	[86]
ent-7-oxo-pimara-8,15-diene-18-ol (98)	*Aldama discolors* (Baker) E.E.Schill. & Panero	*T. b. rhodesiense* (tryp.)	24.3	2.0	[87]
leriifolione (104)	*Salvia leriifolia* Benth.	*T. b. rhodesiense* (tryp.)	1.0	2.6	[89]
12, 16-dideoxy aegyptinone B (105)	*Zhumeria majdae* Rech. F	*T. b. rhodesiense* (tryp.)	3.6	1.7	[90]
11,14-dihydroxy-8, 11,13- abietatrien-7-one (106)	*Zhumeria majdae* Rech. F	*T. b. rhodesiense* (tryp.)	1.8	21.9	[90]
lanugon Q (107)	*Zhumeria majdae* Rech. F	*T. b. rhodesiense* (tryp.)	0.1	15.4	[90]

Table 1. Cont.

Compound [a]	Plant	Parasite (Form) [b]	IC$_{50}$ (μM)	SI	Refs.
miltiodiol (108)	Perovskia abrotanoides Kar.	T. b. rhodesiense (tryp.)	0.5	10.5	[91]
7α-ethoxyrosmanol (109)	Perovskia abrotanoides Kar.	T. b. rhodesiense (tryp.) (trypomastigote)	0.8	14.9	[91]
rosmanol (110)	Perovskia abrotanoides Kar.	T. b. rhodesiense (tryp.)	3.8	1.5	[91]
carnosol (111)	Perovskia abrotanoides Kar.	T. b. rhodesiense (tryp.)	5.4	2.4	[91]
Δ^9-dehydro-ferruginol (112)	Perovskia abrotanoides Kar.	T. b. rhodesiense (tryp.)	7.2	12.3	[91]
11,12-dihydroxy-20-norabieta-5(10),8,11,13-tetraen-1-one (113)	Perovskia abrotanoides Kar.	T. b. rhodesiense (tryp.)	12.0	12.5	[91]
bokkosin (114)	Calliandra portoricensis Hassk.	T. b. brucei ((tryp.)	1.1	246	[92]
8-oxacassa-13,15-dien-7-ol-17-al (115)	Acacia nilotica L.	T. b. brucei (tryp.)	1.4	21.1	[93]
Triterpenes					
ursolic acid (116)	Vitellaria paradoxa C. F. Gaertn	T. brucei (tryp.)	2.4	4.6	[94]
3-O-[α-L-rhamnopyranosyl-(1→2)-β-D-xylopyranosyl]pomolic acid (117)	Vangueria agrestis (Schweinf. ex Hiern) Lantz	T. brucei (tryp.)	11.1	n.d.	[96]
kotschyienone A (122)	Pseudocedrela kotschyi (Schweinf.) Harms	T. brucei (tryp.)	2.5	12.6	[99]
7-deacetyl-7-oxogedunin (125)	Pseudocedrela kotschyi (Schweinf.) Harms	T. brucei (tryp.)	3.18	>31.4	[99]
baurenol acetate (128)	Tabernaemontana longipes Donn.Sm.	T. brucei (tryp.)	3.1	>25.8	[100]
baurenol (129)	Tabernaemontana longipes Donn.Sm.	T. brucei (tryp.)	2.7	>29.6	[100]
polycarpol (134)	Greenwayodendron suaveolens (Engl. & Diels) Verdc.	T. b. brucei (tryp.)	8.1	1.0	[102]
dihydropolycarpol (135)	Greenwayodendron suaveolens (Engl. & Diels) Verdc.	T. b. brucei (tryp.)	8.1	2.4	[102]
cyclovirobuxeine-B (136)	Buxus sempervirens L.	T. b. rhodesiense (tryp.)	1.5	25.0	[103]
cyclomicrophylline-A (138)	Buxus sempervirens L.	T. b. rhodesiense (tryp.)	2.3	42.0	[103]
N-benzoyl-O-acetyl-cycloxo-buxoline-F (141)	Buxus sempervirens L.	T. b. rhodesiense (tryp.)	2.4	30.0	[103]
N20-acetylbuxadine- G (142)	Buxus sempervirens L.	T. b. rhodesiense (tryp.)	1.3	33.0	[103]
O-benzoyl-cycloprotobuxoline-D (146)	Buxus sempervirens L.	T. b. rhodesiense (tryp.)	1.1	12.0	[103]

[a] Some names are not indicated in the corresponding papers; [b] Tryp: trypomastigotes bloodstream forms: n.d.: not defined/not determined.

Table 2. Plant terpenoids with anti-*T. cruzi* activity (2016–2021).

Compound [a]	Plant	Parasite Form	IC$_{50}$ (μM)	SI	Refs.
Monoterpenes and Iridoids					
N-[1-methyl-1-[(1R)-4-methylcyclohex-3-en-1-yl]ethyl]-5-(4-methylphenyl)-1,3,4-thiadiazol-2-amine (1)	n.d	Amastigote	1.3	611.2	[53]
Sesquiterpenes					
mikanolide (31)	*Mikania variifolia* Hieron. and *Mikania micrantha* Kunth	Epimastigote	2.41	31.9	[62]
		Trypomastigote	7.24	10.6	
		Amastigote	15.5	4.3	
deoxymikanolide (32)	*Mikania variifolia* Hieron. and *Mikania micrantha* Kunth	Epimastigote	0.29	992.5	[62]
		Trypomastigote	5.43	54.0	
		Amastigote	22.8	12.5	
		Epimastigote	8.55	5.2	
dihydromikanolide (33)	*Mikania micrantha* Kunth	Trypomastigote	1.03	49.0	[62]
		Amastigote	29.1	1.5	
nobilinon A (39)	*Anthemis nobilis* L.	Intracellular amastigote	2.8	0.5	[64]
nobilinon B (40)	*Anthemis nobilis* L.	Intracellular amastigote	4.2	6.1	[64]
11,13-dihydroxy-calaxin (41)	*Calea pinnatifida* (R. Br.) Less.	Amastigote	8.30	1.88	[65]
enhydrin (42)	*Smallanthus sonchifolius* (Poepp.) H. Rob.	Epimastigote	0.78	n.d.	[66]
uvedalin (43)	*Smallanthus sonchifolius* (Poepp.) H. Rob.	Epimastigote	0.79	n.d.	[66]
polymatin (44)	*Smallanthus sonchifolius* (Poepp.) H. Rob.	Epimastigote	1.38	n.d.	[66]
45	*Scleria striatinux* De Wild.	Amastigote	0.025	0.74	[67]
46	*Scleria striatinux* De Wild.	Amastigote	0.085	1.0	[67]
			19.9	12.9	
eupatoriopicrin (51)	Astearaceae species	Trypomastigote bloodstream form	6.3	40.6	[68]
		Intracellular amastigote			
estafietin (52)	Astearaceae species	Trypomastigote bloodstream form	117	6.8	[68]
		Trypomastigote bloodstream form	33.0	10.4	
eupahakonenin B (53)	Astearaceae species	Trypomastigote bloodstream form	89.3	3.8	[68]
		Intracellular amastigote	21.0	12.8	
minimolide (54)	Astearaceae species	Trypomastigote bloodstream form	25.1	10.7	[68]
		Intracellular amastigote			
tagitinin C (55)	*Tithonia diversifolia* (Hemsl.) A. Gray	Epimastigote	1.15	5.69	
4,15-iso-atriplicolide methacrylate (56)	*Helianthus tuberosus* L.	Trypomastigote	1.6	0.32	[73]
4,15-iso-atriplicolide isobutryrate (57)	*Helianthus tuberosus* L.	Trypomastigote	3.1	0.28	[73]

Table 2. Cont.

Compound [a]	Plant	Parasite Form	IC$_{50}$ (μM)	SI	Refs.
heliantuberolide-8-O-tiglate (58)	Helianthus tuberosus L.	Trypomastigote	5.7	0.68	[73]
(2-methoxy-2,5-epoxy-8-methacryloxygermacra-3Z,11(13)-dien-6,12-olide (59)	Vernonanthura nebularum (Cabrera) H. Rob.	Epimastigote	1.5	>14	[71]
(2-ethoxy-2, 5-epoxy-8-angeloxygermacra-3Z,11(13)-dien-6,12-olide (60)	Vernonanthura nebularum (Cabrera) H. Rob.	Epimastigote	2.1	>14	[71]
8a-methacryloxyhirsutinolide 13-O-acetate (61)	Vernonanthura nebularum (Cabrera) H. Rob.	Epimastigote	2.0	>14	[71]
62	Vernonanthura nebularum (Cabrera) H. Rob.	Epimastigote	3.7	14.3	[71]
66	Vernonanthura nebularum (Cabrera) H. Rob.	Epimastigote	10.7	9.0	[71]
67	Vernonanthura nebularum (Cabrera) H. Rob.	Epimastigote	8.1	13.9	[71]
68	Centratherum puctatum ssp. Punctatum Cass.	Epimastigote	6.8	1.6	[71]
69	Elephantopus mollis Kunth	Epimastigote	4.7	11.5	[71]
eucannabinolide (70)	Urolepis hecatantha (DC.) R.King & H.Rob.	Epimastigote	10	1.5	[72]
santhemoidin C (71)	Urolepis hecatantha (DC.) R.King & H.Rob.	Epimastigote	18	0.83	[72]
goyazensolide (72)	Lychnophora passerina (Mart ex DC) Gardn.	Intracellular amastigote	0.181/24 h 0.020/48 h	52.82/24h 915.0/48h	[73]
hedyosulide (73)	Hedyosmum brasiliense Mart. ex Miq.	Trypomastigote Intracellular amastigote	28.1 21.6	>7 >9	[74]
8-epi-xanthatin-1β,5β-epoxide (75)	Inula viscosa (L.) Greuter	Epimastigote	4.99	3.67	[75]
inuloxin A (76)	Inula viscosa (L.) Greuter	Epimastigote	15.52	3.38	[75]
costic acid (77)	Nectandra barbellata Coe-Teix.	Intracellular amastigote	7.9	>25	[76]
polygodial (80)	Polygonum hydropiper L.	Epimastigote Trypomastigote Amastigote Epimastigote	51.0 68.2 34.4 13.0	n.d	[79]
Polygodial derivative (81)	n.d	Trypomastigote Amastigote Epimastigote	8.4 9.9 12.3	n.d	[79]
Polygodial derivative (82)	n.d	Trypomastigote Amastigote	6.4 6.7	n.d	[79]

Table 2. Cont.

Compound [a]	Plant	Parasite Form	IC$_{50}$ (μM)	SI	Refs.
Polygodial derivative (83)	n.d	Epimastigote	7.2	n.d	[79]
		Trypomastigote	6.9		
		Amastigote	8.3		
epi-polygodial (84)	*Drimys brasiliensis* Miers	Trypomastigote	5.01	>40	[80]
(−)-T-cadinol (85)	*Casearia sylvestris* Sw.	Trypomastigote	18.2	>15	[81]
		Amastigote	15.8		
Diterpenes					
ent-15β-senecioyl-oxy-kaur-16-en-19-oic acid (89)	*Baccharis retusa* DC.	Trypomastigote	3.8	50.0	[84]
taxodione (95)	*Salvia austriaca* Jacq.	Amastigote	7.11	0.27	[86]
7-(20-oxohexyl)-taxodione (96)	*Salvia austriaca* Jacq.	Amastigote	7.76	0.4	[86]
Taxodone (97)	*Salvia austriaca* Jacq.	Amastigote	7.63	0.5	[86]
ent-7-oxo-pimara-8,15-diene-18-ol (98)	*Aldama discolors* (Baker) E.E.Schill. & Panero	Amastigote	15.4	3.0	[87]
ent-2S,4S-2-19-epoxy-pimara-8(3),15-diene-7β-ol (98)	*Aldama discolors* (Baker) E.E.Schill. & Panero	Amastigote	19.4	4.0	[87]
dehydroabietylamine derivative (103)	n.d	Amastigote	0.6	58.0	[88]
Leriifolione (104)	*Salvia leriifolia* Benth.	Amastigote	2.6	0.6	[89]
Triterpenes					
Betulinic acid (118)	n.d	trypomastigote	19.5	18.8	[97]
Betulinic acid derivative (119)	n.d	trypomastigote	1.8	17.3	[97]
Betulinic acid derivative (120)	n.d	trypomastigote	5.0	10.7	[97]
Betulinic acid derivative (121)	n.d	trypomastigote	5.4	5.3	[97]
Perovskone C (130)	*Salvia hydrangea* DC. ex Benth.	Amastigote	3.5	10.7	[101]
perovskone D (131)	*Salvia hydrangea* DC. ex Benth.	Amastigote	3.8	3.6	[101]
Perovskone E (132)	*Salvia hydrangea* DC. ex Benth.	Amastigote	11.5	6.3	[101]
perovskone F (133)	*Salvia hydrangea* DC. ex Benth.	Amastigote	19.8	2.4	[101]
polycarpol (134)	*Greenwayodendron suaveolens* (Engl. & Diels) Verdc.	trypomastigote	1.4	2.0	[102]
dihydropolycarpol (135)	*Greenwayodendron suaveolens* (Engl. & Diels) Verdc.	trypomastigote	2.4	8.1	[102]

[a] Some names are not indicated in the corresponding papers; n.d.: not defined/not determined.

4. Discussion

Human African trypanosomiasis and American trypanosomiasis continue to be a major public health problem, affecting a significant proportion of the world's population, especially in tropical countries. Currently, the drugs used to treat these diseases are scarce and far from being ideal. Therefore, the discovery and development of new drugs and treatments should be a continuous process, and all possible approaches should be explored, mainly focusing on multidisciplinary collaborations. It is also important to stress that the new drugs should be affordable and easy to administer, improving the adherence to the therapeutic protocol, and decreasing the need for patient hospitalization.

Several approaches have been considered for the development of new drugs against these diseases. Due to the high costs and slow pace of new drug discovery, one of the main strategies is the repositioning or repurposing of drugs that were developed and used to treat other diseases. Although several advantages can be addressed, including the lower risk of failing, reduced time frame for drug development, less investment and rapid return [104], drug repositioning have also major drawbacks. These include, for example, the existence of undesirable side effects, problems concerning a different target population, poor stability in conditions of high temperature and humidity, lack of oral bioavailability, and various regulatory issues and intellectual property barriers. Therefore, the development of a new drug that ideally would be suitable for combination therapy, increasing the clinical efficacy, and decreasing side effects and the development of resistance, is a goal of utmost importance [10]. Besides combinatorial chemistry, one of the main strategies for drug discovery is through the phytochemical study of plants or other sources of natural origin. The importance of natural products for the development of drug leads or actual drugs along the last three decades has been reported in various reviews [12].

The evaluation of compounds with anti-parasitic activity is usually performed by two main approaches: the target-based and the phenotypic approaches [10,104]. The target-based methodologies (Sections 2.1.1 and 2.2.1) focus on the specific biochemical pathway of the parasites, and consist of the identification of possible molecular targets (e.g., enzymes) that are significantly involved in the disease and the screening of molecules that possibly interfere with these targets. However, regarding trypanosomiasis, restricted success has been achieved, possibly due to a lack of translation between the activity in the molecular target, and the result on the proliferation of the parasite. In fact, the number of robust and validated molecular targets against these diseases is very limited, and in addition, for several drugs currently used in clinic, the mode of action is not yet completely understood or it comprises several targets [10,104]. By far, the most widely used methodologies to identify anti-trypanosomal drugs are based on the phenotypic methods. They consist of the screening of the compounds directly against the different forms of the parasite, and most of the time, for the bioactive compounds, there is no knowledge regarding their underlying mode of action or their molecular target. Through this screening, the effects on the parasite and the host cell viability (toxicity) can be assessed simultaneously [10].

In this review, 150 terpenic compounds obtained by isolation or derivatization from different plant species, were grouped into four classes of terpenes, namely, monoterpenes and iridoids, sesquiterpenes, diterpenes and triterpenes. The scope of this review was limited to compounds that exhibited in vitro or in vivo activity against the diverse forms of *T. brucei* and/or *T. cruzi*, displaying IC_{50} values in low micromolar range, most of them below 10 µM.

Regarding the anti-*T. brucei* activity, it can be observed that most of the selected compounds were active on the trypomastigote bloodstream form of the parasite (in vitro assays), and several possible hits can be identified. A high number of compounds exhibited very low IC_{50} values (0.05 < IC_{50} < 3.0 µM), when tested against *T. b. rhodesiense* or *T. b. brucei*, also presenting low cytotoxicity on the mammalian cells (SI values higher than 10). Some of the most promising hits are depicted in Figure 16. It is interesting to note that the majority of the bioactive compounds are sesquiterpenes and more specifically, sesquiterpenic lactones. Indeed, the α,β-unsaturated lactone function is very common in biologically active molecules, being responsible not only for their activity but also for the cytotoxicity of the compounds. The presence of this chemical function promotes the Michael-type addition to a suitable nucleophile (for example, the thiol group in proteins), and may irreversibly alkylate critical enzymes and transcription factors that control gene regulation, protein synthesis, cell metabolism, and ultimately, the cell division [105,106]. After the preliminary in vitro studies, two compounds (3 and 7) were further evaluated using in vivo studies on *T. brucei* mouse models achieving very good results.

Concerning *T. cruzi* assays, it is curious to notice that there are much fewer research papers reporting the bioactivity of compounds against this parasite, probably because the in vitro assays using intracellular amastigotes were not so straightforward. Nevertheless, it was possible to select some promising hits that were very active against *T. cruzi* amastigotes, according to the criteria established by DNDi (Figure 17). Some of the most active compounds (**1**, **51**, and **74**) were further evaluated in vivo using a *T. cruzi* mouse model. The best result was obtained for compound **51**, and a significant reduction in parasitemia levels was observed in treated mice (1 mg/Kg/day, for 5 consecutive days), similarly to that obtained with the control group treated with the reference drug benznidazole.

Although most of the reported compounds were remarkably active against some infectious forms of the parasites, some of them also displayed some cytotoxicity on the mammalian cells tested. Furthermore, there is a notorious lack of additional studies on structure-activity relationships (SAR) and on the possible mechanisms of action. In addition, some reasons could be addressed to justify the absence of results for in vivo assays, including that the majority of compounds are isolated in very low amounts, a fact that precludes this type of assay where a large amount of compound is always needed.

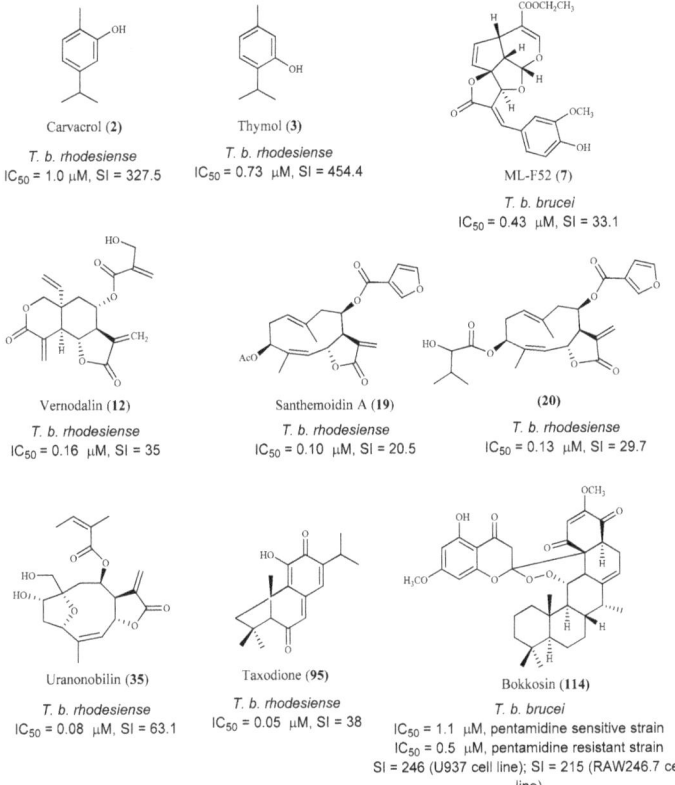

Figure 16. Promising hit compounds for further research into treating Human African Trypanosomiasis.

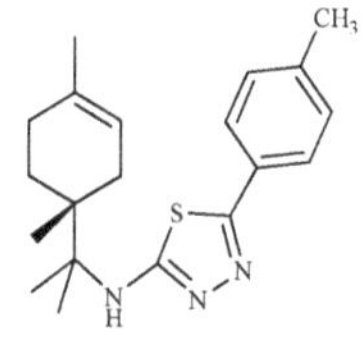

TDZ-2 (1)
IC$_{50}$ = 1.3 µM; SI = 611

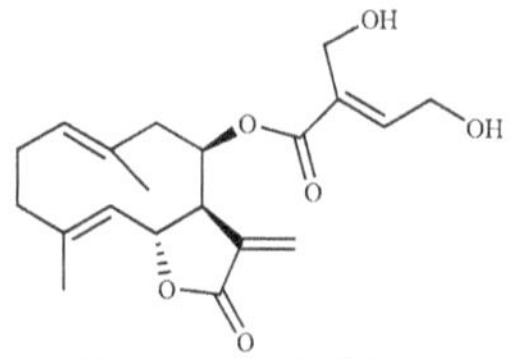

Eupatoriopicrin (51)
IC$_{50}$ = 6.3 µM; SI = 40.6

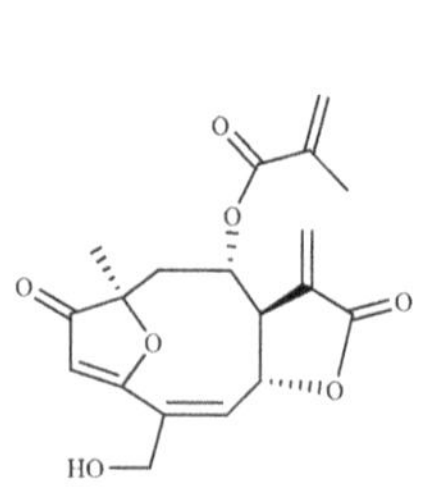

Goyazensolide (72)
IC$_{50}$ = 0.18 µM; SI = 52.8

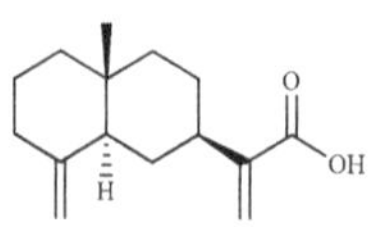

Costic acid (77)
IC$_{50}$ = 7.9 µM; SI = 25

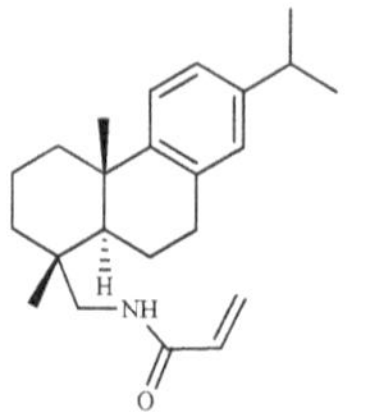

N-(Dehydroabietyl)prop-2-enamide (101)
IC$_{50}$ = 0.6 µM; SI = 58

Figure 17. Promising hit compounds for further research into treating Human American Trypanosomiasis. All the selected compounds were tested against *T. cruzi* intracellular amastigote forms.

5. Conclusions

The data presented in this review gathered the recent scientific research and experimental evidence on the most promising terpenoids derived from plants, and active against *T. brucei* and *T. cruzi* parasites. These data represent the immense efforts of various research groups all over the world, and ultimately the collected information is highly pertinent and can be used, for example, to support the selection of other plants to study, using the chemotaxonomic approach. However, all of these studies are strictly academic and no further translation to drug development has been achieved. There is still a limited collaboration of academic institutions with the pharmaceutical industry, and importantly, obtaining opportunities for research funding is, nowadays, even more challenging. All these aspects have limited or made it difficult for academic researchers to advance promising hits for further development.

In the future, natural products research must be a multidisciplinary process combining phytochemistry with innovative technological resources, in a way that will be significantly different from the past. These technologies must include high-throughput screening and in silico methodologies, as well as new extraction and dereplication procedures, new analytical tools, metabolic engineering, omics-based analysis, informatics, and big data analysis, in order to overcome the constraints of the classic natural products research.

Author Contributions: Conceptualization, N.D.; writing—original draft preparation, R.D. and C.R.; writing—review and editing, N.D., C.R., E.M. and A.M.M. All authors have read and agreed to the published version of the manuscript.

Funding: This research received no external funding.

Institutional Review Board Statement: Not applicable.

Informed Consent Statement: Not applicable.

Conflicts of Interest: The authors declare no conflict of interest.

References

1. World Health Organization. *Ending the Neglect to Attain the Sustainable Development Goals. A Road Map for Neglected Tropical Diseases 2021–2030*; Ntuli, M.M., Ed.; WHO: Geneva, Switzerland, 2021.
2. Hotez, P.J.; Aksoy, S.; Brindley, P.J.; Kamhawi, S. What constitutes a neglected tropical disease? *PLoS Negl. Trop. Dis.* **2020**, *14*, e0008001. [CrossRef] [PubMed]
3. Anisuzzaman; Tsuji, N. Schistosomiasis and hookworm infection in humans: Disease burden, pathobiology and anthelmintic vaccines. *Parasitol. Int.* **2020**, *75*, 102051. [CrossRef] [PubMed]
4. Bhattacharya, A.; Corbeil, A.; Do Monte-Neto, R.L.; Fernandez-Prada, C. Of drugs and trypanosomatids: New tools and knowledge to reduce bottlenecks in drug discovery. *Genes* **2020**, *11*, 722. [CrossRef] [PubMed]
5. Molyneux, D.H.; Asamoa-Bah, A.; Fenwick, A.; Savioli, L.; Hotez, P. The history of the neglected tropical disease movement. *Trans. R. Soc. Trop. Med. Hyg.* **2021**, *115*, 169–175. [CrossRef] [PubMed]
6. World Health Organization. Neglected tropical diseases: Impact of COVID-19 and WHO's response—Maladies tropicales négligées: Impact de la COVID-19 et réponse de l'OMS. *Wkly. Epidemiol. Rec.* **2020**, *95*, 461–468.
7. Cheuka, P.; Mayoka, G.; Mutai, P.; Chibale, K. The Role of Natural Products in Drug Discovery and Development against Neglected Tropical Diseases. *Molecules* **2017**, *22*, 58. [CrossRef] [PubMed]
8. Capela, R.; Moreira, R.; Lopes, F. An overview of drug resistance in protozoal diseases. *Int. J. Mol. Sci.* **2019**, *20*, 5748. [CrossRef] [PubMed]
9. Moreno-Herrera, A.; Cortez-Maya, S.; Bocanegra-Garcia, V.; Banik, B.K.; Rivera, G. Recent Advances in the Development of Broad-Spectrum Antiprotozoal Agents. *Curr. Med. Chem.* **2020**, *28*, 583–606. [CrossRef] [PubMed]
10. Field, M.C.; Horn, D.; Fairlamb, A.H.; Ferguson, M.A.J.; Gray, D.W.; Read, K.D.; De Rycker, M.; Torrie, L.S.; Wyatt, P.G.; Wyllie, S.; et al. Anti-trypanosomatid drug discovery: An ongoing challenge and a continuing need. *Nat. Rev. Microbiol.* **2017**, *15*, 217–231. [CrossRef] [PubMed]
11. Fournet, A.; Munoz, V.; Muñoz, V. Natural products as trypanocidal, antileishmanial and antimalarial drugs. *Curr. Top. Med. Chem.* **2002**, *2*, 1215–1237. [CrossRef] [PubMed]
12. Newman, D.J.; Cragg, G.M. Natural Products as Sources of New Drugs over the Nearly Four Decades from 01/1981 to 09/2019. *J. Nat. Prod.* **2020**, *83*, 770–803. [CrossRef] [PubMed]
13. Schmidt, T.J.; Khalid, S.A.; Romanha, A.J.; Alves, T.M.A.; Biavatti, M.W.; Brun, R.; Da Costa, F.B.; de Castro, S.L.; Ferreira, V.F.; de Lacerda, M.V.G.; et al. The Potential of Secondary Metabolites from Plants as Drugs or Leads Against Protozoan Neglected Diseases—Part II. *Curr. Med. Chem.* **2012**, *19*, 2176–2228. [CrossRef] [PubMed]
14. Tullius Scotti, M.; Scotti, L.; Ishiki, H.; Fávaro Ribeiro, F.; da Cruz, R.M.D.; de Oliveira, M.P.; Jaime Bezerra Mendonça, F. Natural Products as a Source for Antileishmanial and Antitrypanosomal Agents. *Comb. Chem. High Throughput Screen.* **2016**, *19*, 537–553. [CrossRef] [PubMed]
15. Isah, M.B.; Ibrahim, M.A.; Mohammed, A.; Aliyu, A.B.; Masola, B.; Coetzer, T.H.T. A systematic review of pentacyclic triterpenes and their derivatives as chemotherapeutic agents against tropical parasitic diseases. *Parasitology* **2016**, *143*, 1219–1231. [CrossRef] [PubMed]
16. Muschietti, L.V.; Ulloa, J.L. Natural Sesquiterpene Lactones as Potential Trypanocidal Therapeutic Agents: A Review. *Nat. Prod. Commun.* **2016**, *11*, 1569–1578. [CrossRef] [PubMed]
17. Cockram, P.E.; Smith, T.K. Active Natural Product Scaffolds against Trypanosomatid Parasites: A Review. *J. Nat. Prod.* **2018**, *81*, 2138–2154. [CrossRef] [PubMed]
18. Ungogo, M.A.; Ebiloma, G.U.; Ichoron, N.; Igoli, J.O.; de Koning, H.P.; Balogun, E.O. A Review of the Antimalarial, Antitrypanosomal, and Antileishmanial Activities of Natural Compounds Isolated From Nigerian Flora. *Front. Chem.* **2020**, *8*, 1221. [CrossRef]
19. Chan-Bacab, M.J.; Reyes-Estebanez, M.M.; Camacho-Chab, J.C.; Ortega-Morales, B.O. Microorganisms as a potential source of molecules to control trypanosomatid diseases. *Molecules* **2021**, *26*, 1388. [CrossRef]
20. Hzounda Fokou, J.B.; Dize, D.; Etame Loe, G.M.; Nko'o, M.H.J.; Ngene, J.P.; Ngoule, C.C.; Boyom, F.F. Anti-leishmanial and anti-trypanosomal natural products from endophytes. *Parasitol. Res.* **2021**, *120*, 785–796. [CrossRef]
21. Lenzi, J.; Costa, T.M.; Alberton, M.D.; Goulart, J.A.G.; Tavares, L.B.B. Medicinal fungi: A source of antiparasitic secondary metabolites. *Appl. Microbiol. Biotechnol.* **2018**, *102*, 5791–5810. [CrossRef]
22. Nweze, J.A.; Mbaoji, F.N.; Li, Y.M.; Yang, L.Y.; Huang, S.S.; Chigor, V.N.; Eze, E.A.; Pan, L.X.; Zhang, T.; Yang, D.F. Potentials of marine natural products against malaria, leishmaniasis, and trypanosomiasis parasites: A review of recent articles. *Infect. Dis. Poverty* **2021**, *10*, 9. [CrossRef] [PubMed]
23. Lucas, L.A.; Cândido, A.C.B.B.; Santos, M.F.C.; Caffrey, C.R.; Bastos, J.K.; Ambrósio, S.R.; Magalhães, L.G. Antiparasitic Properties of Propolis Extracts and Their Compounds. *Chem. Biodivers.* **2021**, *18*, 310. [CrossRef]
24. Asfaram, S.; Fakhar, M.; Keighobadi, M.; Akhtari, J. Promising Anti-Protozoan Activities of Propolis (Bee Glue) as Natural Product: A Review. *Acta Parasitol.* **2021**, *66*, 1–12. [CrossRef]
25. Simoben, C.V.; Ntie-Kang, F.; Akone, S.H.; Sippl, W. Compounds from African Medicinal Plants with Activities Against Selected Parasitic Diseases: Schistosomiasis, Trypanosomiasis and Leishmaniasis. *Nat. Products Bioprospect.* **2018**, *8*, 151–169. [CrossRef] [PubMed]

26. Naß, J.; Efferth, T. The activity of *Artemisia* spp. and their constituents against Trypanosomiasis. *Phytomedicine* **2018**, *47*, 184–191. [CrossRef] [PubMed]
27. de Morais, M.C.; de Souza, J.V.; da Silva Maia Bezerra Filho, C.; Dolabella, S.S.; de Sousa, D.P. Trypanocidal essential oils: A review. *Molecules* **2020**, *25*, 4568. [CrossRef] [PubMed]
28. Nair, J.J.; van Staden, J. Antiprotozoal alkaloid principles of the plant family Amaryllidaceae. *Bioorg. Med. Chem. Lett.* **2019**, *29*, 126642. [CrossRef] [PubMed]
29. Montesino, N.L.; Schmidt, T.J. Salvia species as sources of natural products with antiprotozoal activity. *Int. J. Mol. Sci.* **2018**, *19*, 264. [CrossRef] [PubMed]
30. da Silva, J.K.; da Trindade, R.; Alves, N.S.; Figueiredo, P.L.; Maia, J.G.S.; Setzer, W.N. Essential Oils from Neotropical Piper Species and Their Biological Activities. *Int. J. Mol. Sci.* **2017**, *18*, 2571. [CrossRef] [PubMed]
31. World Health Organization. Human African Trypanosomiasis (Sleeping Sickness). Available online: https://www.who.int/health-topics/human-african-trypanosomiasis#tab=tab_1 (accessed on 13 January 2022).
32. World Health Organization. Trypanosomiasis, Human African (Sleeping Sickness). Available online: https://www.who.int/news-room/fact-sheets/detail/trypanosomiasis-human-african-(sleeping-sickness) (accessed on 4 March 2021).
33. Drugs for Neglected Diseases Initiative (DNDi) Sleping Sickness. Available online: https://dndi.org/diseases/sleeping-sickness/facts/ (accessed on 7 January 2022).
34. Centers for Disease Control and Prevention (CDC) Parasites—African Trypanosomiasis (also Known as Sleeping Sickness). Available online: https://www.cdc.gov/parasites/sleepingsickness/ (accessed on 6 January 2022).
35. Keiser, J.; Stich, A.; Burri, C. New drugs for the treatment of human African trypanosomiasis: Research and development. *Parasitol. Today* **2001**, *17*, 42–49. [CrossRef]
36. Brand, S.; Norcross, N.R.; Thompson, S.; Harrison, J.R.; Smith, V.C.; Robinson, D.A.; Torrie, L.S.; McElroy, S.P.; Hallyburton, I.; Norval, S.; et al. Lead optimization of a pyrazole sulfonamide series of trypanosoma brucei N-myristoyltransferase inhibitors: Identification and evaluation of CNS penetrant compounds as potential treatments for stage 2 human african trypanosomiasis. *J. Med. Chem.* **2014**, *57*, 9855–9869. [CrossRef] [PubMed]
37. Bijlmakers, M.J. Ubiquitination and the Proteasome as Drug Targets in Trypanosomatid Diseases. *Front. Chem.* **2021**, *8*, e630888. [CrossRef] [PubMed]
38. Kourbeli, V.; Chontzopoulou, E.; Moschovou, K.; Pavlos, D.; Mavromoustakos, T.; Papanastasiou, I.P. An Overview on Target-Based Drug Design against Kinetoplastid Protozoan Infections: Human African. *Molecules* **2021**, *26*, 4629. [CrossRef] [PubMed]
39. Imran, M.; Khan, S.A.; Alshammari, M.K.; Alqahtani, A.M.; Alanazi, T.A.; Kamal, M.; Jawaid, T.; Ghoneim, M.M.; Alshehri, S.; Shakeel, F. Discovery, Development, Inventions and Patent Review of Fexinidazole: The First All-Oral Therapy for Human African Trypanosomiasis. *Pharmaceuticals* **2022**, *15*, 128. [CrossRef] [PubMed]
40. Steketee, P.C.; Giordani, F.; Vincent, I.M.; Crouch, K.; Achcar, F.; Dickens, N.J.; Morrison, L.J.; MacLeod, A.; Barrett, M.P. Transcriptional differentiation of Trypanosoma brucei during in vitro acquisition of resistance to acoziborole. *PLoS Negl. Trop. Dis.* **2021**, *15*, e0009939. [CrossRef] [PubMed]
41. World Health Organization. Chagas Disease (also Known as American Trypanosomiasis). Available online: https://www.who.int/news-room/fact-sheets/detail/chagas-disease-(american-trypanosomiasis) (accessed on 4 March 2021).
42. Dumonteil, E.; Herrera, C. The Case for the Development of a Chagas Disease Vaccine: Why? How? When? *Trop. Med. Infect. Dis.* **2021**, *6*, 16. [CrossRef] [PubMed]
43. Lidani, K.C.F.; Andrade, F.A.; Bavia, L.; Damasceno, F.S.; Beltrame, M.H.; Messias-Reason, I.J.; Sandri, T.L. Chagas disease: From discovery to a worldwide health problem. *J. Phys. Oceanogr.* **2019**, *49*, 166. [CrossRef] [PubMed]
44. Mills, R.M. Chagas Disease: Epidemiology and Barriers to Treatment. *Am. J. Med.* **2020**, *133*, 1262–1265. [CrossRef] [PubMed]
45. Duarte-Silva, E.; Morais, L.H.; Clarke, G.; Savino, W.; Peixoto, C. Targeting the Gut Microbiota in Chagas Disease: What Do We Know so Far? *Front. Microbiol.* **2020**, *11*, 3083. [CrossRef]
46. Onyekwelu, K. Life Cycle of Trypanosoma cruzi in the Invertebrate and the Vertebrate Hosts. In *Biology of Trypanosoma Cruzi*; De Souza, W., Ed.; IntechOpen: London, UK, 2019; ISBN 978-1-83968-204-9.
47. Francisco, A.F.; Jayawardhana, S.; Olmo, F.; Lewis, M.D.; Wilkinson, S.R.; Taylor, M.C.; Kelly, J.M. Challenges in Chagas Disease Drug Development. *Molecules* **2020**, *25*, 2799. [CrossRef]
48. Villalta, F.; Rachakonda, G. Advances in preclinical approaches to Chagas disease drug discovery. *Expert Opin. Drug Discov.* **2019**, *14*, 1161–1174. [CrossRef] [PubMed]
49. García-Huertas, P.; Cardona-Castro, N. Advances in the treatment of Chagas disease: Promising new drugs, plants and targets. *Biomed. Pharmacother.* **2021**, *142*, 112020. [CrossRef] [PubMed]
50. Torrico, F.; Gascón, J.; Barreira, F.; Blum, B.; Almeida, I.C.; Alonso-Vega, C.; Barboza, T.; Bilbe, G.; Correia, E.; Garcia, W.; et al. New regimens of benznidazole monotherapy and in combination with fosravuconazole for treatment of Chagas disease (BENDITA): A phase 2, double-blind, randomised trial. *Lancet Infect. Dis.* **2021**, *21*, 1129–1140. [CrossRef]
51. Don, R.; Ioset, J.-R. Screening strategies to identify new chemical diversity for drug development to treat kinetoplastid infections. *Parasitology* **2014**, *141*, 140–146. [CrossRef] [PubMed]
52. Katsuno, K.; Burrows, J.N.; Duncan, K.; Van Huijsduijnen, R.H.; Kaneko, T.; Kita, K.; Mowbray, C.E.; Schmatz, D.; Warner, P.; Slingsby, B.T. Hit and lead criteria in drug discovery for infectious diseases of the developing world. *Nat. Rev. Drug Discov.* **2015**, *14*, 751–758. [CrossRef] [PubMed]

53. Martins, S.C.; Lazarin-Bidóia, D.; Desoti, V.C.; Falzirolli, H.; da Silva, C.C.; Ueda-Nakamura, T.; de O. Silva, S.; Nakamura, C.V. 1,3,4-Thiadiazole derivatives of R-(+)-limonene benzaldehyde-thiosemicarbazones cause death in Trypanosoma cruzi through oxidative stress. *Microbes Infect.* **2016**, *18*, 787–797. [CrossRef] [PubMed]
54. Tasdemir, D.; Kaiser, M.; Demirci, B.; Demirci, F.; Hüsnü Can Baser, K. Antiprotozoal Activity of Turkish Origanum onites Essential Oil and Its Components. *Molecules* **2019**, *24*, 4421. [CrossRef] [PubMed]
55. Ngahang Kamte, S.L.; Ranjbarian, F.; Cianfaglione, K.; Sut, S.; Dall'Acqua, S.; Bruno, M.; Afshar, F.H.; Iannarelli, R.; Benelli, G.; Cappellacci, L.; et al. Identification of highly effective antitrypanosomal compounds in essential oils from the Apiaceae family. *Ecotoxicol. Environ. Saf.* **2018**, *156*, 154–165. [CrossRef] [PubMed]
56. Kwofie, K.D.; Tung, N.H.; Suzuki-Ohashi, M.; Amoa-Bosompem, M.; Adegle, R.; Sakyiamah, M.M.; Ayertey, F.; Owusu, K.B.A.; Tuffour, I.; Atchoglo, P.; et al. Antitrypanosomal activities and mechanisms of action of novel tetracyclic iridoids from Morinda lucida Benth. *Antimicrob. Agents Chemother.* **2016**, *60*, 3283–3290. [CrossRef] [PubMed]
57. Sut, S.; Dall'Acqua, S.; Baldan, V.; Ngahang Kamte, S.L.; Ranjbarian, F.; Biapa Nya, P.C.; Vittori, S.; Benelli, G.; Maggi, F.; Cappellacci, L.; et al. Identification of tagitinin C from Tithonia diversifolia as antitrypanosomal compound using bioactivity-guided fractionation. *Fitoterapia* **2018**, *124*, 145–151. [CrossRef] [PubMed]
58. Kimani, N.M.; Matasyoh, J.C.; Kaiser, M.; Brun, R.; Schmidt, T.J. Sesquiterpene lactones from Vernonia cinerascens Sch. Bip. and their in vitro antitrypanosomal activity. *Molecules* **2018**, *23*, 248. [CrossRef]
59. Kimani, N.M.; Matasyoh, J.C.; Kaiser, M.; Brun, R.; Schmidt, T.J. Anti-trypanosomatid elemanolide sesquiterpene lactones from Vernonia lasiopus O. Hoffm. *Molecules* **2017**, *22*, 597. [CrossRef] [PubMed]
60. Kimani, N.M.; Matasyoh, J.C.; Kaiser, M.; Brun, R.; Schmidt, T.J. Antiprotozoal Sesquiterpene Lactones and Other Constituents from Tarchonanthus camphoratus and Schkuhria pinnata. *J. Nat. Prod.* **2018**, *81*, 124–130. [CrossRef] [PubMed]
61. Skaf, J.; Hamarsheh, O.; Berninger, M.; Balasubramanian, S.; Oelschlaeger, T.A.; Holzgrabe, U. Improving anti-trypanosomal activity of alkamides isolated from Achillea fragrantissima. *Fitoterapia* **2018**, *125*, 191–198. [CrossRef] [PubMed]
62. Laurella, L.C.; Cerny, N.; Bivona, A.E.; Alberti, A.S.; Giberti, G.; Malchiodi, E.L.; Martino, V.S.; Catalan, C.A.; Alonso, M.R.; Cazorla, S.I.; et al. Assessment of sesquiterpene lactones isolated from Mikania plants species for their potential efficacy against Trypanosoma cruzi and Leishmania sp. *PLoS Negl. Trop. Dis.* **2017**, *11*, e0005929. [CrossRef] [PubMed]
63. Petrelli, R.; Ranjbarian, F.; Dall'Acqua, S.; Papa, F.; Iannarelli, R.; Ngahang Kamte, S.L.; Vittori, S.; Benelli, G.; Maggi, F.; Hofer, A.; et al. An overlooked horticultural crop, Smyrnium olusatrum, as a potential source of compounds effective against African trypanosomiasis. *Parasitol. Int.* **2017**, *66*, 146–151. [CrossRef] [PubMed]
64. De Mieri, M.; Monteleone, G.; Ismajili, I.; Kaiser, M.; Hamburger, M. Antiprotozoal Activity-Based Profiling of a Dichloromethane Extract from Anthemis nobilis Flowers. *J. Nat. Prod.* **2017**, *80*, 459–470. [CrossRef] [PubMed]
65. Lima, T.C.; Souza, R.D.J.; De Moraes, M.H.; Steindel, M.; Biavatti, M.W. A new furanoheliangolide sesquiterpene lactone from Calea pinnatifida (R. Br.) Less. (Asteraceae) and evaluation of its trypanocidal and leishmanicidal activities. *J. Braz. Chem. Soc.* **2017**, *28*, 367–375. [CrossRef]
66. Ulloa, J.L.; Spina, R.; Casasco, A.; Petray, P.B.; Martino, V.; Sosa, M.A.; Frank, F.M.; Muschietti, L.V. Germacranolide-type sesquiterpene lactones from Smallanthus sonchifolius with promising activity against Leishmania mexicana and Trypanosoma cruzi. *Parasites Vectors* **2017**, *10*, 567. [CrossRef] [PubMed]
67. Nyongbela, K.D.; Ntie-Kang, F.; Hoye, T.R.; Efange, S.M.N. Antiparasitic Sesquiterpenes from the Cameroonian Spice Scleria striatinux and Preliminary In Vitro and In Silico DMPK Assessment. *Nat. Products Bioprospect.* **2017**, *7*, 235–247. [CrossRef] [PubMed]
68. Elso, O.G.; Bivona, A.E.; Alberti, A.S.; Cerny, N.; Fabian, L.; Morales, C.; Catalán, C.A.N.; Malchiodi, E.L.; Cazorla, S.I.; Sülsen, V.P. Trypanocidal activity of four sesquiterpene lactones isolated from Asteraceae species. *Molecules* **2020**, *25*, 2014. [CrossRef]
69. Gonçalves-Santos, E.; Vilas-Boas, D.F.; Diniz, L.F.; Veloso, M.P.; Mazzeti, A.L.; Rodrigues, M.R.; Oliveira, C.M.; Fernandes, V.H.C.; Novaes, R.D.; Chagas-Paula, D.A.; et al. Sesquiterpene lactone potentiates the immunomodulatory, antiparasitic and cardioprotective effects on anti-Trypanosoma cruzi specific chemotherapy. *Int. Immunopharmacol.* **2019**, *77*, 105961. [CrossRef] [PubMed]
70. Galkina, A.; Krause, N.; Lenz, M.; Daniliuc, C.G.; Kaiser, M.; Schmidt, T.J. Antitrypanosomal Activity of Sesquiterpene Lactones from Helianthus tuberosus L. Including a new furanoheliangolide with an unusual structure. *Molecules* **2019**, *24*, 1068. [CrossRef]
71. Sosa, A.; Salamanca Capusiri, E.; Amaya, S.; Bardón, A.; Giménez-Turba, A.; Vera, N.; Borkosky, S. Trypanocidal activity of South American Vernonieae (Asteraceae) extracts and its sesquiterpene lactones. *Nat. Prod. Res.* **2021**, *35*, 5224–5228. [CrossRef]
72. Elso, O.G.; Clavin, M.; Hernandez, N.; Sgarlata, T.; Bach, H.; Catalan, C.A.N.; Aguilera, E.; Alvarez, G.; Sülsen, V.P. Antiprotozoal Compounds from Urolepis hecatantha (Asteraceae). *Evid. -Based Complement. Altern. Med.* **2021**, *2021*, 6622894. [CrossRef] [PubMed]
73. Milagre, M.M.; Branquinho, R.T.; Gonçalves, M.F.; de Assis, G.; de Oliveira, M.T.; Reis, L.; Saúde-Guimarães, D.A.; de Lana, M. Activity of the sesquiterpene lactone goyazensolide against Trypanosoma cruzi in vitro and in vivo. *Parasitology* **2020**, *147*, 108–119. [CrossRef]
74. Murakami, C.; Cabral, R.S.A.; Gomes, K.S.; Costa-Silva, T.A.; Amaral, M.; Romanelli, M.; Tempone, A.G.; Lago, J.H.G.; da Bolzani, V.S.; Moreno, P.R.H.; et al. Hedyosulide, a novel trypanosomicidal sesterterpene lactone from Hedyosmum brasiliense Mart. ex Miq. *Phytochem. Lett.* **2019**, *33*, 6–11. [CrossRef]

75. Zeouk, I.; Sifaoui, I.; López-Arencibia, A.; Reyes-Batlle, M.; Bethencourt-Estrella, C.J.; Bazzocchi, I.L.; Bekhti, K.; Lorenzo-Morales, J.; Jiménez, I.A.; Piñero, J.E. Sesquiterpenoids and flavonoids from Inula viscosa induce programmed cell death in kinetoplastids. *Biomed. Pharmacother.* **2020**, *130*, 110518. [CrossRef] [PubMed]
76. Londero, V.S.; Costa-Silva, T.A.; Tempone, A.G.; Namiyama, G.M.; Thevenard, F.; Antar, G.M.; Baitello, J.B.; Lago, J.H.G. Anti-Trypanosoma cruzi activity of costic acid isolated from Nectandra barbellata (Lauraceae) is associated with alterations in plasma membrane electric and mitochondrial membrane potentials. *Bioorg. Chem.* **2020**, *95*, 103510. [CrossRef]
77. Mofidi Tabatabaei, S.; Nejad Ebrahimi, S.; Salehi, P.; Sonboli, A.; Tabefam, M.; Kaiser, M.; Hamburger, M.; Moridi Farimani, M. Antiprotozoal Germacranolide Sesquiterpene Lactones from Tanacetum sonbolii. *Planta Med.* **2019**, *85*, 424–430. [CrossRef]
78. Turner, D.N.; Just, J.; Dasari, R.; Smith, J.A.; Bissember, A.C.; Kornienko, A.; Rogelj, S. Activity of natural and synthetic polygodial derivatives against Trypanosoma cruzi amastigotes, trypomastigotes and epimastigotes. *Nat. Prod. Res.* **2021**, *35*, 792–795. [CrossRef] [PubMed]
79. Bombaça, A.C.S.; Von Dossow, D.; Barbosa, J.M.C.; Paz, C.; Burgos, V.; Menna-Barreto, R.F.S. Trypanocidal activity of natural sesquiterpenoids involves mitochondrial dysfunction, ROS production and autophagic phenotype in trypanosomacruzi. *Molecules* **2018**, *23*, 2800. [CrossRef] [PubMed]
80. Gonçalves, G.E.G.; Morais, T.R.; Gomes, K.d.S.; Costa-Silva, T.A.; Tempone, A.G.; Lago, J.H.G.; Caseli, L. Antitrypanosomal activity of epi-polygodial from Drimys brasiliensis and its effects in cellular membrane models at the air-water interface. *Bioorg. Chem.* **2019**, *84*, 186–191. [CrossRef] [PubMed]
81. dos Santos, A.L.; Amaral, M.; Hasegawa, F.R.; Lago, J.H.G.; Tempone, A.G.; Sartorelli, P. (-)-T-Cadinol—A Sesquiterpene Isolated From Casearia sylvestris (Salicaceae)—Displayed In Vitro Activity and Causes Hyperpolarization of the Membrane Potential of Trypanosoma cruzi. *Front. Pharmacol.* **2021**, *12*, 734127. [CrossRef] [PubMed]
82. Zaki, A.A.; Ashour, A.A.; Qiu, L. New sesquiterpene glycoside ester with antiprotozoal activity from the flowers of Calendula officinalis L. *Nat. Prod. Res.* **2021**, *35*, 5250–5254. [CrossRef] [PubMed]
83. Banerjee, M.; Parai, D.; Dhar, P.; Roy, M.; Barik, R.; Chattopadhyay, S.; Mukherjee, S.K. Andrographolide induces oxidative stress-dependent cell death in unicellular protozoan parasite Trypanosoma brucei. *Acta Trop.* **2017**, *176*, 58–67. [CrossRef] [PubMed]
84. Ueno, A.K.; Barcellos, A.F.; Costa-Silva, T.A.; Mesquita, J.T.; Ferreira, D.D.; Tempone, A.G.; Romoff, P.; Antar, G.M.; Lago, J.H.G. Antitrypanosomal activity and evaluation of the mechanism of action of diterpenes from aerial parts of Baccharis retusa (Asteraceae). *Fitoterapia* **2018**, *125*, 55–58. [CrossRef] [PubMed]
85. Rocha, A.C.F.S.; Morais, G.O.; da Silva, M.M.; Kovatch, P.Y.; Ferreira, D.S.; Esperandim, V.R.; Pagotti, M.C.; Magalhães, L.G.; Heleno, V.C.G. In vitro anti-trypanosomal potential of kaurane and pimarane semi-synthetic derivatives. *Nat. Prod. Res.* **2020**, *36*, 875–884. [CrossRef] [PubMed]
86. Kuźma; Kaiser, M.; Wysokińska, H. The production and antiprotozoal activity of abietane diterpenes in Salvia austriaca hairy roots grown in shake flasks and bioreactor. *Prep. Biochem. Biotechnol.* **2017**, *47*, 58–66. [CrossRef] [PubMed]
87. Nogueira, M.S.; Da Costa, F.B.; Brun, R.; Kaiser, M.; Schmidt, T.J. ent-pimarane and ent-kaurane diterpenes from Aldama discolor (Asteraceae) and their antiprotozoal activity. *Molecules* **2016**, *21*, 1237. [CrossRef] [PubMed]
88. Pirttimaa, M.; Nasereddin, A.; Kopelyanskiy, D.; Kaiser, M.; Yli-Kauhaluoma, J.; Oksman-Caldentey, K.M.; Brun, R.; Jaffe, C.L.; Moreira, V.M.; Alakurtti, S. Abietane-Type Diterpenoid Amides with Highly Potent and Selective Activity against Leishmania donovani and Trypanosoma cruzi. *J. Nat. Prod.* **2016**, *79*, 362–368. [CrossRef] [PubMed]
89. Farimani, M.M.; Khodaei, B.; Moradi, H.; Aliabadi, A.; Ebrahimi, S.N.; De Mieri, M.; Kaiser, M.; Hamburger, M. Phytochemical Study of Salvia leriifolia Roots: Rearranged Abietane Diterpenoids with Antiprotozoal Activity. *J. Nat. Prod.* **2018**, *81*, 1384–1390. [CrossRef] [PubMed]
90. Zadali, R.; Nejad Ebrahimi, S.; Tofighi, Z.; Es-haghi, A.; Hamburger, M.; Kaiser, M.; D' Ambola, M.; De Tommasi, N.; Hadji-akhoondi, A. Antiprotozoal activity of diterpenoids isolated from Zhumeria majdae- absolute configuration by circular dichroism. *DARU J. Pharm. Sci.* **2020**, *28*, 455–462. [CrossRef] [PubMed]
91. Tabefam, M.; Farimani, M.M.; Danton, O.; Ramseyer, J.; Kaiser, M.; Ebrahimi, S.N.; Salehi, P.; Batooli, H.; Potterat, O.; Hamburger, M. Antiprotozoal Diterpenes from Perovskia abrotanoides. *Planta Med.* **2018**, *84*, 913–919. [CrossRef] [PubMed]
92. Nvau, J.B.; Alenezi, S.; Ungogo, M.A.; Alfayez, I.A.M.; Natto, M.J.; Gray, A.I.; Ferro, V.A.; Watson, D.G.; de Koning, H.P.; Igoli, J.O. Antiparasitic and Cytotoxic Activity of Bokkosin, A Novel Diterpene-Substituted Chromanyl Benzoquinone From Calliandra portoricensis. *Front. Chem.* **2020**, *8*, 574103. [CrossRef] [PubMed]
93. Anyam, J.V.; Daikwo, P.E.; Ungogo, M.A.; Nweze, N.E.; Igoli, N.P.; Gray, A.I.; De Koning, H.P.; Igoli, J.O. Two New Antiprotozoal Diterpenes From the Roots of Acacia nilotica. *Front. Chem.* **2021**, *9*, 76. [CrossRef] [PubMed]
94. Catteau, L.; Schioppa, L.; Beaufay, C.; Girardi, C.; Hérent, M.F.; Frédérich, M.; Quetin-Leclercq, J. Antiprotozoal activities of Triterpenic Acids and Ester Derivatives Isolated from the Leaves of Vitellaria paradoxa. *Planta Med.* **2021**, *87*, 860–867. [CrossRef] [PubMed]
95. Labib, R.; Ebada, S.; Youssef, F.; Ashour, M.; Ross, S. Ursolic acid, a natural pentacylcic triterpene from Ochrosia elliptica and its role in the management of certain neglected tropical diseases. *Pharmacogn. Mag.* **2016**, *12*, 319–325. [CrossRef] [PubMed]
96. Osman, A.G.; Ali, Z.; Fantoukh, O.; Raman, V.; Kamdem, R.S.T.; Khan, I. Glycosides of ursane-type triterpenoid, benzophenone, and iridoid from Vangueria agrestis (Fadogia agrestis) and their anti-infective activities. *Nat. Prod. Res.* **2020**, *34*, 683–691. [CrossRef] [PubMed]

97. Meira, C.S.; Barbosa-Filho, J.M.; Lanfredi-Rangel, A.; Guimarães, E.T.; Moreira, D.R.M.; Soares, M.B.P. Antiparasitic evaluation of betulinic acid derivatives reveals effective and selective anti-Trypanosoma cruzi inhibitors. *Exp. Parasitol.* **2016**, *166*, 108–115. [CrossRef]
98. Sousa, P.L.; da Silva Souza, R.O.; Tessarolo, L.D.; de Menezes, R.R.P.P.B.; Sampaio, T.L.; Canuto, J.A.; Martins, A.M.C. Betulinic acid induces cell death by necrosis in Trypanosoma cruzi. *Acta Trop.* **2017**, *174*, 72–75. [CrossRef] [PubMed]
99. Steverding, D.; Sidjui, L.S.; Ferreira, É.R.; Ngameni, B.; Folefoc, G.N.; Mahiou-Leddet, V.; Ollivier, E.; Stephenson, G.R.; Storr, T.E.; Tyler, K.M. Trypanocidal and leishmanicidal activity of six limonoids. *J. Nat. Med.* **2020**, *74*, 606–611. [CrossRef] [PubMed]
100. Carothers, S.; Nyamwihura, R.; Collins, J.; Zhang, H.; Park, H.; Setzer, W.N.; Ogungbe, I.V. Bauerenol acetate, the pentacyclic triterpenoid from Tabernaemontana longipes, is an antitrypanosomal agent. *Molecules* **2018**, *23*, 355. [CrossRef] [PubMed]
101. Tabefam, M.; Farimani, M.M.; Danton, O.; Ramseyer, J.; Nejad Ebrahimi, S.; Neuburger, M.; Kaiser, M.; Salehi, P.; Potterat, O.; Hamburger, M. Antiprotozoal Isoprenoids from Salvia hydrangea. *J. Nat. Prod.* **2018**, *81*, 2682–2691. [CrossRef] [PubMed]
102. Muganza, D.M.; Fruth, B.; Nzunzu, J.L.; Tuenter, E.; Foubert, K.; Cos, P.; Maes, L.; Kanyanga, R.C.; Exarchou, V.; Apers, S.; et al. In vitro antiprotozoal activity and cytotoxicity of extracts and isolated constituents from Greenwayodendron suaveolens. *J. Ethnopharmacol.* **2016**, *193*, 510–516. [CrossRef] [PubMed]
103. Szabó, L.U.; Kaiser, M.; Mäser, P.; Schmidt, T.J. Antiprotozoal nor-triterpene alkaloids from *Buxus sempervirens* L. *Antibiotics* **2021**, *10*, 696. [CrossRef]
104. Pushpakom, S.; Iorio, F.; Eyers, P.A.; Escott, K.J.; Hopper, S.; Wells, A.; Doig, A.; Guilliams, T.; Latimer, J.; McNamee, C.; et al. Drug repurposing: Progress, challenges and recommendations. *Nat. Rev. Drug Discov.* **2018**, *18*, 41–58. [CrossRef]
105. Babaei, G.; Aliarab, A.; Abroon, S.; Rasmi, Y.; Aziz, S.G.G. Application of sesquiterpene lactone: A new promising way for cancer therapy based on anticancer activity. *Biomed. Pharmacother.* **2018**, *106*, 239–246. [CrossRef]
106. Moujir, L.; Callies, O.; Sousa, P.M.C.; Sharopov, F.; Seca, A.M.L. Applications of sesquiterpene lactones: A review of some potential success cases. *Appl. Sci.* **2020**, *10*, 3001. [CrossRef]

MDPI
St. Alban-Anlage 66
4052 Basel
Switzerland
Tel. +41 61 683 77 34
Fax +41 61 302 89 18
www.mdpi.com

Pharmaceuticals Editorial Office
E-mail: pharmaceuticals@mdpi.com
www.mdpi.com/journal/pharmaceuticals

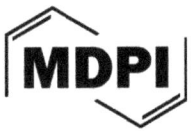

www.ingramcontent.com/pod-product-compliance
Lightning Source LLC
LaVergne TN
LVHW070224100526
838202LV00015B/2088